# Canine
# Behavior

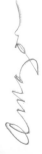

Canine
Behavior

# Canine Behavior

## Insights and Answers

**Bonnie V. Beaver,** DVM, MS, Dipl. ACVB
Professor and Director of Community Practice
Department of Small Animal Clinical Sciences
College of Veterinary Medicine and Biomedical Sciences
Texas A&M University
College Station, Texas

SAUNDERS

ELSEVIER

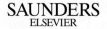

11830 Westline Industrial Drive
St. Louis, Missouri 63146

CANINE BEHAVIOR: INSIGHTS AND ANSWERS, SECOND EDITION

ISBN: 978-1-4160-5419-1

**Library of Congress Cataloging-in-Publication Data**
Beaver, Bonnie V. G., 1944-
Canine behavior : insights and answers / Bonnie V. Beaver. -- 2nd ed.      p. cm.
Includes bibliographical references and index.
ISBN 978-1-4160-5419-1 (pbk. : alk. paper)
1. Dogs--Behavior. I. Title.
SF433.B4 2009

636.7'089689--dc22                                    2008019332

*Vice President and Publisher*: Linda Duncan
*Senior Acquisitions Editor*: Anthony Winkel
*Senior Developmental Editor*: Shelly Stringer
*Publishing Services Manager*: Patricia Tannian
*Senior Project Manager*: Kristine Feeherty
*Designer*: Maggie Reid

Printed in China

Last digit is the print number:  9   8   7   6   5   4   3   2   1

*Veterinarians work to make the lives of animals and people better—it is our passion. We do it as we heal the sick, ensure a safe food supply, protect our country, gather new knowledge, teach the next generation, and tackle behavior problems. Our profession is small in numbers but mighty in accomplishments.*

*Since the last edition of the book, I had the privilege of serving my profession as the Chair of the Executive Board and then President of the American Veterinary Medical Association. It is a long way for a little girl from rural Minnesota to come, especially in an era when she was told that "women cannot be veterinarians." It was an unbelievable journey for which I am truly grateful. I dedicate this book to all my veterinary colleagues. Without your support I could not have accomplished this book nor had my AVMA leadership experiences.*

# Preface

Considering the many recent advances in the understanding and application of behavioral science and modification principles, a revision of *Canine Behavior* is definitely overdue. This second edition is intended to explore the many facets and consequences of behavior in dogs—from normal to abnormal—as it has developed over time. Even though normal behavior does not essentially change, significantly new information is being gathered about our awareness of the complex behaviors of the dog, starting with the dog genome and genetic changes from a wolf-like ancestor to the many varieties of dogs we recognize today. There have also been major strides in knowledge about how to treat a wide range of problem behaviors, which reflect our constantly changing relationships with these magnificent creatures and are specifically addressed in this edition.

It is my aim to meet several goals with this edition. Firstly, the content represents critical and valuable material gleaned from a vast body of classic and newer scientific references. This is intended to help researchers, teachers, veterinarians, and pet owners gain further insights into the dog's communicative, social, sexual, ingestive, eliminative, locomotor, grooming, and sensory behaviors. Secondly, it is designed to provide practical information to veterinarians for the diagnosis and treatments of various behavioral problems. This is accomplished by providing detailed insights into normal dog behavior, how problem behaviors develop, and how they might be prevented and managed successfully and humanely. Lastly, but not least, I hope the book will provide interesting information for fellow dog enthusiasts.

To understand abnormal, it is important to have a clear understanding of normal. The chapters are organized around various large categories of behavior. Within each chapter, normal behaviors are described first, followed by the various types of related behavior problems. Because dogs live in a wide variety of environments, it is impossible to include every scenario of behavior that might occur, but several that have been identified over the years are included. This edition discusses many of the classic normal and abnormal behaviors and expands upon current understandings of major problems such as stereotypies, cognitive dysfunction, and separation anxiety. It also presents the latest insights and applications of behavioral pharmacotherapy as well as practical, rational, and humane approaches to modification techniques for basic and complicated behavioral problems.

Behavior problems result in the death of approximately 10% of the dog and cat population each year—that's more than caused by all infectious diseases. As dogs have changed their habitat from the barnyard to the backyard and into the house, the importance of their behaviors and consequences has been amplified in the lives of their owners.

Veterinarians must be able to advise clients about normal behavior and help prevent and eradicate or minimize problems associated with abnormal behaviors. Only by knowing the natural history of the dog and its innate behavior influenced by the modern realities of domestication can we serve the needs of our canine patients so that they remain valued members of our households and communities for a long time.

**Bonnie V. Beaver, DVM, MS, Dipl. ACVB**

# Acknowledgments

Many people have helped, both directly or indirectly, to ensure the publication of this book. Their support and backing have been important.

My appreciation is expressed to all of my colleagues, particularly Richard Adams, Sandee Hartsfield, Deb Zoran, Nini Hodges, Lore Haug, Patty Hug, and M.A. Crist. Special thanks go to Peppy Shortstockings, Murphy Brown, Rachael Brown, Thelma Beaver, Shirley and Tommy Clem, Larry and Sherry Piper, Lauren and Stan Stephenson, Jean and Nathan Piper, the John Smith family, George and Nyla Rayburn, and the AVMA staff. Finally, I wish to thank the staff at Elsevier for their patience, particularly Maureen Slaten for her ready assistance and her gentle but persistent reminders of important deadlines. I did make it.

# Contents

# Canine Behavior

# Introduction to Canine Behavior

Understanding the dog requires that one understand where it came from, so it becomes necessary to go back to the wolf and beyond. The dog began its association with humans well over 10,000 years ago, a period longer than for any other domestic animal. Since dogs came into our lives, they have filled a number of roles: from companion to food, from alter ego to special sense. It is the great genetic plasticity in *Canis familiaris* that has permitted so much variation in its sizes, colors, and behaviors. In modern times, breeds have been developed for specific purposes, such as herding cattle, retrieving a hunter's kill, and pulling a sled. Although there are behavioral variations between breeds, often related to purpose, the core behaviors of the domestic dog are very similar across breeds and are often similar to those of its closest relative, the wolf. The wolf can serve as a basis for understanding the dog, but it is also important to remember that thousands of years of selective breeding have changed a lot of the behavior too.

## HISTORY OF CANINE DEVELOPMENT

The oldest known ancestor of the domestic dog is the *Miacis*, a small, weasel-sized carnivore that lived approximately 40 million years ago in the Eocene.[60,88,89,211,239] The miacid was probably a forest dweller with a long tail, short limbs, and a plantigrade stance.[60,210] Already at this time, the teeth that would come to be called the *carnassial teeth* had taken on their characteristic shape. By the late Eocene period, the *Cynidictus* had evolved, and it probably gave rise to the *Hesperocyon* (formerly *Pseudocynonsides*).[60,89,182,211] This latest group existed approximately 3 million years ago in the Oligocene and was distinguished by its larger size, longer limbs, better developed carnassial teeth, and

larger brains.[60] The line of ancestors that followed is less clear. Some propose that the *Cynodesmus* of the Miocene gave rise to the *Tomarctus* of the Pliocene, and the *Tomarctus* eventually gave origin to the canids.[60,89] Others theorize that *Hesperocyon* gave rise to the *Leptocyn,* one possible ancestor of the dog, or to the *Tomarctus,* another possible ancestor.[182,211]

Regardless of the exact ancient line, all modern predators (fissipeds) belong to one of three superfamilies: Miacoidea, Feloidea (Aeluroidea), or Canoidea (Arctoidea). Cats, hyenas, and Old World civets belong to the Feloidea. Dogs, wolves, foxes, and jackals belong to the canine subfamily of Canoidea.[60,78]

Even narrowing down the phylogenetic subfamily does not settle another age-old question. What animal is the immediate ancestor of the domesticated dog? Most experts agree that the wolf played a major role in the dog's genetic pool, but there are 32 subspecies of *Canis lupus.*[211] Of the canids, only the wolf, coyote, and jackal have the same number of chromosomes (78) as the dog and can interbreed to produce fertile offspring.[57] A question remains about other common early ancestors or another possible ancestor species.[89,90,318] Dogs and wolves share 71 of 90 behavioral patterns, more than are shared by any other two species.[279] Early DNA tests have provided limited information that the domestic dog, wolf, coyote, and jackal are the most alike among the canids.[69,317,326] Newer isoenzyme genetic distance indicates that the dog is more closely related to the wolf than to other canids.[119,183,314,323]

Assuming the wolf (*Canis lupus*) begot *Canis lupus familiaris*,[211] which begot *Canis familiaris*, which of the many subspecies of wolf started the process? Again, considerable disagreement exists. Some authorities argue for a single origin in northern Eurasia,[278] the Near East,[69] or North America.[119,211] Others argue for the possibility of the occurrence of domestication in different species in diverse locations.[55,57,85,190] How the first dogs gradually changed into the many breeds we have today has been the subject of much speculation over the years. Most people believe that the Arctic breeds probably came first because their physical appearances are very similar to wolves. Others believe that "village dogs" were first.[35,65] These were followed by livestock-guarding dogs and hunting companions, and then by sled dogs, herding and gun dogs, and household dogs.[65] The most current studies of DNA microsatellite subtypes find at least four distinct groupings representing unique "adaptive radiations" (Fig. 1-1).[230] The four groups with similar genetic clusters also tended to share geographic origin, morphology, and/or genetic closeness to the wolf of Southeast Asia, following humans to different parts of the world.[35,230,267] Research into common behaviors also shows some similarities within the four groups. Those closest to wolves show more aggression and less demand for affection than those farthest away.[111]

Exactly when humans started interacting with wolves is difficult to determine. Some of the earliest hominid sites with *Canis lupus* remains were found in Zhoukoudian, China, dating back between 200,000 and 500,000 years; in Kent, England, dating back 400,000 years; and in Nice, France, dating back 125,000 years.[59,211] As evidence of domestication, scientists have pointed to (1) the smaller size of bony remains compared with those of indigenous wolf populations; (2) certain anatomic differences in the skull, mandible, and teeth; and (3) phylogeographic variation. According to these criteria, dogs separated from wolves up to 40,000 years ago. However, DNA evidence for the delineation suggests that dogs originated approximately 135,000 years ago and that occasional wolf backcrosses have occurred.[313]

Domestication probably occurred in more recent history, but exactly when and where is not clear. Burial sites are the most likely source of information, but some researchers question if burials truly indicate early domestication, or if they were

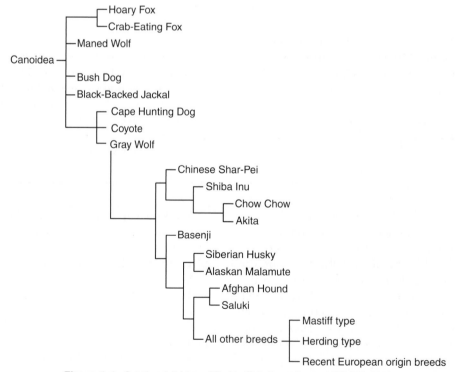

**Figure 1-1.** Genetic subdivisions of Canids. (Data from references 230, 326, 327.)

started somewhat later. A German dog burial site dates back 14,000 years.[58,93,238] Another burial site in Siberia goes back 10,650 years.[93] Evidence of the dog's existence has been found at the Palegawra Cave in Iraq, dating back some 10,000 to 12,000 years,[55,56,211,212] although there is some question about this date.[69] At Ein Mallaha in northern Israel, scientists excavated a tomb dating back to 9350 to 9750 BC that contained a burial of an old human, probably a woman, and a 3- to 5-month-old puppy.[57,59,69,71,190] In China, domesticated dogs have been dated back to 7355 ± 100 BC.[211] The earliest European site is Star Carr in Yorkshire, England, which contained evidence of dogs dating back to 7538 ± 350 BC.[69,211] Swedish and Danish sites date back to 5000 to 6800 BC.[211] In North America, dogs probably accompanied humans over the Bering Strait land bridge from Asia and spread out from there.[165,230,238] Dog burial sites date back 8500 years in western Illinois and 7500 years in Benton County, Missouri.[69,199,210] The ancient Chiribaya dogs of Peru were apparently very prized and recently found mummified bodies date back about 1000 years.[61] Domesticated dogs probably did not exist in Australia more than 12,000 years ago.[57,69] That was the approximate time Tasmania separated from the Australian mainland, and the absence of canids there supports this theory. The dogs that did come to the Australian continent probably did so as recently as 5000 years ago,[70] and eventually reverted to the feral dingo.

How and why domestication of wolves occurred will always be speculative. Some theories about domestication in general suggest that a mutually advantageous relationship between wolves and humans would allow for the loss of such wolf behaviors as self defense and self protection. At the same time, there would be the gain of other behaviors, such as access to food or shelter.[40] Perhaps wolves and humans shared hunting success. Wolves might have followed hunters initially to find game. The wolf that was allowed to share a kill made by its two-legged benefactor would have become somewhat tame.[211] Hunting skills as well as ease of being tamed—traits that benefited the humans—could then have been selectively bred owing to proximity because the most successful wolves took on a favored status and were more apt to be around others with similar traits.

Early humans may actually have taken young cubs from the den to be hand-raised, as was done by Native Americans even into the eighteenth century, and as some people still do.[56,100,182,280] Without a parent to teach hunting skills, the wolf/dog would have become dependent on the humans for food.[40,190] Some probably became scavengers, responsible for keeping the camps clean.[57,90] As suggested by evidence from the Israeli burial site, some wolves may have first shared space with humans simply to provide companionship.[57,69] The relative lack of canid bones at most sites indicates that dogs were probably not a major food source.[69] Other roles these animals could have filled would have been as an occasional "watchdog," religious symbol or sacrifice, draft animal, or source of hides, meat, or warmth at night.[57,90,182,190]

Domestication is a complicated process that involves genetic changes in a large number of animals that are selectively bred over many generations to intensify certain traits and make others secondary. The result is a species that is biologically changed in its morphology, physiology, and behavior.[94,157] The dog became smaller than the wolf, had different colored hair, and was less alert to its environment. Over time the quantitative nature of the various responses change so that rather than a behavioral trait being completely lost, its threshold is heightened or lowered by lack of or consistent exposure to specific stimuli.[249] Many more generations of continued selective breeding modified the dog into a wide variety of shapes, sizes, colors, and behaviors based on the goals and desires of those responsible for mate selection.

The domestication process can occur relatively rapidly in a canid when strict criteria are used.[249] The Russian geneticist D.K. Belvaev was able to create major changes in a group of silver foxes through intense selective breeding only for tameness over approximately 20 generations.[26] By the end of that time, his animals were reported to have sought contact with humans, licked human hands and faces, changed their breeding cycle to twice a year, developed drooping ears and erect tails, and displayed the submissive behaviors of whining and tail wagging.[182,190] In the case of wolf-to-dog evolution, the timeframe was probably much longer than in Belvaev's experiment, because the selection criteria were far less distinct; however, the social structure of the wolf is the closest of any of the wild canids to that of the human, making the wolf the best candidate for domestication.[278]

The physical and behavioral features that tended to be retained in the wolf-to-dog transition were those most associated with juveniles, a phenomenon called *paedomorphosis.*\* In the dog, those wolf cub–like physical features include a smaller size, shorter muzzle, relatively wider cranium or more domed head, reduced tympanic bullae, more convex mandible, larger eyes, smaller teeth, floppy instead of erect ears, and less developed temporalis and masseter muscles. † The retained behavioral characteristics include increased frequency in care-soliciting behaviors, submissive food begging (such as face licking), relative lack of fear, timing of activity periods, curiosity, playfulness, lessened territorialness, and increased seeking of social contacts.[40,87,119]

On the other hand, some distinct differences also developed between wolves and dogs that were unrelated to paedomorphosis. Many of these features were not selected for or against but probably tagged along genetically. The curly tail of some dogs was one of the most obvious early changes. It, in turn, has been followed by a great variation in the size and shape of the tail, its amount of curl, and the position in which it is carried. Unlike other canids, dogs sometimes have the first digit on the rear limbs.[57] The scent gland from the dorsal aspect of the base of the tail is greatly reduced or absent in dogs.[57,94] Reproductively there are differences too. Sexual maturity occurs between 6 and 12 months of age in dogs versus almost 2 years in wolves. Female dogs experience twice as many estrous periods as female wolves in a year, and estrus can occur at any time during the year. Thus, males are reproductively interested throughout the year instead of during a wolf-like 2-month breeding season.[57,278] Dogs have developed better social-cognitive skills than wolves and are able to read human signals, including those that indicate the location of hidden food.[105] Even wolves raised with humans do not show that behavior. Coat colors have increased in dogs. It has been shown in foxes that the change in the color of fur can be related to behavior changes. The amber fox is less aggressive than the gray fox. Also, at least some amber foxes have smaller adrenal and pituitary glands.[57]

Seven thousand years ago, there were specific kinds of dogs. Three thousand years ago heavy hunting dogs, short-legged dogs, and Greyhounds existed.[57,58] Soon dog breeds proliferated. Small dogs share a single insulin-like growth factor I (IGF-I) allele that suggests a specific sequence variant is the major reason for their body size.[298] But dogs now come in a wide variety of sizes, colors, and working skills. Dogs were an integral part of Roman culture and could be found throughout that empire. Probably the first systematic breeding of dogs occurred there. The Romans had fighting dogs, sheepdogs, guard dogs, and small lapdogs.[56,57] As a side note, the *cave canem* signs in Pompeii and Rome were the first "Beware of the Dog" signs; their intent was to warn visitors not to step on the small Italian Greyhounds.[239] Columella, a Roman agricultural authority, is said to have advised the breeding of dogs that did not look like wolves, including black farm dogs that barked at intruders and white sheepdogs.[56]

The licensing of dogs was started by King Henry III of England around the middle of the thirteenth century when he singled out mastiffs.[239] The first competitive dog show was held in 1859 at Newcastle in Britain but was limited to Pointers and Setters. With the start of the shows and the British Kennel Club in 1873, breed standards were gradually tightened until they reached what we know today.[57]

## CURRENT STATUS OF CANIDS

Dogs have been used to meet more human needs than any other domestic species (Table 1-1), and humans keep finding new things for them to do. The original list of four roles animals typically fill—food, clothing, shelter, and transportation—were to be greatly expanded as dogs came to be associated

---

\*References 40, 57, 87, 94, 190, 249.
†References 40, 56, 57, 59, 94, 190.

**TABLE 1-1** Primary roles played by domestic animals throughout history

| Primary roles | Dogs | Cats | Horses | Cattle | Swine | Sheep | Goats | Camels | Reindeer |
|---|---|---|---|---|---|---|---|---|---|
| **Clothing/shelter** | | | | | | | | | |
| Fiber | | | + | | | + | + | + | |
| Hides | + | | + | + | + | + | + | | + |
| **Communication** | + | | | | | | | | |
| **Draft or power source** | + | | + | + | | ± | | | + |
| **Educator** | + | + | + | + | + | + | + | + | + |
| **Extension of human senses** | + | + | | | + | | | | |
| **Food** | | | | | | | | | |
| Meat | + | | + | + | + | + | + | | + |
| Milk | | + | | + | | | + | | |
| Blood | | | | + | | | | + | |
| **Manufacturing** | | | | | | | | | |
| Feces for energy | | | | + | + | | | + | + |
| Feces for feed | | | | + | + | | | | |
| Health products | | | + | | + | + | + | | |
| **Occupation** | + | + | + | + | + | + | + | + | + |
| **Physical health** | | | | | | | | | |
| Poison detection | | + | | | | | | | |
| Exercise | + | | + | | | | | + | |
| **Protection** | + | | | | | | | | |
| **Psychological health** | | | | | | | | | |
| Companionship | + | + | + | + | + | + | + | + | + |
| Extension of ego | + | + | + | + | + | + | + | + | + |
| Recreation | + | + | + | + | + | + | + | + | + |
| Religious figure | + | + | | + | | | | | |
| Therapy | + | + | + | | + | | | | |
| **Research** | + | + | + | + | + | + | + | | |
| **Transportation** | + | | + | | | | | + | + |

with other cultures and time periods. A recognition of the human-animal bond allows for consideration of activities animals do with us, as well as for us. Probably the longest service that dogs have performed is the guiding and guarding of livestock. Even today the use of livestock-guarding dogs is an effective method of managing predation, with 82% of them considered to be an economic asset.[103] Guide dogs for the blind are the most common type of specially trained service dog, extending the sensory capacity of the human with whom they work. But service dogs help humans in much more than the physical sense. They have been shown to provide a tremendous psychologic boost and to facilitate community integration. Their use has been correlated with better attendance at work or school, while reducing the number of human assistance hours needed.[5] Dogs are also an integral part of many search-and-rescue teams.[118] They have served with honor in the military as sentries, smell detectors, early warning systems, and communication go-betweens.[4] Dogs are used as research models and as a child's teacher. Psychologically, they can contribute to good mental health, help bridge social interactions[5,168] and serve as a warm, fuzzy therapist for those who need a feeling heart to listen.

The genomics of dogs is currently a hot research topic, but ultimately the understanding of

| TABLE 1-2 | Genetic associations with temperament or psychic diseases in humans that may relate to similar problems in dogs |
|---|---|
| **Target gene** | **Temperament/psychic disease(s)** |
| 5-HT transporter | Anxiety, harm avoidance, novelty seeking, depression |
| 5-HT$_{2A}$ receptor | Anorexia nervosa |
| 5-HT$_{2C}$ receptor | Reward dependence |
| 5-HT$_6$ receptor | Alzheimer's disease |
| Dopamine transporter | Attention-deficit hyperactivity, novelty seeking |
| Dopamine D$_2$ receptor | Reward dependence, harm avoidance |
| Dopamine D$_3$ receptor | Novelty seeking |
| Dopamine D$_4$ receptor | Novelty seeking, attention-deficit hyperactivity, harm avoidance |
| Catechol-*O*-methyl-transferase | Obsessive-compulsive disorder, attention-deficit hyperactivity |
| Monoamine oxidase A | Impulse aggression, panic disorder |
| Tryptophan hydroxylase | Impulsive aggression, aggression (anger-related traits) |
| Tyrosine hydroxylase | Deliberation, dutifulness |

Modified from reference 300, pp. 356-357.
*HT,* Hydroxytryptamine.

the genetics of behavior will take a lot longer. Behavioral genetic research peaked in the late 1960s and early 1970s and has been spotty since then. It is recognized that there are critical aptitudes, and the military and police in other countries have done some work in using genetics and behavioral selection tools.[43] The heritability of a few traits in hunting dogs has been reported, but these represent only five traits in four breeds.[130,300] Some is known about the interrelationship of certain polymorphic genes as they affect temperament and psychic diseases in humans.[300] We could speculate that there may be a relationship to certain conditions in dogs as well (Table 1-2). Time will tell if any of these relationships exist. Unfortunately, bad genetic traits that can be passed on with desired ones can lead to the culling of working dogs or aggression in pets, as examples.[128,170]

Throughout the world, the cultural views about dogs vary tremendously, and this can be true even within a single country. Where dogs are highly regarded, they may be given human names, allowed to share human beds, and fed human food. At the other end of the spectrum are cultures that consider dogs to be pariahs—social outcasts. In between these two extremes are cultures indifferent to the well-being of dogs.

Although the United States has one of the highest dog ownership rates, it also has a large number of people who refuse to accept any of the responsibility that normally accompanies such ownership. Stray animal populations and euthanasias in animal shelters are statistical proof. For every 415 babies born each hour in the United States, there are 2000 to 3000 new puppies and kittens.[81] That means 60,000 animals must die each day just to maintain a stable population.[81] Surgical sterilization helps, but it is not the solution to the problem of overpopulation.

Exact statistics on dog population in the United States are impossible to get, but over the last 35 years, several groups have made well-researched estimates (Table 1-3). Beginning in 1972, with an estimated dog population of 36.1 million, the numbers rose gradually, reaching 55.6 million dogs in 1983.[131,240] Since 1987 the number of dogs in this country has increased slightly, reaching 61.6 million by 2001.[7,51,52,98,332-334] Even the best efforts to obtain valid data are challenged,[235] so any "data" are really estimates.

Worldwide, there are no reliable canine population data either, but surpluses are a concern everywhere.[156] The United Kingdom had an estimated 6.3 million dogs in 1986, and approximately 700,000 puppies are born there each year.[66,308] Certainly, with the size of the pet food market, manufacturers must have some estimates on dog numbers, but this information is not widely available and the use of manufactured food is not universal.

The number of households having dogs and the average number of dogs for each is another way to look at population statistics (see Table 1-3). In the United States, Australia, Belgium, France, and Ireland, approximately 40% of all homes have at least one dog.[176] In contrast, in Germany, Austria,

**TABLE 1-3**   Estimated U.S. dog population at various times

| Year | 1975 | 1976 | 1981 | 1982 | 1983 | 1987 | 1991 | 1996 | 2001 | 2006 |
|---|---|---|---|---|---|---|---|---|---|---|
| Origin of survey | PFI | AAHA | AAHA | AAHA | AVMA | AVMA | AVMA | AVMA | AVMA | AVMA |
| Dog population (millions) | 41.3 | 43.6 | 48.3 | 48.1 | 55.6 | 52.4 | 52.5 | 52.9 | 61.6 | 72.1 |
| Total number of households (millions) | 67.9 | 72.2 | 79.8 | 82.1 | 85.0 | 113.8 | 112.0 | 98.9 | 104.9 | 115.5 |
| Dog owning households (millions) | 29.1 | 31.3 | 32.7 | 33.3 | 36.1 | 34.7 | 34.6 | 31.2 | 37.9 | 43.0 |
| Percent of households with dogs | 42.9 | 43.4 | 41.0 | 40.5 | 42.5 | 30.5 | 30.9 | 31.6 | 36.1 | 37.2 |
| Dogs per household | 1.41 | 1.39 | 1.47 | 1.43 | 1.54 | 1.51 | 1.52 | 1.69 | 1.63 | 1.7 |

Data from references 7, 51, 52, 98, 240, 310, 330, 334.
*AAHA,* American Animal Hospital Association; *AVMA,* American Veterinary Medical Association; *PFI,* Pet Food Institute.

**TABLE 1-4**   Samples of the American Kennel Club top 10 breeds

| 1973 | 1982 | 1985 | 1992 | 1996 | 2006 |
|---|---|---|---|---|---|
| 1. Poodles | Poodles | German Shepherds | Labrador Retrievers | Labrador Retrievers | Labrador Retrievers |
| 2. German Shepherds | Cocker Spaniels | Labrador Retrievers | Rottweilers | Rottweilers | Yorkshire Terriers |
| 3. Beagles | Doberman Pinschers | Yorkshire Terriers | Cocker Spaniels | German Shepherds | German Shepherds |
| 4. Irish Setters | Labrador Retrievers | Golden Retrievers | German Shepherds | Golden Retrievers | Golden Retrievers |
| 5. Dachshunds | German Shepherds | Cavalier King Charles Spaniel | Poodles | Beagles | Beagles |
| 6. Miniature Schnauzers | Golden Retrievers | Doberman Pinschers | Golden Retrievers | Poodles | Dachshunds |
| 7. | Miniature Schnauzers | Rottweilers | Beagles | Dachshunds | Boxers |
| 8. | Beagles | Cocker Spaniels | Dachshunds | Cocker Spaniels | Poodles |
| 9. | Dachshunds | English Springer Spaniels | Shetland Sheepdogs | Yorkshire Terriers | Shih Tzu |
| 10. | Shetland Sheepdogs | Staffordshire Bull Terrier | Chow Chows | Pomeranians | Miniature Schnauzers |

Data from references 6, 51, 52, 66, 302.

Sweden, and Norway the number is estimated to be between 12% and 15%.[176]

Approximately 2000 distinct dog breeds have existed at varying times throughout history, and there are currently around 400.[230,259] The American Kennel Club recognizes 152 breeds. Slightly over half the dog population in the United States and some European countries are purebred but not necessarily registered.[66,303,330]

Popularity of breeds changes constantly, and only a few breeds account for a large portion of the new puppies (Table 1-4).[52,55,66] The general trend over the past 35 years has been toward large dogs. The success of a dog actor or image can create a sudden demand for a specific breed. Lassie, Rin Tin Tin, Eddie, and the 101 Dalmatians movie have each triggered the extreme popularity of their breed. Unfortunately, the sudden popularity of any individual breed can result in a lot of behavior problems in those dogs. Behaviors, even within breeds, can change over time.[299] The American Cocker Spaniel breed was considered to be a good family dog in the 1950s. At the peak of this popularity, it became an aggressive dog and fell out of favor. Cocker breeders worked hard to get rid of the aggression so by the early 1980s, the breed rose in popularity again. By the middle 1990s, the breed regained a reputation for aggression and fell out of favor once more. Current studies find that correlation between behavior and function of the breed's origins no longer exist, but the behaviors now relate to the breed's current use.[299] There is a positive correlation between use in working dog trials and the playfulness and aggressiveness in the sires, and between dog show use with social and nonsocial fearfulness. A negative correlation exists between dog show use and playfulness, curiosity, and aggressiveness. Popular breeds also have higher sociability and playfulness scores than less popular breeds, which probably relates to why they became popular. Careful selection of breeding animals can be helpful in the overall success of producing consistency in service dogs of certain breeds.[331]

It is logical to expect behavioral and medical disorders to differ somewhat among breeds, because selective breeding tends to concentrate specific traits. Over 350 inherited disorders have been reported in dogs.[230] Breeding for appearance does not take into account the genetics of temperament. Moreover, most books about a breed are written by fanciers of the breed, so there is a tendency for each book to indicate that dogs of that breed are good with children, easy to train, and make wonderful pets. Relatively few authors have approached the subject with a scientific basis and real objectivity.[112,114,115,280]

Veterinarians tend to see a skewed population of dogs, although the patient trends are gradually approaching the norm. In 1983 at least one in four dogs did not visit a veterinarian. By 1997 the number had dropped to approximately one in six dogs.[51,52,301] The average life expectancy for a dog is 13 years,[243] but the mean age of dogs in the United States is about 4 years.[7,329] In fact, over half of all dogs are under 6 years of age.[7,51,52,332] Many dogs die at a young age to balance with the geriatric populations veterinarians usually deal with. The oldest authenticated age worldwide is 29 years and 5 months for an Australian Cattle Dog.[243] At least as evidenced by necropsy data, there is a trend for the mean age of death for neutered dogs to be older than for intact dogs.[36]

Approximately 75% of the dogs that go to veterinary clinics have been spayed or castrated,[1] but over the entire population, only 66% of the animals have been neutered. There is a significant difference between sexes, in that 12% of the males and 47% of the females are neutered.[303,330] Yet estimates, based on owners' responses, run as high as 92% for spayed females and 62% for neutered males. Exact figures are impossible to obtain[175,233]; data suggest that young dogs are less likely to be neutered than older dogs and male dogs less likely than females. Almost one third of dog owners have not neutered their dog because they "just have not gotten around to it."[303]

In this era of genomics, researchers have found that dogs and humans share approximately 25% of their gene sequences.[149] Although that is nowhere close to the shared genes of humans and chimpanzees, it is cause to wonder if this may peak human interest in dogs. The human fascination with and expectations from dogs have been investigated. Results indicate that 68% to 80% of people got the dog for companionship, and about 50% of dog owners say they are emotionally dependent on their animals.[2,7,335] This finding parallels the finding that 76% let their dogs sleep on or by their beds.[2,296] Almost all dog owners talk to their pet and feel that the animal understands them.[296] Studies have shown that people who express little affection for dogs also express little for people. Men who expressed little affection for dogs were also found not to desire attention.[38,168] When dog owners were studied specifically, three to five attitudinal segments were identified.[166,330]

Several years ago the Pet Food Institute did a study of pet owners and described five types of people having a dog. Certainly the distribution within categories has changed over time, but the basic descriptions are still true today. Dog owners categorized as "Companionship Owners" (27% according to the original survey) considered their dogs to be major sources of friendship, companionship, and affection.[330] They usually took their dogs on vacations and generally reported few problems with them. If they had to leave their dogs, these owners would be the most likely to support a pet hotel,[260] or have a pet sitter stay with the dog. This group of owners derives very important psychologic benefits from their dogs.[330] Human names had been given to 52% of the pets, and names of endearment were common, like "Sweetie" and "Baby."[2,96,97] Most dogs with companionship owners have human names, with "Sam," "Max," "Heidi," and "Ginger" being among the most popular.[96] Interestingly enough, 75% of people who have dogs feel that they are more tolerant of the pet's shortcomings than the shortcomings of their spouse or children.[296] Over 50% of companionship owners feed their pets premium brands of food and give them gifts on their birthday or on holidays.[99,193]

"Worried Owners" (24% of the original survey sample) like their dog, but they have a fear that their pets are potentially harmful and that they lack control over them.[330] They often allow their dogs to roam such that they may be gone for a day or two at a time. Worried owners often describe their dogs as "stupid," "dumb," or "spoiled," and they may be embarrassed by their animal's sexual behavior.[330] Veterinarians recognize these owners as they get pulled into or out of the clinic by the dog. Owners subconsciously recognize these dogs because they hate taking the dog for a walk.

For "Valued Object Owners" (19%), the dog is considered an extension of self and given the same quality of care in selection and maintenance as other possessions.[330] Although there is no significant psychologic investment by these owners, neither do they complain about the dog's physical characteristics.[330] With personification of image, castration of male dogs is generally strongly resisted by most of these owners. Even within this group there could be a great deal of diversity, from the aristocratic owner of an Afghan or Pembroke Welsh Corgi, to the black-leather-jacketed owner of an American Pit Bull Terrier or Rottweiler wearing a spiked leather collar. The first group might use regal names like "Sheik" or "Cognac" for their pets, whereas the latter would prefer power names like "Fang," "Brutus," or "Killer."

The fourth group of dog owners from the Pet Food Institute study were those called "Dissatisfied Owners" (19% of the original study population).[330] The general view held by people in this category was that the dog was more trouble than satisfaction. The owners tended to complain about everything from doggy smells and shedding of hair to the dog being a nuisance, overly affectionate, or too expensive. Because any investment in the animal's health was considered too expensive and time consuming, veterinary care was minimal for the dogs of these owners. Interestingly, these owners often had received the animal as a gift or had procured it as a pet for their children.[330] Names chosen for these dogs often reflected the owners' negative or noncommittal attitudes. "Stinky," "Budweiser," and "Dog" were examples.

"Enthusiastic Owners" (17%) were the fifth group identified in the Pet Food Institute study. These people took good care of their dogs and appreciated the friendship and companionship they received.[330] They had few complaints of either physical factors or behavior problems. Though sharing many of the characteristics of the companionship owners, enthusiastic owners were defined as having a less pronounced psychologic commitment to their dogs.[330]

A later study divided pet owners into three groups. The "Pet for Child" owner group (29%) viewed their dogs as guardians and playmates for their children.[166] The "Pet Lovers" (30%) viewed their dogs as companions.[166] The "Pet Dispassionates" (41%) viewed their dogs as serving mainly functional purposes.[166]

People acquire dogs for a number of reasons and from a number of sources. The most common reason for dog ownership seems to be the presence of children between the ages of 6 and 17.[241,250,301,330] The most common sources are breeders, friends, or family members (Table 1-5). When asked why they acquired a specific dog, owners gave a variety of reasons and sometimes more than one. Most (24.0%) chose the dog because of its sex, 17.1% said it was friendly and affectionate, 15.0% cited pity, 14.3% said it was cute, 12.8% liked its color, 12.8% picked

| TABLE 1-5 | Common sources for pet dogs |
|---|---|
| **Source of pet** | **Percentage** |
| Breeder | 30 |
| Friend/family | 20 |
| Pet store | 10 |
| Humane society | 9 |
| Newspaper ad | 8 |
| Animal shelter | 6 |
| Other | 17 |

Data from reference 304.

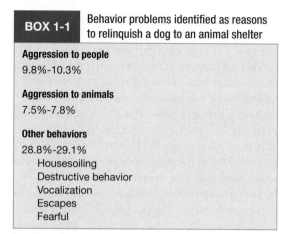

**BOX 1-1** Behavior problems identified as reasons to relinquish a dog to an animal shelter

**Aggression to people**
9.8%-10.3%

**Aggression to animals**
7.5%-7.8%

**Other behaviors**
28.8%-29.1%
    Housesoiling
    Destructive behavior
    Vocalization
    Escapes
    Fearful

Data from references 204, 263, 264.

it for its size, and 13.7% chose it for certain other physical characteristics or appearance in general.[53]

The human-animal bond does have its ups, downs, and "say that agains." One owner euthanized her dog and had it stuffed because she was afraid her son's dog would hurt it![294] Overall, dog owners spend billions of dollars each year on their pets. In Japan, people can actually rent dogs by the hour because owning one is so expensive.[256] Typical expenses of ownership are primarily for food and routine health care, but treatment for illnesses and injuries also requires sizable investments. Of dogs presented for emergency treatment at a large city's teaching hospital, approximately 53% had been hit by a vehicle, and two thirds of those dogs were males. Among owned dogs the number decreases as cities enforce leash laws. Another 10% had been injured in animal interactions, primarily fights with other dogs, and 77% of those dogs were male. Of the 11% admitted because of trauma by a sharp object, two thirds again were male. These dogs overall were significantly younger than those of the typical hospital population, and more of them were male.[154,155]

The source of the pet has been studied relative to development of future health and behavioral problems. In general, the prevalence of problems does not differ according to source of the dog[269]; however, of those adopted from a humane society, fewer were returned by owners who had taken their dogs to a veterinarian.[146] Even when people in that group did return the dog, it was much later and after a more serious effort to solve problems than was the case for owners who never made the veterinary connection.[146]

Dogs that are relinquished to shelters end up there for a variety of reasons. Some owners bring their dogs in requesting euthanasia (16% to 27%), usually because of advanced age, illness, or aggression.[102,144,202] People relinquishing their dogs are often asked to fill out a questionnaire. Confidential questionnaires reveal significantly more behavior problems in the dogs than would be found with nonconfidential questionnaires or in the general dog-owning public.[282,283] Major themes do occur as reasons for surrendering a dog. Lifestyle can make ownership difficult. That can involve everything from working too much to moving (Box 1-1). Certain factors are more apt to predict which dogs will be given up to a shelter. These include an owner who did not participate in an obedience class, lack of veterinary care, sexually intact dogs, a minimum of dog-human shared activities, inappropriate care expectations, at least once weekly episodes of housesoiling, received as a gift or at low cost, and acquired from a shelter.[28,234,264,270]

Older dogs were less likely to be either surrendered to a shelter in the first place or to be returned to the shelter later.[104,205] If the adult dog was rejected, the usual reason given was unacceptable behavior, so it appears that the unsatisfactory placing of dogs is more often due to incompatibility than to disease.[15,104,328] In an effort to decrease the number of dogs returned, shelters give advice to new owners, and some even offer postadoption behavior assistance. Studies show that after the first 12 months 14% to 20% of the adopted dogs are no longer in the home. Of those, 10% were returned, euthanized, or rehomed for behavior reasons.[15,75,232] Overall, 55.4% of adopters reported behavior problems and 54% of those had moderate to severe problems during the first 6 months. During the next 6 months, the actual number reporting minor behavior problems increased, too.[15] Researchers are studying ways to predict which dogs are most likely to develop behavior problems after being placed in a home.[316] The subjective evaluations used in the test predicted 75% of the potential problems and were better than the objective opinions of the animal shelter staff, which predicted only one third.[316] Studies indicate that the most frequent problems in dogs adopted from humane societies included housesoiling, aggression toward human adults, separation anxiety, aggression toward other dogs, car-related problems, pulling on the leash, and disobedience. Other researchers found that dogs that were acquired from shelters, kept in crates, or at least 6 months of age were also at higher risk of being relinquished.[234] In the first month postadoption, 39% to 68% of owners experience a behavior problem with their dog.[177,329] Housesoiling occurs in 51% of the homes and destructive behaviors in 28%.[177] The aggression and separation anxiety problems were the ones most likely to result in the dog being returned. Returns are frequent enough that states have even attempted to legislate the idea of a warranty for buyers of dogs from pet dealers.[244] Retention studies find a better prognosis if the dog and new owners attend a puppy class; the puppy has early handling; the owners use a head halter instead of regular collar; the dog responds to cues; the dog was expensive; there are no children in the home; the dog is female; and the dog sleeps on or near the bed.[75,76,234]

Although *Canis familiaris* has become an important part of our society, only 38% of dog owners keep their pet long term.[244] Every year millions of dogs are disposed of either by sending them to new homes, surrendering them to animal shelters or pounds, or turning them loose to create strays. The stray is defined as a wandering domestic dog that is given unsupervised freedom to travel, either on a regular or intermittent basis.[62,100] The typical

| TABLE 1-6 | Reasons for relinquishment of dogs to animal shelters |
|---|---|
| Reason | Frequency |
| Behavior problems | 46.4% |
| Human housing issues | 30.4%-38.8% |
| Human health/personal issues | 27.1% |
| Request euthanasia | 16.0%-17.7% |
| Human expectations | 14.0%-14.6% |
| Animal housing issues | 12.7% |
| Moving | 12.5% |
| Animal's health | 7.8%-8.2% |
| Human lifestyle | 6.8%-25.4% |
| Animal characteristics | 4.3%-4.5% |

Data from references 202, 206, 265, 270.

reason dogs become strays is because of irresponsible management by dog owners. Evidence indicates the majority of roaming dogs are owned.[200] In this country there are probably few truly feral dogs—ones that have reverted to total self-sufficiency—among the large number of stray dogs.[100] Of the 10 to 17 million dogs entering shelters, 36% to 59% are strays. About 30% are relinquished to the shelter by their owners, and 13% to 20% enter for other reasons.[192,199,201,203,306] Behavior problems are given as the single most common reason for giving up the animal and thus are responsible for up to 70% of the deaths—more than all infectious diseases combined (Table 1-6).[102,129,133,142,162]

The exit rate from shelters is revealing. Approximately 19% to 25% of the dogs leaving the shelter are placed in a new home, 15% are reclaimed by the original owner, and 55% to 66% are euthanized.* Of owners who returned their dog to the shelter, 89.7% did so because of an undesirable behavior.[328] Shelters are looking for better ways to predict success of dogs adopted. Some provide counseling. Others are looking for behavioral or endocrine tests that are significant.[121] The perfect answer seems a long way off, however. The annual euthanasia rate is 10% to 20% for the overall U.S. dog population; 4 to 9 million dogs are killed in U.S. animal shelters and pounds each year.†

---

*References 129, 169, 192, 201-203, 265, 295.
†References 8, 12, 141, 198, 213, 233, 241, 295, 307.

The causes of dog overpopulation are numerous and complex, and this book is not intended to address all the possibilities. In general terms, though, excess dogs mean more puppies are being born than there are homes available. It has been estimated that 1000 to 2000 puppies are born every hour in this country.[24] That means that 70,000 puppies are born each day, compared with 10,000 human babies.[306] A single intact bitch can directly and indirectly give rise to 67,000 dogs over a 6-year period.[306,307] The lifetime rate of production for a female dog is only slightly lower for spayed females than for intact ones, because 20% of all neutered animals have been allowed to reproduce before being neutered.[175,213]

If each dog litter averaged five puppies, it would be necessary to terminate 1 to 2 million pregnancies each year to prevent an excess of puppies.[213] Although spay/neuter programs have reduced the degree of the overpopulation problem, at least in certain areas, these surgical procedures would be most effective if they occurred before any litters were sired or whelped.[142] It has been argued that the cost of surgical neutering is a deterrent, but studies show that to be true only about 5% of the time.[303] The irony is that the rate of intact animals increases in direct relationship with the income of the owners.[175,273] More than surgery is needed to control dog numbers. It may take education of the next generation of dog owners and regulation of the demand.[142,273]

Stray dogs pose several problems for society. In addition to the unpleasant aesthetics of mass euthanasias, there are public health and nuisance problems.[62,306,307] Stray dogs account for 20% of dog bites to humans.[20] They can carry zoonotic diseases, especially rabies. Stray dogs can be traffic hazards, and they can be predators of livestock and wildlife populations, even upsetting the ecologic balance. Finally, roaming dogs foul the environment by tipping over garbage cans and leaving excreta. The estimated 61.6 million dogs in the United States weigh an average of 14.5 kg and produce 40 ml of urine per kilogram of body weight per day.[191] The result is 35.73 million liters of urine deposited by dogs each day. These same dogs produce 20.94 million kilograms of feces per day, assuming each dog eliminates 0.34 kg of feces.[25] If 144 flies can hatch from each defecation;[25] there is a potential for 17.7 billion flies hatching daily.[20]

## ANIMAL BEHAVIOR IN THE VETERINARY PRACTICE

There is a strong tendency to think of veterinary behavior in the realm of a treatment, rather than as a list of preventive services that can be offered to dog owners. Preventing problems is even more important than treating them. A practice can offer a number of services that help strengthen the human-animal bond, generate revenue, and do not require large amounts of time,[33] and all members of the staff can contribute to the success of the programs. For new pet owners, a clinic team can help with preselection consultations, preventive behavior counseling, puppy socialization classes, community-related events like vaccination fairs or National Pet Week parties, and recommending preventive management products and services.[159,223]

### Preselection Consultations

Preselection consultations can take a number of different forms and can be available to specific clients or to the public as a whole. The most obvious form of these consultations would be to offer appointments for individuals and families who are seriously considering getting a dog and want to be sure they are selecting the right breed for their family and lifestyle. How to make this service known is the biggest challenge, because most puppies are obtained as spur-of-the-moment purchases. Technology is increasing our ability to reach potential pet owners. By putting general information on clinic websites and in client newsletters, writing a column for a local newspaper, or hosting a local radio or television public service show, veterinarians can educate the whole public, not just current clients. Then specific questions can be dealt with during a preselection consultation targeted to a particular family's concerns. There are a number of subjects that potential dog owners should consider before getting a dog. The most obvious is the breed, although they often have their minds already made up. However, they need to think of things like anticipated yearly costs for dog food, veterinary care, preventive medicines, and grooming; care when the owner is gone; requirements for obedience training, specific elimination areas, and exercise; amount of time available to interact with the dog; and amount of shedding, brushing, and upkeep. Future owners should then put their expectations up against the actual characteristics of the breed or breeds they are considering to see if they fit. Books like *The Perfect Puppy*[114] are nice additions for future dog owners to see. It is important that books recommended are unbiased as to the traits of a breed.

## Preventive Behavior Consultations

Preventive behavior counseling begins the first time the new dog enters the clinic. Because most people have one dog at a time,[303] many of the basics should be covered. Those basics include what to feed, vaccinations schedules, parasite control information, housetraining and crate training techniques, proper socialization procedures, basic puppy obedience training, and techniques to help the dog successfully view the owners as its leaders. With the large amount of information that needs to be shared, most veterinary practices find that handouts help emphasize points mentioned in the clinic. This information can also be made available through a lending library of books and videos, and with website information. It is also helpful to have a checklist in the record so that information can be spread out over several visits and for consistency between the various staff who may interact with the puppy.

## Puppy Socialization Classes

Puppy socialization classes complement preventive behavior counseling. It allows a time to reinforce the lessons of the regular clinic visits, provide more in-depth information that regular puppy appointments cannot accommodate, provide new material, and start puppy obedience lessons. In addition, clinic-sponsored socialization classes provide a safe environment for puppies to socialize with other dogs and with people of all types. For those practices interested in providing puppy socialization/kindergarten classes, special sources are available that detail how to establish and run such classes.[137,196,313]

## Products to Help Prevent Behavior Problems

Clinics can sell or recommend a wide variety of products that help prevent behavior problems. Of these, most will fall into four categories. Crates and exercise pens keep the dogs confined when owners cannot actually watch them. In addition, once the puppy gets used to these products, it will often spend part of the day in them without coaxing. This makes the crate or pen a nice product for traveling with the dog by taking along the smell of home and the familiar surroundings in a safe environment. The second category of product that helps prevent behavior problems is the head halter. Even 6- to 8-week old puppies can learn correct behavior and simple obedience lessons with the head halter. This is a humane way to hold a puppy's attention, without putting pressure on the trachea or forcing prongs into the neck. More is discussed on this topic in Chapter 2. Chew toys, the third category, that can dispense food treats give mental stimulation to puppies. In some of these toys, the center is hollowed out so that a food treat like cream cheese or peanut butter can be smeared inside. These keep the puppy busy trying to get all the treat out. When frozen, it takes even longer to get out. Other forms of the hollow-center toy allow the owner to put in kibble, which is then dispensed slowly as the puppy rolls the ball around. A low-cost variation of this would be to put some kibble into an empty 2-liter soda bottle that has been flattened. Other chew toys allow food treats in the crevices of the surface or simply allow the puppy to chew on them. The fourth category included other types of toys that can encourage human-puppy interactions and puppy exercise. Ropes with which the puppy can play tug-of-war with the owner, tennis balls for chasing, and Frisbees to catch are examples. Articles in each of these categories will decrease the opportunity and need for puppies to get into trouble with destructive chewing.

It is also important to ask each time the dog is seen if there are any undesirable behaviors that the owner has noticed. Early identification can prevent long complicated behavior workups later and greatly decrease the time needed to diagnose and treat a particular problem. Some basic questions can be added to the admission form or to routine history-taking, or special behavior questionnaires can be added to preadmission information.[224] Approximately two thirds of pet owners feel that their animal is well behaved, but 85% report specific problem behaviors.[242] As with similar studies in the past, problems noted tended to be nuisance ones (barking/growling 17%, jumping on people 13%, begging for food 11%, digging 8%, running away 6%, destructive behavior 5%).[242]

## INTRODUCTION TO EVALUATING BEHAVIOR PROBLEMS

Within the last 30 years, veterinarians have become more comfortable in working up animal behavior problems. Many recognize their obligation in this discipline because of their responsibilities in diagnosing mental conditions in addition to physical ones, appreciating the interconnection between behavior and medical conditions,[33] and ability to modify behavior with psychotherapeutic drugs. Much of this need to help dogs with behavior problems reflects the change in society's major role for the dog, from a working farm animal or backyard inhabitant to a four-legged family member. Approximately 90% of owners surveyed feel that the dog is or is almost a family member.[10] An equal number want help managing a pet's behavior problems.[197] An animal is not capable of seeking help alone or describing its problem[16]; it takes an owner, too. Unfortunately, owners may not know what is normal canine behavior or may have unrealistic expectations of the dog,[82] because they have known individual dogs only as family members and have not observed the more universal aspects of dog behaviors. But when a behavior is considered problematic, pet owners agree it can have a big impact on their lives.[207]

Animals show behaviors based on their reflexes, instincts, and learning, although it is usually a combination of all three.[245] Exactly what behavior is shown will depend on external factors, such as environmental stimuli, and internal factors, such as mood, hormones, physical capabilities, previous experience, and sensory capabilities. Even such things as the presence or absence of the owner in the examination room influences the physiology and behavior.[229] Usually when an owner is present, heart rates are lower and aggressive behaviors are significantly more common. Animal behavior problems can be related, then, to the biology of the species and to its environment.[266] Another aspect is important in veterinary medicine too—the role of pathologic processes.[186]

A full understanding of animal behavior problems may not be possible until we understand its deepest-level biologic interactions, in descending order from phenotype, neuroanatomy, neurophysiology/neurochemistry, molecular, genotype, or the levels of "causality."[221,226] But behaviorists have come a long way from the days of tranquilizers and euthanasia solutions. Today we recognize many of the complexities that contribute to behavior problems and can proactively work to make things better.

The scope and severity of behavior problems vary greatly. In general, 70% to 75% of dissatisfactions pet owners have with their animals are classified as nuisances rather than serious or dangerous problems.[9,10] The most common nuisances are territorial defensive behavior, overprotection of the owner, and excessive vocalization.[22] Destructive behaviors, barking, overexcitement, rushing at people or dogs, and jumping on people are also common complaints.* Veterinarians can proactively work to prevent those behaviors from developing. The veterinary behaviorist sees problems that are more serious, with more than half related to aggression,[14,72] and visits to a behavioral specialist are often a last-ditch effort by the owner to avoid euthanizing an animal. Euthanasia is the leading cause of death of companion animals, and behavior problems are the leading cause of euthanasia.[24] Thus, a behavior problem can be viewed as a "terminal disease" and correcting it as the only way to save the animal's life.[312,322]

Aggression, separation anxiety, and housesoiling are the most common behavior problems seen as referral cases.[22,72,336] Among breeders of purebred dogs, abnormal temperaments were listed as one of

---

*References 3, 47, 153, 157, 261, 315.

the top 12 important issues.[120] More than 35 years ago, the veterinary profession was encouraged to deal with behavior problems by breeders and dog owners, making animal behavior a unique specialty that grew from the public asking for help.[45]

At least 40% of pet owners take their animal to a veterinarian once or twice a year, and another 32% make three to four visits.[1] Just over half the owners say they have discussed a behavior problem with the veterinarian,[1,297,335] and 78% would seek help for a developing problem from the veterinarian.[303] Of owners who had adopted their dog from an animal shelter, 89% felt it was helpful to have an office visit just to discuss behavior.[122] Because early intervention is best, veterinarians should include questions at the yearly visits to screen for the development of problems.[126] Questions could cover areas such as presence of unruly behavior, development of signs of aggression (protection of objects or food), housesoiling, and other areas that are commonly associated with behavior problems.

Different researchers have looked at different ways to categorize animal behavior problems.[27,132] Perhaps the most descriptive uses three large categories and then subdivides those (Box 1-2).[27] It may be helpful to use these broad categories to think of appropriate questions to ask during routine examinations to be sure early signs of behavior problems are not already showing up. Under each of the three categories described in Box 1-2, more is known about the owners most likely to make the complaints. For aggressive dogs, owners who complained were likely not to consider themselves to be the primary caregiver, and the dogs were more likely to have come from pet shops or shelters.[28] Dogs that were considered to be disobedient were more likely to be associated with homes having more family members, men, and owners not having previous experience with dogs. The dogs were more likely to be considered purebred and small in size.[28] The complexity of responses about the reactive behaviors made it difficult to find common factors among owners.

Obedience training is a common recommendation to make for owners of new dogs, but its relationship to the development of behavior problems is confusing. Some studies suggest it has no relationship with the development of problems,[324,325] but others suggest there is.[54,138] Agility class attendance is significantly correlated with a reduced number of behavior problems.[29] Formal obedience training at home is negatively correlated, perhaps because it is more likely to be associated with punishment rather than rewards.[29] It is appropriate to recommend obedience training classes for all dog owners, but there are important things that need to be part of that recommendation. First, and most important, is that the owner be the person working the dog. It should *never* be sent off for training, even if the owner then comes to work with it for a few days. In the best case, the dog learns how to obey the trainer, but in the worst case bad things happen. Obedience classes are more about training the owner than the dog, so the owner must be part of the lessons. The second factor is that the trainer uses only positive training methods. Telling a dog "no" may stop a behavior, but it does not show the correct or expected response. Shaping a behavior by allowing only the desired outcome and rewarding that outcome is more satisfying to the owner and not stressful for the dog. Heavy leash corrections, shouting, and swatting are not good training techniques. They only vent frustrations.

| BOX 1-2 | Major classifications of dog behavior problems |
|---------|-----------------------------------------------|

**Reactive behavior**

Overexcitement (62.6%)
Distressed in house (16.7%)
Apprehensive with animals (7.9%)
Behavior of natural drives (7.9%-24.4%)
Destructive behavior (5.3%)
Noise-related (2.6%)

**Disobedient behavior**

In house with human (15.8%)
In public with human (7.9%)
In public with owner aggravation (7.9%)
In house with owner aggravation (2.6%)

**Aggressive behavior**

In house with human (3.1%-11.4%)
In public with animals (8.8%)
In house with animals (2.6%)

Data from references 27, 28, 153.

Behavior problems can present a dilemma for the practitioner, because it can take a long time to adequately work up a case. In some cases, owners may view it as being easier to get rid of the dog than have to work up or treat the problem. For early and simple problems, like a puppy defecating in the house, the time required for the history, diagnosis, and recommendations may be only 15 minutes. But for the adult dog that is showing aggression, the history-taking alone may require 2 hours.

Handling the behavior case adequately can take excessive amounts of time if the situation is not well planned. The shorter and simpler problems may be handled successfully during a routine office call, but for those where more time is needed, the client should be asked to return when an appropriate number of appointment times can be merged. In this way, the veterinarian can devote proper attention to the client. The client, in turn, would be expected to pay for the time required, just as if the veterinarian's time were involved in performing an ultrasound or surgical procedure.[50]

## Signalment

For any veterinary case, the first information acquired should be the signalment. Alone it can provide a great deal of information for a behavior case, as it can for a medical case. The age of the dog can be helpful, particularly if the dog is very young or very old. For example, a case of housesoiling by a 3-month-old puppy would be worked up and treated differently than one involving a geriatric patient. Incomplete or improper housetraining is the highest differential for the puppy. Medical problems, including neurologic changes, head the list for the senior. Similar variations according to age can also apply in cases of aggression and other behavior problems. The typical dog presented for a problem is a young adult, around 3 years of age.[336]

The sex of the dog can vary the list of differentials for a problem. Dominance aggression, intermale aggression, and roaming are much more likely to occur in intact male dogs. Maternal-protective aggression is characteristic of bitches with puppies. More than 50% of dogs presented for behavior problems are intact males.[317,321,336] This fact suggests that testosterone may be important in the development of behavior problems. The effects of neutering and the relationship of gender to various problems will be discussed in later chapters.

Breed differences do occur in regard to behavior. Problems with a particular breed, however, may vary according to its popularity, its general location, and over time. National trends do occur, but the fact that a certain breed ranks high on a list of problem dogs may not be significant. Popular breeds (see Table 1-4) will necessarily be represented in higher numbers for any given problem. Only when the rate of a certain problem in that breed is higher than the distribution of the breed in the canine population can it be considered a breed-specific problem. As an example, if excessive barking is considered, 10 owners of Rat Terriers complain and three owners of Beagles complain. It is easy to assume that barking is a bigger problem for Rat Terriers. But, if you knew that there are 100 Rat Terriers (incidence of barking = 10%) and five Beagles (incidence of barking = 40%), you would view the problem differently.

The relative incidence of a specific behavior problem in a breed can vary by location.[162] One reason is that sometimes a breed is more popular in one area than in others. Another reason is that a particularly popular sire can spread a genetically based problem, establishing a regional emphasis or occasionally a national one. In a few cases, the breeder chooses to ignore or at least not acknowledge the presence of the problem, allowing it to become well established within a breed.

The incidence of a behavior problem within a breed can change over time. Not too long ago, American Cocker Spaniels, which were extremely popular, became known for various types of aggression.[19,162] An interesting contrast can be made with the same breed 50 years ago, when Scott and Fuller chose to breed the Cocker Spaniel as the model for nonaggressiveness in their 13-year behavioral genetics study.[280] After a breed loses its popularity, conscientious dog breeders continue to select dogs carefully to mate using more rigorous criteria. The people who were trying to make a fast dollar through indiscriminate breeding selection have moved on to other breeds.

One clue to behavior problems may be the pet's name. The name of the dog can provide an interesting insight as to its role within the family. Endearing and human names are probably most common when the dog is considered to be a family member. Noncommittal or derogatory names may indicate a neutral or negative relationship. These relationships could be contributing to the development of the problem behavior and will likely determine the willingness of the owner to participate in achieving a successful outcome.

## Case History

For most behavior cases, the majority of information will come from the history, so the importance of history-taking cannot be overemphasized. The main goal is to obtain an accurate description of all important aspects of the problem, including relevant information about the pet, the associated humans, and the environment.[134,320,323] It is important to not let owners use judgmental descriptions because of their biases.[30,167] "The dog is guilty" or "he did it to get even" are examples. Another goal is to identify the immediate consequences of the behavior, understand the development of the behavior, and uncover other related problems that may be present.[323] There is evidence linking the owner's relationship to the dog and the development of behavior problems.[209] Dominance aggression has been tied to the anthropomorphic involvement of the owner. Owner anxiety can be related to overexcitement and displacement activities in their dog, but not to the development of phobias.

General background information should be part of an inclusive history for dogs with behavior problems because, in many cases, past events can direct future actions. Specific information would include where they got the dog; how well was it socialized; how much, when, and what type of food/treats it gets; how much and what type of training it has had; other animals in the household; and people in the household and their general schedules. The medical history needs to be included as well. A dog not current on its rabies vaccination that is presented for problems with aggression has some significant liability issues. Those with chronic diseases may require lessons on how to be frequently medicated, may have chronic pain that increases their aggressive tendencies, or may be on medications that limit the choices for psychotherapeutic agents.[287] An early puppyhood history may not be available for dogs adopted from animal shelters or rescued, and that can make understanding the depth of the problem difficult. Food and treat information is very useful, because both can be used as rewards during behavior modification sessions. In fact, using different treats during both the history-taking and treatment discussion sessions can provide information about how successful food rewards will be. The goal is to find a treat the dog "would die for" so that very tiny pieces can be offered as rewards. Because eating also satiates hunger, training sessions are best timed to occur before a meal rather than after. Many owners describe their dogs as moderately well trained, but then go on to say it will only respond to "sit" commands, while on leash, about 50% of the time. Dogs that have been obedience trained will have a different incidence of behavior problems than will dogs without training.[54] Note, however, that although this information is important historically, no statistical correlation exists between either obedience training or spoiling and the incidence or type of any behavior problem.[324,325] Information about other animals and people in the household can be useful for problems involving the social behaviors.

For some practitioners, a history form is useful to be sure that all pertinent data are obtained (see the Appendix).[23,134,150] Others prefer an open format wherein owners are invited to discuss their perspectives first, and additional questions by the practitioner elicit missing information. For the recently developed but less serious types of problems, a structured questioning style may be suitable. In a referral setting, however, the owners will usually want to describe the problem as they see it. Having them fill out a form before the visit can provide useful information. It also can be useful to start discussions by asking owners where they got the pet and if they know anything about its parents. Then ask for a description of the pet's life history up to the present day. It is often necessary to refocus a discussion to get owners to describe the actual behaviors, rather than provide their interpretation of what the animal is doing or why.[30] It is also important to clarify vague descriptions. "The dog is destroying the sofa because I don't spend enough time with him" needs to be divided into information about the sofa (how, when, where, what parts) and what is the human-dog interaction schedule. Other vague descriptors, like "all the time," "a lot," "alpha," and "tried everything," must be better defined.

The writing of the history for the patient's record can tax even the fastest note taker, but this technique gathers a lot of information that might otherwise be missed, assures the owner of the veterinarian's interest in the pet, and helps the owner focus on particular events when more specific questioning follows. Newer techniques can include making a video record of the session. Questions during the owner's narrative can be asked, but for clarification of a point or to redirect the narrative as the owner continues. After the owner has completed his or her segment, it is appropriate to ask for more details about specific episodes.[320] Some practitioners choose to ask about the latest episode first.[68,320] Others want the descriptions to occur in the order of occurrence. It should also be noted that different owners may have different perspectives about the problem or memories of the events. For this reason, it can be helpful to have all the people involved present for this visit, if possible.[68]

The six general questions to be answered in any history-taking session involve what, how, where, when (two different "when" questions), and who. We will look at each of these questions next.[18,23] Based on the answers to these questions, many more-specific questions can help focus on the total scope of the problem.

1. *What exactly happens?* This is the first question to ask. It is necessary to understand the entire problem, and that is the purpose of this question. When an owner complains that the dog is "doing it" in the living room, he or she could be referring to urination, defecation, masturbation, biting, digging, or any of dozens of other behaviors. Another dog may be said to leave "presents," meaning it is defecating in inappropriate locations. Eliminative and sexually related behaviors seem to be the most difficult for owners to discuss, but a nonjudgmental use of proper

descriptive terminology allows the owners to be more specific about the problem. As part of the "what" set of questions, the veterinarian should determine if there is a trigger stimulus and if that trigger needs to be a certain intensity, proximity, or duration. As an example, a dog may be presented for aggressively lunging at people while on walks. Does this happen for every person it sees or only for those closer than 5 feet? 20 yards? Or more?

2. *How does it happen?* If the owner has actually seen the problem behavior, a detailed description of the behavior is appropriate. If they have not actually seen the behavior, they can set up a video recorder. Just as with seizures, the owner's description of how long each event lasts can be exaggerated, so careful questioning is indicated. It is also important to know whether the owner has tried to or can interrupt or stop the undesired behavior. If he or she can interrupt the behavior, the specific technique used is an important piece of information because it may actually be rewarding the undesired behavior.

3. *Where does it occur?* For some behaviors, the "where" may be a specific place, such as in the car, outdoors, in the house, or on the owner's foot. Many times, however, the answer is "all over the house." In these cases, careful questioning will often narrow down the location to one or two spots. To the owner, the smell of urine or feces may seem to be all over the house, but the actual site of elimination could be limited to one chair in the living room. A drawing of the floor plan of the house or layout of the yard may be helpful to envision the extent of the problem. The answer to "where" can provide insight to causes. Destruction of the carpet or wall near the door through which the owner usually exits is indicative of separation anxiety. A chair used by a recent house guest may be the target of urine marking. Also determine if there are possible distracters nearby that might be triggering the behavior. Children playing after school could trigger barking episodes on weekday afternoons, for example.

4. *When did the problem start?* The answer to this question can be helpful in two ways. The

beginning of the behavior may be associated with a specific event—a visiting guest, a new baby, a new job. Or the behavior may be associated with certain events that the owner has not thought about. For example, the Christmas holidays are often associated with major changes in schedules for pet owners and consequently for pets as well. A few days of cold, rainy weather often are associated with the start of a housesoiling problem. Veterinarians need to consider calendar and weather-related triggers for problem behaviors, because owners usually do not make these connections. Owners might not consider how sensitive a dog can be to an owner's longer work hours, on-the-job stresses, marital strife, loss of a loved one, or upcoming marriage. The length of time a problem has existed also helps from a prognostic standpoint for estimating how long it will take to correct the problem.

5. *When does the problem occur?* Some problems occur at certain times of the day. Others are related to either the presence or absence of the owner. Knowing the schedule of dog and owner helps put this information into perspective. The schedules also may explain variations in the pattern of frequency and intensity.[217] The answer to this "when" question may suggest a therapeutic plan as simple as having the owner leave when the behavior starts. Additional information under the "when" heading will include frequency and duration of the average bout.[217] In some cases, owners describe the behavior as totally unpredictable but then go on to describe what triggers the behavior. What they are really saying is that the behavior is truly predictable and therefore avoidable, but the danger is in the not predicting.[214]

6. *Who is involved?* The "who" question can provide a lot of information. It is important to determine who the target of the behavior is, or if there is one. Rather than asking directly, because the dog is usually viewed as "doing it to get even with me," ask questions about who usually sits in the destroyed chair or whose dirty clothes are urinated on instead. When a behavior occurs, are certain people always present? A behavioral history also should get information about the dog and the people with which it normally interacts. This includes learning who can successfully interrupt the behavior, as well as who cares for and trains the dog.

A seventh question, *"Why does it happen?"* is more one of academic curiosity. Although owners may ask why, they usually mean "why me?" In a few situations, the "why" question answers itself. For example, the dog urinates on the carpet about 8:00 every evening because its bladder is too full and the owners are not providing the opportunity to get outdoors. In some situations, however, the "why" will not really be answered until we understand brain function at the cellular level.

Another important part of history-taking is to determine what steps the pet's owner has already taken to try to solve the problem.[68] The knowledge that a specific therapy has already been appropriately tried means it need not be done again. In some cases, this information also can rule out certain possibilities on a list of differential diagnoses. If a therapy was tried but discontinued too quickly, or if compliance with accepted protocol was poor, it can be tried again with emphasis on the correct methods.

Determining how bothered owners are about the problem behavior provides insight into how hard they are willing to work to make a change. The dog that keeps the owner awake at night has a highly motivated owner. The dog that barks all day while the owner is gone has an owner who is mad at the neighbor for complaining, but is not really motivated to change the dog's behavior. Directly asking how much effort owners are willing to make can be helpful to get them to actually voice their commitment to change.

## Physical Examination

Because behaviors do not exist in isolation, it is important to examine and treat the whole animal. So, the next step is a thorough physical examination. As is normally done, the animal is evaluated in regard to body weight, temperature, respiration, and pulse. The abdomen is palpated and the thorax ausculted. Particular emphasis may need to be placed on a neurologic evaluation, eye examination, musculoskeletal evaluation, prostatic examination, and evaluation of any skin lesions or anal sacs. Physical problems should be noted and evaluated in their total contexts. Medical conditions can be common risk factors in dogs presented for behavior problems.[23,138,228] Common sense is also necessary here. Every practitioner will encounter some very aggressive dogs that cannot be carefully examined. A behavior practice often collects more than its share of such animals. The highest priority must be human safety. It may not be possible to do a detailed physical examination on some of these aggressive dogs.

With a behavior case, the physical examination becomes broader in scope. It includes how the dog interacts with other dogs, new humans, and the hospital environment. Subtle cues like excessive alertness, aggression toward anything that moves, tail posture, owner-dog interaction, abnormal gait, and reluctance to break eye contact provide a wealth of information that complements other information. Special situation trials can be set up to look at reactions. Walking one dog past another, staring at the dog, and putting down food can be tried. Even allowing the nonaggressive dogs to roam the exam room can provide insight into how they behave and how their owners react.[46]

## Special Tests

In working up a behavior problem, the veterinarian will use different tests to rule in or rule out the differential diagnoses chosen. In some cases, the final diagnosis is made on the basis of response to therapy. In others it is solely dependent on the historical findings. Usually it lies somewhere in between, and then special tests become important. Identifying disease-related causes of behavior problems may require that additional information be obtained through special tests, or the tests may be needed to be sure a certain medication is appropriate.

A complete blood count, biochemical profile, and urinalysis are the most common tests. They are appropriate for any geriatric patient but particularly one presented for housesoiling[135] or one that will be put on medication. Other chemical tests, such as pre-eating and posteating bile acid, thyroid hormone, and canine trypsin-like immunoreactivity (cTLI) concentrations might be appropriate. Radiographs with or without special contrast media,

ultrasonograms, electroencephalograms, electroretinograms, fundic exams, nuclear scans, computerized tomograms, and magnetic resonance imaging are needed in certain cases.

As with traditional medical problems, potential behavioral problems can be ruled out based on the test results, with a resulting shift of the rank on the differential list. The veterinarian and client can work together to determine how deeply to examine a problem and in what order any tests should be done.

## Diagnosis

As with any case worked up by a veterinarian, it is important to consider all differentials to make the specific diagnosis.[311] It should also be expected that the list of differential diagnoses will combine medical and behavior problems. For example, a list of differentials for a dog urinating in the house could include urinary tract infection, kidney disease, diabetes mellitus, diabetes insipidus, hyperadrenocorticism, psychogenic polydipsia, unavailability of access to normal eliminative locations, marking behavior, and separation anxiety.

Behaviors can be classified in broad terms by etiology, description, or function.[31] According to *etiology,* the behavior would be classified as normal—either instinctive or learned—or abnormal. If it is abnormal, it could be (1) pathophysiologic, either hereditary or acquired; (2) experiential, that is, learned from early experience; or (3) psychosomatic. To illustrate the difference between normal and abnormal, consider that grooming would be a normal behavior even if the owner did not appreciate the associated noise when it occurred during the night. In contrast, acral lick dermatitis is the result of excessive grooming as an abnormal behavior.

Another perspective of normal versus abnormal behavior is that behavior can be (1) normal for the animal and acceptable to the owner; (2) normal for the animal but unacceptable to the owner; (3) abnormal for the animal but acceptable to the owner; or (4) abnormal for the animal and unacceptable to the owner.[23,151] The four scenarios could also be stated as (1) normal–no problem; (2) normal-problem; (3) abnormal–no problem; and (4) abnormal-problem.

The *descriptive* classifications of behavior name the behavior activity.[31] These classifications would include urination, destructive chewing, digging, excessive barking, and many others. Most veterinary behaviorists use this scheme as the primary one. Aggression is the main exception because it is usually subdivided by function for more specific treatments.

*Functional* classifications involve relationships between the animal, its behavior, and its environment.[31] Diagnoses under this classification can relate to a stimulus-response relationship such as separation anxiety, a disease such as hypothyroid aggression, a physiologic state such as fear biting, or other factors like genetics or developmental conditions.

The diagnostic approach used most commonly is a mixture of classification schemes. As an example, separation anxiety is functional, whereas the urination, defecation, whining, digging, and destructive chewing that contribute to the overall behavior resulting from separation anxiety are descriptive.

Another approach to establishing a diagnosis is to categorize the problem behavior as being genetic, social, medical, or stress-related so that therapies can be more generalized.[21,23] Behavioral *genetics* is a difficult field to relate to dogs.[80] The 13-year study by John Scott and John Fuller at the Jackson Laboratory points out many of the difficulties in doing such research.[280] Expense alone probably means a similar effort will never occur again. On the other hand, the frequency of a certain behavior within a dog breed may be a stimulus for a dog club to sponsor research into the associated genetics. Certain behaviors have been shown to be genetically based within certain breeds. An emotionally unstable line of Pointers is one example.[195] Other behaviors seen frequently in specific breeds have not been proved to be genetically based but have a high index of suspicion. Behaviors such as flank sucking, fear biting, leash fighting, and showing a fear of loud noises can have a genetic component.[19,257] Still other behaviors have been proved to be programmed and are elicited by certain situations. Submissive urination, urine marking, and pseudopregnancy are examples.[106, 319] Even breed-specific behaviors can have genetic variation and be influenced by the puppy's size, age, maternal influence, and sex.[173,215] As the specifics of the dog genome are sequenced and studied and as test prices are reduced, the genetic causes of certain problems will be better understood.

*Improper socialization* and early handling of a puppy can result in significant social behavior problems in an older dog. These dogs may not relate well to other dogs, humans, or different environments. In affected animals, aggression or shyness can be exaggerated when the animal is forced into uncomfortable situations.

*Medical* causes of behavior problems occur in dogs. Examples include aggression associated with seizures or hypothyroidism, polydipsia associated with hyperadrenocorticism, and aphagia associated with cervicovertebral malformations that make it painful to lower the head to eat. In some cases, the connection between the behavior and medical problem is obvious. Other times, discerning the medical relationship becomes a diagnostic challenge.[117] In the DAMN IT (degenerative; anomalous; metabolic; neoplastic, nutritional; infectious/inflammatory, immune-mediated; traumatic, toxin) scheme for evaluating differential diagnoses, every category has medically based conditions that must be included as causes of abnormal behavior.[161] Although not always the highest priority in a differential list, medical problems certainly should be considered if there is a sudden change in behavior or if the response to behavior therapy alone is poor.[136] More behavior problems will shift into this category as neurotransmitters are better understood. Obsessive-compulsive and stereotypic disorders are medical conditions.

The fourth major category is *stress-related* (frustration) behaviors. How a dog reacts to stress depends on its breed and the environment. This is the largest category of behavior problems and one receiving a lot of attention today because of the concurrent emphasis on drug therapy. Despite the current attention on psychopharmacology, behavior modification can still be successfully used alone or in combination with drugs to manage stress.

## Treatment

Successful treatment depends on an accurate diagnosis, appropriate therapeutic protocol, a cooperative owner, and follow-up to fine tune the therapy as needed. The more work owners must do, the less likely they are to comply fully. And, part of what determines their willingness to comply is the amount of trust they have left in their pet.[214] The therapeutic management of a behavior case may involve appropriate treatment of concurrent/contributing medical problems; client education about what is happening, what needs to be done, and what to expect; environmental management to minimize repetition of the behavior; behavior modification; and/or drug therapy. These will be discussed in the next section.

## Prognosis

Owners want to know the prognosis for a behavior problem and how long it will take for their pet to be "cured." Before a prognosis can be given or even a therapeutic plan devised, it is important to determine the level of owner commitment.[134,163] For that, it is helpful to ask owners what their feelings are about their dogs[320] and what their goals are for the behavior-treatment program. If the "therapeutic plan" will involve a major commitment of time and effort, the owners need to know that up front rather than figure it out later and possibly become discouraged. They must be not only willing but able to make the program work.[163]

Factors in the prognosis for behavior therapy include the etiology, duration, and type of problem, plus the response to therapy.[42] In regard to *etiology,* the easiest behavior problems to treat are normal behaviors or simple, learned ones of an individual dog. The toughest are abnormal, complex, unlearned problems involving several dogs.

The *duration of the problem* often determines how long it will take to treat it. This is especially true when learning is involved, because the animal will have to unlearn the unacceptable behavior in addition to learning the desired behavior. If it is of long duration, the unacceptable behavior will take longer to unlearn.

The *type of problem* dictates how treatable the condition is. Certainly, past successes dealing with similar problems give the behaviorist a better chance to be successful and a better prognostic perspective. Also, the simpler the solution is, the greater the likelihood of an acceptable outcome. Distrust or fear of the dog complicates the prognosis. When owners become fearful, as often happens with aggression,

they may never trust the dog again, even though the actual type of aggression would otherwise be treatable. Client and public safety are factors that must be considered, and euthanasia may be the only "treatment" that is appropriate.

Many things influence the *response to a therapeutic plan.* Assuming a correct diagnosis, variation among individual dogs can affect an outcome. Another critical factor is owner compliance. When the therapy is a pill a day, compliance is reasonable. The more involved a behavior modification plan becomes, the lower the overall success rate will be. Owner expectations are also important. Some people are grateful for a small improvement, whereas others expect miracles overnight.

## Follow-up

The follow-up of a behavior case is important for the best treatment success. Studies show that clients do not consistently follow the recommendations even though they understand the rationale behind the protocols.[92] Compliance is approximately 60%.[164] By establishing a specific follow-up procedure, the veterinarian provides extra incentive to owners to carry out the therapeutic protocol,[164] and the results provide valuable information to better learn how to manage various types of cases. Follow-up calls allow the veterinarian and client to fine tune treatment protocols. If left to clients to call back, approximately 40% never do so after the appointment and less than 15% will call back more than five times.[247] For cases in which medications are prescribed, the client is significantly more likely to follow up than when pets are not medicated. Clients are also more likely to call back if the dog is younger or if they have owned the dog only for a short period.[247] Clients who receive follow-up contacts are more likely to feel that the treatment has had a positive effect and are more willing to seek help again if needed.[251] One of the hardest parts of evaluating treatment outcomes is to learn if there really is improvement, so researchers have looked for objective methods to do so.[123] The use of a scale of 1 to 5 or of 1 to 10 can be helpful if applied before and after a consulting visit. Although most clients report less than great results, they still are generally pleased with the consultation and more likely to keep the animal.[92]

# INTRODUCTION TO BEHAVIOR THERAPY

Once a diagnosis has been made for a behavior problem, an appropriate therapeutic regimen must be designed. It is common to look for the "magic pill," or ultimate solution. Everyone wants a quick fix. In the real world, such solutions are seldom available. The situation may require client education, environmental management, behavior modification, drug therapy, or some combination. Numerous studies in human and veterinary medicine have shown that the more involved a treatment protocol is, the lower the compliance rate. Therefore, it may be necessary to lay out a stepwise treatment plan instead of implementing everything at one time, or to tackle one problem at a time.

## Client Education

Client education has always been an important part of veterinary medicine. Relative to behavior problems, the approach becomes threefold. In the first part, it is important to educate dog owners about how the problem developed and things that caused it to escalate in severity. The educated owner is more willing to follow instructions for treating the condition or to understand why there is no instant cure.

The second type of education helps owners to treat their pet's condition properly. That might be instructing them about how many pills should be given and when, or it might be about how much to feed or exercise the dog. In behavior, client education can include the hows and whys of environmental management and various types of behavior modification.

The third type of owner education involves teaching owners about normal behavior. Because one category of dog-owner interactions is normal behavior that is unacceptable to the owner, the veterinarian often is required to educate the owner about what is normal for a dog. Because a dog cannot change a normal species-specific behavior, the owner may have to change expectations or find an alternative that allows both owner and pet to have their way. If a dog disturbs the owner at night by jumping on and off the bed, for example, the owner may want to make the dog lie still. Because it would be difficult to get a dog to change this behavior, other alternatives may be acceptable. Some owners will learn to ignore the disturbances once they find out that they cannot make it stop. Others, not willing to tolerate the restless behavior, may choose to have the dog sleep in another part of the house. A few would absolutely insist that the dog must continue to sleep in the bedroom. For these owners, keeping the dog in a crate or tethered at night would be an alternative. Teaching the client about what is normal for a dog provides a service that can be particularly valuable as preventive medicine, as well as being therapeutic.

## Environmental Management

Changing a behavior often involves changing or enriching the environment.[46] This technique can prevent the development of problems in the first place, and it is important for problems because it prevents the reinforcement of the unacceptable behavior. Intermittent reinforcement of a problem behavior can strengthen the behavior. So, tight control to prevent the behavior from happening at all is critical, especially if behavior modification also is being used. For example, it might be necessary to remove a chair that is the frequent target of urine marking or to change a time schedule for improved interactions between owner and dog. As another example, consider the fact that barking at night is commonly triggered by the barking of other dogs. Therefore, letting the dog stay in the garage or house at times when barking is expected may muffle the noise of the far-off bark enough to keep the resident dog quiet.

Environmental management allows normal behavior to continue but in a way that is acceptable to the owner. In the example of a loud grooming lick at night that is bothersome to an owner, a simple solution can be offered. Letting the dog sleep in another part of the house does not stop the grooming; it just moves the sound farther away. Similarly, adding a wading pool for an overheated dog or keeping it in the air conditioned home allows the dog to cool off without digging up the flower beds. Changing the environment, then, can change some behaviors, or at least the perception that a behavior is a problem. Enriching the environment also gives the dog something to do (Fig. 1-2). There are a number of

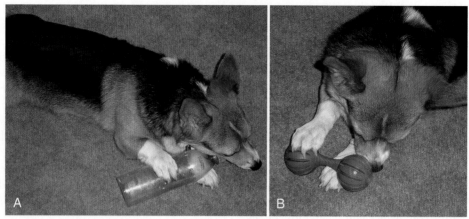

**Figure 1-2.** Environmental enrichment can be as simple as **(A)** an empty plastic bottle or more elaborate, like a commercial food dispensing toy **(B)**.

devices that are commercially available,[158] with new ones coming into the market all the time.

## Behavior Modification

Behavior modification is the use of the principles of learning to effect a change in an individual. How an animal learns will be discussed in greater detail in Chapter 2, but the various methods of behavior modification that can be used will be discussed here. For purposes of this section, any type of reward or punishment will be called a *reinforcer,* whether it positively or negatively reinforces a specific behavior.

### Conditioning

Conditioning is a process in which the dog learns to respond in a specific way when presented with a specific stimulus. For example, the dog is conditioned to assume a sitting position whenever the owner says "sit." This lesson could come through a number of different types of learning, but the general connection between the "sit" stimulus and the physical response is what is important. Reinforcers are usually used along with conditioning to modify behavior.

### Counterconditioning

The opposite of conditioning is counterconditioning. Here, learning is used to replace an unacceptable behavior with an acceptable one in response to the same stimulus. The owner first finds a highly

prized reinforcer, often a food treat, occasionally a play toy.[127] The owner will then have the dog focus on the prize reinforcer while a mild stimulus for the unacceptable behavior occurs. The dog should not be allowed to react negatively. The purpose is for the dog to come to associate the prized treat with the stimulus so that the unacceptable behavior is no longer shown. Suppose a dog goes out into the muddy backyard and gets covered in mud each morning during a particularly wet season. The owner is unhappy because as soon as the dog comes into the house, it will dash from room to room spreading mud everywhere. By teaching the dog to sit on command for a prized food reward, the owner can make the dog sit as soon as it enters the house. This gives the owner time to reward the appropriate response and wipe the mud off the paws. Another example would be to gradually teach a dog that did not like to ride in a car to want to go for a ride. In this case the dog is taught to "heel" and "sit" first. It is walked a short way toward the car and asked to "sit." That acceptable response is reinforced with a food treat. Gradually over several sessions, the dog will "heel" and "sit" closer and closer to the car. Then the door is opened and closed without entering while the dog "sits." Next the dog gets in, "sits," and immediately exits. Eventually the car is started and turned off, backed up 5 feet and driven forward again, then 10 feet, a short trip, and finally to some fun place. Gradually the not wanting to go for a ride is replaced with a "cannot wait" attitude. Counterconditioning is often coupled with desensitization if the dog's behavior is associated with fear or excessive sensitivity.

### Desensitization

When a dog shows an excessive amount of fear, sensitivity, or reactivity to a stimulus, it can be desensitized to that stimulus through learning. Desensitization (also called systematic desensitization) introduces the stimulus but in such a small amount that no reaction occurs. Gradually the amount of stimulus is increased, but never so fast as to elicit a response. The dog that is afraid of thunder can be desensitized by playing recordings of the sound very softly in a nonthreatening environment. The volume is increased very slowly. Desensitization like this can be coupled with counterconditioning by adding a play or eating stimulus at the same time that the volume is being increased.

### Habituation

Habituation is a learning technique in which the reaction-provoking stimulus is repeated until it no longer elicits a response. For the dog that runs barking to a door in response to a ringing doorbell, the bell can be rung repeatedly until the dog stops barking.

### Extinction

Another technique for behavior modification is extinction. Certain behaviors can be extinguished by removing all reinforcers. Dogs quickly learn that they can get attention from an owner for a specific behavior, and getting that attention reinforces the behavior. By simply stopping the attention, the owner can cause the behavior to gradually stop, too. For example, the dog that barks at night often gets yelled at by the owner. The dog learns that barking will result in interaction with the owner, and perhaps even the owner will appear or let the animal into the house. The simplest way to stop the barking is for the owner to ignore it. Initially that can be difficult, and the dog may actually bark more. Once the pet learns that the desired response is not going to happen, the amount of barking decreases to normal levels.

### Flooding

Flooding is a learning technique that can make a problem significantly worse if not done properly, so it is usually not a technique recommended for owners. In this method, the dog is exposed to the stimuli continuously until there is a major improvement in its reactions. The key words here are *continuously* and *major*. If a dog is afraid of people, the owner could bring together several friends and have them sit in a circle with the dog physically restrained in the center. The people remain in that circle until the dog noticeably relaxes, however long that might be. Each successive trial becomes shorter in duration until the animal is no longer fearful of being in the company of people.

## Drug Therapy

The use of drugs to treat behavior problems is nothing new, yet it remains a hot topic. Probably one reason drug therapy is popular is that both veterinarians and owners want to fix problems quickly and without a great deal of effort or time investment, so a "magic pill" would be nice. Owners often perceive improvement in a pet's problem just because they are doing something. Giving a pill is the easiest approach they can take. The placebo effect shown in well-controlled pain studies in dogs was 56%, even though it has been said to be as low as 26%.[109,180] Also, veterinarians are used to the medical-treatment paradigm, as opposed to the mental-management one—prescriptions feel more comfortable. A third reason for the popularity of drug therapy could be that many practitioners are not comfortable with behavior modification. Regardless of the cause of the interest in drug use for behavior problems, a great deal remains to be learned, and most drug use for behavior problems is still extra-label, so owner consent is recommended.

Historically, the first drugs used to treat behavior problems probably were those used for euthanasia. Even today the euthanasia solution remains the one most used for behavior problems when animal-shelter dogs are included in statistics. Fortunately, there have been a number of advances in neuropharmacology, and several more are currently being worked on (Box 1-3). Today euthanasia can be a last resort, not a first one.

| BOX 1-3 | Classification scheme for various psychotherapeutic drugs |
|---|---|

**Antianxiety drugs**

| *Sedative-automatic* | *Sedative-hypnotic* |
|---|---|
| Antipsychotics | Barbiturates |
|   Acetophenazine |   Butabarbital |
|   Haloperidol |   Phénobarbital |
|   Trifluoperazine | Benzodiazepines |
| Azapirones |   Alprazolam |
|   Buspirone |   Chlordiazepoxide |
|   Gepirone |   Clonazepam |
|   Ipsapirone |   Clorazepate dipotassium |
| Diphenylmethane |   Diazepam |
|     antihistamines |   Hafazepam |
|   Diphenhydramine |   Lorazepam |
|   Hydroxyzine |   Oxazepam |
| Tricyclic antidepressants | Glycerol derivatives |
|   Amitriptyline |   Meprobamate |
|   Doxepin |   Tybamate |

**Antidepressant drugs**

| | |
|---|---|
| Adrenergic stimulants | Sympathomimetic |
|   Salbutamol |     stimulants— |
| Aminoketones |     amphetamines |
|   Bupropion |   Dextroamphetamine |
| Benzodiazepines |   Levoamphetamine |
|   Alprazolam | Sympathomimetic |
| Bicyclics |     stimulants— |
|   Zimeldine |     amphetamine |
| Clomipramine |     surrogates |
| Lithium |   Magnesium pemoline |
| Monoamine oxidase |   Methylphenidate |
|     inhibitors (MAOIs) |   Pipradrol |
|   Isocarboxazid | Tetracyclics |
|   L-Deprenyl |   Maprotiline |
|   Phenelzine | Tricyclics |
|   Tranylcypromine |   Amineptine |
| Nomifensine |   Amitriptyline |
| Phenylpiperazines |   Butriptyline |
|   Nefazodone |   Clomipramine |
|   Trazodone |   Desipramine |
| Selective serotonin |   Doxepin |
|     reuptake inhibitors |   Imipramine |
|     (SSRIs) |   Maprotiline |
|   Citalopram |   Nortriptyline |
|   Fluoxetine |   Protriptyline |
|   Fluvoxamine |   Trimipramine |
|   Paroxetine | Unusual tricyclics |
|   Sertraline |   Amoxapine |

| **Antipsychotic drugs** | **Beta-blocking drugs** | **Hypnotic drugs** | **Narcotic antagonists** | **Progestins** |
|---|---|---|---|---|
| Benzoquinolizine | Propranolol | Antihistamines | Naloxone | Medroxyprogestrone |
|   Tetrabenazine | |   Chlorpheniramine | Naltrexone |   acetate |
| Butaclamol | |   Diphenhydramine | | Megestrol acetate |
| Butyrophenones | |   Methpyriline | | |
|   Droperidol | | Barbiturates | | |
|   Haloperidol | |   Pentobarbital | | |
| Dibenzodiazepine | |   Secobarbital | | |
|   Clozapine | |     sodium | | |
| Dibenzoxazepine | | Benzodiazepines | | |
|   Loxapine | |   Flurazepam | | |
| Diphenylbutylpiperidenes | |   Nitrazepam | | |
|   Penfluridol | |   Temazepam | | |
|   Pimozide | |   Triazolam | | |
| Indolic derivative | | Glutarimides | | |
|   Molindone | |   Glutethimide | | |
| Phenothiazines | |   Methyprylon | | |
|   Acepromazine | | Halogenated | | |
|   Acetophenazine | |     hydrocarbons | | |
|   Acetylpromazine | |   Chloral hydrate | | |
|   Butaperazine | | Higher alcohols | | |
|   Chlorpromazine | |   Ethchlorvynol | | |

| BOX 1-3 | Classification scheme for various psychotherapeutic drugs—cont'd |
|---|---|

| **Antipsychotic drugs—cont'd** | **Hypnotic drugs—cont'd** |
|---|---|
| Fluphenazine | Quinazolones |
| Mesoridazine | Methaqualone |
| Perphenazine | |
| Piperacetazine | |
| Promazine | |
| Thioridazine | |
| Trifluoperazine | |
| Phenylpiperazine | |
| Oxypertine | |
| Reserpine | |
| Thioxanthenes | |
| Chlorprothixene | |
| Flupenthixol | |
| Thiothixene | |

A few years ago there was a rush to try the tricyclic antidepressants and selective serotonin reuptake inhibitors. Veterinarians began prescribing a number of drugs for a wide variety of behavior problems. Unfortunately, in many cases, a specific diagnosis is never determined. Consequently, even with improvement of the animal's behavior, it is difficult to predict what situations are best suited for that drug. In veterinary medicine, there has always been a tendency to try a new behavior drug to treat all types of problem behaviors. In the past, however, there was usually only a single drug to try. Today there are a large number of human psychotropic drugs available from a variety of pharmacologic classifications. Progress in behavioral pharmacology comes when drug trials occur after a specific diagnosis is determined.

The first question that should be asked is whether drug therapy is even appropriate for the case. Drugs do not help a normal behavior that is considered undesirable. Many factors need to be considered before a specific drug is chosen.[185]

When a behavior problem is related to a specific medical entity, appropriate treatment may be obvious. Hypothyroid aggression, irritable aggression from chronic pain of hip dysplasia, tail chasing or aggression during a seizure, and poor learning resulting from hydrocephalus are just a few examples. Other drugs used in neuropharmacology should be looked at a little more closely. Except for specific medical causes of behavior changes, drug therapy is seldom sufficient to eliminate the problem.[110] They can be useful to augment the other treatments. The summary of drug doses for small animals as currently cited in the literature is found in the Appendix. This information, the reader is cautioned, continually changes as new knowledge is gained.

The ideal drug would be one that effectively eliminates the behavior problem, works on all patients, has no side effects, has a rapid onset of action,[124,258] has a wide margin of safety,[124,258] will not impair normal motor or mental functions,[125] has an intermediate half-life,[258] and has a defined therapeutic blood level.[258] Unfortunately, the ideal drug does not exist. Yet the percentage of binding, active metabolites, half-life, and site of action for many drug groups are being identified and allow a better understanding of how therapeutic responses occur (Table 1-7). Most drugs currently used in behavioral therapy undergo hepatic metabolism and are either substrates for or affect cytochrome P450 enzymes.[37,288] This has implications for patients on other medications.

This section of the chapter is intended to be an introduction to drugs used as part of a treatment plan for behavior problems. Space prevents it from being all inclusive, so the reader is directed to other sources for more in-depth and newer information.[67,74,288]

| TABLE 1-7 | Pharmacokinetic parameters for various drugs in veterinary medicine, including half-life and active metabolites | | | |
|---|---|---|---|---|
| Drug | Tl/2b (hr) | Protein binding (%) | Active metabolites | Tl/2b (hr) |
| **Benzodiazepines** | | | | |
| Chlordiazepoxide | 7-15 | 93 | Desmethyl-demoxepam | 14-46 |
| Diazepam | 14-90 | 94-98 | Nordiazepam | 30-200 |
| Halazepam | | 98.6 | Nordiazepam | 30-200 |
| Clorazepate | | 98.6 | Nordiazepam | 30-200 |
| Prazepam | | 98.6 | Nordiazepam | 30-200 |
| Flurazepam | | | Desmethyl | 40-100 |
| | | | Hydroxyethyl | 6-7 |
| **Tricyclics** | | | | |
| Imipramine | 9-24, 28 | 76-95 | Desipramine | 20-40 |
| Amitriptyline | 31-46, 21 | 82-96 | Nortriptyline | |
| Nortriptyline | 18-93, 36 | 93-95 | 10-Hydroxy | 21-57 |
| Desipramine | 14-62, 21 | 73-90 | Hydroxy | 22-59 |
| Protriptyline | 54-198, 78 | | | |
| Doxepin | 8-24, 17 | | Desmethyl | 9-33 |
| Clomipramine | 22-84, 23 | | Desmethyl | 7-20 |
| Maprotiline | 36-108, 43 | | | |
| **Antipsychotics** | | | | |
| Chlorpromazine | 8-35 | 98-99 | 7-Hydroxy | |
| Thioridazine | 9-30 | 99 | Mesoridazine | |
| Butaperazine | 10-15 | | Sulforidazine | |
| Perphenazine | 8-21 | | | |
| Fluphenazine | 14-24 | | | |
| Haloperidol | | 92 | | |
| **Antidepressants** | | | | |
| Fluoxetine | 87 | | | |
| Sertraline | 26 | | | |
| Paroxetine | 21 | | | |
| Fluvoxamine | 19 | | | |
| Bupropion | 15 | | | |
| Trimipramine | 13 | | | |
| Amoxapine | 8 | | | |
| Venlafaxine | 3.6 | | | |
| Trazodone | 3.5 | | | |
| Nefazodone | 3 | | | |
| **Others** | | | | |
| Lithium | 20 | 0 | None | |

Data from references 125, 258.

All five major monoamine neurotransmitters (acetylcholine, dopamine, gamma-aminobutyric acid, norepinephrine, and serotonin) work at the various synaptic transmission sites through several different modes of action using presynaptic or postsynaptic mechanisms. Presynaptic sites can be affected in seven ways.[208] The first is availability of the precursors for the making of a neurotransmitter. This can be altered when (1) precursors are administered directly, as with tyrosine or L-dopa for dopamine; (2) transport of the precursor to the brain is altered, as when the blood-brain barrier is changed; or (3) the precursor delivery into the neuron is changed.

Synthesis of the various neurotransmitters is a second way to affect presynaptic transmission. Monoamine neurotransmitters are usually made in nerve terminals and can more readily respond to activity changes in the neuron. The slower-responding peptide neurotransmitters are larger proteins or prohormones that must come from the ribosomes in the cell body to the terminals. Drugs or metabolites that affect the synthesis of either neurotransmitter can then affect behavior. Once made, neurotransmitters are stored in neurotransmitter-specific vesicles. These storage vesicles can be inhibited from forming or can be made to release their contents—a third area for presynaptic involvement.

The fourth mechanism affects the release of the contents of the storage vesicles. This mechanism requires the entrance of calcium into the nerve terminal and a fusion of the vesicle wall with the presynaptic nerve membrane. Some drugs cause a leakage of the neurotransmitter from the vesicles out of the terminal. The amount of the neurotransmitter may be so low that the postsynaptic receptor is unaffected, but through feedback mechanisms, it will still reduce the synthesis or release of additional amounts of that neurotransmitter.

The fifth site for presynaptic effects is the specific reuptake system for each neurotransmitter. Reuptake is an important method to stop synaptic actions, and blocking the system can prolong the effect of the neurotransmitter. Catabolic enzymes metabolize neurotransmitters, but if they are inhibited, the synaptic actions are also enhanced—a sixth mechanism.

Finally, presynaptic transmission can be affected by the makeup of the various neurotransmitters within a neuron. Each type or combination of types can be released by a different stimulus frequency.

Postsynaptic events also can alter the reaction to neurotransmitters.[208] The first postsynaptic event has to do with the receptors for each neurotransmitter. There are two families of receptors.[208] One family, like gamma-aminobutyric acid-A (GABA-A) and nicotinic receptors, incorporates an ion channel into its structure. The second family uses guanine nucleotide-binding proteins (G proteins) to alter intracellular function. Within each of these two families, there also can be multiple receptor subtypes for each neurotransmitter. Multiple subtypes have been identified for serotonin[63,64,101,285] and several others for acetylcholine.[208] In addition, a single neuron can have more than one subtype for each neurotransmitter, and receptors can vary in sensitivity in different areas of the brain.[174]

A second postsynaptic event can affect the various intraneuronal chemical components that are activated by neurotransmitters. These components include the G proteins, cyclic adenosine monophosphate, inositol phospholipid-specific phospholipase C, and protein phosphorylation. Increasing or decreasing the sensitivity of postsynaptic responses is also possible.

With all the different locations at a synapse that react with the various neurotransmitters in so many ways, understanding normal brain function, much less that of the abnormal brain, is extremely difficult. Even more complicated is the fact that there are species variations, too. With the advent of psychopharmacology, drug actions on the central nervous system are becoming better understood. Drugs are also being designed to target specific neurotransmitters by actions at presynaptic and postsynaptic sites (Table 1-8). Currently a number of human drugs are being tried for behavior problems in animals, but a wide spectrum remains to be tried. An understanding of the broad categories and of some representative drugs can result in a more rational selection.

Serotonin processing can be used as an example. It is formed from tryptophan and degraded by monoamine oxidase. In addition to being found in the brain, serotonin can be found in other cells of the body, including the platelets and the intestinal wall.[285] After it is released into the interneuronal space, it is again picked up by the cell to be used once more. Tricyclic antidepressants inhibit this reuptake, resulting in a prolonged effect.[285] Psychotropic drugs can have a number of side effects, and some are worse than others. In general, they can potentiate cardiac arrhythmias, bring on seizures, affect thyroid hormone levels, and induce hepatic enzymes.[221] Weight gain can also occur through an increase in thirst and appetite.[221]

### Antianxiety (Anxiolytic) Drugs

Anxiety is even more difficult to quantify in animals than in humans, but as in humans, the threat that generates anxiety in dogs seems to come from within, unlike the case with fear, which is related

| **TABLE 1-8** | Comparative properties of various antidepressants | | | | | |
|---|---|---|---|---|---|---|
| Drug | Selectivity for blocking uptake serotonin over norepinephrine | Potency of dopamine uptake blockage | Affinity for H1-receptor blockade | Affinity for muscarinic receptor blockade | Affinity for α1-adrenoceptor blockade | Affinity for dopamine D2-receptor blockade |
| Amitriptyline | 0.36 | 0.043 | 91 | 5.6 | 3.7 | 0.1 |
| Amoxapine | 0.0094 | 0.053 | 4 | 0.1 | 2 | 0.62 |
| Bupropion | 0.15 | 0.16 | 0.015 | 0.0021 | 0.022 | 0 |
| Clomipramine | 5.2 | 0.056 | 3.2 | 2.7 | 2.6 | 0.53 |
| Desipramine | 0.0026 | 0.019 | 0.91 | 0.5 | 0.77 | 0.03 |
| Doxepin | 0.068 | 0.018 | 420 | 1.2 | 4.2 | 0.042 |
| Fluoxetine | 23 | 0.062 | 0.016 | 0.05 | 0.017 | 0.015 |
| Fluvoxamine | 71 | 0.02 | 0.00092 | 0.0042 | 0.013 | 0.13 |
| Imipramine | 0.31 | 0.02 | 9.1 | 1.1 | 1.1 | 0.05 |
| Maprotiline | 0.0022 | 0.034 | 50 | 0.18 | 1.1 | 0.29 |
| Nefazodone | 4.2 | 0.042 | 0.0044 | 0.0091 | 2.1 | 0.11 |
| Nortriptyline | 0.015 | 0.059 | 10 | 0.67 | 1.7 | 0.083 |
| Paroxetine | 45 | 0.059 | 0.0045 | 0.93 | 0.029 | 0.0031 |
| Protriptyline | 0.0035 | 0.054 | 4 | 4 | 0.77 | 0.043 |
| Sertraline | 64 | 0.39 | 0.0041 | 0.16 | 0.27 | 0.0093 |
| Trazodone | 26 | 0.0071 | 0.29 | 0.00031 | 2.8 | 0.026 |
| Trimipramine | 0.2 | 0.029 | 370 | 1.7 | 4.2 | 0.56 |
| Venlafaxine | 5.4 | 0.019 | 0 | 0 | 0 | 0 |
| Amphetamine | | 1.2 | | | | |
| Diphenhydramine | | | 7.1 | | | |
| Atropine | | | | 42 | | |
| Phentolamine | | | | | 6.7 | |
| Chlorpromazine | | | | | | 5.3 |

Data from references 95, 258.

to a specific external event.[125] Panic attacks are described as acute anxiety of rapid onset, with a crescendo of symptoms of sympathetic overactivity.[284] They can last a few minutes to several hours.

### Sedative-Hypnotics

Antianxiety drugs have been around for many years. They can be grouped in two ways based on general actions (see Box 1-3).[125] The *sedative-hypnotics* produce effects that start with sedation and progress toward sleep or hypnosis as the dose is increased. Other effects of these drugs include muscle relaxation, anticonvulsant action, and development of tolerance and dependence.[125] Common examples of sedative-hypnotics used in veterinary medicine would include the barbiturates and the benzodiazepines.

The barbiturates are used most because of their antiseizure properties. They affect the GABA receptor-benzodiazepine receptor-chloride ion channel complex.[225] These drugs can negatively affect cognition and are well recognized for hepatotoxicity when used long term.

The *benzodiazepines* have come to be the most popular of the antianxiety drugs for humans, because they have more desirable attributes and fewer undesirable effects when compared with other antianxiety drugs. The mechanism of action may account for this. Postsynaptic benzodiazepine-specific receptors are functionally linked to GABA-A receptors and to an associated chloride ion channel.[125,143,284,286,288] The benzodiazepines augment the GABA, as an inhibitory neurotransmitter, to open the chloride ion channel, letting chloride into the neuron to cause hyperpolarization and decreased firing.[125,140,187] Low doses alleviate anxiety, agitation, and fear by actions on receptors in the limbic system. Moderate doses are more anxiolytic and facilitate social interactions, and high doses are associated with confusion via the hippocampus and cerebral cortex.[140,143,290] Side effects relate to the metabolites and can include sedation, cortical depression, ataxia, increased appetite, paradoxical excitement, memory deficits, and muscle relaxation in both humans and dogs, provided there is no history of seizures.[288,290] These drugs disinhibit behaviors, including aggression.[288] They can also interfere with learning and memory, so they are not helpful where learning must occur. Alprazolam is also an antipanic drug that helps dissociate fearful events, such as thunderstorms, from long-term memory. Amnestic effects lasting 15 to 30 minutes are associated with these drugs when they are given intravenously.[271]

### Sedative-Autonomics

The second subgroup of antianxiety drugs are the *sedative-autonomics*. These affect the peripheral autonomic nervous system, as with anticholinergic blocking. The sedation produced is qualitatively different than with the sedative-hypnotics, at least in humans.[125] In addition, these drugs tend to increase muscle tone, lower seizure thresholds, and minimize development of tolerance or dependence.[125] Habituation is nevertheless a problem, partially because of the long half-lives and the active metabolites.[263] As with many drugs with long half-lives, abrupt withdrawal of sedative autonomics should be avoided, even in animals.

Of the sedative-autonomics, the *azapirone* buspirone has been used the most. In humans it is considered to be about as effective in generalized anxiety disorders as the benzodiazepines, although its onset of activity is longer.[64,290] Azapirones differ from benzodiazepines by being less sedative, having minimal impairment on central sensory processing, and being ineffective in treating panic disorders or obsessive-compulsive problems.[32,64,140,284,290] The mechanism of action is as a serotonin$_{1A}$ partial agonist at the serotonin$_{1A}$ subtype postsynaptic receptor[64,140,231,290] and as a full agonist at the presynaptic autoreceptors.[284,286,288] Azapirones also interact with dopamine and noradrenergic neurotransmitter systems,[63,64,187,286] but most clinical effects are probably because of the serotonin activity.[63] As a partial serotonin$_{1A}$ agonist, onset takes 1 to 3 weeks.[187] Buspirone, the primary drug in this group, has been shown to be most useful in fearful cats during intercat aggression and has not been commonly used in dogs.

The most commonly used anxiolytic drugs in veterinary medicine from this group have been phenobarbital and diazepam. Use of these two is complicated somewhat because both drugs are narcotics and neither is a particularly good antianxiety agent in dogs. Phenobarbital is useful as an antiseizure medication and therefore useful to treat behavioral manifestations of seizures. Diazepam works fairly well in species other than the dog, leaving one to wonder whether the neurotransmitter systems may be somewhat different between species. Liver problems have been associated with diazepam, mainly in the cat, probably because of its long half-life. Tricyclic antidepressants and selective serotonin reuptake inhibitors are receiving more attention as anxiolytic drugs at this time.

### Antidepressant Drugs

A number of drugs classified as antidepressant are currently receiving attention for their effect on behavior problems in animals, especially the tricyclics and selective serotonin reuptake inhibitors. Often, however, depression is not the specific problem being treated by antidepressants. In general, these drugs are used for their anxiolytic properties.[94,293] As a class, antidepressant drugs primarily affect levels of the monoamine neurotransmitters via glutamate.[246]

### Lithium

*Lithium* is a human antidepressant drug that has been tried in animals with behavior problems.[255] It is thought to accelerate the presynaptic destruction of catecholamines, inhibit neurotransmitter release at the synapse, and reduce the sensitivity of the postsynaptic receptor.[125,140] Antimanic effects may be associated with lithium blocking the supersensitivity of dopamine neurons.[125] Its regulation of serotonin activity is complex, although well studied. Its ability to stabilize serotonin levels may result in mood stabilization.[125] Its chemical similarities with calcium and magnesium might increase membrane permeability and thus affect various enzyme systems.[125] As newer and safer drugs have become available, lithium has lost its popularity in human medicine. Its role in veterinary medicine has been superficially explored, but potential side effects can be serious and there is a narrow margin of safety.

### Tricyclic Antidepressants

The *tricyclic antidepressant drugs* are structurally related to phenothiazine and are classified as mixed serotonin and norepinephrine reuptake inhibitors.[44,187,222,288] Drugs of this class probably work by attaching to and inhibiting the presynaptic serotonin transporter protein, thus inhibiting reuptake.[140,143,222,225,289] They also block acetylcholine, dopamine, and norepinephrine, which accounts for many of the side effects.[39,140] Because they block histamine receptors, they also have antipruritic properties.[219] The tricyclic drug metabolites can be more potent inhibitors of norepinephrine uptake than is the parent compound.[222] Amitriptyline and clomipramine have been used the most in veterinary medicine. Physicians prescribe the tricyclics to treat anxiety, anxiety plus depression, panic disorders, and obsessive-compulsive disorders.* Veterinarians use them for housesoiling cats in whom interstitial cystitis might be involved, separation anxiety in dogs, generalized anxiety, obsessive-compulsive disorders, and neuropathic pain. The effects of the tricyclics in treating obsessive-compulsive disorders may relate to cells in the dorsal horn of the spinal cord being modulated by the drug before stimulation, implicating an aberrant sensation.[219]

The various tricyclics differ most in the degree of sedation they produce. Imipramine and clomipramine produce low levels of sedation, and amitriptyline produces a high level of sedation.[125,216] Changing from one to another is of limited value. Failure to get a response to two tricyclics probably indicates the need to try a different class of drugs.[125]

Side effects of tricyclics are associated with their anticholinergic properties and include mild sedation (especially during the first week), mydriasis, arrhythmia, tachycardia, dry mouth, constipation, hypotension, and urinary retention.* Nausea, sexual dysfunction, seizures, potentiation of concurrent thyroid conditions, and agranulocytosis have also been reported.[83, 187, 219, 288] There are no reports of cardiac abnormalities developing in healthy dogs placed on these drugs.[248, 253, 254] It has been shown by electrocardiograms that the P wave had a significant negative correlation with the serum concentration of amitriptyline and a significantly positive one with the serum concentration of clomipramine.[227] Renal and liver values did not change when followed over a long term,[227] and there is a wide margin of safety.[252] Owners should be warned that the tricyclics can be associated with a bitter taste, although the veterinary-approved form of clomipramine avoids that problem. There is competitive metabolism with phenothiazine, and metabolism of the tricyclics is stimulated with the concurrent use of barbiturates.[187] Cimetidine may inhibit the antidepressant mechanism and increase the risk of toxicity.[187] A dose of 15 mg/kg can be fatal to a dog.[187]

A steady-state concentration in the blood occurs within 4 days for clomipramine,[147] but the onset of action can be as long as 2 to 6 weeks because of time needed for serotonin to build up in the interneuron synapse.[284] Even with that, an animal's owner may report a change in the pet's behavior within a few days.[178] Long-term use of the tricyclics apparently increases the sensitivity of postsynaptic serotonin receptors, in part because of the increased number of serotonin$_{1A}$-binding sites.[174] The time it takes for this effect to occur is consistent with the delay in onset of action relative to depression.[174] The long duration of onset has to do with serotonin buildup at the neurotransmitter level, not to the drug's half-life. Over time, the increased presence of serotonin leads to a remodeling of the synapse to enhance transmission efficiency and ultimately stimulate elements essential to cellular learning and memory.[225] Drug treatment should last at least 6 weeks before it is abandoned as a failure. Drug therapy should be ended by gradual withdrawal rather than abrupt

---

*References 83, 86, 219, 231, 284, 305.

*References 140, 178, 187, 216, 218, 222, 254, 284, 285, 289.

stoppage,[148] and some owners report that they now see the drug was actually making a difference. Onset had been too gradual to make an obvious difference.

### Monoamine Oxidase Inhibitors

*Monoamine oxidase inhibitors* (MAOIs) are also classified as antidepressants but are infrequently used. Monoamine oxidase (MAO) is found in many body tissues, so most of the inhibitor drugs are nonspecific. In addition, several of these drugs inhibit MAO in a way that is irreversible, so they are potentially very toxic.[44,140] In presynaptic neurons, MAO is a mitochondrial enzyme involved in the deamination of catecholamines. This deamination in turn reduces production of the neurotransmitter.

Within the brain there are two naturally occurring types of MAOs: type A for norepinephrine and serotonin, and type B for dopamine and phenylethylamine.[125,140,263,288] Both types share dopamine and tyramine as substrates. MAO-A selectively metabolizes or, if present in large amounts, blocks serotonin and norepinephrine. MAO-B selectively metabolizes benzylamine and β-phenylethylamine, or both.[125,263,285] The newer MAOIs have a higher affinity for either type A or type B. Most antidepressant effects are targeted for MAO-A.[285] L-Deprenyl is said to be more specific for MAO-B, but it is also metabolized to L-amphetamine and L-methamphetamine.[288] Phenylethylamine also increases in the central nervous system, which can also result in amphetamine-like effects.[288] These could theoretically account for some of its effects.[183,263] By day 5, plasma levels are undetectable.[184] It decreases the free radical load, both by reducing their production and by facilitating their removal.[160] In addition, L-deprenyl mitigates the breakdown of phenylethylamine, dopamine, tyramine, and norepinephrine; enhances catecholaminergic activity; and slows the progression of neurodegenerative disease associated with normal age-related MAO-B increases.[116] In humans, L-deprenyl is a Parkinsonian drug and helps with major depression, where it has been used transdermally.[181] In geriatric dogs, it is used as a treatment for cognitive disorders.[261,262] Increased locomotion is another effect reported, which would be considered desirable in geriatric patients.[291] Side effects include atropine-like responses, weight gain,

hypotension, restlessness, and, rarely, liver damage.[285] Extreme caution must be exercised if the dog has been on other medications. There are long interdrug times if the dog has been on narcotics, antidepressants, or other MAO inhibitors.[160]

### Selective Serotonin Reuptake Inhibitors

*Selective serotonin reuptake inhibitors* (SSRIs) are drugs that work at presynaptic sites. This newer group of psychoactive drugs is often compared to the tricyclics. The two types of drugs are approximately equal in their antidepressant effects,[188,284,285] although the SSRIs provide an advantage in treating anxiety combined with depression.[188] Lower than normal amounts of the neurotransmitter serotonin is involved in depression, irritability, hostility, and mood regulation.[143,188] It is no surprise, then, that the SSRIs have been reported to affect a number of behaviors and conditions, including separation anxiety, dominance aggression, and obsessive-compulsive disorders.[120,288,292] In general, all SSRIs work to enhance serotonin at the synaptic area, so there is no advantage to switching drugs within the group if one does not work. SSRIs inhibit CYP2D6 of the P450 enzyme group, so they can react with the tricyclics.[37] This can lead to the "serotonin syndrome," which is characterized by agitation or depression; altered muscle tone or neuromuscular activity (myoclonus, hyperreflexia, tremors, ataxia, and seizures); hyperthermia; and diarrhea.[11] Although antidepressants are known to lower circulating thyroid hormone levels, research in humans suggests that supplementing triiodothyronine (t3) can enhance the effects of the SSRIs.[194]

Side effects of SSRIs in humans include nausea, muscle rigidity, anxiety, sexual dysfunction, insomnia, anorexia, diarrhea, nervousness, and headaches.[140,285,289,292] The drug clomipramine works as an SSRI.[220] Generally, however, it is not included in the SSRI group because it is also a norepinephrine reuptake inhibitor.[188] Fluoxetine, the SSRI drug used most often in veterinary medicine, now comes in a palatable form as a treatment for separation anxiety. It is being tried for a wide variety of problems in dogs, including compulsive behaviors and depression. Fortunately for dogs, the research leading to the veterinary formulation provided a great deal of information about its pharmacokinetics in this species. As with other drugs that take time to achieve serotonin buildup in the synapses, there will be eventual remodeling of the postsynaptic neuron.[225] If the drug is to be stopped, it should be done gradually.[225]

### Sympathomimetic Stimulants

*Sympathomimetic stimulants* are classified as antidepressant drugs, even though they are not considered to be particularly good ones. They are used in veterinary behavior therapy for the treatment of hyperkinesis.[23,41] Children with attention deficit hyperactivity disorder are the human models. For them primary medications used are stimulants like amphetamine or methylphenidate. Secondary medications for those who do not tolerate the stimulants are usually tricyclic antidepressants.[309] Amphetamines work in part by being taken up into the vesicles of the nerve terminals where they replace the stored norepinephrine.[263] The psychostimulant effects of this class of drugs are mediated at the dopamine synapse.[79,272]

## Antipsychotic Drugs

As a group, antipsychotic drugs block dopamine receptors, particularly subtype $D_2$.[187,288] Side effects are common and include seizures, sedation, and motor restlessness.[187] They are used in human obsessive-compulsive patients who are not responding to conventional therapies.

### Phenothiazines

The *phenothiazines* are the most commonly used of the drugs that have antipsychotic and hypnotic effects in veterinary medicine, In general, however, the phenothiazines are not particularly effective in behavior therapy except as a hypnotic. The dose is the primary determinant of how hypnotic the effect is.

Acepromazine, promazine, and chlorpromazine are the most commonly used phenothiazines. They are prescribed to be given before long trips and to minimize destructive behavior that might occur during thunderstorms or separation from the owner. There are better choices, however, because it is the sedation that is helpful rather than the effect on learning or memory.[41,216] The side effects can be serious and must be considered before use is started. Differences in response to any of the antipsychotic drugs, especially to oral doses, are largely the result of differences in individuals.[125] These include idiosyncratic reactions of excitement, lowering of the seizure threshold, and hypotension.[178,288] At least some of these drugs are noncompetitive blockers that work at the nicotinic acetylcholine receptors[13] as dopamine agonists.[178,281] The phenothiazines decrease the initiation of motor activity at the basal ganglia of the brain.[41]

Haloperidol is an antipsychotic drug frequently used in humans. It is a dopamine receptor antagonist.[189] There is no reliable dose in animals, and side effects can be serious.[172] Chronic blockage of dopamine $D_2$ receptors downregulate $D_1$ receptors, producing severe memory impairment.[49] It is rarely used by veterinary behaviorists.

## Beta-Blocking Drugs

The noradrenergic antagonists that are beta-adrenergic receptor blocking drugs first came into vogue as antipsychotic medications and were used to treat schizophrenia. These drugs may also serve as a membrane-stabilizing agent in higher doses.[125] Controlled studies indicate onset of action may be extremely prolonged.[48] In humans, beta blockers such as propranolol have also been used to treat situational anxiety because they tend to reduce somatic manifestations like tremors and sweaty palms.[178,187,288] Propranolol has been shown also to be an antagonist and partial agonist at the serotonin$_{1A}$ receptors.[288] It has been used with mild success for situational fears, such as firecrackers and acquired fear associated with the show ring, even after 3 to 4 days of therapy. There may be better success if the drug is combined with pindolol, which may disinhibit the serotonin neurons, or with phenobarbital.[187,288] Potential problems include excessive sedation, hypotension, bradycardia, and heart failure.[187]

## Hypnotic Drugs

A number of different types of drugs are classified as hypnotic because of their properties of inducing or approaching the induction of sleep. Most drugs in this group that are significant to veterinary medicine are discussed elsewhere relative to their other uses in psychotherapy. Some members of this list tend to be slightly more hypnotic than others in their group.

### Antihistamines

The *antihistamines* have received some interest in veterinary medicine, but controlled studies have not been performed to evaluate which, if any, behaviors are most positively affected by their use. The sedative effect on the central nervous system can be useful for situations that cause mild apprehension, such as car trips. In humans, histaminergic neurons are characterized by the presence of numerous markers for other neurotransmitter systems, making it difficult to study their specific functions. Researchers have identified three histamine receptor subtypes—$H_1$, $H_2$, and $H_3$. Most of the antihistamines currently available are $H_1$-receptor antagonists, which affect the cortical activation and arousal mechanisms.[274] Several antidepressants and antipsychotic drugs also have a high affinity for $H_1$ receptors, probably accounting for their sedative properties.[274] Contraindications for use of the antihistamines would be related to their anticholinergic or atropine-like effects. Caution is needed if certain problems exist, like hyperthyroidism, urinary retention, or glaucoma.[216] Newer drugs in this group are being designed to minimize their $H_1$ affinity.

### Opiate Antagonists

Neurologically, three subtypes of opiate receptors have been identified—μ, δ, and κ.[34,263,268] Although distribution of the various receptors varies throughout the brain, it has been shown that opiates generally work on multiple receptor subtypes. Most agonist analgesics work on the μ receptor, and naloxone will displace the compound from that site.[268] As with other psychotherapeutic drugs, opiate antagonists are used to block the receptors; but here too, chronic use can result in an antagonist-induced receptor upregulation. Apparently over time there is an increase in the number of receptors, primarily μ, which is expressed behaviorally as a supersensitivity to the actions of opioids.[34] It has been well documented that opiates facilitate stimulation within the brain, perhaps by their actions on dopaminergic neurons.[314]

Narcotic antagonists have been used in veterinary medicine to reverse the effects of narcotic drugs used as sedatives. They have also been used to try to control stereotypic behaviors, under the theory that the behavior is self-rewarding via the release of naturally occurring opioids (endorphins, enkephalins).[216] It is known that high doses of amphetamine-like drugs are associated with a stereotyped syndrome.[145] Because the currently available narcotic antagonists have short durations of action, they are most helpful as diagnostic aids rather than as long-term therapies for animals. Pentazocine, a mixed narcotic agonist/antagonist, and naltrexone, a pure opioid antagonist, have been used when longer action is desired.[216] In humans, naltrexone has a short half-life but an extended action because one of its active metabolites has a long duration.[171] Because dogs metabolize the drug differently and do not form this metabolite, naltrexone should not be particularly useful when long duration is needed.[171]

### Progestins

The exact mechanism of the progestins is not understood, but it has been speculated that they mimic the action of progesterone, inhibiting the brain mechanisms responsible for male behavior[113] or lowering serum testosterone levels. They also have an antianxiety calming effect. For those reasons they have proved most useful for controlling undesirable male sexually dimorphic behaviors and behavior problems in which stress is a factor. The down side of their use is a high incidence of serious side effects with long-term use. The total incidence of side effects is 22%.[139] A number of different side effects must be considered when making a decision to use oral progestins. Because injectable products cannot be withdrawn from the body and so can be active for long periods, their use is not recommended. Of the many side effects, an increase in appetite can be desirable.[107,113,152] Because food intake in dogs is controlled by the owner, weight gain does not have to occur if it is undesirable. The more serious side effects include mammary nodules/hyperplasia/neoplasia,* uterine hyperplasia/pyometra[108,152,216,236,237] depression of corticosteroid output,[73,107,108,113] diabetes mellitus,† and acromegaly.[73,77,152]

---

*References 41, 73, 91, 108, 113, 152.
†References 41, 107, 108, 113, 152, 216, 237.

## Other Drugs

### Melatonin

*Melatonin* is a neurohormone produced by the pineal gland from tryptophan. Synthetic formulations have become popular in efforts to minimize the effects of jet lag. It does have well-documented antioxidant properties.[204] In veterinary medicine, the use of melatonin and an effective dose remain to be studied in controlled tests. This drug has been used for generalized anxiety and in geriatric patients who have a day/night shift. In humans, melatonin levels in the blood are highest before bedtime,[204] so dosing is recommended before bedtime. No controlled studies on behavioral effects have been done in dogs.[288]

### Synthetic Pheromones

*Synthetic pheromones* are being used to try to calm animals. DAP (dog-appeasing pheromone) is described as the synthetic version of the pheromone associated with the mammary gland region of a lactating bitch. However, there is considerable variation in reaction to the use of this product, and well-controlled studies are yet to be done. Some dogs are described as choosing to selectively rest near the product diffuser. Some are neutral to its presence, and a few become agitated, apparently from the product.

### Tryptic Alpha-S1 Caseine Hydrolysate

*Tryptic alpha-S1 caseine hydrolysate* is a biopeptide from milk that has been patented under the name Lactium for use as an anxiolytic.[17] A double-blinded, placebo-controlled study in 47 dogs showed a statistically reduced anxiety level compared with placebo. It will be interesting to see long-term results and results from larger, independent studies. This product is not currently available in the United States.

### N-Methyl-d-Aspartate Receptor Antagonists

*N-methyl-D-aspartate* (NMDA) *receptor antagonists* alter glutamatergic neurotransmission, which is thought to be associated with obsessive-compulsive disorders.[179] This class of drugs has selective action on the glutamate system and seems to complement fluoxetine to improve results.[179] Memantine and dextromethorphan are members of this group.

## Psychoactive Herbs

The use of herbs in the prevention of or treatment for behavior problems has become big business, and the use of these materials in pets parallels their popularity in humans. It is beyond the scope of this book to go into what is known about each one, so readers are directed to other sources.[84, 275-277]

## References

1. AAHA pet owner survey results. Trends Mag 1993; IX(2):32.
2. AAHA's fourth annual pet survey looks at human-animal bond. Trends Mag 1995; XI(2):30.
3. Adams GJ: The prevalence of behavioural problems in domestic dogs: A survey of 105 dog owners. Aust Vet Pract 1989; 19(3):135.
4. After 50 years, war dogs should find home. J Am Vet Med Assoc 1993; 203(12):1663.
5. Allen K, Blascovich J: The value of service dogs for people with severe ambulatory disabilities: A randomized controlled trial. J Am Vet Med Assoc 1996; 275(13):1001.
6. American Kennel Club: AKC dog registration statistics: 2006 rank. http://www.akc.org/reg/dogreg_stats.cfm, 3/9/2007.
7. American Veterinary Medical Association: U.S. Pet Ownership and Demographics Sourcebook. Schaumburg, IL: AVMA, 2007.
8. Anchel M: Overpopulation of Cats and Dogs: Causes, Effects, and Prevention. New York: Fordham University Press, 1990.
9. Anderson RK: Demographic characteristics of dogs: Their owners and reported dog behavior problems. American Veterinary Society of Animal Behavior meeting, Atlanta, GA, July 20, 1986.
10. Anderson RK, Vacalopoulos A: Demographic characteristics of dogs, their owners and reported dog behavior problems. Am Vet Soc Anim Behav Newsletter 1987; 10(1):3.
11. Antidepressant treatment of canine behavioral problems. Vet Forum November 2000:25.
12. Arkow P: New statistics challenge previously held beliefs about euthanasia: A new look at pet overpopulation. Latham Letter 1993; XIV(2):1.
13. Arneric SP, Sullivan JP, Williams M: Neuronal nicotinic acetylcholine receptors: Novel targets for central nervous systems therapeutics. In Bloom FE, Kupfer DJ (eds): Psychopharmacology: The Fourth Generation of Progress. New York: Raven Press Ltd, 1995, p. 95.
14. Association of Pet Behaviour Counsellors: Annual Review of Cases 2000. http://www.apbc.org.uk/2000/report.htm, 4/9/2001.
15. Bailey GP, Hetherington JD, Sellors J: Successful rescue dog placement in combination with behavioral counseling. Waltham Focus 1998; 8(3):17.

16. Beata C: The challenge of dealing with the human dimension. In Landsberg G, Mattiello S, Mills D (eds): Proceedings of the 6th International Veterinary Behaviour Meeting & European College of Veterinary Behavioural Medicine-Companion Animals European Society of Veterinary Clinical Ethology. Brescia, Italy: Fondazione Iniziative Zooprofilattiche e Zootechinche, 2007, p. 79.

17. Beata C, Lefranc C, Desor D: Lactium: A new anxiolytic product from milk. In Mills D, Levine E, Landsberg G, et al (eds): Current Issues and Research in Veterinary Behavioral Medicine. West Lafayette, IN: Purdue University Press, 2005, p. 150.

18. Beaver BV: Behavioral histories. Vet Med Small Anim Clin 1981; 76(4):478, 480.

19. Beaver BV: The genetics of canine behavior. Vet Med Small Anim Clin 1981; 76(10):1423.

20. Beaver BV: The role of veterinary colleges in addressing the surplus dog and cat population. J Am Vet Med Assoc 1991; 198(7):1241.

21. Beaver BV: Feline Behavior: A Guide for Veterinarians. Philadelphia: Saunders, 1992.

22. Beaver BV: Owner complaints about canine behavior. J Am Vet Med Assoc 1994; 204(12):1953.

23. Beaver BV: The Veterinarian's Encyclopedia of Animal Behavior. Ames, IA: Iowa State University Press, 1994.

24. Beaver BV: Human-canine interactions: A summary of perspectives. J Am Vet Med Assoc 1997; 210(8):1148.

25. Beck AM: The Ecology of Stray Dogs: A Study of Free-Ranging Urban Animals. Baltimore: York Press, 1973.

26. Belyaev DK: Destabilizing selection as a factor in domestication. J Heredity 1979; 70:301.

27. Ben-Michael J, Vossen JMH, Felling JA, et al: The perception of problematic behavior in dogs: Application of multi-dimensional scaling and hierarchical cluster analysis. Anthrozoös 1997; 10(4):198.

28. Bennett PC, Rohlf V: Owner-companion dog interactions: Relationships between demographic variables, potentially problematic behaviours, training engagement and shared activities. Appl Anim Behav Sci 2007; 102(1-2):65.

29. Blackwell EJ, Twells C, Seawright A, et al: The relationship between training methods and the occurrence of behaviour problems in a population of domestic dogs. In Landsberg G, Mattiello S, Mills D (eds): Proceedings of the 6th International Veterinary Behaviour Meeting & European College of Veterinary Behavioural Medicine-Companion Animals European Society of Veterinary Clinical Ethology. Brescia, Italy: Fondazione Iniziative Zooprofilattiche e Zootechinche, 2007, p. 51.

30. Borchelt PL, Tortora DF: Animal behavior therapy: The diagnosis and treatment of pet behavior problems. AAHA Proceedings 1979:3.

31. Borchelt PL, Voith VL: Classification of animal behavior problems. Vet Clin North Am [Small Anim Pract] 1982; 12(4):571.

32. Boulenger JP, Squillance K, Simon P, et al: Buspirone and diazepam: Comparison of subjective, psychomotor and biological effects. Neuropsychobiology 1989; 22:83.

33. Bower C: The role of behavioural medicine in veterinary practice. In Horwitz DF, Mills DS, Heath S (eds): BSAVA Manual of Canine and Feline Behavioural Medicine. Quedgeley, Gloucester, England: British Small Animal Veterinary Association, 2002, p. 1.

34. Brady LS: Opiate receptor regulation by opiate agonists and antagonists. In Hammer RP (ed): The Neurobiology of Opiates. Boca Raton, FL: CRC Press Inc, 1993, p. 125.

35. Brisbin Jr IL, Risch TS: Primitive dogs, their ecology and behavior: Unique opportunities to study the early development of the human-canine bond. J Am Vet Med Assoc 1997; 210(8):1122.

36. Bronson RT: Variation in age at death of dogs of different sexes and breeds. Am J Vet Res 1982; 43(11):2057.

37. Brösen K: Differences between the SSRI. Eur Neuropsychopharmacology 1995; 5(3):174.

38. Brown LT, Shaw TG, Kirkland KD: Affection for people as a function of affection for dogs. Psychol Rep 1972; 31:957.

39. Bruhwyler J, Chleide E, Rettori MC, et al: Amineptine improves the performance of dogs in a complex temporal regulation schedule. Pharmacol Biochem Behav 1993; 45(4):897.

40. Budiansky S: A special relationship: The coevolution of human beings and domesticated animals. J Am Vet Med Assoc 1994; 204(3):365.

41. Burghardt Jr WF: Using drugs to control behavior problems in pets. Vet Med 1991; 86(11):1066.

42. Burghardt Jr WF: Formulating a prognosis for behavioral therapy. American Veterinary Medical Association meeting, Minneapolis, July 18, 1993.

43. Burghardt Jr WF: Behavioral aspects of selective breeding in working dogs. http://www.avma.org/conv/cv2002/cvnotes/CAn_AnB_BAS_BuW.asp, 7/3/2002.

44. Burke MJ, Preskorn SH: Short-term treatment of mood disorders with standard antidepressants. In Bloom FE, Kupfer DJ (eds): Psychopharmacology: The Fourth Generation of Progress. New York: Raven Press Ltd, 1995, p. 1053.

45. Campbell WE: Dr. Antelyes, touché. Mod Vet Pract 1973; 54(4):5.

46. Campbell WE: Environmental changes. Mod Vet Pract 1977; 58(3):275.

47. Campbell WE: Effects of training, feeding regimens, isolation and physical environment on canine behavior. Mod Vet Pract 1986; 67(3):239.

48. Casey DE: Tardive dyskinesia: Pathophysiology. In Bloom FE, Kupfer DJ (eds): Psychopharmacology: The Fourth Generation of Progress. New York: Raven Press Ltd, 1995, p. 1497.

49. Castner SA, Williams GV, Goldman-Rakic PS: Reversal of antipsychotic-induced working memory deficits by short-term dopamine D1 receptor stimulation. Science 2000; 287:2020.

50. Catanzaro TE: Behavior management as an income center. Vet Forum May 1994:50.

51. Center for Information Management. U.S. Pet Ownership and Demographics Sourcebook. Schaumburg, IL: AVMA, 1993.

52. Center for Information Management. U.S. Pet Ownership and Demographics Sourcebook. Schaumburg, IL: AVMA, 1997.

53. Chapman B, Voith V: Dog owners and their choice of a pet. American Veterinary Society of Animal Behavior meeting, Atlanta, GA, July 20, 1986.

54. Clark GI, Boyer WN: The effects of dog obedience training and behavioural counselling upon the human-canine relationship. Appl Anim Behav Sci 1993; 37(2):147.

55. Clutton-Brock J: Man-made dogs. SCI 1977; 197:1340.

56. Clutton-Brock J: Domesticated Animals from Early Times. Austin, TX: University of Texas Press, 1981.

57. Clutton-Brock J: Dog. In Mason IL (ed) : Evolution of Domesticated Animals. New York: Longman, 1984, p. 198.

58. Clutton-Brock J: Origins of the dog: Domestication and early history. In Serpell J (ed): The Domestic Dog: Its Evolution, Behaviour, and Interactions with People. Cambridge, England: Cambridge University Press, 1885, p. 7.

59. Clutton-Brock J, Jewell P: Origin and domestication of the dog. In Evans HE (ed): Miller's Anatomy of the Dog, 3rd ed. Philadelphia: Saunders, 1993, p. 21.

60. Colbert EH: Evolution of the Vertebrates: A History of the Backboned Animals Through Time, 3rd ed. New York: John Wiley & Sons, 1980.

61. Collyns D: Mummified dogs uncovered in Peru. http://news.bbc.co.uk/2/hi/americas/5374748.stm, 9/25/2006.

62. Coman BJ, Robinson JL: Some aspects of stray dog behaviour in an urban fringe area. Aust Vet J 1989; 66(1):30.

63. Coop CF, McNaughton N: Buspirone affects hippocampal rhythmical slow activity through serotonin$_{1A}$ rather than dopamine D$_2$ receptors. Neuroscience 1991; 40(1):169.

64. Coplan JD, Wolk SI, Klein DF: Anxiety and the serotonin$_{1A}$ receptor. In Bloom FE, Kupfer DJ (eds): Psychopharmacology: The Fourth Generation of Progress. New York: Raven Press Ltd, 1995, p. 1301.

65. Coppinger R, Coppinger L: Differences in the behavior of dog breeds. In Grandin T (ed): Genetics and the Behavior of Domestic Animals, New York: Academic Press, 1998, p. 167.

66. Council for Science and Society: Companion Animals in Society. New York: Oxford University Press, 1988.

67. Crowell-Davis S, Murray T: Veterinary Psychopharmacology. Ames, IA: Blackwell Publishing, 2006.

68. Danneman PJ, Chodrow RE: History-taking and interviewing techniques. Vet Clin North Am [Small Anim Pract] 1982; 12(4):587.

69. Davis SJM: The Archaeology of Animals. New Haven, CT: Yale University Press, 1987.

70. Dayton L: On the trail of the first dingo. Science 2003; 302(5645):555.

71. Davis SJM, Valla FR: Evidence for domestication of the dog 12,000 years ago in the Natufian of Israel. Nature 1978; 276(5688):608.

72. Denenberg S, Landsberg GM, Horwitz D, et al: A comparison of cases referred to behaviorists in three different countries. In Mills D, Levine E, Landsberg G, et al (eds): Current Issues and Research in Veterinary Behavioral Medicine. West Lafayette, IN: Purdue University Press, 2005, p. 56.

73. Dodman NH, Shuster L: Pharmacologic approaches to managing behavior problems in small animals. Vet Med 1994; 89(10):960.

74. Dodman NH, Shuster L (eds): Psychopharmacology of Animal Behavior Disorders. Malden, MA: Blackwell Science, 1988.

75. Duxbury MM, Jackson JA, Line SW, et al: Puppy socialization class attendance and other factors related to postweaning handling: The association with retention of dogs in their homes. AVSAB Annual Symp Anim Behav Res 2002 Meeting Proc, 2002:4.

76. Duxbury MM, Jackson JA, Line SW, et al: Evaluation of association between retention in the home and attendance at puppy socialization classes. J Am Vet Med Assoc 2003; 223(1):61.

77. Eigenmann JE, Venker-van Hargen AJ: Progestogen-induced and spontaneous canine acromegaly due to reversible growth hormone overproduction: Clinical picture and pathogenesis. J Am Anim Hosp Assoc 1981; 17(5):813.

78. Eisenberg JF: The Mammalian Radiations: An Analysis of Trends in Evolution, Adaptation, and Behavior. Chicago: The University of Chicago Press, 1981.

79. Ernst M, Zarnetkin A: The interface of genetics, neuroimaging, and neurochemistry in attention-deficit hyperactivity disorder. In Bloom FE, Kupfer DJ (eds): Psychopharmacology: The Fourth Generation of Progress. New York: Raven Press Ltd, 1995, p. 1643.

80. Fält L: Inheritance of behaviour in the dog. In Anderson RS (ed): Nutrition and Behaviour in Dogs and Cats. Oxford, England: Pergamon Press, 1984, p. 183.

81. Faulkner LC: Pet population problem. Calif Vet 1973; 27(6):19.

82. Feddersen-Petersen D: Social behavior of wolves and dogs. Vet Q 1994; 16(51):515.

83. Feinberg M: Clomipramine for obsessive-compulsive disorder. Am Fam Physician 1991; 43(5):1735.

84. Feldman S: Psychotropic herbal medications: Potential for use in companion animals. ACVB Annual Symp Anim Behav Res 2002 Meeting Proc, 2002:77.

85. Fiennes R, Fiennes A: The Natural History of the Dog. London: Weidenfeld and Nicolson, 1968.

86. Flament MF, Rapoport JL, Berg CJ, et al: Clomipramine treatment of childhood obsessive-compulsive disorder: A double-blind controlled study. Arch Gen Psychiatry 1985; 42:977.

87. Fox MW: Canine Behavior. Chicago: University of Chicago Press, 1965.

88. Fox MW: Behaviour of Wolves, Dogs, and Related Canids. New York: Harper and Row, 1971.

89. Fox MW: Understanding Your Dog. New York: Coward, McCann & Geoghegan, Inc, 1972.

90. Fox MW: The Dog: Its Domestication and Behavior. New York: Garland STPM Press, 1978.

91. Frank DW, Kirton KT, Murchison TE, et al: Mammary tumors and serum hormones in the bitch treated with medroxyprogesterone acetate or progesterone for four years. Fertil Steril 1979; 31(3):340.

92. Frank D, O'Connor JM: Comprehension, compliance, outcome and satisfaction: A retrospective survey of 49 clients with dogs (Canis familiaris) treated for behavior problems. In Mills D, Levine E, Landsberg G, et al (eds): Current Issues and Research in Veterinary Behavioral Medicine. West Lafayette, IN: Purdue University Press, 2005, p. 189.

93. From predator to pal. Science February 3, 2006; 311:587.

94. Fuller JL, Fox MW: The behaviour of dogs. In Hafez ESE (ed): The Behavior of Domestic Animals, 2nd ed. Baltimore: Williams & Wilkins, 1969, p. 438.

95. Fuller RW, Wong DT: Serotonin reuptake blockers in vitro and in vivo. J Clin Psychopharmacol 1987; 7(6)Suppl:36S.

96. FYI. DVM 1987; 18(6):54.

97. FYI. DVM 1987; 18(9):26.

98. Gehrke BC: Results of the AVMA survey of U.S. pet-owning households on companion animal ownership. J Am Vet Med Assoc 1997; 211(2):169.

99. Geisler J: New AAHA study: Veterinary clients treat their pets more and more like people. DVM 1996; 27(1):16S.

100. Gentry C: When Dogs Run Wild: The Sociology of Feral Dogs and Wildlife. Jefferson, NC: McFarland & Company Inc, 1983.

101. Glennon RA, Dukat M: Serotonin receptor subtypes. In Bloom FE, Kupfer DJ (eds): Psychopharmacology: The Fourth Generation of Progress. New York: Raven Press Ltd, 1995, p. 415.

102. Gorodetsky E: Epidemiology of dog and cat euthanasia across Canadian prairie provinces. Can Vet J 1997; 38(10):649.

103. Green JS, Woodruff RA: Breed comparisons and characteristics of use of livestock guarding dogs. J Range Manage 1988; 41(3):249.

104. Griffiths BCR: Studies from the Birmingham Dogs' Home: (1) The problem of resettling strays and unwanted animals. J Small Anim Pract 1975; 16(11):717.

105. Hare B, Brown M, Williamson C, et al: The domestication of social cognition in dogs. Science 2002; 298(5598):1634.

106. Hart BL: Anthropomorphism: Two perspectives. Canine Pract 1978; 5(3):12.

107. Hart BL: Problems with objectionable sociosexual behavior of dogs and cats: Therapeutic use of castration and progestins. Compend Contin Educ [Small Anim] 1979; 1:461.

108. Hart BL: Progestin therapy for aggressive behavior in male dogs. J Am Vet Med Assoc 1981; 178(10):1070.

109. Hart BL, Cliff KD: Interpreting published results of extra-label drug use with special reference to reports of drugs used to correct behavior in animals. J Am Vet Med Assoc 1996; 209(8):1382.

110. Hart BL, Cooper LL: Integrating use of psychotropic drugs with environmental management and behavioral modification for treatment of problem behavior in animals. J Am Vet Med Assoc 1996; 209(9):1549.

111. Hart BL, Hart L: Breed-specific profiles of canine *(Canis familiaris)* behavior. In Mills D, Levine E, Landsberg G et al (eds): Current Issues and Research in Veterinary Behavioral Medicine. West Lafayette, IN: Purdue University Press, 2005, p. 107.

112. Hart BL, Hart LA: Selecting the best companion animal: Breed and gender specific behavioral profiles. In Anderson RK, Hart BL, Hart LA (eds): The Pet Connection: Its Influence on Our Health and Quality of Life. St. Paul, MN: Center to Study Human-Animal Relationship and Environments, 1984, p. 180.

113. Hart BL, Hart LA: Canine and Feline Behavioral Therapy. Philadelphia: Lea & Febiger, 1985.

114. Hart BL, Hart LA: The Perfect Puppy: How to Choose Your Dog by Its Behavior. New York: WH Freeman and Company, 1988.

115. Hart BL, Miller MF: Behavioral profiles of dog breeds. J Am Vet Med Assoc 1985; 186(11):1175.

116. Heath S: Behaviour problems in the geriatric pet. In Horwitz DF, Mills DS, Heath S (eds); BSAVA Manual of Canine and Feline Behavioural Medicine. Quedgeley, Gloucester, England: British Small Animal Veterinary Association, 2002, p. 109.

117. Heath SE: The challenge of medical differentials. In Landsberg G, Mattiello S, Mills D (eds): Proceedings of the 6th International Veterinary Behaviour Meeting & European College of Veterinary Behavioural Medicine-Companion Animals European Society of Veterinary Clinical Ethology. Brescia, Italy: Fondazione Iniziative Zooprofilattiche e Zootechinche, 2007, p. 81.

118. Hebard C: Use of search and rescue dogs. J Am Vet Med Assoc 1993; 203(7):999.

119. Hemmer H: Domestication: The Decline of Environmental Appreciation. New York: Cambridge University Press, 1990.

120. Heninger GR: Indoleamines: The role of serotonin in clinical disorders. In Bloom FE, Kupfer DJ (eds): Psychopharmacology: The Fourth Generation of Progress. New York: Raven Press Ltd, 1995, p. 471.

121. Hennessy MB, Voith VL, Mazzei SJ, et al: Behavior and cortisol levels of dogs in a public animal shelter, and an exploration of the ability of these measures to predict problem behavior after adoption. Appl Anim Behav Sci 2001; 73(3):217.

122. Hetts S: Behavior Rx: Is a behavior wellness program for you? Trends Mag 2000; XVI(2):14.

123. Hewson CJ, Luescher UA, Ball RO: Measuring change in the behavioural severity of canine compulsive disorder: The construct validity of categories of change derived from two rating scales. Appl Anim Behav Sci 1998; 60(1):55.

124. Hodgman SFJ: Abnormalities and defects in pedigree dogs. I. An investigation into the existence of abnormalities in pedigree dogs in the British Isles. J Small Anim Pract 1963; 4:447.

125. Hollister LE: Clinical Pharmacology of Psychotherapeutic Drugs, 2nd ed. New York: Churchill Livingstone, 1983.

126. Horwitz D: Integrating behavioral medicine into veterinary practice. Appl Anim Behav Sci 1994; 39:187.

127. Horwitz DF: Classical counterconditioning in the treatment of behavior problems. Am Vet Med Assoc Conv Proc July 2006.

128. Houpt KA: Behavioral genetics of cats and dogs. 138th Annual AVMA Convention-Convention Notes. http://www.avma.org/noah/members/convention/conv01/notes/04010101.asp, 6/11/2001.

129. Houpt KA, Honig SU, Reisner IR: Breaking the human-companion animal bond. J Am Vet Med Assoc 1996; 208(10):1653.

130. Houpt KA, Willis MB: Genetics of behaviour. In Ruvinsky A, Sampson J (eds): The Genetics of the Dog, New York: CABI Publishing, 2001, p. 371.

131. How Many Dogs and Cats in the U.S.? Latham Letter, 1985; VI(2):21.

132. Hsu Y, Serpell JA: Development and validation of a questionnaire for measuring behavior and temperament traits in pet dogs. J Am Vet Med Assoc 2003; 223(9):1293.

133. Huff PE: Euthanasia and animal shelters. Oreg Vet Med Assoc Anim Wel Forum 1990:8.

134. Hunthausen W: Collecting the history of a pet with a behavior problem. Vet Med 1994; 89(10):954.

135. Hunthausen WL: Rule out medical etiologies first in geriatric behavior problems. DVM 1991; 22(7):24.

136. Hunthausen W, Whiteley HE, Landsberg G, et al: Ask the board: Behavior. Vet Forum June 1994:16.

137. Jackson J, Anderson RK: Early Learning for Puppies. Falcon Heights, MN: Animal Behavior Consulting, 1999, p. 87.

138. Jagoe A, Serpell J: Owner characteristics and interactions and the prevalence of canine behavioural problems. Appl Anim Behav Sci 1996; 47:31.

139. Joby R: The control of undesirable behaviour in male dogs using megestrol acetate. J Small Anim Pract 1984; 25:567.

140. Julien RM: A Primer of Drug Action: A Concise Non-technical Guide to the Actions, Uses, and Side Effects of Psychoactive Drugs, 7th ed. New York: WH Freeman and Company, 1995.

141. Kahler S: Stalking a killer: The "disease" of euthanasia. J Am Vet Med Assoc 1992; 201(7):973.

142. Kahler S: Forum urges commitment to resolving overpopulation. J Am Vet Med Assoc 1993; 202(2):183.

143. Kamerling SG: Drugs and animal behavior. 138th Annual lAVMA Convention-Convention Notes. http://www.avma.org/noah/members/convention/conv01/notes/04050101.asp, 6/11/2001.

144. Kass PH, New Jr JC, Scarlett JM, et al: Understanding animal companion surplus in the United States: Relinquishment of nonadoptables to animal shelters for euthanasia. J Appl Anim Welfare Sci 2001; 4(4):237.

145. Kelly PH: Drug-induced motor behavior. In Iversen LL, Iversen SD, Snyder SH (eds): Handbook of Psychopharmacology: Vol 8, Drugs, Neurotransmitters, and Behavior. New York: Plenum Press, 1977, p. 295.

146. Kidd AH, Kidd RM, George CC: How can pet adoptions be more successful? New research examines veterinarian's role. Latham Letter 1992; Xlll(4):9.

147. King JN, Maurer MP, Altmann BO, et al: Pharmacokinetics of clomipramine in dogs following single-dose and repeated-dose oral administration. Am J Vet Res 2000; 61(10):80.

148. King JN, Overall KL, Appleby D, et al: Results of a followup investigation to a clinical trial testing the efficacy of clomipramine in the treatment of separation anxiety in dogs. Appl Anim Behav Sci 2004; 89(3-4):233.

149. Kirkness EF, Bafna V, Halpern AL, et al: The dog genome: Survey sequencing and comparative analysis. Science 2003; 301(5641):1898.

150. Knol BW: Behavioural problems in dogs. Problems, diagnoses, therapeutic measures and results in 133 patients. Vet Q 1987; 9(3):226.

151. Knol BW: Social problem behavior in dogs: Etiology and pathogenesis. Vet Q 1994; 16(51):505.

152. Knol BW, Egberink-Alink ST: Treatment of problem behavior in dogs and cats by castration and progestagen administration. A review. Vet Q 1989; 11(2):102.

153. Kobelt AJ, Hemsworth PH, Baranett JL, et al: A survey of dog ownership in suburban Australia—Conditions and behaviour problems. Appl Anim Behav Sci 2003; 82(2):137.

154. Kolata RJ, Johnston DE: Motor vehicle accidents in urban dogs: A study of 600 cases. J Am Vet Med Assoc 1975; 167(10):938.

155. Kolata RJ, Kraut NH, Johnston DE: Patterns of trauma in urban dogs and cats: A study of 1000 cases. J Am Vet Med Assoc 1974; 164(5):499.

156. König J: Surplus dogs and cats in Europe. In Allen RD, Westbrook WH (eds): The Handbook of Animal Welfare. New York: Garland STPM Press, 1979, p. 81.

157. Kretchmer KR, Fox MW: Effects of domestication on animal behaviour. Vet Rec 1975; 96(2):102.

158. Landsberg G: Products for preventing or controlling undesirable behavior. Vet Med 1994; 89(10):970.

159. Landsberg G: Providing behavior services to clients. Friskies PetCare Symposium: Small Animal Behavior Proceedings 1998:32.

160. Landsberg G: Behavior problems in the geriatric dog and cat. Friskies PetCare Symposium: Small Animal Behavior Proceedings 1998:37.

161. Landsberg GM: Veterinarians as behavior consultants. Can Vet J 1990; 31(3):225.

162. Landsberg GM: The distribution of canine behavior cases at three behavior referral practices. Vet Med 1991; 86(10):1011.

163. Landsberg GM: Techniques for solving behavior problems. American Veterinary Medical Association meeting, Minneapolis, July 17, 1993.

164. Lane JR, Bohon LM: Effect of telephone follow-up on client compliance in the treatment of canine aggression. In Mills D, Levine E, Landsberg G, et al (eds): Current Issues and Research in Veterinary Behavioral Medicine. West Lafayette, IN: Purdue University Press, 2005, p. 192.

165. Leonard JA, Wayne RK, Wheeler J, et al: Ancient DNA evidence for Old World origin of New World dogs. Science 2002; 298(5598):1613.

166. Levine BN: Practice today: Small animal pet population trends and demands for veterinary service. Trends Mag 1985; I(3):24.

167. Levine ED: How I treat nuisance behaviors in dogs. Am Vet Med Assoc Convention Proceedings, 2007.

168. Lockwood R: The influence of animals on social perception. In Katcher AH, Beck AM (eds): New Perspectives on Our Lives with Companion Animals. Philadelphia: University of Pennsylvania Press, 1983, p. 64.

169. Lord LK, Wittum TE, Ferketich AK, et al: Demographic trends for animal care and control agencies in Ohio from 1996 to 2004. J Am Vet Med Assoc 2006; 229(1):48.

170. Lorenz JR, Coppinger RP, Sutherland MR: Causes and economic effects of mortality in livestock guarding dogs. J Range Manage 1986; 39(4):293.

171. Luescher A: Personal communication, October 31, 2002.

172. Luescher AU: Compulsive behaviour. In Horwitz DF, Mills DS, Heath S (eds): BSAVA Manual of Canine and Feline Behavioural Medicine, Quedgeley, Gloucester, England: British Small Animal Veterinary Association, 2002, p. 229.

173. Mackenzie SA, Oltenacu EAB, Houpt KA: Canine behavioral genetics—A review. Appl Anim Behav Sci 1986; 15(4):365.

174. Maes M, Meltzer HY: The serotonin hypothesis of major depression. In Bloom FE, Kupfer DJ (eds): Psychopharmacology: The Fourth Generation of Progress. New York: Raven Press Ltd, 1995, p. 933.

175. Manning AM, Rowan AN: Companion animal demographics and sterilization status: Results from a survey in four Massachusetts towns. Anthrozoäs 1991; V(3):192.

176. Marchand C, Moore A: Pet populations and ownership around the world. Waltham International Focus 1991; 1(1):14.

177. Marder A: Behavior problems after adoption. Am Vet Soc Anim Behav Proc 2001:2.

178. Marder AR: Psychotropic drugs and behavioral therapy. Vet Clin North Am [Small Anim Pract] 1991; 21(2):329.

179. Maurer BM, Dodman NH: Animal behavior case of the month. J Am Vet Med Assoc 2007; 231(4):536.

180. McMillan FD: The placebo effect in animals. J Am Vet Med Assoc 1999; 215(7):992.

181. Mertens P: Transdermal selegiline: FYI. AVSAB Discussion List November 11, 2002.

182. Mestel R: Ascent of the dog. Discover, October 1994:90.

183. Milgram NW, Ivy GO, Head E, et al: The effect of L-deprenyl on behavior, cognitive function, and biogenic amines in the dog. Neurochem Res 1993; 18(12):1211.

184. Milgram NW, Ivy GO, Murphy MP, et al: Effects of chronic oral administration of L-deprenyl in the dog. Pharmacol Biochem Behav 1995; 51(2/3):421.

185. Mills D: The challenge of selecting medication. In Landsberg G, Mattiello S, Mills D (eds): Proceedings of the 6th International Veterinary Behaviour Meeting & European College of Veterinary Behavioural Medicine-Companion Animals European Society of Veterinary Clinical Ethology. Brescia, Italy: Fondazione Iniziative Zooprofilattiche e Zootechinche, 2007, p. 85.

186. Mills DS: Medical paradigms for the study of problem behaviour: A critical review. Appl Anim Behav Sci 2003; 81(3):265.

187. Mills DS, Simpson BS: Psychotropic agents. In Horwitz DF, Mills DS, Heath S (eds): BSAVA Manual of Canine and Feline Behavioural Medicine, Quedgeley, Gloucester, England: British Small Animal Veterinary Association, 2002, p. 237.

188. Montgomery SA: Selective serotonin reuptake inhibitors in the acute treatment of depression. In Bloom FE, Kupfer DJ (eds): Psychopharmacology: The Fourth Generation of Progress. New York: Raven Press Ltd, 1995, p. 1043.

189. Moon BH, Feigenbaum JJ, Corson PE, et al: The role of dopaminergic mechanisms in naloxone-induced inhibition of apomorphine-induced stereotyped behavior. Eur J Pharmacol 1980; 61:71-8.

190. Morey DF: The early evolution of the domestic dog. Am Scientist 1994; 82(4):336.

191. Morgan RV (ed): Handbook of Small Animal Practice. New York: Churchill Livingstone, 1988.

192. Moulton C, Wright P, Rindy K: The role of animal shelters in controlling pet overpopulation. J Am Vet Med Assoc 1991; 198(7):1172.

193. Move over Cindy Crawford—Fido has more clout! Trends Mag 1996; XII(2):37.

194. Moyer P: Thyroid supplementation enhances antidepressant response. http://www.medscape.com/viewarticle/544942_print, 10/6/2006.

195. Murphree OD, Dykman RA: Litter patterns in the offspring of nervous and stable dogs. I: Behavioural tests. J Nerv Ment Dis 1965; 141(3):321.

196. Myers WS: How to start puppy kindergarten classes. Vet Pract News 2001; 13(5):19.

197. Myers WS: On good behavior. Vet Pract News 2001; 13(10):34.

198. Nassar R, Fluke J: Pet population dynamics and community planning for animal welfare and animal control. J Am Vet Med Assoc 1991; 198(7):1160.

199. Nassar R, Mosier JE: Canine population dynamics: A study of the Manhattan, Kansas, canine population. Am J Vet Res 1980; 41(11):1798.

200. Nassar R, Mosier JE, Williams LW: Study of the feline and canine populations in the greater Las Vegas area. Am J Vet Res 1984; 45(2):282.

201. National Council on Pet Population Study and Policy: The shelter statistics survey, 1994-97. http://www.petpopulation.org/statsurvey.html, 2/13/2006.

202. National Council on Pet Population Study and Policy: The top ten reasons for pet relinquishment to shelters in the United States. http://www.petpopulation.org/topten.html, 2/13/2006.

203. National shelter census results revealed. J Am Vet Med Assoc 1997; 210(2):160.

204. Natural Standard Patient Monograph: Melatonin. http://www.mayoclinic.com/print/melatonin/NS_patient-melatonin/DSECTION=all&METOD=print, 3/19/2007.

205. New Jr JC, Salman MD, King M, et al: Characteristics of shelter-relinquished animals and their owners compared with animals and their owners in U.S. pet-owning households. J Appl Anim Welfare Sci 2000; 3(3):179.

206. New Jr JC, Salman MD, Scarlett JM, et al: Moving: Characteristics of dogs and cats and those relinquishing them to 12 U.S. animal shelters. J Appl Anim Welfare Sci 1999; 2(2):83.

207. Notari L, Gallicchio B: Owners' perceptions of behaviour problems and behaviour therapists in Italy: A preliminary study. In Landsberg G, Mattiello S, Mills D (eds): Proceedings of the 6th International Veterinary Behaviour Meeting & European College of Veterinary Behavioural Medicine-Companion Animals European Society of Veterinary Clinical Ethology. Brescia, Italy: Fondazione Iniziative Zooprofilattiche e Zootechinche, 2007, p. 35.

208. Nutt JG, Irwin RP: Principles of neuropharmacology: Synaptic transmission. In Klawans HL, Goetz CG, Tanner CM (eds): Textbook of Clinical Neuropharmacology and Therapeutics, 2nd ed. New York: Raven Press Ltd, 1992, p. 15.

209. O'Farrell V: Owner attitudes and dog behaviour problems. Appl Anim Behav Sci 1997; 52(3-4):205.

210. Oldest American dog. DVM 1993; 24(2):49.

211. Olsen SJ: Origins of the Domestic Dog: The Fossil Record. Tucson: University of Arizona Press, 1985.

212. Olsen SJ, Olsen JW: The Chinese wolf, ancestor of New World dogs. Science 1997; 197:533.

213. Olson PN, Johnston SD: New developments in small animal population control. J Am Vet Med Assoc 1993; 202(6):904.

214. Overall K: The success of treatment outcomes. APDT Newsletter 2001:11.

215. Overall KL: Preventing behavior problems: Early prevention and recognition in puppies and kittens. Purina Specialty Review: Behavioral Problems in Small Animals 1992:13.

216. Overall KL: Practical pharmacological approaches to behavior problems. Purina Specialty Review: Behavioral Problems in Small Animals 1992:36.

217. Overall KL: Part 1: A rational approach: Recognition, diagnosis, and management of obsessive-compulsive disorders. Canine Pract 1992; 17(2):40.

218. Overall KL: Part 2: A rational approach: Recognition, diagnosis, and management of obsessive-compulsive disorders. Canine Pract 1992; 17(3):25.

219. Overall KL: Part 3: A rational approach: Recognition, diagnosis, and management of obsessive-compulsive disorders. Canine Pract 1992; 17(4):39.

220. Overall KL: Use of clomipramine to treat ritualistic stereotypic motor behavior in three dogs. J Am Vet Med Assoc 1994; 205(12):1733.

221. Overall KL: Understanding repetitive stereotypic behaviors: Signs, history, diagnosis, and practical treatment. AVMA Convention Proceedings, Pittsburgh, PA, July 1995.

222. Overall KL: The role of pharmacotherapy in treating dogs with dominance aggression. Vet Med 1999; 94(12):1049-1052.

223. Overall KL: Early intervention & prevention of behavior problems. Step 1: The owner and pet must match. Vet Forum May 2001:42.

224. Overall KL: Early intervention & prevention of behavior problems. Step 2: Routine screening unveils pet misbehaviors. Vet Forum August 2001:42.

225. Overall KL: Noise phobias in dogs. In Horwitz DF, Mills DS, Heath S (eds): BSAVA Manual of Canine and Feline Behavioural Medicine. Quedgeley, Gloucester, England: British Small Animal Veterinary Association, 2002, p. 164.

226. Overall KL: Evaluation and management of behavioral conditions. http://www.ivis.org/special_books/braund/overall/chapter_firm.asp?LA=1, 9/17/2002.

227. Overall KL, Dunham AE: Effects on renal and hepatic values of long-term treatment with tricyclic antidepressants and selective serotonin reuptake inhibitors. AVSAB Annual Symp on Anim Behav Res 2002 Meeting Proc 2002:73.

228. Owren T, Matre PJ: Somatic problems as a risk factor for behavior problems in dogs. Vet Q 1994; 16(51):505.

229. Palestrini C, Baldoni M, Riva J, et al: Evaluation of the owner's influence on dog's behavioural and physiological reactions during the clinical examination. In Mills D, Levine E, Landsberg G, et al (eds): Current Issues and Research in Veterinary Behavioral Medicine. West Lafayette, IN: Purdue University Press, 2005, p. 277.

230. Parker HG, Kim LV, Sutter NB, et al: Genetic structure of the purebred domestic dog. Science 2004; 304:1160.

231. Pato MT, Pigott TA, Hill JL, et al: Controlled comparison of buspirone and clomipramine in obsessive-compulsive disorder. Am J Psychiatry 1991; 148:127.

232. Patronek GJ, Beck AM, Glickman LT: Dynamics of dog and cat populations in a community. J Am Vet Med Assoc 1997; 210(5):637.

233. Patronek GJ, Glickman LT: Development of a model for estimating the size and dynamics of the pet dog population. Anthrozoös 1994; VII(1):25.

234. Patronek GJ, Glickman LT, Beck AM, et al: Risk factors for relinquishment of dogs to an animal shelter. J Am Vet Med Assoc 1996; 209(3):572.

235. Patronek GJ, Rowan AN: Determining dog and cat numbers and population dynamics. Anthrozoös 1995; 8(4):199.

236. Pemberton PL: Feline and canine behavior control: Progestin therapy. In Kirk RW (ed): Current Veterinary Therapy. VII Small Animal Practice. Philadelphia: Saunders, 1980, p. 845.

237. Pemberton PL: Feline and canine behavior control: Progestin therapy. In Kirk RW (ed): Current Veterinary Therapy. VIII Small Animal Practice. Philadelphia: Saunders, 1983, p. 462.

238. Pennisi E: A shaggy dog history. Science 2002; 298(5598):1540.

239. Perlson J: The Dog: An Historical, Psychological and Personality Study. New York: Vantage Press, 1968.

240. Pet estimates vary. The NACA News 1984; 6(3):1.

241. Pet overpopulation. Canine Pract 1994; 19(2):21.

242. Pet owners blissfully ignorant, survey says. Vet Pract News 2000; 12(11):8.

243. Pet pause. Advantage 1991; 1(1):2.

244. Pet warranties. AVMA News from Washington, November 1, 1998.

245. Polsky RH: Ethology: A foundation for treating behavior problems. Vet Med 1994; 89:192.

246. Popoli M, Gennarelli M, Racagni G: Modulation of synaptic plasticity by stress and antidepressants. Bipolar Disord 2002; 4:166.

247. Posage JM, Lindsay M, Marder A, et al: Client follow-up after initial pet behavior consultation. AVSAB Annual Symposium on Anim Behav Res 2002 Meeting Proc 2002:60.

248. Pouchelon J-L, Martel E, Champeroux P, et al: Effects of clomipramine hydrochloride on heart rate and rhythm in healthy dogs. Am J Vet Res 2000; 61(8):960.

249. Price EO: Behavioral aspects of animal domestication. Q Rev Biol 1984; 59(1):1.

250. Profile of the dog owner. Bull Inst Study Anim Prob 1979; 1(2):4.

251. Radosta-Huntley LA, Reisner IR, Shofer FS: Comparison of 24 cases of canine fear-related aggression with structured, clinician-initiated follow-up and 42 cases with unstructured client-initiated follow-up. In Mills D, Levine E, Landsberg G, et al (eds): Current Issues and Research in Veterinary Behavioral Medicine. West Lafayette, IN: Purdue University Press, 2005, p. 42.

252. Rann R: Target animal safety in dogs and cats with clomipramine. AVSAB Newsletter 1997; 19(2):3.

253. Reich MR, Ohad DG, Overall KL, et al: Electrocardiographic assessment of antianxiety medication in dogs and correlation with serum drug concentrations. J Am Vet Med Assoc 2000; 216(10):1571.

254. Reich M, Overall KL: Assessment of anti-anxiety medication on canine and feline patients: Potential for cardiac side effects and correlation with intermediate metabolite levels. Am Vet Soc Anim Beh meeting presentation, Baltimore, MD, July 27, 1998.

255. Reisner I: Use of lithium for treatment of canine dominance-related aggression: A case study. Appl Anim Behav Sci 1994; 39:190.

256. Reitman V: Hi, Rover! Fetch the Ball, Rover! Now Beg, Rover! Bye-Bye, Rover! The Wall Street Journal, June 23, 1994:B1.

257. Reuterwall C, Ryman N: An estimate of the magnitude of additive genetic variation of some mental characters in Alsatian dogs. Hereditas 1973; 73(2):277.

258. Richelson E: Pharmacology of antidepressants—Characteristics of the ideal drug. Mayo Clin Proc 1994; 69:1069.

259. Riser WH: The Dog: His Varied Biological Makeup and Its Relationship to Orthopaedic Diseases. AAHA/ALPO Pet Foods, Inc, 1985.

260. Room at the top. Mod Vet Pract 1976; 57(4):326.

261. Ruehl WW: Rationale to develop the investigational drug L-deprenyl for use in pet dogs. Am Vet Soc Anim Behav Newsletter 1993; 15(1):4.

262. Ruehl WW, DePaoli AC, Bruyette DS: L-Deprenyl for treatment of behavioral and cognitive problems in dogs: Preliminary report of an open label trial. Appl Anim Behav Sci 1994; 39:191.

263. Ryall RW: Mechanisms of Drug Action on the Nervous System, 2nd ed. New York: Cambridge University Press, 1989.

264. Salman MD, Hutchison J, Ruch-Gallie R, et al: Behavioral reasons for relinquishment of dogs and cats to 12 shelters. J Appl Anim Welfare Sci 2000; 3(2):93.

265. Salman MD, New Jr JG, Scarlett JM, et al: Human and animal factors related to the relinquishment of dogs and cats in 12 selected animal shelters in the United States. J Appl Anim Welfare Sci 1998; 1(3):207.

266. Sambranus HH: Applied ethology—its task and limits in veterinary practice. Appl Anim Behav Sci 1998; 59(1-3):39.

267. Savolaminen P, Zhang Y, Luo J, et al: Genetic evidence for an East Asian origin of domestic dogs. Science 2002; 298(5598):1610.

268. Sawyer DC: Pain control in small-animal patients. Appl Anim Behav Sci 1998; 59(1-3):135.

269. Scarlett JM, Saidla JE, Pollock RVH: Source of acquisition as a risk factor for disease and death in pups. J Am Vet Med Assoc 1994;204(12):1906.

270. Scarlett JM, Salman MD, New Jr JG, et al: Reasons for relinquishment of companion animals in U.S. animal shelters: Selected health and personal issues. J Appl Anim Welfare Sci 1999; 2(1):41.

271. Scharf MB, Sachais BA: The pharmacology of disordered sleep. In Klawans HL, Goetz CG, Tanner CM (eds): Textbook of Clinical Neuropharmacology and Therapeutics, 2nd ed. New York: Raven Press Ltd, 1992, p. 307.

272. Schatzberg AF, Schildkraut JJ: Recent studies on norepinephrine systems in mood disorders. In Bloom FE, Kupfer DJ (eds): Psychopharmacology: The Fourth Generation of Progress. New York: Raven Press Ltd, 1995, p. 911.

273. Schneider R: Observation on overpopulation of dogs and cats. J Am Vet Med Assoc 1975; 167(4):281.

274. Schwartz J-C, Arrang J-M, Garbarg M, et al: Histamine. In Bloom FE, Kupfer DJ (eds): Psychopharmacology: The Fourth Generation of Progress. New York: Raven Press Ltd, 1995, p. 397.

275. Schwartz S: Use of herbal remedies to control pet behavior. In Houpt KA (ed): Recent Advances in Companion Animal Behavior Problems, International Veterinary Information Service. http://www.ivis.org, 8/7/2000.

276. Schwartz S: Psychoactive Herbs in Veterinary Behavior Medicine. Ames, IA: Blackwell Publishing, 2005, p. 400.

277. Schwartz S, Weymouth S: Medicinal herbs for treatment of behavior problems in dogs and cats. http://www.avma.org/conv/cv2002/cvnotes/CAn_AnB_MHT_ScS.asp, 7/3/2002.

278. Scott JP: The effects of selection and domestication upon the behavior of the dog. J Natl Cancer Inst 1954; 15(3):739.

279. Scott JP: The evolution of social behavior in dogs and wolves. Am Zool 1967; 7:373.

280. Scott JP, Fuller JL: Canine Behavior: The Genetic Basis. Chicago: University of Chicago Press, 1965.

281. Seeman P: Dopamine receptors. In Bloom FE, Kupfer DJ (eds): Psychopharmacology: The Fourth Generation of Progress. New York: Raven Press, Ltd, 1995, p. 295.

282. Segurson SA, Serpell JA, Hart BL: Evaluation of a behavioral assessment questionnaire in animal shelters. In Mills D, Levine E, Landsberg G, (eds): Current Issues and Research in Veterinary Behavioral Medicine. West Lafayette, IN: Purdue University Press, 2005, p. 179.

283. Segurson SA, Serpell JA, Hart BL: Evaluation of a behavioral assessment questionnaire for use in the characterization of behavioral problems of dogs relinquished to animal shelters. J Am Vet Med Assoc 2005; 227(11):1755.

284. Shader RI, Greenblatt DJ: The pharmacotherapy of acute anxiety: A mini-update. In Bloom FE, Kupfer DJ (eds): Psychopharmacology: The Fourth Generation of Progress. New York: Raven Press Ltd, 1995, p. 1341.

285. Shanley K, Overall K: Rational selection of antidepressants for behavioral conditions. Vet Forum November 1995:30.

286. Shull-Selcer EA, Stagg W: Advances in the understanding and treatment of noise phobias. Vet Clin North Am [Small Anim Pract] 1991; 21(2):353.

287. Simpson BS: Behavioral considerations of chronic disease states. Am Vet Med Assoc Convention Proceedings, 2007.

288. Simpson BS, Papich MG: Pharmacologic management in veterinary behavioral medicine. Vet Clin North Am [Small Anim Pract] 2003; 33(2):365.

289. Simpson BS, Simpson DM: Behavioral pharmacotherapy Part I. Antipsychotics and antidepressants. Compend Contin Educ [Small Anim] 1996; 18(10):1067.

290. Simpson BS, Simpson DM: Behavioral pharmacotherapy Part II. Anxiolytics and mood stabilizers. Compend Contin Educ [Small Anim] 1996; 18(11):1203.

291. Siwak CT, Gruet P, Woehrlé F, et al: Comparison of the effects of adrafinil, propentofylline, and nicergoline on behavior in aged dogs. Am J Vet Res 2000; 61(11):1410.

292. Sommi RW, Crismon ML, Bowden CL: Fluoxetine: A serotonin-specific, second-generation antidepressant. Pharmacotherapy 1987; 7(1):1.

293. Stein DJ, Borchelt P, Hollander E: Pharmacotherapy of naturally occurring anxiety symptoms in dogs. Res Communications Psych Behav 1994; 19(1-2):39.

294. Stuffed dog. Anthrozoös 1994; Vll(2):147.

295. Suttell RD: Animal supporters continue their fight against overpopulation. DVM 1994; 25(6):10.

296. Survey reveals bond between owners and pets. J Am Vet Med Assoc 1996; 209(12):1985.

297. Survey shows disparity between veterinarians, clinic staff. Vet Pract News 2003; 15(6):11.

298. Sutter NB, Bustamante CD, Chase K, et al: A single *IGF1* allele is a major determinant of small size in dogs. SCI 2007; 316(5821):112.

299. Svartberg K: Breed-typical behaviour in dogs—Historical remnants or recent constructs? Appl Anim Behav Sci 2006; 96(3-4):293.

300. Takeuchi Y, Houpt KA: Behavior genetics. Vet Clin North Am [Small Anim Pract] 2003; 33(2):345.

301. Teclaw R, Mendlein J, Garbe P, et al: Characteristics of pet populations and households in the Purdue Comparative Oncology Program catchment area, 1988. J Am Vet Med Assoc 1992; 201(11):1725.

302. Tedor JB, Reif JS: Natal patterns among registered dogs in the United States. J Am Vet Med Assoc 1978; 172(10):1179.

303. The state of the American pet: A study among pet owners, prepared for Ralston Purina. http://www.purina.com/institute/survey.asp, October 2000.

304. Third annual pet owner survey fetches results. Trends Mag 1994; X(1):44.

305. Thorén P, Åsberg M, Cronholm B, et al: Clomipramine treatment of obsessive-compulsive disorder: I. A controlled clinical trial. Arch Gen Psychiatry 1980; 37:1281.

306. Thornton GW: The welfare of excess animals: Status and needs. J Am Vet Med Assoc 1992; 200(5):660.

307. Thornton GW: Pet overpopulation: Why is a solution so illusive? Urban Animal Management Discussion Papers 1993:18.

308. Thrusfield MV: Demographic characteristics of the canine and feline populations of the UK in 1986. J Small Anim Pract 1989; 30(2):76.

309. Towbin KE, Leckman JF: Attention deficit hyperactivity disorder in childhood and adolescence. In Klawans HL, Goetz CG, Tanner CM (eds): Textbook of Clinical Neuropharmacology and Therapeutics, 2nd ed. New York: Raven Press Ltd, 1992, p. 323.
310. Troutman CM: Dog owners and their use of veterinary services. J Am Vet Med Assoc 1988; 193(9):1056.
311. Turner DC: Treating canine and feline behaviour problems and advising clients. Appl Anim Behav Sci 1997; 52 (3-4):199.
312. Tynes VV: This doctor says it's time to offer behavior counseling. Vet Econ 1995; 36(6):64.
313. Ultimate Puppy Kit. http://www.premier.com, 4/9/2007.
314. Unterwald EM, Kornetsky C: Reinforcing effects of opiates—Modulation by dopamine. In Hammer RP (ed): The Neurobiology of Opiates. Boca Raton, FL: CRC Press Inc, 1993, p. 361.
315. Vacalopoulos A, Anderson RK: Canine behavior problems reported by clients in a study of veterinary hospitals. Appl Anim Behav Sci 1993; 37(1):84.
316. Van der Borg JAM, Netto WJ, Planta DJU: Behavioural testing of dogs in animal shelters to predict problem behaviour. Appl Anim Behav Sci 1991; 32(2-3):237.
317. Vilà C, Savolainen P, Maldonado JE, et al: Multiple and ancient origins of the domestic dog. SCI 1997; 276(5319):1687.
318. Voith VL: Clinical animal behavior. Calif Vet 1979; 33(6):21.
319. Voith VL: Functional significance of pseudocyesis. Mod Vet Pract 1980; 61(1):75.
320. Voith VL: Anamnesis. Mod Vet Pract 1980; 61(5):460.
321. Voith VL: Profile of 100 animal behavior cases. Mod Vet Pract 1981; 62(6):483.
322. Voith VL, Borchelt PL: Introduction to animal behavior therapy Vet Clin North Am [Small Anim Pract] 1982; 12(4):565.
323. Voith VL, Borchelt PL: History taking and interviewing. Compend Contin Educ [Small Anim] 1985; 7(5):432.
324. Voith VL, Wright JC, Danneman PJ: Is there a relationship between spoiling a dog, treating it like a person, obedience school, and behavior problems? Am Vet Soc Anim Behav Newsletter 1987; 10(1):9.
325. Voith VL, Wright JC, Danneman PJ: Is there a relationship between canine behavior problems and spoiling activities, anthropomorphism, and obedience training? Appl Anim Behav Sci 1992; 34(3):263.
326. Wayne RK: Molecular evolution of the dog family. Trends Genet 1993; 9(6):218.
327. Wayne RK, Benveniste RE, Janczewski DN, et al: Molecular and biochemical evolution of the carnivore. In Gittleman JL (ed): Carnivore Behavior, Ecology and Evolution. Ithaca, NY: Comstock Publishing Associates, 1989, p. 465.
328. Wells DL: A review of environmental enrichment for kenneled dogs. *Canis familiaris*. Appl Anim Behav Sci 2004; 85(3-4):307.
329. Wells DL, Hepper PG: Prevalence of behaviour problems reported by owners of dogs purchased from an animal rescue shelter. Appl Anim Behav Sci 2000; 69(1):55.
330. Wilbur RH: Pets, pet ownership, and animal control: Social and psychological attitudes, 1975. Proceedings of the National Conference on Dog and Cat Control. Denver, CO, February 3-5, 1976:21.
331. Wilsson E, Sundgren P-E: The use of a behaviour test for the selection of dogs for service and breeding. II. Heritability for tested parameters and effect of selection based on service dog characteristics. Appl Anim Behav Sci 1997; 54(2-3):235.
332. Wise JK: Veterinary health care market for dogs. J Am Vet Med Assoc 1984; 184(2):207.
333. Wise JK: Veterinary health care market for miscellaneous pets. J Am Vet Med Assoc 1984; 184(6):741.
334. Wise JK, Yang J-J: Veterinary service market for companion animals, 1992. Part 1: Companion animal ownership and demographics. J Am Vet Med Assoc 1992; 201(7):990-992.
335. Woodbury D: Risking life or limb for Fido. Trends Mag 1999; XV(2):30.
336. Wright JC, Nesselrote MS: Classification of behavior problems in dogs: Distributions of age, breed, sex and reproductive status. Appl Anim Behav Sci 1987; 19(1-2):169.

## Additional Readings

Akil H, Watson SJ, Young E, et al: Endogenous opioids: Biology and function. Ann Rev Neurosci 1984; 7:223.
Althaus T: The development of a harmonic owner-dog relationship. J Small Anim Pract 1987; 28(11):1056.
Baillie JR: The behavioural requirements necessary for guide dogs for the blind in the United Kingdom. Br Vet J 1972; 128:477.
Baldessarini RJ, Frankenburg FR: Clozapine: A novel antipsychotic agent. N Engl J Med 1991; 324(11):746.
Bardens JW: Combined estrogen-androgen steroid therapy in canine practice. North Am Vet March 1957; 38:93.
Beata C, Beaumont E, Diaz C, et al: Comparison of the effect of alpha-casozepine (tryptic hydrolysate of alpha S1-caseine) and selegiline chlorhydrate in the treatment of anxious disorders in dogs. In Landsberg G, Mattiello S, Mills D (eds): Proceedings of the 6th International Veterinary Behaviour Meeting & European College of Veterinary Behavioural Medicine-Companion Animals European Society of Veterinary Clinical Ethology. Brescia, Italy: Fondazione Iniziative Zooprofilattiche e Zootechinche, 2007, p. 118.
Beaver BV: Solving animal behavior problems. Proc Am Anim Hosp Assoc 1982:3.
Beaver BV: Canine behavior problems. Proc Am Anim Hosp Assoc 1986:18.
Beaver BV: Fear biting in dogs. The Friskies Symposium on Behavior 1994:1.
Beck AM, Loring H, Lockwood R: The ecology of dog bite injury in St. Louis, Missouri. Public Health Rep 1975; 90:262.
Blackshaw JK: Abnormal behaviour in dogs. Aust Vet J 1988; 65(12):393.
Bowen J: The challenge of behavioural modification. In Landsberg G, Mattiello S, Mills D (eds): Proceedings of the 6th International Veterinary Behaviour Meeting & European College of Veterinary Behavioural Medicine-Companion Animals European Society of Veterinary Clinical Ethology. Brescia, Italy: Fondazione Iniziative Zooprofilattiche e Zootechinche, 2007, p. 83.
Budge RC, Spicer J, St. George R, et al: Compatibility stereotypes of people and pets: A photograph matching study. Anthrozoös 1997; 10(1):37.

Budiansky S: The ancient contract. U.S. News and World Report, March 20, 1989:75.

Burghardt Jr WF: Behavioral medicine as a part of a comprehensive small animal medical program. Vet Clin North Am [Small Anim Pract] 1991; 21(2):343.

Campbell WE: The case history method. Mod Vet Pract 1975; 56(9):648.

Campbell WE: A rapid approach to animal behavior problem solving. Mod Vet Pract 1977; 58(10):879.

Campbell WE: Veterinary ethology: The challenge. Mod Vet Pract 1977; 58(12):1035.

Campbell WE: The prevalence of behavioral problems in American dogs. Mod Vet Pract 1986; 67(1):28.

Cancela LM, Artinián J, Fulginiti S: Opioid influence on some aspects of stereotyped behavior induced by repeated amphetamine treatment. Pharmacol Biochem Behav 1988; 30(4):899.

Coffey DJ: Ethology and canine practice. J Small Anim Pract 1971; 12:123.

Cornick JL, Hartsfield SM: Cardiopulmonary and behavioral effects of combinations of acepromazine/butorphanol and acepromazine/oxymorphone in dogs. J Am Vet Med Assoc 1992; 200(12):1952.

Crowell-Davis S: Veterinary animal behavior: Where did it come from? What problems does it face? Where is it going? Equine Pract 1987; 9(3):26.

Crowell-Davis SL: Psychopharmacology Part I. AAHA Scientific Proceedings 2001:12.

Crowell-Davis SL: Psychopharmacology Part II. AAHA Scientific Proceedings 2001:16.

Daniels TJ, Bekoff M: Feralization: The making of wild domestic animals. Behav Process 1989; 19:79.

Delgado PL, Charney DS, Price LH, et al: Serotonin function and mechanism of antidepressant action. Arch Gen Psychiatry 1990; 47:411.

Fatjó J, Amat M, Ruiz de La Torre JL, et al: Small animal behavior problems in a referral practice in Spain. AVSAB Annual Symposium on Anim Behav Res 2002 Meeting Proc 2002:55.

Fatjó J, Ruiz de la Torre JL, Manteca X: Epidemiology of small animal behavior problems in Spain. Am Vet Soc Anim Behav Proc 2001:24.

Fava M, Rosenbaum JF: Suicidality and fluoxetine: Is there a relationship? J Clin Psychiatry 1991; 52:108.

Feldmann BM, Carding TH: Free-roaming urban pets. Health Serv Rep 1973; 88(10):956.

Fielding WJ, Mather J: Stray dogs in an island community: A case study from New Providence, The Bahamas. J Appl Anim Welfare Sci 2000; 3(4):305.

Fisher GT, Volhard W: Puppy personality profile. Purebred Dog AKC Gazette March 1985:36.

Futuyma OJ, Slatkin M: Coevolution. Sunderland, MA: Sinauer Associates Inc, 1983.

Gerber HA, Jöchle W, Sulman FG: Control of reproduction and of undesirable social and sexual behaviour in dogs and cats. J Small Anim Pract 1973; 14:151.

Giros B, Jaber M, Jones SR, et al: Hyperlocomotion and indifference to cocaine and amphetamine in mice lacking the dopamine transporter. Nature 1996; 379:606.

Godbout M, Palestrini C, Beauchamp G, et al: Puppy behaviour during physical examination at the veterinary clinic: A pilot study. In Landsberg G, Mattiello S, Mills D (eds): Proceedings of the 6th International Veterinary Behaviour Meeting &

European College of Veterinary Behavioural Medicine-Companion Animals European Society of Veterinary Clinical Ethology. Brescia, Italy: Fondazione Iniziative Zooprofilattiche e Zootechinche, 2007, p. 27.

Godbout M, Palestrini C, Beauchamp T, et al: Puppy behavior at the veterinary clinic: A pilot study. J Vet Behav 2007; 2(4):126.

Goddard ME, Beihartz RG: Genetic and environmental factors affecting the suitability of dogs as guide dogs for the blind. Theor Appl Genet 1982; 62:97.

Hallinan L: Behavior training boosts practice, helps pets. Vet Pract News 2000; 12(1):31.

Hannah HW: Property rights in dogs. J Am Vet Med Assoc 1976; 168(7):580.

Hart BL: Behavioral interaction between dogs and people. Canine Pract 1974; 1(4):6.

Hart BL: Genetics and behavior of the dog. Canine Pract 1975; 2(6):10.

Hart BL: Successive approximation: The key to behavioral therapy. Canine Pract 1978; 5(5):8.

Hart BL: Drugs and shows. Canine Pract 1979; 6(4):12.

Hart BL: Behavioral indications for phenothiazine and benzodiazepine tranquilizers in dogs. J Am Vet Med Assoc 1985; 186(11):1192.

Hart BL, Hart LA: Selecting the best companion animal. Kalkan Forum 1985; 4(2):40.

Hart BL, Hart LA: Selecting pet dogs on the basis of cluster analysis of breed behavior profiles and gender. J Am Vet Med Assoc 1985; 186(11):1181.

Hart BL, Eckstein RA, Powell KL, et al: Effectiveness of buspirone on urine spraying and inappropriate urination in cats. J Am Vet Med Assoc 1993; 203(2):254.

Hart BL, Murray SRJ, Hahs M, et al: Breed-specific behavioral profiles of dogs: Model for a quantitative analysis. In Katcher A, Beck A (eds): New Perspectives for Our Lives with Animal Companions. Philadelphia: University of Pennsylvania Press, 1983, p. 47.

Hewson C, Ball RO, Luescher UA, et al: The effect of clomipramine on monoamine metabolites in the normal canine brain. Am Vet Soc Anim Behav Newsletter 1995; 17(4):4.

Holliday TA, Cunningham JG, Gutnick MJ: Comparative clinical and electroencephalographic studies of canine epilepsy. Epilepsia 1970; 11:281.

Is bigger better? Mod Vet Pract 1975; 56(6):438.

James R: Greyfriars Bobby. Dog Fancy April 1977:10.

Jenike MA, Baer L: An open trial of buspirone in obsessive-compulsive disorder. Am J Psychiatry 1988; 145(10):1285.

Jones BA, Beck AM: Unreported dog bites and attitudes towards dogs. In Anderson RK, Hart BL, Hart LA (eds): The Pet Connection: Its Influence on Our Health and Quality of Life. Minneapolis: Center to Study Human-Animal Relationship and Environments, 1984, p. 355.

Jones RD: Use of thioridazine in the treatment of aberrant motor behavior in a dog. J Am Vet Med Assoc 1987; 191(1):89.

Kennes D, Ödberg FO, Bouquet Y, et al: Changes in naloxone and haloperidol effects during the development of captivity-induced jumping stereotypy in bank voles. Eur J Pharmacol 1988; 153:19.

Kleiman DG, Eisenberg JF: Comparisons of canid and felid social systems from an evolutionary perspective. Anim Behav 1973; 21:637.

Lange KE: Wolf to woof: The evolution of dogs. Natl Geo January 2002:2-31.

Lehner PN, McCluggage C, Mitchell DR, et al: Selected parameters of the Fort Collins, Colorado, dog population, 1970-1980. Appl Anim Ethol 1983; 10:19.

Ley JM, Bennett P: Measuring personality adjectives to measure personality in dogs *(Canis familiaris):* Report on a pilot study. In Mills D, Levine E, Landsberg G, et al (eds): Current Issues and Research in Veterinary Behavioral Medicine. West Lafayette, IN: Purdue University Press, 2005, p. 114.

Lucidi P, Bernabò N, Panunzi M, et al: Ethotest: A new model to identify (shelter) dogs' skills as service animals or adoptable pets. Appl Anim Behav Sci 2005; 95(1-2):103.

Mandelker L: Clinical use of piperacetazine to modify behavior in dogs and cats: A practitioner's viewpoint. Vet Med Small Anim Clin 1079; 74(4):505.

Mandelker L: Uncovering many new psychotherapeutic agents. Vet Forum August 1990:28.

Marder A: Pushing Prozac. Animals 1994; 127(6):14.

Markway D, Cornick-Seahorn J: Using $a_2$-adrenergic agonists without aggression from the patient. Vet Forum December 2001:26.

Marshall MA, Hart BL: Behavior modification technique. Canine Pract 1979; 6(4):8.

Martson LC, Bennett PC: Reforging the bond—Towards successful canine adoption. Appl Anim Behav Sci 2003; 83(3):227.

Milgram NW, Racine RJ, Nellis P, et al: Maintenance on L-deprenyl prolongs life in aged male rats. Life Sci 1990; 47:415.

Miller DO, Staats SR, Partlo C, et al: Factors associated with the decision to surrender a pet to an animal shelter. J Am Vet Med Assoc 1996; 209(4):738.

Mills JHL, Nielsen SW: Age, breed, and sex distribution in Connecticut dogs. J Am Vet Med Assoc 1967; 151(8):1079.

Miolo A, Re G: Emerging role of polyphenols ginkgo biloba and resveratrol as neuroprotectors in brain aging of dogs and cats: A review. In Landsberg G, Mattiello S, Mills D (eds): Proceedings of the 6th International Veterinary Behaviour Meeting & European College of Veterinary Behavioural Medicine-Companion Animals European Society of Veterinary Clinical Ethology. Brescia, Italy: Fondazione Iniziative Zooprofilattiche e Zootechinche, 2007, p. 129.

Muller G: Postoperative use of clomipramine (Clomicalm ND): Preliminary results. Proc Third International Cong Vet Behav Med 2001:203.

Nassar R, Mosier J: Canine population dynamics. J Am Vet Med Assoc 1981; 178(5):478.

Nassar R, Mosier J: Projections of pet populations from census demographic data. J Am Vet Med Assoc 1991; 198(7):1157.

Notari L, Goodwin D: A survey of behavioural characteristics of pure-bred dogs in Italy. Appl Anim Behav Sci 2007; 103: 118.

Overall KL: Prescribing Prozac means taking thorough medical, behavioral history. DVM 1996; 27(11):2S,4S.

Paul ES, Serpell JA: Obtaining a new pet dog: Effects on middle childhood children and their families. Appl Anim Behav Sci 1996; 47(1-2):17.

Pickar D, Vartanian F, Bunney WE, et al: Short-term naloxone administration in schizophrenic and manic patients. Arch Gen Psychiatry 1982; 39:313.

Polsky RH: Companion animal behavior from the viewpoint of an ethologist. Companion Anim Pract 1989; 19(6-7):3.

Polsky RH: The misbehavior of owners. Vet Pract Staff 1993; 5(4):3.

Polsky RH: The steps in solving behavior problems. Vet Med 1994; 89(6):504.

Polsky RH: Methods used in behavior therapy. Vet Med 1995; 90(6):524.

Polydorou K: Stray-dog control in Cyprus: Primitive and humane methods. Int J Study Anim Probl 1983; 4(2):146.

Posage JM, Bartlett PC, Thomas DK: Determining factors for successful adoption of dogs from an animal shelter. J Am Vet Med Assoc 1998; 213(4):478.

Raskind MA: Alzheimer's disease: Treatment of noncognitive behavioral abnormalities. In Bloom FE, Kupfer DJ (eds): Psychopharmacology: The Fourth Generation of Progress. New York: Raven Press Ltd, 1995, p. 1427.

Robinson GW: Characterization of several canine populations by age, breed, and sex. J Am Vet Med Assoc 1967; 151(8):1072.

Robinson GW: A comparison of licensed and hospital dog populations. J Am Vet Med Assoc 1968; 152(9):1383.

Rooney NJ, Bradshaw JWS: Breed and sex differences in the behavioural attributes of specialist search dogs—A questionnaire survey of trainers and handlers. Appl Anim Behav Sci 2004; 86(1-2):123.

Roth BL, Meltzer HY: The role of serotonin in schizophrenia. In Bloom FE, Kupfer DJ (eds): Psychopharmacology: The Fourth Generation of Progress. New York: Raven Press Ltd, 1995, p. 1215.

Rudorfer MV: Challenges in medication clinical trials. Psychopharmacol Bull 1993; 29(1):35.

Schaffer CB, Phillips J: The Tuskegee behavior test for selecting therapy dogs. Appl Anim Behav Sci 1984; 39:192.

Scott DW: Clinical use of piperacetazine in dogs and cats. Vet Med Small Anim Clin 1974; 69(6):723.

Seksel K: Learning and training as they relate to behaviour disorders. Proceedings of 75th Jubilee New Zealand Veterinary Association, Massey University Publication No. 185, 1998:11.

Serpell JA: The influence of inheritance and environment on canine behaviour: Myth and fact. J Small Anim Pract 1987; 28(11):949.

Serpell J (ed): The Domestic Dog: Its Evolution, Behaviour and Interactions with People. Cambridge, England: Cambridge University Press, 1995.

Shakesby AC, Anwyl R, Rowan MJ: Overcoming the effects of stress on synaptic plasticity in the intact hippocampus: Rapid actions of serotonergic and antidepressant agents. J Neurosci 2002; 22(9):3638.

Shanley K, Overall K: Psychogenic dermatosis. In Kirk RW, Bonagura JD (eds): Current Veterinary Therapy Xl. Philadelphia: Saunders, 1992, p. 552.

Sokolowski JH: False pregnancy. Vet Clin North Am [Small Anim Pract] 1982; 12(1):93.

Stabenfeldt GH: Physiologic, pathologic and therapeutic roles of progestins in domestic animals. J Am Vet Med Assoc 1974; 164(3):311.

Stein DJ, Dodman NH, Borchelt P, et al: Behavioral disorders in veterinary practice: Relevance to psychiatry. Comp Psychiatry 1994; 35(4):275.

Straatmant I, Hanson EKS, Edenburg N, et al: The influence of a dog on male students during a stressor. Anthrozoös 1997; 10(4):191.

Tanquary J, Masand P: Paradoxical reaction to buspirone augmentation of fluoxetine. J Clin Psychopharmacol 1990; 10(5):377.

Tedor JB, Reif JS: Natal patterns among registered dogs in the United States. J Am Vet Med Assoc 1978; 172(10):1179.

Tuber DS, Hothersall D, Voith VL: Animal clinical psychology: A modest proposal. Am Psychol 1974; 29:762.

Turek IS, Ota KY, Bohm M, et al: Piperacetazine vs. chlorpromazine in the treatment of schizophrenia. lnt Pharmacopsychiatr 1970; 4:239.

Uhde TW, Stein MB, Post RM: Lack or efficacy of carbamazepine in the treatment of panic disorder. Am J Psychiatry 1988; 145:1104.

Urmanski A: Canine acral lick dermatitis. Soc Vet Hosp Pharm Newslett 1995; 14(3):1.

Voith VL: Multiple approaches to treating behavior problems. Mod Vet Pract 1979; 60:651.

Voith V, Borchelt P: Fears and phobias in companion animals. Compend Contin Educ [Small Anim] 1985; 7(3):209.

Voith VL, Borchelt PL: The fearful dog. Vet Tech 1985; 6(9):435.

Wise JK, Yang J-J: Dog and cat ownership, 1991-1998. J Am Vet Med Assoc 1994; 204(8):1166.

Woodbury D: Fido's no longer in the doghouse. Trends Mag 1998; XIV(2):42.

Worden AN: Abnormal behaviour in the dog and cat. Vet Rec 1959; 71:966.

Wright JC, Nesselrote MS: Classification of behavior problems in dogs: Distributions of age, breed, sex, and reproductive status. Appl Anim Behav Sci 1987; 19(1-2):169.

Zohar J, Insel TR, Zohar-Kadouch RC, et al: Serotonergic responsivity in obsessive-compulsive disorder: Effects of chronic clomipramine treatment. Arch Gen Psychiatry 1988; 45:167.

# Canine Behavior of Sensory and Neural Origin

The nervous system is responsible, either directly or indirectly, for all behaviors. The brain processes the input from the senses, develops a response, and ultimately drives appropriate motor functions. This chain of input-processing-output can be affected by several factors, including hormonal state, previous experiences, alertness, "mood," health, environment, and sensory capability. Understanding the input to output components helps us understand behaviors, both normal and abnormal.

## THE SENSES

Because the range of detection capabilities for each of the senses varies tremendously among species, human limitations make it very difficult to appreciate the sensory ranges of animals. These limitations make developing sensitive equipment and appropriate experiments for other species difficult. They also complicate interpretation of the results. Being aware of these limitations is therefore an important asset for a veterinarian.

### Sense of Vision

For most humans, vision is the primary sense, and we are surprised to learn that it is not necessarily that important to other species. It can also be difficult to imagine how animals with visual capabilities different from our own see the world around them. For dogs, the sense of vision is based on what might be needed for a hunter. The development of the canine visual system is incomplete at birth, as evidenced by the sealed eyelids of a neonate. The palpebral reflexes are present at birth, but most of the other protective responses do not appear until later (Table 2-1). Even after the eyes open, development continues. Although we typically think of the palpebral reflex as the only one for eye protection, dogs also have a vibrisso-palpebral

reflex, so that they blink if the vibrissae are touched.[120]

Like most predators, the dog has a visual field with a relatively large amount of binocular vision and a large blind spot behind the head (Fig. 2-1). The dog's binocular field is 60 to 116 degrees versus 140 to 160 degrees for humans.[290,366] Each eye has an additional monocular field of 86 to 90 degrees, resulting in a total visual field of 240 to 290 degrees.* In humans, the visual field is approximately 180 degrees.[366,457] The extreme variation in head shapes among the breeds allows for tremendous variation in the extent of the blind area, from 70 to 120 degrees. Contrast the eye placement of a Borzoi with that of a Pekingese (see Fig. 2-1). Head shape also affects eye placement somewhat. In general, the eyes are placed at the front of the head with a slight angle of divergence varying from 15 to 52 degrees, depending on the head shape.†

Visual deprivation during the first 5 weeks of life does not affect myelinization of the visual cortex, but it does result in significant structural, biochemical, and electrophysiologic changes.[130,132] If a puppy has one eyelid fixed so that it never sees from that eye, later tests show that normal vision will not occur when the lid is unsealed.[397] Suppose a puppy's right eyelid is sealed past the normal time after birth. The pup's normal left eye would have a visual field from approximately 120 degrees to the left to 30 degrees to the right of the midline, or the normal 150-degree range. The deprived right eye, however, would see only the 90 degrees farthest to the right and would not see in the forward binocular area.[397] Thus, there would be a full range of vision, but it would be monocular.

---

*References 34, 196, 290, 366, 397, 457.
†References 108, 196, 290, 366, 367, 411, 457.

**TABLE 2-1**  Sensory response development in puppies

|  | Age behavior appears | Age behavior is adult-like | Age behavior disappears |
|---|---|---|---|
| **Audition** | | | |
| Auditory-evoked cortical potentials | 12-14 days | 4-5 weeks | |
| Auditory orienting | 18-25 days | | |
| Auditory startle | 12-14 days | 15-24 days | |
| Ears opening | 12-14 days | 5 weeks | |
| Sound recognition | 1 day | | |
| **Electroencephalographic activity** | Birth | 16 weeks | |
| **Equilibrium** | | | |
| Blindfolded righting | 25-28 days | | |
| Negative geotaxis | 4 days | | |
| Vestibular head righting | 1 day | 5 weeks | |
| Vestibular placing reflexes | 3 weeks | | |
| **Gustation** | | | |
| Gustation | Birth | | |
| Lick/swallow reflex from dry mouth | 3 weeks | | |
| Solid food ingestion | 2-3 weeks | | |
| Sucking reflex | Birth | | 21-35 days |
| **Olfaction** | | | |
| Olfaction | Birth | | |
| Olfactory-defense reflex | 15-21 days | | |
| **Touch** | | | |
| Anogenital reflex | Birth | | 21-28 days |
| Auriculonasocephalic reflex | Birth | | 25-42 days |
| Crossed-extensor reflex | Birth | | 2.5-4 weeks |
| Cutaneous pain | Birth | | |
| Dermal (temperature) reflex | 17-21 days | | |
| Galant's reflex | Birth | | |
| Head retraction | Birth | | 28 days |
| Panniculus reflex | Birth | | |
| Pinna and head shake | 1-2 days | | |
| Positive thigmotaxis | Birth | | |
| Rooting reflex | Birth | | 25 days |
| Scratch (ear-scratch) reflex | 2 days | 4-5 weeks | |
| Tactile placing, pelvic limb | 5-9 days | | |
| Tactile placing, thoracic limb | 2-6 days | | |
| Toe-pinch reflex (nociceptive withdrawal) | Birth to 19 days | | |
| Touch | Birth | 3 weeks | |

*Continued*

| TABLE 2-1 | Sensory response development in puppies—cont'd | | |
|---|---|---|---|
| | Age behavior appears | Age behavior is adult-like | Age behavior disappears |
| **Vision** | | | |
| Corneal-blink reflex | 10-16 days | | |
| Depth perception | 28 days | | |
| Electroretinographic activity | 10 days | 28 days | |
| Eyes opening | 10-16 days | | |
| Light-blink (photomotor) reflex | Birth | 5 weeks | |
| Palpebral reflex | Birth | | |
| Positional nystagmus | 10-16 days | | |
| Pupillary reflex | 2-3 weeks | 4-5 weeks | |
| Vibrisso-palpebral reflex | Birth to 3 days | | |
| Vision | 10-16 days | 3-4 weeks | |
| Visual-evoked cortical potentials | 10 days | 5 weeks | |
| Visual-defense reflex | 27-35 days | | |
| Visual for finding food | 22-25 days | | |
| Visual orienting | 20-25 days | 4-5 weeks | |

Data from references 31, 46, 119, 120, 122, 123, 126, 148, 207, 455.

The development of cells within the brain also is affected by early visual deprivation. If the right eye has been covered, the cells of the right geniculate dealing with monocular vision for that eye will be normal, but lamina A cells in the right geniculate will be 40% larger than normal, and those in the lamina $A_1$ layer will be smaller than normal.[397] Cells in the left geniculate will be normal for the monocular area, smaller in the left lamina A layer, and 17% larger than normal in the left lamina $A_1$ layer.[397] Compensatory hypertrophy in the auditory and somatosensory cortex can also occur.[130]

Internal anatomic features indicate several differences between canine and human vision. The amount of fiber decussation in the optic nerves is an indication of the relative amount of binocular vision. In dogs, one fourth of the fibers decussate at the optic chiasm. In humans, one half do.[108,457] In dogs, the lens of the eye is large relative to the globe of the eye. In humans, the lens-to-globe ratio is 1:18, but in the dog it is 1:10.2.[411] The retinal magnification factor, a function of axial length, is 0.19 mm per degree, for an axial length of 19 mm.[196]

Dogs may not focus as well as humans. At least five factors suggest that conclusion. First, both the fovea centralis and macula lutea are areas that enhance visual acuity in the human eye. The canine retina lacks the macula lutea.[206,366,411] Second, dogs tend to be hypermetropic (farsighted), with images focusing behind the retina at 0.25 to 1.5 diopters (D).[290,411] If 20/40 vision means a person sees at 20 feet what a person with normal sight would see at 40 feet, it is estimated that the visual acuity for dogs is 20/50 to 20/100.[290] Functionally, this farsightedness is insignificant for canine hunters, because dogs with a lens size of 0.75 to 1.5 D have no diminution of their ability to find and chase rabbits.[411] Motion is probably more important to canine vision than detailed images. Of interest is a breed predisposition for myopia (nearsightedness). German Shepherds have a 53% incidence of myopia, and Rottweilers have a 54% incidence.[290] Astigmatism is rare in dogs, occurring in only 4.2%.[290]

The third reason dogs may not focus as well as humans is related to their enhanced ability to see at night. The tapetum reflects light that enters, causing it to be bounced around and magnifying its effects. This gives the dog a light collection factor of 5.6 × $10^5$ compared with a high in other night-hunting species of 1 × $10^6$.[196] The minimum threshold for light is approximately four to five times lower for dogs than for humans.[290] As a result of the reflected

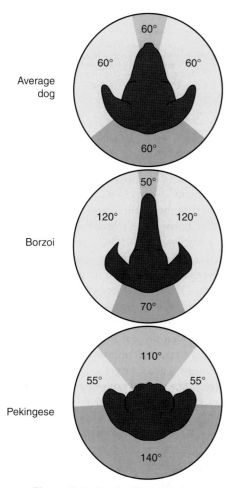

**Figure 2-1.** The visual field of the dog.

An estimate of canine visual acuity is 1.3 to 2 times that reported for cats and 0.2 to 0.4 times that of primates tested under similar conditions.[321] Also supporting the concept of reduced visual acuity are the canine histologic features of unadjusted central ganglion cell densities and lower numbers of optic nerve fibers (Table 2-2).[321]

In repeating patterns, like the alternating light and dark bars of a grate, the visual-evoked cortical potentials (VECP) and pattern-evoked retinal potentials (PERR) help evaluate how thick the lines must be to be perceived as distinct when viewed from different distances and at different intensities of illumination. These are measures of fundamental spatial frequency.[321] The mean VECP for dogs is 12.5 cycles per degree. The mean PERR is 11.61 cycles per degree.[321]

Most dogs do not watch television, probably for other reasons than the quality of the shows available. Although certain sounds tend to draw a dog's attention, the poor form recognition of their vision may make the picture insignificant. It has also been suggested that the scanning rate of the gun in the picture tube, which updates the screen 60 times per second, is too slow to keep a full picture for a dog, which sees only a flicker.[290] In support of this supposition, dogs can discriminate individual flickers of light at rates much higher than humans can.[72] Whereas humans can usually detect 50 to 60 Hz, dogs can detect 80+ Hz.[290]

The histologic makeup of the retina indicates some of the differences between canine and human vision. In addition to the presence of a tapetum, as already mentioned, dogs have a different distribution of rods and cones. Even though the central 25-degree area of each retina has the densest population of cones,[229] in the dog's eye the area is still predominantly rods.[290] In humans, the area has significantly more cones.[290] The rod photopigment, rhodopsin, in dogs has a peak light sensitivity to wavelengths of 506 to 510 nm, as is typical for night-adapted species.[290] The cone sensitivity for humans is around 496 nm, and this pigment regenerates much faster in humans after being exposed to bright light.[290]

It is generally believed that dogs have some ability to see color, but whether dogs actually use color

light, the dog can see better in dark environments but the trade-off is a fuzzier retinal image.

Limited accommodation is a fourth reason dogs do not focus well. Dogs have an accommodative range of 2 to 3 D and are unable to accurately focus on objects closer than 33 to 50 cm.[290] A fifth reason that dogs have reduced focusing ability compared with humans is that behaviorally they have less need for it. Their activities do not require fine discrimination of static forms, but rather are more dependent on the motions, sounds, and smells of potential prey.[148] The image seen by the generic dog is like a general form without a lot of details. This image has been equated to what a person sees near sunset,[355] having less form and pattern than a view in full sun.[148]

| **TABLE 2-2** | Comparison of visual acuity in dogs, cats, and primates | | |
|---|---|---|---|
| | **Dog** | **Cat** | **Primate/Human** |
| Estimated acuity (cycle per degree) | 12.59 | 2.5-9.0 | >30 |
| Retinal ganglion cell density (mm$^2$) | 7000 | 6000 | |
| Retinal ganglion cells | 1.7 × 10$^5$ | | |
| Optic nerve fibers | 1.5 × 10$^5$ | 1.2 × 10$^5$ | 1.2 × 10$^6$ |

Data from references 13, 14, 321.

in their daily activities has been the subject of much debate. It has been argued that the mere presence of cones in the retina signify color vision. This may or may not be true,[5] but other research provides more information.

Within the eye of a dog, cones have two classes of photopigments. One peaks at 429 to 435 nm (violet) and the other at 555 nm (yellow-green).[206,290,314] The middle range for humans, 475 to 485 nm (blue-green), may appear to dogs as gray.[290] This characteristic compares favorably to the dichromatic characteristic in animals, giving them a yellow, bluish, black, white, and gray discrimination. Humans have a total range of violet-to-red (350 to 700 nm) spectrum of visible light.

Among studies to determine if dogs can distinguish one color from another, 10 of 17 concluded that dogs had this ability.[205,290] Some of these studies strongly indicated that form and brightness were more significant than color.[5,457] In a few studies, care was taken to negate the intensity of reflected light as an inadvertent cue. Results, even from these studies, also suggest some color vision is present. Two behavioral reasons lend support to the conclusion that color vision is used at least minimally by dogs.[314] Dogs can be trained in color-discrimination tests. This quality is in contrast to many other dichromatic species. In addition, once trained in color discrimination, a research dog will tend to ignore obvious brightness cues in favor of color choices. This tendency, too, distinguishes the dog from other dichromatic species.

The detection of motion is extremely useful to a canine hunter. Experimentally, dogs could recognize moving objects at 810 to 900 m and stationary ones at 585 m.[290,457] Determining clinically how much vision an individual dog has is difficult. Tests

currently available include the menace response, an ophthalmologic exam, an electroretinogram (ERG), a pattern electroretinogram (PERG), a visual-evoked response (VER), preferred looking, and the optokinetic nystagmus (OKN) technique.[305,323]

Preferred-looking tests present the dog with a preference test between figures with irregular contours. The OKN reflex is based on the natural response in which the eyes and head move to follow the direction of motion of a visual stimulus. A special unit can present specific visual target grids of various sizes, and responses can be monitored to determine when a target's size is too small to be perceived. The normal range for the OKN response in dogs is a 5.04' to 5.75' arc,[305] and normal dogs perform better on visual acuity tests at a distance of 30 cm.[110] In normal dogs, the PERG visual resolution limit is 6.9 ± 2.6 minutes of arc/phase in the center 15 degrees of the retina and 11.8 ± 2.3 minutes of arc/phase peripheral to that.[323]

The optic nerves carry retinal information to the brain. The mean number of nerve fibers in each optic nerve of a dog is 153,712.[13,14,321] At the intersection of the right and left nerves, there is decussation of approximately one fourth of the fibers.[108,457] Within the brain, the occipital lobes are responsible for vision. Bilateral ablation causes object blindness but not the loss of the ability to discriminate light intensities.[366]

The tapetum, something so visible in adult dogs, does not develop until after birth.[362] It is common to notice its absence during ophthalmologic exams of 6- to 8-week-old puppies presented for vaccinations, but to see it present by 12 weeks. Eye color, too, changes from the blue in most young puppies to its adult color during the first several weeks of life. The final color has not been found to correlate with reactivity to environmental stimuli.[243]

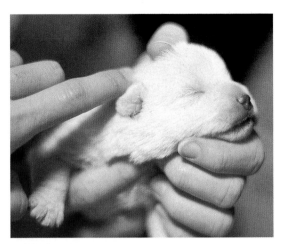

**Figure 2-2.** Ear canals and eyes are physically sealed in newborn puppies.

## Sense of Audition

The auditory system, like the visual system, is incomplete at birth and continues to undergo maturation in the postnatal puppy (Fig. 2-2). The ear canals begin to open around 12 to 14 days of age. Although this opening seems to occur in a few days, the canal actually continues to widen for approximately 5 weeks.[46] Associated responses, such as auditory startle and auditory-evoked cortical potentials, also appear about the time the ears first open (see Table 2-1). Auditory-evoked responses develop rapidly and expand toward the high frequencies during the first 3 weeks and are relatively mature by the fourth or fifth week.[129,363]

The ability to hear a particular tone is actually dependent on two factors: the frequency of the tone and its intensity (loudness). In theory, then, very low or high frequencies could be heard if the volume were loud enough. Frequency plotted against intensity would produce a U-shaped curve. Practically, however, human hearing usually ranges from a low of 13 to 20 Hz (cycles per second) to a high of 16,000 to 20,000 Hz-—about seven octaves.* Audiologists say that humans hear best between 1000 Hz and 4000 Hz, and the average person can distinguish 2000 pitches. The average conversational voice has a pitch of approximately 120 Hz for the male human and 250 Hz for the female, with the typical range varying from 300 to 4000 Hz.[22] The intensity for auditory testing is approximately 20 decibels (db), about the loudness of a whisper.

The auditory range of dogs is somewhat greater than that of humans. The region of maximum peripheral sensitivity, or best hearing, is 200 to 15,000 Hz.[357] At the low frequencies of 20 to 250 Hz, dogs and humans hear with the same acuity.[104,134] Above 250 Hz, the dog has a lower intensity threshold to response,[134,252] and its best sensitivity with lowest intensity is at approximately 8000 Hz.[177,178] The upper limit of the canine audible frequency range varies considerably by researcher, from 26,000 Hz to between 44,000 Hz and 100,000 Hz.* At an intensity of 60 db, dogs can hear as high as 41,000 to 47,000 Hz.[22,177]

Behaviorally, frequencies above 35,000 Hz are probably insignificant because of the intensity necessary.[108] Based on possible upper limits of dog auditory abilities, ultrasonic devices may not actually be ultrasonic. For example, the ultrasonic flea collars use pulses of 30,000 to 50,000 Hz, and 73% of dogs show a response to these devices, including distress responses.[375] As would be expected from this test and others using pulses ranging from 14,000 to 45,000 Hz at up to 75 db, no device tested so far can be detected by nor repel all dogs.[41] Tests have shown that dogs are more likely to show increased motor activity and a "come" response to short-duration notes of high frequency than to longer notes of lower frequency. The latter work better for "sit" and "stay" responses.[275]

The general cortical areas for audition are similar in most species and are best studied in cats.[33] Frequencies of 100 to 400 Hz concentrate on the anterior ectosylvian gyrus, and those of 8000 to 16,000 Hz go to the intermediate and posterior ectosylvian gyrus, over the sylvian gyrus and middle ectosylvian sulcus.[439] Each ear is represented by a similar but not identical pattern on the right and left cerebral cortices, but the pattern is more strongly present on the contralateral side.[439,440]

---

*References 22, 104, 163, 177, 181, 252.

*References 53, 104, 108, 134, 148, 178, 355, 357.

Partial hearing loss is difficult to determine, and even complete deafness can go unnoticed for a long time. Preyer's reflex, the pricking of the ears in response to a sound, is the basis of a behavioral test for hearing, but this reflex is very inconsistent in dogs at frequencies below 8000 Hz.[305] Behavioral responses to pure-tone stimuli also provide a good estimation of the dog's hearing ability.[403] The most common test for hearing loss is the brainstem auditory-evoked reflex (BAER). The BAER does not develop until after 2 weeks of age and then matures gradually until puppies are 4 to 7 weeks old.[46,220] Deafness, whether congenital or drug induced, does not produce brainstem-evoked potentials.[220,226,227,299] Incomplete hearing losses result in intermediate responses.[421]

Mobility of the pinna allows a dog to place the source of a sound to within approximately 4 degrees of its location.[158] Even though there are differences among individual dogs in interaural distance variations and the size of the tympanic membranes, neither type of difference affects hearing ability.[175,177]

Studies also have shown that dogs can categorize different sounds. Based on their reactions, they seem to classify them as natural dog sounds and as nondog sounds.[178]

## Sense of Gustation

The sense of taste in dogs is apparently very similar to that in humans, although palatability is very different. Dogs are capable of responding to substances that taste like acid, bitter, salt, and sweet to humans when tested by nerve responses.[108,456] It has been argued that carnivores do not need to taste sweet, and that the sweet response is minimal in carnivores because they do not eat fruit.[108]

Whereas various papillae of the tongue develop at different ages in the fetal puppy, taste buds are first seen on the forty-seventh fetal day.[115] Neonates have the ability to show taste preferences; the neonate's nerve responses to six different sugars are identical to those of an adult.[115,116] The gustatory system continues to mature somewhat after birth, and the olfactory contribution to taste is learned with various experiences.[26,115] Studies of dogs trained to validate specific flavors show their selections are made primarily by the sense of smell instead of taste.[193]

Clinical tests to evaluate the presence or absence of taste are rare. It is important to distinguish between taste and taste preferences.[31] Palatability tests really evaluate preference and olfaction more than the degree of gustatory function. One test, behavioral gustometry, has been proposed as a clinical test that might have applicability in veterinary medicine.[305] The test takes advantage of a dog's innate lick response when presented with a novel flavor, and this same response occurs to intravenous solutions. In rats, it is even possible to produce taste aversions with intravenous solutions.[305] Appropriate licking responses to different concentrations of various sweet and bitter substances have been shown to occur in dogs. Concern about the potential for adversive osmolarity and pH effects has meant salt and sour solutions have not been tried.[305] In dogs, the normal range of behavioral gustometry response to sucrose is between −15 and −7 molar concentration in Ringer's solution.[305]

## Sense of Olfaction

Dogs have long been recognized as having an outstanding sense of smell. Their ability to use this sense has been tapped for tracking, drug detection, locating accelerants in suspected arson, and even finding people buried under avalanches, water, or building rubble. Understanding the extremes of canine smell has been a difficult task for scientists because limited human olfactory capabilities make experimental design difficult. For example, one study attempted to determine whether dogs could be trained to be living smoke detectors. Behavior was shaped so that a dog would push a lever if smoke was detected at the test site and not press it if smoke was not smelled. The dogs were then taught to check a specific location in each of three rooms. A problem occurred in that when the dogs smelled smoke in either the first or second room, they responded with a positive response in all rooms thereafter.[225] It was ultimately decided that those results would be considered acceptable, because in a real-life situation, if one room was on fire it would not matter whether the others were.

To appreciate the olfactory sense, it is useful to make anatomic comparisons between dogs and humans. The total surface area of olfactory epithelium is 2.0 to 11.5 cm$^2$ in humans and 75 to 150 cm$^2$

in dogs.[53,134,148,422,423] Humans have 5 to 20 $\times$ $10^6$ cells in the olfactory bulb, and dogs have 2.8 $\times$ $10^8$ cells.[53,134,148] Differences in the structure of the olfactory bulbs in dogs and cats as compared with humans include more surface area (the cat has 13.9 $cm^2$),[423] a cribriform plate that wraps around the bulbs instead of being flat, and olfactory nerve fibers entering from the sides, above, and below instead of just the front.[368] These types of differences suggest an early specialization toward a sophisticated sense of smell.[368] From the olfactory bulbs, impulses travel through the olfactory tracts, olfactory tubercle, pyriform area, and hippocampus to the amygdala.[187]

The importance of early stimulation by various odors is not well studied in newborn puppies, although it has been shown that they are capable of smelling specific odors within the first 15 minutes after birth.[463] Studies in rats have shown that surgical closure of one of the external nares for the first month after birth results in a 25% reduction in size of the ipsilateral olfactory bulb.[142]

The ability of dogs to detect dilutions of various odors has been researched. In interpreting the results of any such study, however, it is important to realize that a dog can respond to the primary odor via cranial nerve I or through the chemoreceptors of the ethmoid and palatine branches of cranial nerve IV.[304] Odors that have been shown to stimulate only the olfactory nerve include cloves, lavender, anise, asafetida, benzol, and xylol.[6] The odor of lavender has been successfully used as aromatherapy to reduce travel-induced excitement.[461] Lavender and chamomile in animal shelters result in apparently calmer behaviors.[159] The odors that trigger responses of both the olfactory and trigeminal nerves include camphor, eucalyptus, pyridin, butyric acid, phenol, ether, and chloroform.[6] Amylacetate works only on the olfactory nerve at low concentrations, but it will trigger the trigeminal as well at higher levels.[231]

Whereas humans can detect odor concentrations at $10^{-4.5}$ molar (M) to $10^{-5.0}$ M, and most animals can detect concentrations of $10^{-6}$ M to $10^{-9}$ M, dogs can detect some concentrations at $10^{-17}$ M.[162,231,353] Dogs are at least 2 to 4 $\log_{10}$ units more sensitive to odors than humans.[231,301] Odor-detection studies have covered a wide variety of chemicals, both in solutions and as vapors (Table 2-3). As might be expected, the level of detectability is directly related to molecular size, at least for straight-chain fatty acids.[15]

Humans have harnessed the olfactory capabilities of dogs to extend our own abilities. We typically

**TABLE 2-3**  Molar concentrations of chemicals detectable by canine

| Detectable chemicals | Solutions (in molars) | Vapors (in molars) |
| --- | --- | --- |
| Acetic acid | $10^{-2.5}$ to $10^{-3.838}$ | $10^{-7.383}$ to $10^{-15.08}$ |
| Alpha-ionone | | $10^{-6}$ to $10^{-17.68}$ |
| Amylacetate | | $10^{-5.7}$ to $10^{-9.43}$ |
| Benzaldehyde | | $10^{-6}$ to $10^{-14}$ |
| Butyric acid | $10^{-4.38}$ to $10^{-5.082}$ | $10^{-11.25}$ to $10^{-16.78}$ |
| Caproic acid | $10^{-3.56}$ to $10^{-4.875}$ | $10^{-9.82}$ to $10^{-16.18}$ |
| Caprylic acid | $10^{-4.25}$ to $10^{-6.298}$ | $10^{-12.11}$ to $10^{-16.08}$ |
| Eugenol | | $10^{-8}$ to $10^{-16}$ |
| Heptanoic acid | $10^{-3.87}$ | |
| Heptylic acid | $10^{-6.122}$ | $10^{-11.27}$ to $10^{-14.318}$ |
| Isobutyric acid | $10^{-4.916}$ | $10^{-11.199}$ |
| Oenanthic acid | $10^{-3.8}$ | |
| Pentanoic acid | $10^{-3.5}$ to $10^{-5.082}$ | $10^{-11.83}$ |
| Propionic acid | | $10^{-9.78}$ to $10^{-15.38}$ |
| Sulfuric acid | $10^{-7}$ | |
| Valeric acid | $10^{-3.29}$ to $10^{-5.294}$ | $10^{-9.82}$ to $10^{-16.28}$ |

Data from references 15, 134, 148, 231, 300, 301, 305, 353, 422.

think of the Bloodhound and German Shepherd breeds as the scent-tracking and drug-detection dogs, but other breeds are used by federal and state agencies, as well as by private firms. A military working-dog study found small breeds could also be successfully trained for odor detection of drugs and explosives and could be useful where limited space was a problem.[81] Recent studies are focusing on the canine olfactory capability to detect various diseases in humans, including bladder, lung, melanoma, and breast cancers.[276,360] Also, with the advent of gene research, the relationship between success in detector trained dogs and their genetic makeup is under study.[324]

The ability of dogs to identify and track people is certainly the best known use of their sense of smell. Dogs have been used to identify criminals in scent lineups with approximately 75% accuracy.[389] Trained dogs can easily distinguish among the odors of different individuals, unless the people are identical twins.[215,414] Even identical twins can be differentiated if the scents of both are available for comparison.[214] Interestingly, clothing from human infants was indistinguishable to the dogs in one study if the infants were on the same breast-fed milk diet.[414] Dogs that are cross-trained to find either live people or cadavers do not do as well at finding live people compared with dogs trained to find the living only when both live and cadaver scents are present.[253]

Studies using a chromatogram differentiated over 200 peaks in four fractions for human body odor. Dogs apparently use scents in the second and third fractions.[414] Although individual aptitude and day-to-day performance can vary, the body location for odor source usually does not make a difference in matching success for dogs, even though such odors may be very different to a human nose.[48,49,215,396]

Actual tracking success by experienced dogs can be as high as 93.3% under general conditions and 100% when the dogs are given the scent with the same article of clothing actually used to lay the track.[432] Tracking behavior occurs in three phases.[429] The initial searching phase is when the dog is seeking the particular scent. Once located, the track is investigated to determine direction—the deciding phase. Here the dog moves about half as fast as before and sniffs for a much longer period. Sniffing greatly increases the contact of odor molecules with olfactory mucosa. Up to 10,000 times greater concentration occurs at the mucosa than in the air.[304] Nasal flow rate is an important factor in determining the response to odors.[433] During the tracking phase, direction of travel is apparently determined by comparing odor strengths from consecutive footprints and following those that have increasing intensity.[420] Male dogs and younger dogs tend to be more accurate.[462]

Under field conditions, dogs may use more than just the human odor cue. Smells from crushed vegetation and the compression of earth may provide additional information.[134] Optimal tracking time occurs when the ground temperature is a little higher than the air temperature and there is a moderate amount of moisture, making early evening and early morning favorite hunting times for many keen-scenting carnivores.[108,187] Although little correlation was shown between climate changes and performance scores in studies, there is experimental evidence that certain outdoor conditions can result in the loss of odor on a glass object in 3 weeks.[224] This loss of odor did not occur when the glass object was kept indoors. It has also been found that when dogs overheat, they may not work as well.[152] The need to pant diverts air from the olfactory epithelium.

In addition to tracking, dogs have been trained to detect many types of odors. Dogs have the ability to sniff out truffles because of the odor of the δ-16 sex hormone steroid present in them, as well as in other plants like celery and parsnips.[20] They are also capable of differentiating between the feces from different species, such as various bears, wolves, coyotes, and foxes.[410] Their success in this search increases after castration.[20] Dogs are used daily in airports, in schools, and on border check stations throughout the United States to sniff out drugs and explosives. Efforts to hide or mask odors from a well-trained dog are rarely successful, even with multiple layers of insulation, different light intensities, or strong, unpleasant smells.[82,153,215]

Dogs have also been successfully trained to identify estrous cows by scents in milk samples, vaginal mucus, and other body fluids. The dogs were able to detect pre-estrous cows within 1 to 2 days of estrus in 64% of the milk-sample trials.[173] They were 83% correct during estrus but responded to only 8% of cows in the luteal phase.[173] Accuracy in detecting estrus from swabs of the vulva and vestibule was 97%, from deep vaginal fluid 86%, and from voided urine 86%.[223]

Attempts to alter the olfactory capabilities of dogs have centered on various types of drugs. Steroids appear to elevate the threshold values, at least to eugenol and benzaldehyde, as measured by an electroencephalogram (EEG) and by innate behavior responses.[109] Amphetamines, alone or with caffeine or bromine, have been shown to result in a sharpened sense of smell in trained police dogs, an increase in intensity during searching activity, and improved tracking and selection skills.[232] Prolonged use, however, has the opposite effect.[232] A 3.5% zinc sulfate solution infused into the nasal cavity will result in a peripheral anosmia lasting at least 6 weeks.[193,194,309] (The use of an inflatable cuff on a tracheostomy tube prevents the animal from inhaling air over olfactory mucosa and can be used as another method to produce reversible anosmia.)[194]

All mammals have a vomeronasal organ as part of a second chemoreceptive olfactory system.[422] Anatomically, each palatine duct connects the incisive papilla in the mouth to the ipsilateral vomeronasal organ at the base of the nasal septum. Cilia are present on the vomeronasal receptor cells in dogs, although not in other animals.[163] The vomeronasal nerve consists of bipolar neurons that leave the organ to penetrate the cribriform plate and terminate in the glomerular layer of the accessory olfactory bulb.[162,163] Because the palatine ducts are narrow, they must be actively opened to allow substances to enter and be moved by the cilia up the 50- to 60-mm duct to the vomeronasal organ.[2]

Flehman behavior, licking, and tongue flicking will open the ducts to allow nonvolatile, high-molecular-weight substances and pheromones access to the vomeronasal organ.[163,304] Many of the individual neurons are very selective for either male or female urine, and the firing rates increase dramatically in the vomeronasal nerve.[188] Unlike classic olfactory neurons, those of the vomeronasal organ do not adapt to prolonged stimulus exposure.[188] The result mediates endocrinologic and behavioral responses to sex-related odors. Flehman behavior, although obvious in horses and cattle, is inconspicuous in dogs because the philtrum and pendulous lips limit the mobility of the upper lip. Instead, dogs tend to hold their mouths open with their heads slightly extended. Dogs can also be seen using a slow licking motion to introduce substances like horse or cow urine into the mouth to taste or smell. In dogs, there is also a connection between the palatine duct and the ipsilateral nasal cavity, so appropriate odors can come that way too.[2]

Dogs use olfaction to gather part of their information about individuals they encounter. The canine-specific greeting of sniffing the nose of the least familiar dogs and the flank or perineal area of those they know are examples of this. Similarly, dogs sniff familiar adult persons with more interest in the thighs and perineum and less interest in the thorax and arms.[117] The interest in body odors of unfamiliar children is directed toward the anogenital area, just the opposite of the interest in adult humans.[291] Duration of sniffing familiar and unfamiliar people is the same, however.[117]

Olfactory problems are common complaints in veterinary practice, so it is helpful to be able to assess function. About 85% of owners of hunting dogs will complain about an olfactory problem in their dog at some time.[187,305] Several conditions can produce temporary or partial anosmia in any dog, including canine distemper, canine parainfluenza, some seizures, hyperadrenocorticism, diabetes mellitus, hypothyroidism, nasal tumors, head trauma, modified live canine distemper vaccinations, and car exhaust.* There is unpublished data suggesting there is some reduction in a dog's sense of smell around 10 years of age, but there are also many individual exceptions.[306] Clinical tests to evaluate a dog's ability to smell include electro-olfactography (also known as EEG olfactometry, electroolfactogram, or behavioral olfactometry). Behavioral responses of avoidance, approach, sniffing, and licking are used to determine when and if

---

*References 187, 304, 305, 307, 308, 402.

the dog detects gradually increasing concentrations of a particular odor.[304,305] Although normal threshold values have been determined for eugenol, benzaldehyde, amylacetate, cyclohexanone, and cocaine HCl, only eugenol does not affect the trigeminal nerve as well as the olfactory and would therefore be useful in such a test.[304,309]

## Sense of Touch

### External Tactile Development

Touch is a sense that is generally well developed at birth to protect the canine neonate and help it find food (see Table 2-1). Physical contact with the bitch has a calming effect on distressed puppies, and they respond with the rooting reflex, pushing the head into a warm object (Fig. 2-3). This reflex helps a blind neonate, which is still unable to thermoregulate on its own, keep close to its mother and siblings. That is also the purpose of Galant's reflex and the auriculonasocephalic reflexes. When the puppy's flank is touched, Galant's reflex causes it to respond by turning its head and neck toward that same side (Fig. 2-4). The auriculonasocephalic reflex is a turning of the head when the side of the face is touched. Young puppies will show distress if put on a cold surface and will sleep when the surface is warm,[143,210] but it will be 2.5 to 3 weeks before they are able to identify the touch of a hot object. The crossed extensor reflex is usually considered an abnormal one in an adult dog; however, it is normal in a puppy up to 28 days of age (Fig. 2-5).[126]

Pain perception varies in individual dogs, but certain behaviors are associated with it. These behaviors can include aggression, excessive activity, fear, hyperexcitability, immobility, self-mutilation, vocalization, hiding, relative lethargy, or unusual responses to the owner.[387,398] Early experience can affect pain perception. Puppies raised in isolation

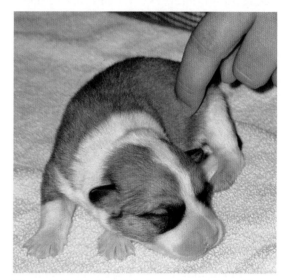

**Figure 2-4.** Galent's reflex is shown when this 3-day-old puppy turns toward the side it is touched on.

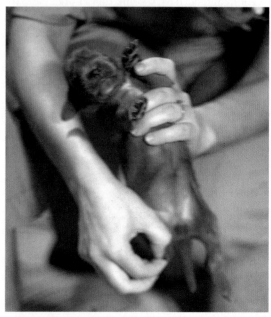

**Figure 2-5.** The crossed extensor reflex is normal up to 28 days of age in puppies.

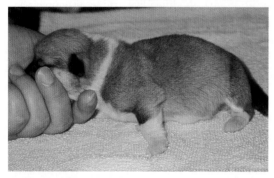

**Figure 2-3.** The rooting reflex is expressed when the puppy pushes into a warm object.

do not seem to know how to avoid painful stimuli and apparently perceive pain differently, too.[280] Tail docking is one of the main painful elective procedures a newborn puppy may encounter. Intense vocalizations, on average 24, last only during the actual procedure.[319] Puppies are generally asleep again in 3 minutes.[319]

One other touch-related reflex is the head retraction (jaw-jerk) reflex, where a tap to the maxilla just below the nose results in a quick, involuntary, backward jerk of the head.[119,120] Accompanying the head retraction is an elevation of the forelimbs.

### Tactile Vibrissae

Dogs use tactile information from their facial whiskers (vibrissae) to help navigate in confined spaces and low-light environments. Although the coloring of vibrissae may vary among individual dogs, the general distribution is similar for all (Fig. 2-6). The prominent vibrissae above each eye make up the superciliary tufts. The slightest movement of these produces a reflex blink, probably originally needed to help protect the eyes of hunting dogs.[4] The vibrissae on each cheek are the genal tufts, and there can be one or two sets. The upper genal tuft is caudal to the eye, whereas the lower one is caudal to the angle of the mandible.[4] The mystacial tufts are located on the rostral portion of the upper lips.

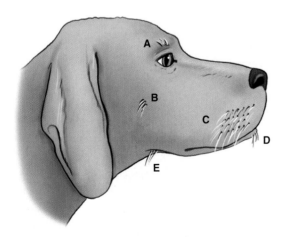

**Figure 2-6.** Tactile vibrissae of the dog. **A,** Superciliary tufts; **B,** genal tufts; **C,** mystacial tufts; **D,** mandibular tuft; **E,** intermandibular tuft.

These vibrissae are arranged in four or five rows on each side. The unpaired mandibular, or submental, tuft covers the chin as a V-shaped double row of vibrissae. The unpaired, circular intermandibular, or interamal, tuft is located more caudally. Movement of these vibrissae contributes to facial expressions. They usually stand out in aggressive behaviors and are folded backward in submissive ones. There may also be a tuft beneath the eye called the subocular, or suborbital, tuft.[4]

### Unexplained Senses

At times, dogs may show unusual behavior immediately before an earthquake occurs.[53,255] Not all dogs show these behavior changes, and the dogs that do may not show changes before every quake. These findings are consistent with evidence of physical precursors that are associated with some earthquakes and detectable by and significant to some dogs.[255] Similarly, some dogs are capable of detecting the onset of a seizure or heart attack before the victim is aware that it is about to happen. We are not exactly sure how the dogs do this, but it could be through the detection of a unique scent or very subtle changes in body postures.

Dogs also seem to have an uncanny ability to tell time.[59] Owners often relate stories of the dog that starts barking at a certain time or becomes a canine alarm clock. Some of the behaviors continue because of owner rewards, but some do not. There is no question that dogs are very sensitive to schedules, so changes are probably best made gradually.[59]

Owners often describe incidents of their dog being able to detect when the person is about to arrive home before they actually arrive. Studies do not confirm that this actually occurs,[470] so most cases are more likely to be a matter of timing instead.

## CANINE PLAY BEHAVIOR

Play is a behavior mainly associated with the young of a species, and it can be done alone or with another individual. The young show the greatest variations in play and spend the most time devoted to it. The purposes of play have been debated for a long time.[37,111] For any individual, play behavior probably has many purposes. For the individual puppy, much learning occurs through play, and that is why it is being discussed in this chapter. The purposes may change over time and in different environments. One of the earliest theories of the purpose of play is that it allows the infant to acquire the motor skills and coordination necessary for long-term survival. A puppy practices various portions of adult behaviors, such as stalking, mounting (Fig. 2-7), or fighting, and perfects them in play. Usually the pup does not go through the entire adult-like behavior sequence and will exaggerate portions or display behaviors out of sequence. Play helps polish the behavioral performance. The endless variety of combinations used in play allows greater flexibility in the eventual behavioral repertoire of the adult dog. Physical exercise is a third reason for play behaviors.

The reasons for play behavior mentioned so far would apply in cases of individual or social play. Those that follow are special benefits of social interactions among puppies or occasionally with humans. For the domestic dog, learning to control the intensity of its bite is one of the most significant lessons of play. Normally, littermates bite and paw each other. In one study, biting was involved in 87.2% of these encounters. Biting included the head shaking in 4.2% of the encounters, face biting in 39%, scruff biting in 6.4%, and bites to other parts of the body in 37.6%.[37] Of the remaining playful interactions, 12.8% were face pawing and 4.2% involved side-to-side head shakes with a bite.[37]

The significance of the biting behaviors comes with its lessons. When the pressure causes pain, the hurt pup will yelp and stop the interaction (Fig. 2-8). The lesson learned is that the amount of pressure used was enough to get a pain reaction. Unfortunately for owners who play with a solitary puppy, they may teach it the wrong lesson by tolerating hard bites to their hands (Fig. 2-9). Puppies learn to moderate play based on feedback that causes them to quit playing, escalate to serious aggression, or vocalize for help from a third party.[444] The "light touch" or "soft mouth" comes from early lessons in which light pressure is enough to end the play bout.

Social play can help in the socialization of a puppy to its own species or to humans; however, play is not necessary for socialization to occur. Socialization is discussed in greater detail in Chapter 4. Social relationships between individuals can be built and maintained through play, eliminating the need for the more dangerous aggressive encounters, as could happen during the establishment of dominance rankings among puppies. For dogs, this use of social play is more common than it is for their wolf and coyote relatives.[37] Social play also allows puppies to become more adept at giving and understanding subtle body language. Dog-to-dog play does not decrease the amount of play that

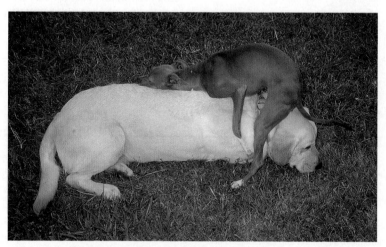

**Figure 2-7.** A play mount by a puppy is not always appropriately oriented.

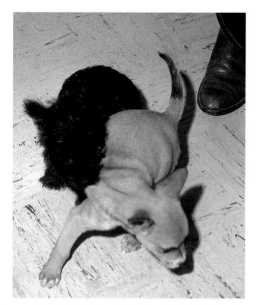

**Figure 2-8.** A play bite results in the victim's trying to get away from the interaction.

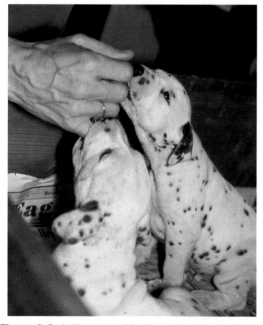

**Figure 2-9.** Letting a puppy bite a human hand teaches that the behavior is acceptable. (From Beaver BV: Early training of puppies. Vet Med Small Anim Clin 1983; 78:862. Used with permission of Veterinary Medicine Publishing Group.)

occurs between the dog and its owner, and the type of play behaviors in each situation are structurally different.[191,376]

Another reason for the existence of play behavior is hard to quantify. Play could be a pleasurable experience performed for the intangible enjoyment of the behavior.[37]

Play forms vary considerably among species. This variation is mainly the result of anatomic differences and a substantial genetic component.[38] Social play bouts between dogs are typically preceded by a play-solicitation signal that can be very subtle or very obvious. The classic dog posture, the play bow, is a rear-end-up and front-end-down posture. The exaggerated approach (play rush, gamboling) is a loose, bouncy gait at a speed faster than a walk, with head and shoulders swinging in a side-to-side manner.[37] Approach/withdrawal is a third type of play-solicitation behavior.[37] One dog approaches the second and then either rocks back and forth as if to withdraw or backs away varying distances before repeating the approach. Face pawing or the pawing intention of a rapid forelimb movement while too far away for contact is another signal used.[37] In leap-leap solicitations, puppies show two rearing behaviors in a row.[37] Barking and other general body movements can also be used to solicit play. Subtle changes such as a head movement, rolling of the eyes, stalking, approach, or withdrawal may trigger playful interactions.[37]

Social play is seen in all canids to some degree and represents a combination of competition and cooperation. Beagle puppies show play seven times more often than young coyotes do and three times more often than wolf cubs.[37] Solicitations for play in puppies are usually first seen between 21 and 23 days of age.[37] The success rate of a solicitation behavior being followed by a play bout varies from 56% to 96% (mean = 77%) according to one study.[37] In theory the various aspects of social play should be shared equally between the participants. However, that is not the case. Role reversals do occur about equally in chase and tackles, but not in mounts, muzzle bites, or muzzle licks.[27] These might be early clues as to future social orders between the puppies.

Parts of the various adult behaviors can be seen as play. Owners generally accept the growling, stalking, and chasing. Mounting, clasping, and thrusting, however, are sexual behaviors that are difficult for many owners to accept in a play context. These behaviors do occur occasionally as play in puppies, starting around day 27 (Fig. 2-10).[37] More than 80% of the time, these behaviors are shown by male puppies, with females usually showing only clasping when they do use the behaviors in play.[37] Roughness during play, however, does not have a sex distinction.[37]

Individual play rarely occurs when a dog is individually housed.[37] Instead, it appears most when play solicitation is unsuccessful or social play is blocked for some reason.[37] An example of this in a home environment is the dog that has a lot of toys but seems to play with them only when the owner is present. Laboratory dogs will spend 24% of their time interacting with toys when other dogs are housed with them.[195]

Toys are seldom used by dogs when they are alone; instead, they are more commonly associated with play solicitation. Puppies are likely to chew to explore their environment and in play, so it is important that they have oral toys, such as those they can hold, shake, bite, or carry.[208] Owners can actually couple toys with several roles, including cue for calmness, reduction of separation anxiety, reduction of overactivity, cleaning the teeth, indicator of general health, and possible way to offset cognitive decline.[191] They must also keep in mind that some dogs can destroy any toy.

## CANINE LEARNING

The Russian scientist Ivan Pavlov pioneered the field of learning, and much of his work has led to our current understanding of the basic principles. Learning, by definition, is a process that modifies an individual's behavior or knowledge as the result of interaction with the environment.[34] Because dogs are capable of independent thought, they are capable of learning all day, every day. Channeling this ability to learn results in a pet that is more desirable, and if done for dogs in an animal shelter, it makes the dog more likely to be adopted.[263] Dogs, like other animals, learn in two general ways: classic (respondent or Pavlovian) learning and operant (instrumental) learning. Operant learning has several subdivisions. Dogs show various types of learning, although the existence of some types is more difficult to prove than that of others.

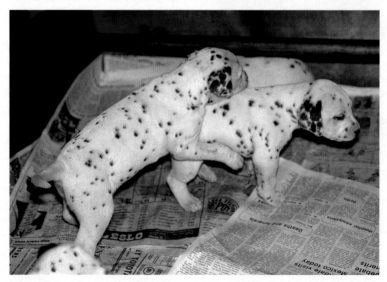

**Figure 2-10.** Play mounting is a normal play behavior in puppies rather than a sexual behavior.

## Classic (Respondent, Pavlovian) Conditioning

In classic, or respondent, or Pavlovian conditioning, an *unconditioned stimulus* (UCS) results in an *unconditioned response* (UCR), which is often associated with a glandular or smooth-muscle action. Food is a UCS because when it is presented to a hungry dog, the dog responds by salivating, salivation being the UCR. This conditioning requires no training and is a predictable outcome: UCS → UCR. Now if a *neutral stimulus* (NS) is added immediately before or at the same time as the UCS, the NS alone has no effect on the dog, but the UCS + NS → UCR because of the UCS. A ringing bell (the NS) does not result in salivation, but if it rings as food is presented, the dog will salivate because of the food and eventually will make the connection between the ringing of the bell and the food presentation. Soon the dog will salivate at the sound of the bell. The shorter the interval is between the UCS and the NS, at least in avoidance learning, the faster the learning, the greater the resistance to extinction, and the shorter the time to the avoidance response.[217] At this point, the NS becomes a conditioned stimulus (CS) because alone it can produce the same result as the UCS. The response is called a conditioned response (CR) when it results from the learned stimulus.[320,416,441,443]

Classic conditioning can take many forms in dogs. In the example of the ringing bell, substitute the sound of a can opener or a cupboard door squeak and consider the number of pet dogs drooling on their owners' shoes as the dogs' dinners are prepared. Many fears and phobias also start this way and grow gradually worse through the UCS + NS pairing. Teaching word commands is another example. The word "sit" is an NS but when used in connection with a food treat slowly moved back over a dog's head to get the appropriate physical response, the word gradually becomes a CS. In this way dogs can be trained by classic conditioning to retrieve specific objects by command. When asked to retrieve one of three available objects, a dog is able to do so with 83% to 92% accuracy.[473] The ability to form a quick, rough understanding of a new word, based on a single exposure, is called "fast mapping."[218] It has been shown in dogs that were able to infer the names of novel items and correctly identify those novel items at least 1 month later.[218]

## Operant (Instrumental) Conditioning

Thorndike's law of effect holds that a behavior is primarily influenced by its effect.[416] In other words, if a behavior is followed by a satisfactory result, it is likely to be repeated. If the result is negative, the act is less likely to be repeated, The response is acquired as the result of reinforcement.[441,443] Trial-and-error learning is equated with this law of effect, but habituation, imprint, insight, latent, and observational learning would be other forms as well.[34]

### Trial-and-Error Learning

In *trial-and-error learning,* the first occurrence of a behavior is purely a random occurrence, but the immediate rewarding of the behavior increases the likelihood that it will occur again. Subsequent occurrences of the behavior are closer together because each is rewarded, Eventually, all the occurrences do not have to be rewarded for the behavior to continue, as long as there is intermittent reinforcement. A dog barks one night because it hears something, and the owner is awakened. To stop the barking, the person yells at the dog. The dog gets a brief reward of social contact. Each time it barks, the dog gets additional verbal contact with the owner, and the amount of barking increases dramatically. The tired owner, fearing that the dog will also bother the neighbors, lets the dog into the house when it barks. The dog now gets the physical form of social contact as well as verbal.

### Habituation Learning

*Habituation learning* involves the repetition of a stimulus until a response no longer occurs. In this case, the reinforcement is the recognition that nothing happens. A gun dog learns to accept the sharp noise of a gunshot through hearing repetitive firing. This type of learning can be used diagnostically for hyperactivity and hyperkinesis, and therapeutically for problems such as dogs that attack a ringing telephone.

## Imprint Learning

*Imprint learning* occurs in multiple forms but is restricted to a sensitive period. The young of a species imprint to a mother figure, usually the first thing around them. This is what they follow and bond to. Mothers imprint to their newborns, often by smell and sight. This two-way bonding process gives the young its best chance for survival, food, and emotional security. Each animal gets an internal reinforcer with some intrinsic value.

## Insight Learning

*Insight learning* is often equated with thinking. Its presence is difficult to prove in animals, but it probably does occur in dogs. Evidence is only anecdotal that dogs can think into the future, but it provides a hint of what canine capabilities might be. For example, laboratory beagles were being tested daily through the various patterns of the Hebb-Williams maze at Texas A&M University. On one occasion, a dog known for running pell-mell through all trials suddenly stopped. He looked left, looked right, looked left again, and took off at a run to the left. It appeared as if he were deciding which way to run.

Another example of apparent insight learning involved a dog that would climb up on a wood pile next to a fence to jump out of the yard. After the family discovered how the escapes occurred, they moved the wood pile to the center of the yard. A few days later the dog had again escaped. The family noticed a small pile of wood by the fence but assumed one of the children had assembled it. Then one day the family watched the dog carry one stick at a time to the fence. Rewards for insight learning come with the achievement of a goal.

## Latent Learning

*Latent learning* is learning that is hidden or not immediately obvious. That means the reinforcer may not be obvious either. A number of studies have looked at the development of young puppies that were handled versus those that were isolated or those with enriched versus barren environments, before 16 weeks of age.*

---

*References 132, 137-139, 146, 270, 279, 358, 392, 453, 471.

Clear differences were found in the vestibular neuron layer and gamma-amino-butyric acid (GABA), glutamine, threonine, alanine, and esterases in the central nervous system of the stimulated versus nonstimulated dogs. Stimulated puppies also had larger adrenals, better coordination, more exploratory behaviors, more sociability toward people, better problem-solving ability, higher social dominance, less emotional arousal in novel situations, less random activity, and faster maturing brains as shown on EEGs. Differences in heart rates were observed for the two groups. Yet, young puppies are apparently very plastic in their ability to develop normally. Those raised in isolation, with only two 10-minute breaks in isolation each week, were nevertheless essentially normal.[146]

## Observational Learning

*Observational learning* is a sixth type of operant learning. In some cases, a dog can watch another successfully perform a problem-solving behavior and then copy its behavior, accomplishing the same feat more rapidly than if it had used trial-and-error learning only. These types of studies often use food as the reinforcer, but not always. As an example, puppies that stayed with their mother and watched her successfully work in narcotic detection trials were significantly better at learning the same task than were puppies that did not watch.[408] Social cognition, discussed in Chapter 4, is another variation of observational learning. Maturation of visual function and motor coordination sets the lower age limit for the appearance of observational learning.[3]

## Genetics and Learning

Many internal and external variants have a direct influence on a dog's ability or desire to learn. Genetics has been shown to be one of these influences. The importance of genetics in behavior and personality was recognized by Pavlov.[77] In studies comparing the dog with the wolf, the cubs were seen to perform better on problem-solving tasks such as detour tests in which insight learning would occur.[141] Other tests in puppies suggested only that the genetic mechanism for performance on this type of test was not clearly defined.[391] In part, genetics can influence the innate patterns of reactivity,[102,303] tolerance of frustration,[145] physiologic effects from emotion-provoking stimuli,[303,316,391] response to punishment,[144] and reaction to isolation.[146] However, there are probably greater differences in learning ability between individual dogs than between dog breeds as a whole. Tests on various breeds do not show significant differences between them.[364]

## Motivation and Learning

The learning of tasks is more dependent on emotional and motivational factors than on ability factors.[9] In addition to the animal's being in the right mood and having the capability to learn, the reinforcement or punishment must be appropriate in type, intensity, and timing. In other words, the motivation must be appropriate. When prevented from getting food and then having a barrier placed between them and the person, dogs that can see the person through the barrier leave the food alone. Those that can get to the food undetected will do so.[45] Studies in mice indicate that feeding them immediately after aversive training sessions enhances memory retention via the vagus nerve.[118] This correlation has not yet been made in dogs. It is interesting to speculate on its possibility, especially in highly food-motivated dogs. Of 17 variables studied, five were identified as significant for learning.[9] They include activity and impulsiveness; docility, or responsiveness to the human trainer; manipulation; visual observation; and persistence of positional habits.[9]

The motivation to continue or stop a behavior depends on reinforcement or punishment. Understanding what they are and how to use them is critical in animal behavior. Reinforcers can be internal, positive, or negative. *Internal reinforcers* are mainly associated with endorphin release that comes from an accomplishment. This means behaviors that have an internal reward are the most difficult to stop. Dogs that chase cars are rewarded because the car goes away. *Positive reinforcers*, often thought of as rewards like food or praise, are most associated with training. Primary reinforcers involve a reward that consists of something necessary for survival. This could be food, water, or shelter. Secondary reinforcers, like praise, are desirable but not necessary. In young puppies, primary reinforcers are usually the most appropriate type to use. As the dog gets older, a secondary reinforcer can become important by pairing it with a primary one using classic conditioning. Dogs trained only with positive reinforcement show fewer behavior problems than those trained any other way.[42]

It has been debated whether social interaction and petting are primary or secondary reinforcers for dogs. This point is still open to debate, but it is possible that for some dogs these rewards are truly primary ones, whereas for others they are much less significant. Response to even a passive person, for some dogs, can be strong following prolonged deprivation.[16] These dogs would be most affected by *time-out* discipline following a misbehavior. Sending them immediately to a barren room without food, water, or social interactions for 3 to 5 minutes may be helpful for discouraging some socially related behaviors like aggression and excessive owner-protection behavior.[318]

*Negative reinforcement* is not punishment. Instead, the reward in negative reinforcement comes from the removal of a negative, aversive stimulus contingent on a specific behavior.[34,43] Suppose a fearful dog hides under the bed, and the owner starts to crawl under to pull the dog out. The dog growls out of fear, and the surprised owner backs away. In this case, the human's withdrawal becomes the negative reinforcer for the growling behavior, because the aversive stimulus goes away, which results in a reduction of the dog's fear.

*Punishment* involves the use of an aversive stimulus during or immediately after a particular behavior, thus lowering the probability that the behavior will occur again. Punishment based on the substrate of affection is more effective than pure punishment in establishing an internalized code of obedience in a dog.[145] Positive punishment is the application of something the dog considers to be negative—a firm "no," a slap, or a kick. The negative punishment is the withdrawal of something that is desirable, such as social withdrawal or removal of a toy being played with. As with reinforcers, the value of a punisher must be considered from the individual animal's perspective.[43] Punishments, too, come in many forms, and individual dogs vary as to what they consider punishment. If the end result of a punishment is not a decreased incidence of the behavior, then the technique is not truly a punishment to that dog.[43] For a punishment to be effective, it must be immediate, occur every time the behavior occurs, be of appropriate intensity and duration, be appropriate for the context of the behavior, and permit an alternative response from the animal.

Some dogs will react to a raised voice with roll-over submissive behavior. Pain, as from the slap of a hand, would not faze a Rottweiler, may be too severe for a Poodle, and would provoke aggression from a Boston Terrier. The intensity of the punishment relative to the individual and to the motivation is as important as the timing of its application. It must be strong enough to be considered a punishment by the dog, but not so strong as to be excessive or dangerous.[43] A punishment can evoke a sympathetic fight-or-flight response, such as aggression, fear, or submission, and it can interfere with the lesson intended or with the human-dog relationship.[43,165] On the other hand, if the punishment is too mild to begin with and is gradually increased, the effective level will have to be much higher than would have been needed initially.[43]

Punishment is most effective if the dog experiences it immediately in the context of the event rather than in the presence of the owner, unless the problem directly affects the owner. That often means the punishment must occur when the owner is not present. Remote punishment equates the performance of a particular behavior with a negative result. If pushing a door open to get into a forbidden room results in a string of cans noisily landing near the dog, the unacceptable behavior of opening the door is immediately punished. Other forms of remote punishment include mousetraps or a shocking device that is activated when the dog jumps onto the sofa, a motion-activated switch that will turn on a hair dryer to blast a dog with air if it attempts to jump on a specific chair, and no-bark collars. The variety of remote punishment devices is limited only by the imagination. Many monitors and devices are available commercially,[233] and more are becoming available all the time. Their use, however, must be guided by the same concepts as for any other punishment: The application must immediately follow the act,[167] it must be directly related to the stimulus,[167] and it must occur every time a behavior is attempted.[43] Habituation can occur if a low-level punishment is used too often.[43]

One punishment technique that can be useful is a *conditioned* punisher, a stimulus that becomes associated with punishment so that punishment is anticipated just with the use of the stimulus.[43] A firm, sharp "no" can be associated with a leash correction for a dog that wants to sniff a fire hydrant. Eventually the verbal "no" alone stops the inappropriate behavior. A noise that occurs a second before a shock can take on the same significance as the shock. As the animal's motivation increases relative to the degree of punishment expected, the conditional punisher becomes less effective. Thus, attempts to go to a fire hydrant may easily be controlled verbally, but a rabbit that suddenly runs can be too great a temptation.

The use of time-out as a punishment has been described as the equivalent of "time-out from positive reinforcement."[43] The owner takes the dog to the location where the brief isolation is to occur. Attempts to use time-out may actually reward the unacceptable behavior because of owner interaction and because it may take too long for the dog to connect the behavior with the punishment. Ignoring the dog's deed and making eye contact may be more effective punishment than a time-out.

Dogs trained only with punishment are more likely to have poor obedience and show fear to other dogs than are dogs trained with reinforcement.[42,430]

No standardized protocol of reinforcers or punishments will work for all dogs. Techniques must be tailored for the individual. It has been shown that puppies younger than 9 days old can learn to avoid aversive stimuli such as a blast of cold air,[17,418] but we typically do not rely on learning at that age. It is inappropriate to start punishment at a low intensity and increase it if the response is not appropriate. Animals are capable of adjusting so that later on, even high-intensity similar punishments are meaningless.[43] Conversely, a punishment that is too harsh may evoke fear, aggression, or submission instead of the desired response.[43] Punishment used too often can also become meaningless through habituation.[43] Behaviors with a strong genetic tendency, ones that may serve as their own reward, and ones the animal is highly motivated to do are probably least likely to be suppressed by punishment.[233]

Reinforcement schedules for rewards or punishment are important factors in speed and retention of learning. A schedule of reinforcement can be immediate or delayed, continuous or intermittent. If intermittent, the schedule can be fixed or variable, by ratios or intervals.[443] The lesson is learned faster if the reinforcement (or punishment) is given immediately after each occurrence.[165,441] Continuous use of punishment usually works better than intermittent use, because when the threat of punishment disappears, the behavior reappears.[165] Unfortunately, owners tend to be inconsistent with punishment, which means the schedule is intermittent.

An immediate reward schedule is more important for animals than for humans, because we cannot discuss a learning issue with the animal. As the period between performance of behavior and receipt of reward gets longer, the dog tends to miss the connection between the two events. In fact, the dog may actually start a second behavior and come to associate the reward or punishment with the wrong behavior. The ideal interval between a behavior and its reinforcement is no more than 0.5 second,[411,443] with a 30-second delay losing its effectiveness in about one third of the animals.[459] The ability to *remember* something that was learned in the past is different from the ability to *learn* about something that happened in the past.[43] The "guilty" look is simply a submissive body posture, often interpreted incorrectly by owners.

Once the lesson has been learned, an intermittent reinforcement schedule of rewards tends to be most effective. This intermittent schedule can be fixed or variable by either ratios or intervals.[416] Using *ratios,* the reward could be given after every specific number of occurrences, like every third or eighth. This schedule would use a *fixed ratio* (FR) of intermittent reinforcement of FR3 or FR8. If the ratio varied each time but maintained a certain average, such as rewarding the third occurrence, then the fifth, then the second, then the sixth, the ratio would be *variable* (VR). This illustration would be VR4, because the average is four occurrences.

Time is the other factor that can be used. When the dog is rewarded for the next occurrence of a behavior after a specific time has elapsed from the last reward, the reinforcement is by a fixed interval. The "sit" response to an appropriate command could be rewarded at least 10 minutes after the last reward regardless of the number of correct responses in between (FI10). If the time frame changes between rewards, such as from 10 minutes to 5 minutes to 20 minutes, the reinforcement is by variable intervals (VI9).

The amount and type of motivation required for a dog to enact a behavior varies considerably according to the individual, the surrounding environment, and the relative satisfaction attained from the behavior. In some cases, the reward for a particular behavior can be controlled by the owner. A special food reward for sitting on command and a pat on the head for coming when called are examples. Many times, however, it is the situation that is rewarding, so the types of rewards are variable.[165] Chasing a jogger or a car is rewarded by "making" the object go away. Barking results in attention or being let in the house. Digging gives the dog a cooling hole or an escape route. Regardless of what the specific behavior problem is, it is important to evaluate the situation to determine if some situational reward is involved.

Environmental enrichment by way of intellectual problem solving can be very useful in preventing or stopping behavior problems.[95] Most dogs do not get to use their minds much and will spend considerable time figuring out how to get food out of a puzzle (Fig. 2-11). Adding novel items to the environment is another way to enrich it. Dogs show more interest in and interaction with new objects.[219]

If rewards play a role in an undesirable behavior, diversion from that behavior can be rewarded instead. The dog that jumps up to get attention can be told to sit instead for the same attention. The dog that guards its food bowl from the owner can learn instead that the owner's approach means it will get small food rewards for good behavior. Diverting the barking dog's attention provides a brief period of silence that can be rewarded.

A bridging stimulus can be helpful in shaping new behaviors. Using classical conditioning, an NS like the sound of a clicker is paired with the food

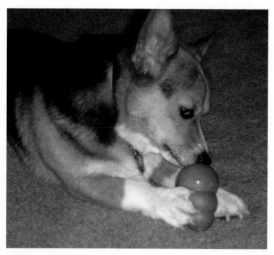

**Figure 2-11.** Food puzzles and toys are environmental enrichment aids.

or praise-positive reinforcement for an appropriate response. Eventually the dog learns that a clicker sound will be followed shortly by the actual reward. This gives the owner a little extra time to present the primary reinforcer for a correct response and it gives the dog immediate feedback of a correct response. The click bridges the time of response to reinforcer.

*Extinction* of a learned behavior means the behavior no longer occurs, just as if it had never been learned. Extinction occurs fastest if the initial reinforcement or punishment schedule is continuous rather than intermittent.[165,441] Although extinction is best accomplished by eliminating the reinforcement that has been occurring for the undesirable behavior, punishment may work when that is not possible.[165] A dog that has learned to bark to get attention will gradually stop the behavior if it no longer gets any attention while barking. Traumatically acquired behaviors would be the exception, such as a fear of noise that developed because at one time firecrackers were tied to the animal's tail. This type of behavior maintains a marked resistance to extinction even without continued reinforcement.[413]

## Dog Collars, Head Halters, and Harnesses

A number of different types of restraint devices are available on the market. Most dogs will wear a standard type of flat or rolled collar made out of leather or nylon strapping adjusted by a buckle. For training, however, the standard collars may not work well because the dog learns how to lean into it much like a draft horse leans into the collar to pull its load. This leads to increased intraocular pressure that could be harmful, at least to certain dogs.[354] Choke chains and prong collars have been used as training aids and for control during walks for a long time. Dogs can still learn how to lean into them and ignore the pain. Injuries can result if they are not used correctly. More recently the head halters (head collars) have become popular. The Gentle Leader (originally called the Promise) head halter was the first, and several other types have come on the market to try to emulate the Gentle Leader's success. Most fall short.[172] The advantage of the head halter as a training and management tool is apparent, because there is almost instant recognition by the dog that it is now under control of the holder of the leash. For some dogs, that simply means lowering their head—a trick owners often equate with depression. Others will paw at the nose piece or try to exaggerate their pulling. The bottom line is if the head cannot go, neither can the body. The owner now has control without pain or struggle. Owners also feel more confident in allowing some slack in the leash because a quick, mild tug brings compliance. Studies show that despite the reaction shown, a dog wearing a head halter is no more stressed than one wearing a regular collar.[325]

Head halters also are very useful for handling aggressive dogs because of the head control. Although the dog can still bite, it is possible to control the motion of the head. A person can also enforce a command by grabbing a leash attached to the head halter, far away from the mouth.

A few dogs do not seem to be able to adjust to wearing a head halter, but they usually do fine with some of the no-pull harnesses now available. These usually put some pressure across the chest or shoulders as the leash is tightened. That pressure is released as the pulling forward is slowed.

## Intelligence and Learning

Two questions most dog owners want answered are, "How smart is my dog?" and "How smart are dogs compared with other animals?" Breeds of dogs have been ranked for "obedience and working intelligence."[75,221] IQ tests also have been devised by several people to test individual dogs,[73,75] some of which result in the majority of dogs being ranked as "above the average."[73] Aristotle considered the dog, elephant, and a few other mammals to have a mental level of a human child, whereas Descartes considered nonhuman species to have little or no intelligence.[458] Others have ranked the dog somewhere below primates but above ungulates.[458]

The difficulty with the whole issue of intelligence is that there is no standardized definition, and in fact, multiple kinds of intelligence are now recognized. Some consider general intelligence to be related to the ability to learn anything, but others have specified seven types of intelligence in humans: bodily-kinesthetic, interpersonal, intrapersonal, linguistic, logical-mathematical, musical, and spatial.[75] It has been proposed that dogs have three types of intelligence: adaptive, working (or obedience), and instinctive.[75]

*Adaptive intelligence* is that involved in learning and problem solving. *Learning ability* is defined here as the number of experiences needed to create relatively permanent memory.[75] *Problem solving* is the ability to overcome obstacles by using previous knowledge in new ways and piecing together information to create solutions in novel situations.[75] In tests in which a dog must pull a string to get a food reward, the dog is only successful if the food and string are perpendicular to him. The dog is not successful if the string angles to the food and will pick the wrong string if two strings are crossed.[330] The second type of intelligence proposed for dogs is *working intelligence* or *obedience intelligence,* a term that is self-explanatory. The third is *instinctive intelligence,* so called because it consists of the genetically determined abilities and behavioral predispositions that are known as instincts.[75]

Without a standard definition of intelligence in general, it is impossible to set up a universally accepted test to measure it. The great variety of genetic diversity among dogs makes it even more difficult to measure intelligence. Capacities that increase the ability of a particular breed or type of dog to learn in a special situation may, in fact, limit that dog's range of adaptability in other situations.[123,391]

If, then, it is difficult to measure intelligence within a single species, it is even more difficult to compare the intelligences of different species. Newer studies have found quantitative and qualitative differences among species insufficient for ranking nonhuman vertebrates.[265,266] The testing of single paradigms can result in a ranking across species, but these rankings are the measure of genetic predispositions rather than true comparisons. If a response must be made by a pelvic limb kicking backward for example, porpoises and horses would score high, but parrots, dogs, and snakes would not be considered very intelligent. When the nose-push response is used, porpoises and horses would again score high, and so would dogs and parrots. Perhaps the appropriate response to the question, "How smart is my dog?" is "As smart as you want to believe."

## Age-Related Learning

Puppies are capable of learning within the first few days of life. They are able to learn to differentiate wire from cloth between days 2 and 6.[417] In testing appetitive and aversive conditioning using sucking strength as a measure of the response to milk, no fluid, or a quinine solution, puppies ages 3 to 10 days show the expected responses.[419] They can reach the 50% criterion level as early as 15 days and the 90% level by 19 days of age.[76]

Reversal learning is present in Beagles before 2 weeks of age.[18] CRs involving body movements come later, paralleling the development of motor skills. Stable conditioned reflexes to sound, light, and odor stimuli appear between 18 and 21 days of age, and conditioned avoidance response comes after 20 days.[147] The earliest age of a conditioned orientation is 21 days.[209] Conditioned body movements are first seen at 22 days, and specific CRs of the forelimb appear at 30 days.[209]

Stable learning begins at 8 to 9 weeks in puppies, which is their most sensitive time.[125,132] Traumatic experiences (i.e., traumatic from the dog's perspective) at this stage of life are not forgotten and can adversely affect social relations in later life.[125,132] The basic learning capacity is developed by 3 months of age, but poor motor skills, a short attention span, and emotional excitability can make traditional learning methods ineffective.[60,393] If puppies are placed in isolation at this age, there is a deterioration of their capacity to learn new behaviors and decreased retention of some previously learned behavior.[246] Enriched environments provide for better emotional growth than do restricted ones[246,279,467,471] and are valuable for kenneled dogs as well as in-home pets.[460] Early environmental enrichment has been shown to affect information processing and plasticity-related neural effects, such as neurogenesis, synapse formation, and dendritic branching.[114] By 4 months, the speed of formation of the conditioned reflexes begins to slow down, perhaps because previous learning begins to interfere with new learning.[393] Dogs that are treated as companions by their owners have lower problem-solving skills and are more socially dependent than working dogs.[434] This probably reflects the fact that their ability to learn is not encouraged and does not reinforce the "learning to learn" trait.

Diets can affect learning in young puppies, just as in young children. Defects are most obvious in severely deprived puppies, but studies are looking for nutritional components that improve the ability to learn. One ingredient that has been identified to improve learning is decosahexaenoic acid (DHA).[184] It is a long-chain polyunsaturated fatty acid, normally present in a bitch's milk, organ meat, cold water fish, and eggs, and it is synthesized in the liver.[184] From there, it accumulates in the retina and gray matter of young animals.

Traditional obedience training is often deferred until 6 months of age or more. However, very young puppies are capable of learning short, focused lessons before that. Standard obedience techniques are based on a World War I training manual using a choke collar and leash technique that is not appropriate for younger puppies.[60] The military now purchases older dogs and requires approximately 70 days to train them successfully.[52]

At the other end of the age spectrum, geriatric dogs take more time to learn various tasks involving several different types of learning and they have working memory deficits.[*] Improvement is possible. Something as simple as the diet can significantly improve a geriatric dog's ability to learn, and yet that same diet has no effect on younger, adult dogs.[283] Other studies have looked at the effect of estrogen in aged dogs. Estrogen has been shown to improve learning, particularly in female dogs, but it impairs memory in both sexes.[427] There also is significant concern about the dangerous side effects of estrogen administration.

## PUPPY SELECTION AND TEMPERAMENT TESTS

Selecting the right puppy that will grow up to be an important part of the family has long been the goal for new dog owners and breeders alike. Unfortunately, selection is usually done on a spur-of-the-moment impulse and is based on physical attractiveness. Behavior and personality often do not become important until later, especially if the dog chosen does not turn out to have a personality that suits its owner. A very dominant dog can control the household when the owner has a meek personality. Conversely, the dominant owner is often unhappy with a timid, shy dog. Guidelines for puppy selection are therefore desirable. Such guidelines are particularly valuable when there is a desire to know which puppy in a litter has the potential to become the best obedience, field-trial, or guide dog. As a result, several different puppy selection tests have been developed, primarily for the 5- to 7-week-old dog.[*]

Five basic tests for puppy selection involve social attraction (attempting to have the puppy come), following (seeing if the puppy will follow), restraint (response to being held on its back), social dominance (response to touching the top of its shoulders), and elevation dominance (response to being held off the ground). The results aim to predict basic personality/temperament types so as to help prevent an inappropriate selection; however, no correlation has been proven between test results and adult personalities.[†]

Situational fear and anxieties are common in puppies as they learn about their new environment.

---

*References 1, 88, 283, 285, 326, 428.

*References 25, 55, 56, 61, 64, 65, 75, 105, 332, 335, 450, 452.
†References 25, 29,157, 334, 343, 469.

Without careful management, these can escalate. Recent work shows these anxieties can be reduced with the use of a Dog Appeasing Pheromone collar.[96] Puppy interaction and play increases, to improve overall socialization.

Certain personality traits do remain stable over time, so knowing about them might help puppy selection or early training in some situations. Playfulness, the tendency to chase moving objects, sociability, and boldness are traits that remain stable.[425] Follow-up studies on how these traits predicted later behaviors had some surprising results. Chase-proneness correlated to a human-directed play interest and nonsocial fear rather than the predatory behavior.[424] Playfulness corresponded to the puppy's interest in playing with people. Sociability corresponded with the attitude toward strangers, and curiosity continued in its form into adulthood.[424] The tendency to show exploratory behavior may increase over time. In potential guide dogs, fearfulness at 3 months of age has some predictive value for adult fearfulness. Accuracy of the predictions improves only with increased age of testing.[155] Even when a special breeding program is designed to maximize early experiences and to help minimize fearfulness,[156] a potential guide dog is most apt to fail in the training program not by some factor that can be measured but because it does not take responsibility for the blind person.[358] An estimate of the heritability of temperament is 0.51 in German Shepherds.[264] However, some police dog programs have been able to successfully predict which puppies will succeed in their program between 2 and 9 months of age.[409] Because so many environmental influences can shape a puppy's personality between the time of a temperament test and adulthood, the main benefit from applying such a test might be to provide "flags" for the potential development of certain problems.[25,332,334,335]

## ADULT DOG PERSONALITIES AND TEMPERAMENT

When owners are polled about their adult dog's personality, 48% describe the dog as stable. Another 30% describe their pet as fearful, 13% say their dog is dominant or aggressive, and 9% call the dog reactive to sensory stimuli.[274] Over half the dogs described by their owners as having a temperament problem might be helped with appropriate behavior therapy. Many behaviors have a genetic component but as was shown in an extensive research project, the relationship of genetics to behavior is rarely simple.[393]

Temperament has been studied and described in many ways over the years. Most of the descriptions are based on results of some type of test in an attempt to bring objectivity to the study; however, individual dog traits, breed prototypes done by experts, and observational tests have also been reported.[212] Even though most of these tests were done on adult dogs instead of puppies, the biggest shortcoming remains the same—the tests were not validated.[212] Recent work with behavior tests questionnaires regarding service dogs is coming closer.[395,468,469] Although these are highly desirable to help increase the success of the dogs actually trained for these purposes, it is not likely to be very helpful to the general dog owner.

Certain personality traits have a genetic component, but what we often forget is that undesirable traits can also be inherited. A line of nervous Pointers showed less friendly behaviors and lower responsiveness in serum creatine phosphokinase levels and heart rate to atropine or isoproterenol[315] than other Pointers. They also failed to improve with chronic imipramine treatment.[426] Even intensive handling of these puppies did not result in a normal-acting Pointer.[438] These data suggest the possibility of hypothalamic coordination of the brain and autonomic nervous system with pituitary-adrenal gland interactions.[315]

## NEUROLOGIC ORIGINS OF BEHAVIOR

At the time of birth, a newborn German Shepherd puppy's brain is 8 $cm^3$.[190] Development of the brain and nervous system continues after birth, but at a slower rate than before.[74] The morphologic changes in the puppy brain over the first 8 weeks of neuronal changes include increasing brain size to 80 $cm^3$ and sulci development.[121,123,124,135,190] Physiologic changes are also taking place. Some of these physiologic changes show in the appearance or disappearance of the various reflexes already discussed. Some are discussed in connection with neuromuscular function in Chapter 9. Another indication of continued neurologic development can be seen in changes associated with the EEG. In puppies younger than 18 days of age, low amplitudes with random low-frequency patterns on EEGs do not distinguish wakefulness and sleep.[70,127] At 18 to 20 days, a difference starts to appear, and by 4 to 5 weeks, the difference is marked.[70,127] By 3 weeks, all the differentiations of wave patterns of quiet sleep, active sleep, and wakefulness have appeared, and by day 25, it is rare for a puppy to go from wakefulness to REM sleep directly.[127] At 29 to 35 days, it becomes possible to differentiate alert, drowsy, slow-wave sleep, and REM sleep on the basis of the EEG.[128]

At 5 to 8 weeks of age, four characteristic patterns are seen on puppy EEGs.[70] The first is a fast-activity, low-amplitude pattern during excitation. A pattern of medium frequencies and amplitude of resting occurs at 8 to 14 cycles per second. Deep sleep has a low-frequency, high-amplitude pattern. A fourth pattern of intermediate waves with mixed frequency and amplitude, is typical of neither wakefulness nor sleep.[70] Thus, the EEG results indicate a relatively mature brain after 5 weeks[133] and an adult-like one at 8 weeks of age,[70] even though the adult size of approximately 120 cm$^3$ is not reached until 16 weeks.[190]

Early stress can speed up maturation of the brain as shown on an EEG.[130] Later in life, EEG activity is secondary to changes in arousal but unrelated to specific performance of behaviors.[437] Evoked potentials of the auditory and visual cortex develop rapidly for the first 3 weeks and are relatively mature in another 1 to 2 weeks.[129] This development parallels the development of the related senses. Dogs raised with social and partial sensory deprivation have abnormal EEGs and short-latency visual-evoked potentials that correlate with their overt behavioral abnormalities.[130]

Oxygen consumption and resistance to circulatory arrest by the neonate's brain also parallel the changes in the EEG. During the first 7 weeks, the metabolic rate proceeds rostrally from the medulla to the caudate nucleus.[183] Even in the adult, oxygen needs are higher in the newer phylogenetic layers, a possible explanation for the resistance to anoxia in young puppies.[183] The neonate's respiratory center will function 17 times longer than that of an adult after complete circulatory arrest, but this response decreases gradually until it becomes adult-like by 4 months of age.[214]

Myelinization of the central nervous system also continues after birth. During the first 3 weeks after birth, myelinization of the spinal cord continues causally from the cervical cord to the motor roots and then to the sensory roots.[130,133,136] In the fourth week, myelin appears in the somatosensory neocortex.[130,133] At 6 weeks, there is continued myelinization of the visual and auditory cortex.[130,133]

Although all the brain is related to some aspect of behavior, the part most strongly implicated is the limbic system. Most of our information about the brain and limbic system involvement has been acquired from rat, cat, and primate studies. The specific structures considered to be part of the limbic system vary somewhat according to different researchers, but most agree that the limbic system consists of the limbic lobe and associated subcortical structures. The limbic lobe consists of the cingulate gyri, dentate gyri, hippocampus, parahippocampal gyri, and subcallosal gyri. Associated structures include the amygdaloid complex, epithalamus, hypothalamus, rostral thalamic nuclear areas, and septal nuclei.

Specific areas of the limbic system have been associated with certain behaviors. We still only have a partial understanding of their relationship to specific neurotransmitters and their metabolites. For example, increased amounts of 3-methoxy-4-hydroxyphenylglycol in the cerebrospinal fluid of certain men have been statistically correlated to their history of aggressive behavior, but 5-hydroxyindoleacetic acid has not.[51] The prefrontal area of the brain is partially related to memory, and dopamine has been implicated in the cognitive process of the working memory.[466] Ultimately, real breakthroughs in psychopharmacologic management will come from an understanding of which neurotransmitters work at which locations to result in which behaviors. For now, understanding the functions of the various areas is an important first step.

The hypothalamus is one of the best-studied areas of the brain. Several aspects of behavior are controlled there, including appetite, water balance, predation, sexual behavior, the sleep-wake cycle, and the emotions of fear, aggression, anger, and rage. The hunger center is in the lateral hypothalamus, and the satiety center is in the anterolateral part.[20] The amygdala is also involved with the learning of fear. It has been hypothesized that fear is at least partially caused by a chronic overreaction of the amygdala or to its failure to turn off after a threat has passed.[342] Bilateral lesions in the anterior hypothalamic-medial preoptic regions can reduce juvenile mounting and eliminate copulatory behavior in male dogs.[164,166,171] In self-stimulation trials, these general areas were predominant.[386] Behaviors associated with self-stimulation were sniffing, salivation, urination, defecation, and licking movements.[386]

The hippocampus is also broad in its behavior ties and is complex in its relationships. This area has been associated with attention mechanisms, emotions, internal physiologic changes, personality, psychomotor seizures, recent memory, and submissive behavior patterns. The amygdaloid complex modulates the activity of the hypothalamus, especially as related to agonistic behavior, activity patterns, water consumption, and food intake. Bilateral lesions of the amygdala have been clinically helpful for extremely nervous dogs with no or only minor tendencies for aggression.[10] Amygdala-hippocampal-pyriform lesions result in a dog that is extremely submissive to people.[149]

Septal nuclei moderate sensory emotional responses to prevent overactivity, and they moderate water consumption. They can suppress aggressive behavior of hypothalamic or amygdaloid origin. Removal of the septal area can result in increased aggression or irritability.[166] The thalamus regulates the state of consciousness and the hypothalamus, as well as integrating sensory input. Temporal lobe lesions change dominant personalities by making the dog less responsive, as well as by reducing aggression.[149] The neocortex makes up 84% of the adult dog brain versus 96% of the human brain.[164]

Another area of the brain, the locus caeruleus, has been shown to be related to behavior. Dysregulation is apparently related to the development of phobias and panic.[216,342] Because it is the primary nonadrenergic nucleus of the human brain and directly supplies the limbic system, pharmacologic manipulation works well in truly affected people.[342]

Body temperature regulation is a brain-controlled function that matures after birth. Newborn puppies have a very limited ability to respond to environmental temperature changes. In comfortable temperatures, around 30° C, neonates remain relaxed and fall asleep. Contact with the bitch's mammary region will bring the core temperature of a newborn puppy to within 1° of the mother's.[83] As the environmental temperature rises above 31° C, signs of distress appear in the puppy, whose core body temperature increases.[365] Below an environmental temperature of 27.5° C, puppies again become distressed and respond by increased alertness, vocalization, hypernoea, and restlessness because they cannot shiver.[83,365] If put in an ambient temperature of 1 to 6° C, a 1-day-old puppy will lose heat at the same rate as will a beaker of saline of the same weight.[211] During the first 10 days, puppies become better able to tolerate falling environmental temperatures, but not rising temperatures.[83,365] By 3 weeks of age, a puppy can maintain body temperatures even in hot or cold extremes.[211]

Emesis, as controlled by the chemoreceptive emetic trigger zone (CTZ) and the vomiting center (VC), is another behavior that matures after birth. The VC can be activated by the second day after birth.[359] Its reactivity increases markedly until the fifth day, when it stabilizes.[359] The CTZ is first responsive on day 5, becomes rapidly more responsive during the next 5 days, and then continues a slow increase in reactivity until the end of the first month.[359]

The neurotransmitters of the brain remain a topic of research interest. Interspecies differences have been discovered, mainly in neurotransmitters' differences by location. However, it will be a long time before we really understand specifics relative to these substances and their various sites of action in dogs. As with the anatomic brain, changes still occur postnatally in the development of the neurotransmitters, as evidenced by the increased levels of amino acids during the first several weeks.[99]

The receptors for different neurotransmitters affect behavior in several ways.[216] Activation of dopamine receptors in the mesolimbic pathway mediates reward, incentive, motivation, and speed of learning and response. $D_1$ receptor activation is related to the maintenance of movement, whereas activation of $D_2$ receptors in the nigrostantal pathway affects the initiation and repetition of movement. $D_2$ receptors are probably also involved in stereotypies. Increased aggression is associated with increased dopamine release, and abnormally high dopamine levels have been associated with stereotypies, schizophrenia, and psychotic depression. Serotonin has a number of subtypes of receptors, of which some have known functions (Table 2-4). Low turnover of serotonin has been connected with a variety of conditions, including anxiety, anorexia, impulsivity, offensive aggression, schizophrenia, and suicidal depression. Norepinephrine and noradrenergic receptors mediate reward, arousal, and fear response. Excessive activity results in mania, whereas insufficient activity results in depression. Because GABA is a universally inhibitory neurotransmitter, activation of GABA receptors reduces movement and anxiolytic states. Group 1 neurotransmitters are synthesized from amino acids and include several of current interest (Box 2-1).[20] The neuropeptides in Group 2 are composed of short-chain peptides that also come from amino acids. The third group includes specific amino acids like glycine, glutamate, and aspartate, plus GABA.

Of interest in regard to the relationship of aggression and diet is the transport of tryptophan across the blood-brain barrier and the eventual production of serotonin. Diets with a high meat component are rich in tryptophan and other amino acids, including tyrosine and leucine.[20] These three amino acids use the same transport mechanism across the barrier, but tryptophan is in the lowest concentration in the blood, so it loses out to tyrosine and leucine for transport sites.[20] The result is actually a lowering of serotonin production after a meat meal.[20]

A newer area of behavior is psychoneuroimmunology. It has been shown that dogs with behavior problems as adults were more likely than normal dogs to have been sick as puppies. Problem behaviors included in the association to early illness were dominance aggression, aggression to strangers, fear of strangers, fear of children, separation-related barking, and sexual mounting of people.[100] It is theorized that the cytokine released during the illness may result in neurotoxins that lead to neuronal dysfunction and cell death.[100]

## SENSORY AND NEURAL BEHAVIOR PROBLEMS

Problems relating to the brain and its sensory and learning abilities can be very broad in scope and difficult to diagnose. Some, like seizures, may be

| TABLE 2-4 | Conditions affected by serotonin (5HT) subtype receptors |
| --- | --- |
| **Receptor** | **Condition affected/controlled** |
| $5HT_{1A}$ | Psychomotor responses |
| $5HT_{2A}$ | LSD-like hallucinatory behavior |
| $5HT_{2B}$ | Vasoconstriction, migraines |
| $5HT_{2C}$ | Anxiety, appetite |
| $5HT_3$ | Pain, anxiety, gastrointestinal motility, emesis |

Data from reference 216.

| BOX 2-1 | Common neurotransmitters and related amino acids |
| --- | --- |

| **Group 1 neurotransmitters (and related amino acids)** | **Group 2 neurotransmitters** | **Group 3 neurotransmitters** |
| --- | --- | --- |
| Tryptophan → 5-hydroxytryptophan → **serotonin** | **Several neuropeptides** from various amino acids | Gamma-amino-butyric acid |
| Tyrosine → DOPA → **dopamine** → **noradrenaline** → **adrenaline** | | Glycine |
| Lecithin → choline ↔ **acetylcholine** | | Glutamate |
| Histidine → **histamine** | | Aspartate |

Data from reference 20.

unusual in their presentation but controllable with drug therapy. Others are being studied as possible models for human disease. Canine cognitive dysfunction is one example. Still others remain a frustrating challenge to understand and treat, such as the fear of thunder.

Many organic conditions can affect a dog's behavior, as illustrated in Boxes 2-2 and 2-3. Behavioral signs typically associated with organic disease can be broad, ranging from circling to aimless pacing, head pressing, disorientation, depression or lethargy, seizures, appetite changes, elimination pattern changes, or nonrecognition.[352] It is beyond the scope of this text to discuss all the various neurologic problems, such as epilepsy and postdistemper encephalitis. Some neurologic conditions do, however, deserve attention in connection with the subject of this text, such as stereotypies and obsessive-compulsive disorders. They will be discussed here, although current understanding of

---

**BOX 2-2**  **Organic causes of behavior changes**

Canine cognitive dementia/senility
Cauda equine lesions
Central nervous system reticulosis
Cerebral anoxia
Cerebral vascular accident
Dancing Doberman syndrome
Drugs
    Anticonvulsants
    Antiparasiticides levamisole/ivermectin in Collies
    Hallucinogenic drugs
    Mood-altering drugs
    Over-the-counter drugs: ibuprofen
    Sedatives/tranquilizers/anesthetics
Encephalitis—acute/post
    Bacterial
    Fungal
    Immune-mediated
    Parasitic
    Protozoal
    Rickettsial
    Viral
        Canine distemper
        Parainfluenza
        Rabies
        Vaccination-induced
Fever
Hepatic encephalopathy
Hydrocephalus
Hyperactivity
Hyperkinesis
Hyperthyroidism
Hypoglycemia
Hypothyroidism
Inherited metabolic deficiencies
    Copper toxicosis
    Fucosidosis
    Lethal acrodermatitis
    Lysosomal enzyme deficiency
    Multisystem neuronal degeneration

Insecticides
    Chlorinated hydrocarbons
    DEET
    Fenvalerate
    Organophosphates
    Pyrethrins
Meningitis
    Chronic granulomatous
    Intracranial
    Spinal
    Steroid-responsive
Mental-lapse aggression syndrome
Metabolic diseases
    Diabetes mellitus
    Hepatic disease
    Hyperadrenalism
    Renal disease
Narcolepsy/atypical narcolepsy
Necrosis of or around nerves/spinal cord
Neuronal axoid lipofuscinosis
Ocular disease
    Cataracts
    Glaucoma
    Progressive retinal atrophy
Seizure disorders
    Postictal effects
Thiamine deficiency/thiamine toxicity
Toxicity
    Ethylene glycol
    Lead
Trauma
Tumor
    Brain
    Spinal cord
Vasculitis

Data from references 34, 198, 238, 351, 352.

| BOX 2-3 | Conditions that might be confused with behavior problems |
|---------|----------------------------------------------------------|

Abscesses
Anal sac
    Impaction
    Inflammation
Arthritis
    Autoimmune
    Hip dysplasia
Blindness
    Cataracts
    Glaucoma
    Progressive retinal atrophy
    Retinal detachment
Deafness
Diabetes
    Insipidus
    Mellitus
Estrous behavior
Hyperadrenocorticism
Hypoadrenocorticism
Hypocalcemia
Hypoglycemia
Misinterpretations of normal behavior
Myositis
    Polymyositis
    Temporomasseter
Pain
    Disk disease
    Trauma
    Vertebral instability
Pruritis
    Atopy
    Flea allergy
    Food allergy
Puberty
    Behavioral
    Reproductive
Renal medullary washout

Data from references 238, 351, 352.

these two behaviors in particular is still relatively rudimentary. Only after additional research will we be able to appreciate the complex role of neurotransmitter systems in the behaviors, both normal and abnormal, of various species.

## Seizures

Behavioral seizures in dogs take a number of forms, depending on the area of the brain affected. It has been shown experimentally that damage to relatively small neural areas can result in fairly dramatic behavioral changes. Also, irritative lesions, such as occur in brain scarring, can produce these changes with only unilateral damage.[166] In some dogs, a behavioral change may precede or follow the more classic, generalized tonic-clonic seizure.[186] Behavioral seizures that are not associated with the generalized pattern are more difficult to diagnose.[47] Histories may indicate staring into space,[47,84] flank sucking,[366] head bobbing,[352] flank biting,[47] voracious appetite,[166] vomition,[47] diarrhea,[47] aggression (including growling),[47,166,310] fearful behavior,[147,166] excessive restlessness,[84,85,166,310] jaw chomping,[166] snapping at imaginary flies,[85,228,268] inappropriate barking,[166,310] tail chasing,[97] and circling.

Seizures are repetitive, paroxysmal, and associated with an excessive neuronal discharge. Diagnosis based on EEG recordings would necessitate catching the dog during an actual seizure.[47] In some cases, abnormal EEG activity, such as spikes or sharp waves, also may be present at times other than during an actual seizure.[66] Special imaging, as with computerized tomography or magnetic resonance imaging, may show abnormal structures.[310]

Treatment of behavioral seizures can be as difficult as treatment for the more traditional seizures. Both typically involve the use of anticonvulsants, such as phenobarbital. As many of the seizural behaviors are neither long in duration nor harmful to the animal—nor dangerous to others—treatment may not be indicated. It is probably also inappropriate to medicate an animal if it will be impossible to evaluate whether the medication is helping to control the problem. Some neurologists, however, advocate treatment for any dog that has seizures, so whether to treat remains a decision between the veterinarian and client. The biggest dilemma regarding treatment occurs when the seizure is expressed as an aggressive behavior. Idiopathic epilepsy may have a heritable component,[90,186] so breeding an affected dog is not recommended.

## Fly (Air) Snapping

Some dogs appear to be watching something and then suddenly leap up and snap at the imaginary object. The behavior is sudden, directed, and intermittent. This fly (or air) snapping, mentioned already as one type of behavioral seizure, can have several other etiologies. It has been blamed on diseases of the eyes, such as remnants of fetal blood vessels, and it has been diagnosed at necropsy to have diffuse gliosis of the optic tracts and lateral geniculates.[67] Fly snapping also occurs in dogs without ocular disease or seizures. Other differential diagnoses include an attention-getting, learned behavior[168] or an obsessive-compulsive behavior.

Other than the actual behavior for fly snapping, clinical presentations vary considerably. Age of onset can be anywhere from 1 year to more than 10 years.[67] Frequency of the fly snapping behavior can be as high as 30 times per hour or as low as once daily or even once weekly on average.[67] Spontaneous remissions also have been reported, lasting from 1 week to 5 months, with active periods of 1 week to 2 years before another remission occurs.[67] In addition, more than half these dogs show at least one other type of behavior change at about the same time, such as feet licking, aggression, or pica.[67]

Successful treatment, if treatment is warranted, depends on the etiology. As should be expected, not all cases respond to phenobarbital,[228] and of those that do, there is still the issue of spontaneous remission that may actually be responsible for the "positive" results.[67] Dogs that have learned fly-snapping behavior usually exhibit it only in certain situations and are usually easy to distract.[268] For these dogs, the owner can ignore the behavior instead of rewarding it with attention, punish the behavior, or ask for a substitute behavior, such as having the dog sit, that can be rewarded. If, on the other hand, the behavior of fly snapping is directly related to specific stressful stimuli, the owner needs to modify the environment and perhaps use anti-anxiety drugs. Phenothiazine drugs have helped in at least one complicated case.[213] Compulsive behaviors will be discussed later in this chapter.

## Cognitive Dysfunction

For several years there was a debate as to whether there were behavioral changes associated with aging in dogs or whether changes were really just manifestations of osteoarthritis or other diseases. It is generally accepted now that behavior changes can occur independent of other conditions. Because of the identification of a condition in which neuropathology was identified, we have also learned a lot about other age-related behavior changes.[406] Two geriatric groups exist—age impaired and age unimpaired—although, with increasing age comes a greater likelihood of one or more behavioral changes.[174,285,313] Cognitive dysfunction is defined as "age-related or senior onset behavior changes that are not attributable to a general medical condition."[189,385] In dogs, aging has a greater effect on learning,[326] curiosity, exploration, and responses to novel stimuli than on locomotor activities. Several terms, including senility,[272] senile dementia,[113] senile cerebral dysfunction,[281] and cognitive dysfunction,[384] have been suggested for a series of clinical signs that are not associated with general medical problems; *cognitive dysfunction* is the term that is typically applied. Although many behaviors can be involved, typical ones are reduced reactivity to stimuli with decreased perception, changes in the sleep-wake cycle, deficits in memory for familiar places or people, spatial disorientation and confusion, forgetfulness of learned behaviors and habits, anxiety, irritability, inability to negotiate stairs in the absence of musculoskeletal problems, apparent hearing impairment, reduced activity and attention, reduced cognitive function, such as the ability to learn, and loss of housetraining.* Many of these signs are hard to quantify and can be very subtle to an owner, making accurate diagnosis difficult. Attempts have been made to develop a diagnostic score sheet,[349] but most behaviorists rely on identifying the major changes instead. By looking at four of the parameters—housetraining, orientation in the home and yard, sleep-wake cycle, and social interactions—researchers were able to identify at least one impairment in 28% of dogs at 11 to 12 years of age.[189,241,242,313] By 14 years, 48% had some impairment,[19] and by 16 years of age, 68% showed impairment in at least one category.[241,242,313] There can also be differences between sexes and breeds. Intact male dogs are less likely to show cognitive impairment by 14 years of age and are significantly less likely than neutered dogs of either sex to progress from mild to severe impairment in

---

*References 113, 176, 197, 234, 235, 247, 272, 281, 379, 381, 382, 384.

18 months.[170] Beagles were affected differently than age-matched mix breed dogs.[285]

Neuropathologic changes do occur in affected dogs, as do changes in neurotransmitters and in the hypothalamic-pituitary-adrenal axis.[241,383] The activity of the cholinergic neurotransmitter system appears to decrease, causing reduced cerebral perfusion, serotonin levels fall, and monoamine oxidase-B levels appear to increase to cause a reduction in dopamine.[113,197,234,281] There is increased production and decreased clearance of free radicals.[234,407] Dogs and humans both show age-related accumulations of neuromelanin in the substantia nigra, possibly as a by-product of catecholamine metabolism.[287] Old dogs also have Lafora-like bodies and Aβ42 amyloid plaques in the frontal and entorhinal cortices, and perhaps in the hippocampus, of the brain.[88,89,247,287] In addition, there is ventricular dilation, meningeal thickening, meningeal calcification, demyelination, reduced number of neurons, neuroaxonal degeneration, increased number of apoptic bodies, lipofuscin, vascular changes, and gliosis.[241,346] The amount of oxidative damage on amyloid load correlates to the severity of cognitive dysfunction.[241] In rats, handling and environmental manipulation for the young results in an increased concentration of glucocorticoid receptors in the hippocampus.[278] This can offset the glucocorticoid response to stress that would otherwise result in hippocampal neuron death, cognitive impairments, and a cascade of other aging changes.[278,369]

Medical conditions are common in geriatric pets, so a complete workup is necessary to rule out medical causes of the signs. Diagnostic workups eliminate other causes and determine if treatment options are possible. In addition to the typical complete blood count, biochemical panel, serum electrolytes, and urinalysis, abnormal functioning of the pancreatic, thyroid, and adrenal glands must be ruled out.[113] Metabolic disorders that can also reduce cortical function include hypothyroidism, diabetes mellitus, hyperadrenocortism, hepatic encephalopathies, hypoglycemia, and renal disease.[399] Neoplasia and encephalitis must also be ruled out.

Treatment options for cognitive dysfunction generally fall into one of four categories: dietary management, environmental enrichment, supple-

ments, and pharmacologic therapies.[236] Antioxidants and diets rich in antioxidants have been shown to result in significant improvement of signs,[283,476] and special diets are now commercially available. Antioxidants that are used include vitamins C, E, and B$_6$, beta carotene, selenium, and various flavonoids and carotenoids. The L-carnitine and dl-α-lipoic acid enhance mitochondrial function, and omega-3 fatty acids promote cell membrane health and possibly have antiinflammatory effects.[11,12,236] They help learning, but not memory.[11]

Environments that encourage exercise and contain novel toys and situations actually help minimize mental decline.[202,236,284,286] Those dogs that have enriched environments and special diets show the best results.[202,236,286,289]

Supplements, which have become a popular option for humans, are now being used in dogs to help stop, and potentially reverse, signs of cognitive dysfunction. The nutriceuticals contain a variety of substances, including phosphatidylserine, *Ginkgo biloba*, resveratrol, and vitamins C, E, and B$_6$. Tests are limited but suggest marked improvement is possible.[237,328,329] Phosphatidylserine, a phospholipid that is a major building block of cell membranes, prevents neuronal apoptosis and improves cognitive function in humans and dogs.[236,328] *Ginkgo biloba* may be helpful in several ways. It inhibits monoamine oxidase-A and B to increase dopamine levels, has phosphatidylserine-like activity, stimulates cholinergic and serotonergic systems, improves cerebral blood flow, increases neuronal glucose bioavailability, and may protect neurons against apoptosis.[236,296] Resveratrol rescues hippocampal neurons from oxidative damage and reduces beta-amyloid secretion.[296] Vitamins are associated as cofactors in neurotransmitter synthesis, may compliment the actions of other products, and may neutralize free radicals.[236]

The drug selegiline (L-deprenyl) has been approved for cognitive dysfunction and will improve the clinical signs.[176,380,382,384] Dogs will do better on tasks that have positive reinforcement, but take longer if no reward is presented.[288,294] As a monoamine oxidase-B inhibitor that reduces the reuptake of dopamine and as a drug that reduces the deleterious effects of free radicals, selegiline offers hope for improved activity levels and quality of life in some of the affected dogs.[236,247,381,384,404] Drugs that increase blood flow to the brain, nicergoline and propentofylline, have had mixed results.[176,405] Estrogen supplementation has been reported to significantly improve learning and memory tasks, especially in female dogs,[427,428] but the potential side effects do not make this a good therapeutic option. Testosterone may be a neuroprotectant, at least in humans.[236] Adrafinil is a new class of narcolepsy drug available in Europe that is showing promising results in treating cognitive dysfunction.[405]

## Response to Fever

Illness caused by various agents results in a febrile response, which in turn sets off a chain reaction of secondary responses to help the animal survive the insult.[169] Fever, through the promotion of interleukin-1, works on various brain nuclei to cause depression, anorexia, increased sleepiness, decreased grooming, and decreased water intake. These behaviors conserve energy, which is needed because of the decreased food intake and the increased metabolic rate. The secondary effect is to reduce the intake of dietary iron. Because many pathogens need iron and a certain temperature for optimal growth, increased body temperature and reduced plasma iron concentrations tend not to support their growth.

## Hyper Syndrome

Dogs that continually show excessive activity (the *hyper syndrome*) may do so for a number of reasons. A thorough history, complete diagnostic workup, good observational skills, and perhaps a drug trial may be necessary to establish the diagnosis. The hyper syndrome can be divided into five categories: overactivity, food sensitivities, hyperkinesis, hyperactivity, and "other." Excessive excitability, unruliness, and hyper behaviors were the fourth largest category of behavior problems seen in three practices, constituting 6.3% of all cases.[98,239] Because owners often think of and probably represent these behaviors as "normal" for young dogs, it is likely that many cases are missed.

## Overactivity

High energy levels can be present for many reasons and the animal can still be normal. Certain dogs have a lot of natural energy, some because of a genetic predisposition and some as an individual variation. Dogs from working breeds that were developed to go all day seem to be most predisposed to overactivity. Others do not get enough exercise for the energy levels they have, especially those on high-energy diets.

## Food Sensitivity

In human medicine, a connection has been made between multiple food allergies, atopy, and hyper behavior. In veterinary medicine, a few dogs show excessive energy because of food sensitivity. Usually the problem is suspected because of an accidental change in diet, but it should be considered in any case of excessive energy. An eliminative food trial should use a unique meat source or one of the special commercial allergy diets for 6 weeks in an appropriate trial. The dog should not get rawhides or other treats during this trial. If this diet is successful in solving the problem behavior, commercial hypoallergenic diets can be used for maintenance. Sometimes inappropriate responses occur to high dietary protein levels. A corresponding low level of carbohydrates may contribute to the high-protein problem.[445] Dietary change may be the solution here too.

## Hyperkinesis

In humans, the terms *hyperkinesis, hyperactivity,* and *attention-deficit hyperactivity disorder* (ADHD) are used interchangeably. In dogs, however, hyperactivity and hyperkinesis can be separated based on the dog's response to therapy, and thus probably by cause. Differentiation of ADHD into multiple conditions is just beginning in human medicine as noninvasive brain scan technology becomes more sophisticated.[7] In children, hyperkinesis is manifested by a high level of locomotor activity (fidgeting and squirming), profound deficits in the behavioral suppression capacity (talking excessively, blurting out answers before the question is completed), disappearance of behavior patterns essential to survival (reduced social and sexual behavior, increased aggressiveness), learning deficits, and deficits in attention (being easily distracted) and thought processes.[58,78,245,436] In novel environments, however, the child may appear normal. Human studies strongly implicate a decrease in the dopaminergic neurotransmitter system[107,245,436] in the anteromedial frontal cortex and, to a lesser extent, in the nucleus accumbens.[245] Mice that lack the gene encoding the plasma membrane dopamine transporter have elevated dopaminergic tone, are hyper, have impaired spatial cognitive function, and respond with reduced locomotion to pyschostimulants.[150] They suggest possible causes of ADHD as genetic and/or defective neurotransmitters. Treatment of affected children usually involves psychotherapy, pharmacotherapy, and structured educational programs.[436] Drug therapy involves the use of a stimulant, such as methylphenidate, amphetamine, dextroamphetamine, or magnesium pernoline,[78,106,436] with methylphenidate being most commonly used.

Samuel Corson[58,61] did much of the pioneering work regarding hyperkinesis in dogs, starting with a 1-year-old Cocker Spaniel-and-Beagle-mix male named Jackson. During the initial study, Jackson changed from an uncontrollable, aggressive dog that refused to be contained in a Pavlovian conditioning apparatus to a friendly, docile dog while on amphetamine treatment. Corson's laboratory and others subsequently developed a spontaneous canine model for hyperkinesis.

In dogs, clinical signs of hyperkinesis include a poor ability to respond with appropriate behavior, impaired learning (often these dogs are obedience school failures), sustained tachycardia, persistent hyperpnea, excessive salivation, increased energy metabolism, vasopressin-type antidiuresis, inability to stop a behavior sequence but reacting to new ones, impaired attention span, restlessness, hypervigilance, lack of bite control in a puppy, and poor habituation learning.* They may be presented for problems other than "hyper behavior" and the owner never include it as a problem. In humans, coexisting problems are common.

Treatment protocols for affected dogs are similar to those for children. The hyperkinetic dog calms down with a stimulant such as amphetamine or methylphenidate, the latter of which lasts longer.* Methylphenidate should be started at a low dose and increased gradually if it produces no initial behavior change. Increased irritability or activity, or the appearance of atypical behaviors after administration of the drug, would indicate the dog is not hyperkinetic.

Because methylphenidate is a classified drug, it is recommended that predrug and postdrug activities be evaluated periodically. A video recording of the dog before treatment starts or a 15- to 30-minute log of activities will provide objective comparative data on whether the drug is making a difference. Repeat the activity check, and take the dog off medication every 6 months or so to be sure it still needs medication. On days when activity levels do not matter, the dog can be left unmedicated without harm.

Once the hyperkinetic dog is responding to the medication, the owners should begin working to correct any undesirable behaviors that remain and to reinforce desirable behaviors. Before medication, a learning disability exists from nonadaptive hyperactivity.[40] Lessons learned under the influence of the medication are retained. Over time, the dose of medication should be reduced to find the minimum amount needed to retain the desired effect.

Both amphetamine and dextroamphetamine are relatively short acting, which necessitates frequent dosing, and there is concern for the possibility of amphetamine abuse by humans. As a result, methylphenidate is most commonly used in veterinary medicine. It is recommended that the veterinarian rule out medical and dietary causes of hyper behaviors to narrow down the differential diagnoses to hyperkinesis, hyperactivity (discussed next), and idiopathic hyper syndrome. If the dog fails to respond to a trial therapy of acepromazine, the owners should make a video recording of the dog's behavior, or the animal can come into the clinic again for verification of its behavior by video

---

*References 23, 24, 57, 64, 78, 269.

*References 34, 57, 58, 78, 79, 200, 444, 449.

or a count of various activities (such as jumping, barking, or movement) over a 15- to 30-minute period. Then a trial therapy of methylphenidate is started for a 1- to 2-week period, beginning with a low dose and increasing as needed over the next few days. If improvement is seen, the activity levels should again be objectively evaluated before a longer use prescription is written. Reevaluation by activity-level monitoring, first while the dog is on the drug and then 24 to 48 hours after withdrawal of the drug, is indicated at 6-month intervals.

Studies in normal people and in hyperkinetics suggest that dextroamphetamine and methylphenidate will reduce activity levels in both groups.[254,370,371,412,475] However, meta-analysis across studies of three different drug categories did show that the stimulants are the most effective treatment of ADHD.[112] Unlike people, normal experimental animals will respond to stimulants with increased brain and motor activity. Affected animals show no increase but instead have a 68% clinical response rate of normalized behavior.[107] Dogs that respond this way have higher peak blood levels of amphetamine and its active metabolite, *P*-hydroxyamphetamine, than do nonresponders.[24] Their level of improvement also parallels amphetamine blood levels. Responders have lower levels of norepinephrine, dopamine, and homovanillic acid in the brain tissue, as well as lower levels of homovanillic acid in the cerebrospinal fluid.[23]

The incidence of spontaneous recovery from hyperkinesis in dogs has not been documented. Among children, half can eventually discontinue medication, but up to 60% will retain this problem into adulthood, needing years of medication.[378,465] Owners have often coped with a very restless dog for well over a year before they seek veterinary help, thinking the dog is just going through a normal puppy-growth phase. In some cases, they have found ways to cope with the behavior, such as by having the dog live outdoors. Other owners who are familiar with normal dog behavior have recognized the excessive restlessness as abnormal but have tried the increased-exercise, obedience-class route, without success. What the effect of delayed treatment may be for long-term success is not known.

If the dog responds favorably to the drug therapy trial, it is maintained on the drug at that dose for the first 6 months. It may be possible to reduce the dose after each 6-month evaluation, because a dog will generally need less over time and eventually may not need continued medication. In addition, the dog should be worked by the owner in obedience classes when drug therapy has rendered it capable of learning. Regular work in obedience classes and appropriate training in the home may be useful in helping to reduce the amount of medication needed. "Drug holidays" are possible on days when the excessive activity and accompanying behaviors do not matter. Jackson, the dog studied by Samuel Corson,[64] needed medication for only a few weeks; by then, he had learned self-control and what behaviors were acceptable. That is not typical for most cases.

### Hyperactivity

The clinical presentation of hyperactivity is exactly the same as that for hyperkinesis. The dog demonstrates an excessive degree of restlessness, inability to learn, poor habituation, and difficulty adjusting to new surroundings. After other medical and dietary causes of hyper behavior have been ruled out, the diagnosis of hyperactivity can be made based on response to therapy. The dog will calm down to a normal level of activity after medication with a tranquilizer, typically acepromazine at a low to moderate dose. If the dog does not calm down, if there is a paradoxical reaction, if motor activity is affected before the behavior, or if the normal activity level lasts only a few hours, then the dog is probably not hyperactive. To the owners, the difference in behavior is very clear. A response of "maybe a little change" really indicates no change and a need to try another possible diagnosis.

For dogs that respond in a desired way to the tranquilizer, they should be maintained on the lowest dose needed. The dog should be started in an obedience class, because it can now learn acceptable behaviors. As with treatment for hyperkinesis, learning seems to reduce the amount of drug therapy needed by dogs with hyperactivity, so trial reductions in the tranquilizer dose should be attempted on a regular basis. After an initial response, some dogs will need an upward adjustment in the dose of the tranquilizer. This upward dose may be needed because of induction of the liver enzyme system. Eventually, though, drug therapy for many dogs can gradually be eliminated. On days when hyper behavior does not matter, it is appropriate to not medicate the dog.

### "Other" Category of Excessive Activity

The fifth category of excessive activity is "other." Several types of medical conditions would be included here, like hyperthyroidism and increased estrogen levels.[446] An occasional dog is both hyperactive and hyperkinetic, making treatment particularly difficult. Some owners reward the wrong behavior,[446] inadvertently encouraging the unruliness or excessive levels of play.[444] Idiopathic hyper behavior must be included as a possibility, too, because some dogs do not respond to known treatments.

### Stereotypic Behavior

A stereotypy is an intentional repetitive behavior—a nonfunctional, noninjurious, highly predictable sequencing of actions, often performed in a specific and rhythmic manner.* As an example, stereotypic pacing is the rhythmic walk to one side of an enclosure, the flip of the head while turning, and the walk to the other side before repeating the turn. This is the most common stereotypy associated with carnivores. Motion is not always a part of stereotypy, however. One stereotypy is a motionless staring from a frozen body posture.[262]

Evidence suggests that the adoption of such stereotypic behaviors may be a coping mechanism to deal with stress or suboptimal environments, at least when first developed.† A genetic predisposition for a particular stereotypy, or at least a lower tolerance to some stressors, may exist.[277] Stereotypies can also represent a ritualized behavior shown in situations of mental conflict.[464] Debate continues as to whether stereotypies are harmful or helpful, but it is generally accepted that it would be better if they were not needed by the animal in the first place.[34]

The development of a stereotypy is divided into four stages,[464] with a progressive narrowing of the behavioral repertoire until only self-directed behavior remains.[92,262] In the first stage, an animal in conflict will make many attempts at escape or aggression. Exhaustion results in immobility—stage 2. In stage 3, the animal repeats the fight/flight trials until, in stage 4, it develops a specific, repeatable pattern, perhaps even losing its orientation to the external stimulus.

The behavior may strengthen because of positive feedback, perhaps involving endogenous opioid peptides.[92] Experimentally, both amphetamine and apomorphine can be used to induce certain stereotypies,[50,230,258,298] but they can inhibit others, even in low doses.[230] Naloxone, a narcotic antagonist, can partially inhibit drug-induced stereotypies,[230,277,298] suggesting that dopamine may be involved in stress-induced, but not in drug-induced stereotypies.[92,230] The interconnection between the opioids and dopamine is probably related to highly localized opioid receptors in the striatal and limbic structures innervated by the dopaminergic neurons in the ventral mesencephalon.[92] Brain opioid peptides are released under stress and activate dopaminergic neurons, so stereotypies are related to opiate receptor blockers and dopamine antagonists.[262]

A number of theories have been proposed as to why stereotypies occur. First, it is thought that the environment may produce a state of hyperarousal, as can occur in a conflict situation, and that this hyperarousal is dissipated by performance of the stereotypy.[92,262] The second theory is that the environmental situation instead produces a low arousal level that the animal finds aversive. The animal then performs the stereotypy to increase the level of arousal.[92] Although the first theory has the widest acceptance, reduced plasma cortisol levels support the second.[92]

Others describe the causes of stereotypies as pathophysiologic or experiential.[257,262] Pathophysiologic theory suggests that there might be a genetic predisposition to stereotypies, perhaps because of a heightened sensitivity to stressors, or that they might be acquired by way of infections, trauma, or toxins.[262] Experiential theory subdivides stereotypies into those resulting from early experiences,

---

*References 34, 92, 131, 257, 262, 271, 277, 292, 464.
†References 34, 35, 54, 262, 271, 292, 464.

those that are reactively abnormal as the result of an inadequate environment, those that are conditionally abnormal as the result of certain rewards and learning, and those resulting from iatrogenic causes, as when they are drug induced.[262]

Stereotypies are difficult to treat because they are complicated in their etiologies and expression. It is not appropriate to physically prohibit the behavior without addressing the cause and providing therapy. If trigger stimuli can be identified, it will be important to eliminate them and to desensitize the dog to them. Enrichment of the environment is also important. That includes increasing ways to and amounts of exercise, food puzzles, and games with the owner. It is impossible to know if the performance of the stereotypy is self-rewarding, thus having an internal endorphin reinforcement, or whether there is a different internal drive. Appropriate drug therapy may come from trial-and-error. Serotonergic drugs, primarily clomipramine or the selected serotonin reuptake inhibitors, are generally the most successful, but it can take several weeks to appreciate any changes. For those dogs that do not respond, it is then reasonable to rule out the endorphin-based problems with a narcotic antagonist like naltrexone or naloxone. Unfortunately, only naltrexone comes in an oral form. In humans, its metabolite 6-β naltrexol is the active endorphin antagonist, but this metabolite is not formed in dogs.[259] Response with these may also take time as the animal comes to realize that the behavior is no longer associated with the desired response; because of the short duration of appropriate drug levels, it is difficult to maintain therapeutic levels.

## Obsessive-Compulsive Disorders

In some situations, a stereotypy can progress to become an obsessive-compulsive disorder; however, a distinction should be made between the two conditions. Not all stereotypies are obsessive-compulsive conditions, and not all obsessive-compulsive behaviors are stereotypies. The American Psychiatric Association defines an *obsession* as a persistent idea, thought, impulse, or image that is experienced as intrusive or senseless.[8,34] A *compulsion* is a repetitive, purposeful, and intentional behavior performed in a stereotyped fashion in response to an

obsession.[8,34,477] The behaviors are thought to be a method to cope with stress, frustration, or conflict and, over time, develop into compulsions.[258,259] The compulsive behavior is not pleasurable; it is just anxiety reducing.[185] The behaviors can involve either mental or physical rituals that are out of context and they are excessive in duration, frequency, and intensity.[346]

Various studies in humans with obsessive-compulsive disorders indicate abnormalities in the inferior prefrontal cortex and ventricle-to-brain ratio; in blood flow to the orbital areas of the frontal cortex, dorsal parietal cortex, and caudate nuclei; and in glucose metabolism in the cerebral hemispheres, caudate nuclei, and orbital gyri.[28,282] Although more than 90% of human patients have both obsessive and compulsive components to their affliction, some have only one of the two.[185] Those suffering from compulsions without obsessions tend to have higher ventricle-to-brain ratios than do those having both parts of the disorder. Differences have been found in the brains of those with childhood onset of obsessive-compulsive disorders versus those with adult onset.[28] For people who respond to drug therapy, abnormal positron emission tomography (PET) scans tend to normalize during therapy.[28,282]

Dogs may show specific repetitive behaviors to the exclusion of and interfering with other, more normal behaviors,[336] but it is impossible to know whether there is an obsessive component in dogs similar to that in humans. Sophisticated diagnostics like PET scans have not been used to study problem dogs. The dilemma is therefore presented of whether dogs and other domestic animals really experience the equivalent of human obsessive-compulsive disorder or only a compulsive disorder. For purposes of discussion here, the term *obsessive-compulsive disorder* will be used.

Obsessive-compulsive disorders are among the newest classification categories for abnormal behaviors, and scientists are only beginning to understand their complexities. One theory suggests that the output of the medial orbital region, mainly glutamate, may drive a person's obsessive-compulsive circuits in the caudate nucleus, resulting in increased inhibition of GABA output from the globus pallidus. This GABA reduction makes the thalamus vulnerable to glutamate and results in a self-sustaining cycle.[19] Other researchers believe there is an aberrant serotonin mechanism, perhaps with an abnormal endorphin metabolism.[282,336]

Computerized tomography implicates abnormalities in the basal ganglia, especially in the region of the caudate nucleus, in humans with obsessive-compulsive disorders.[336] Various drugs with selected serotonin reuptake inhibiting activity have been used in humans, with 60% to 80% showing improvement.[185,356] Those used most commonly have been clomipramine and fluoxetine.[331,361,372,415] Physical thwarting of the behavior is considered inappropriate because it does not address the cause,[262] and it only increases the tensions until expression of the behavior is again possible.

In dogs, it has been suggested that chronic, unresolved conflicts, frustrations, or stress could eventually lead to the development of an obsessive-compulsive disorder.[203,240,260] Using acral lick dermatitis as a model, there is strong evidence supporting this relationship.

Human behaviors associated with obsessive-compulsive disorders occur in 2% to 3% of the population.[338] In dogs, the incidence is reported to be about the same.[98,339] Human traits can include depersonalization, anorexia nervosa, trichotillomania (hair pulling), Tourette's syndrome (tics), sexual compulsions, hypochondriasis, compulsive personality disorders, and delusional disorders.[185,336]

Behavior patterns in dogs that may represent an obsessive-compulsive disorder include excessive grooming, flank sucking, leg/foot chewing, tail chasing, whirling/spinning, freezing, pacing, fence running, floor scratching, growling at self, polyphagia, polydipsia, fixation on or staring at shadows or objects, jumping in place, circling, "fly" or air biting, chasing real or imaginary objects, vocalizations, excessive grooming or hair chewing, self-mutilation, and licking or eating (pica) of atypical objects.* Obsessive-compulsive disorders appear at social maturity and they may be sporadic or heritable (Table 2-5).[240,260,347] If there is a genetic

*References 66, 239, 256, 257, 259, 261, 262, 336, 345, 347.

| TABLE 2-5 | Obsessive-compulsive disorders associated with specific breeds |
|---|---|
| Breed | Obsessive-compulsive condition |
| Australian Cattle Dogs | Tail chasing |
| Border Collie | Staring at shadows, chasing lights |
| Doberman Pinscher | Flank sucking |
| English Bull Terrier | Whirling, freezing, sticking head under/between objects |
| German Shepherd | Tail chasing |
| Miniature Schnauzer | Freezing, checking rear end |
| Staffordshire Bull Terrier | Spinning, circling |

Data from references 256, 258, 259, 260, 261.

component, then purebred animals could provide an exciting potential for learning more about obsessive-compulsive disorders,[336, 338] especially relative to canine genomics. The condition does not appear to be associated with the lack of training, stimulation, or social interactions.[347]

Studies indicate that brain physiology may change over time.[257] This evidence is supported clinically in dogs that develop chronic problems with acral lick dermatitis,[338,372] a problem discussed further in Chapter 10. In the early stages, most dogs can be treated for acral lick dermatitis by giving them increased exercise and behavior modification alone, after the initial wound has been appropriately treated. Other cases of a more chronic nature can be controlled by a narcotic antagonist, with behavior modification added for long-term results. A third group will respond with complete or partial regression of signs to psychopharmacologics that increase serotonin levels at the neurosynapses, mainly tricyclic antidepressants and selected serotonin reuptake inhibitors.[338,372] A few that do not respond well to these drugs will show improvement if an $N$-methyl-D-aspartate (NMDA) receptor antagonist is added to act on glutamatergic neurotransmission.[273] Unfortunately, there remains a fourth group that fails to respond to any of the treatment protocols and serves to illustrate that the complete pathophysiology of compulsive behavior is not known.[257]

In some dogs, obsessive-compulsive disorders may coexist with, be related to, or develop from other medical problems such as dermatitis, epilepsy, and metabolic disorders. At least in some of these dogs, the apparent compulsive behavior may be the clinical manifestation of the hyper syndrome, and its treatment can eliminate or significantly decrease the repetitive behavior. This phenomenon can explain why clinical response is occasionally seen with other drugs, such as anticonvulsants that can also have an anxiolytic or sedative effect.[222,262] A number of differential diagnoses for an obsessive-compulsive disorder must be considered. These can include allergies/atopy, anxiety, attention seeking, boredom, conflicts, learned, lack of environmental stimulation, hyperactivity/hyperkinesis, infectious diseases, metabolic conditions, neurologic disease, neuropharmacologic activity, sensory neuropathies, separation anxiety, and tick-borne pathogenic diseases.[260,261,336,337]

The differentials list demonstrates the importance of a good physical examination and laboratory workup of suspected causes. It has been reported that in 63 cases of obsessive-compulsive disorders, there was a significant increase found in the packed cell volume (PCV), blood hemoglobin (Hb) and mean corpuscular volume (MCV), and a significant decrease in the white blood cell count (WBC) and mean corpuscular hemoglobin concentration (MCHC).[203] The relationship of these values to the problem behavior is not known at this time.

Treatment protocols for obsessive-compulsive disorders can be complicated because of various triggers for the behaviors, acute or chronic states, presence or absence of an internal reward, degree of obsession, and presence or absence of a genetic influence. It is important for the management of these cases to first identify specific triggers of the behavior, and then to ensure that those triggers can no longer occur when the dog is present. Desensitization can be used for specific triggers if long term management is not possible, but this is less than desirable. Drug therapy offers some hope for affected animals as an aid to behavior modification.

Clomipramine and fluoxetine have both been well studied.[182,204,240,256,260] Although drug therapy may not stop the problem behavior, it is often helpful in reducing the clinical manifestations enough that the owners are satisfied.[261]

Other general recommendations for environmental enrichment including exercise and techniques that will give the mind something to do. It is also important to be sure that the owners do not use punishment. A study in humans that involved the person reminding themselves that the obsessive thought was "some garbage thrown up by a faulty circuit" compared before and after brain scans of activity in the orbital frontal cortex.[36] The dramatic decrease in posttreatment activity for thought therapy only was exactly the same as for patients on drug therapy alone.[36] This suggests that behavior modification and environmental enrichment are very appropriate components in a therapeutic protocol for dogs with an obsessive-compulsive disorder.

## Anxiety, Fears, and Phobias

*Anxiety* is the feeling of apprehension due to the anticipation of some unidentified threat or danger. For most dogs, this means a temporary stressor is present and recovery occurs quickly. There are some dogs, however, that seem to be constantly anxious, and generalized anxiety may result in that animal being overly sensitive to threats.[160] *Fear* is a feeling of apprehension from the presence of an object, individual, or situation.[346] It is an adaptive response that prompts an individual to remove or protect itself from a real danger or noxious stimuli and thus increase its chances for survival.[66,312,400,446] The level of fear is proportionate to the intensity of the stimulus.[286] By way of contrast, a *phobia* is an intense fear response to a stimulus that is out of proportion—excessive for the degree of threat in a given situation.[302,400,442,446,448] It will interfere with normal functioning. In a laboratory setting, phobias tend to require repeated exposure to a stimulus to develop, and then they can be extinguished easily.[400] Naturally occurring phobias, however, can develop after a single exposure and are usually directed to a specific stimulus. They can generalize to other stimuli over time and often get worse with repeated exposures.[312,400] Owner anxiety is not associated with a higher incidence of phobias in dogs, although the phobia may cause more anxiety in the owner.[322] *Pseudophobias* are attention seeking behaviors that have been reinforced to the point they are almost automatic for a specific stimulus and may become stereotypies.[302]

Dogs commonly develop fears about certain situations, so veterinarians must be able to adequately advise owners on how to deal with such problems. One study indicated that 0.8% of pet owners had discussed fearful behavior as a problem with their veterinarians, but the actual incidence of fear in dogs has not been established. In part, this is because the term "fear" can be defined in many ways, and owners may not recognize the early signs of a fear-based problem. Of those patients seen in practices that do behavioral counseling, 5.9% to 14.5% of the cases were related to fears or phobias.[68,98,239]

Each species is programmed genetically to respond fearfully to particular stimuli and in certain ways.[66] The natural fear-evoking stimuli would be expected to be predators, environment, associated events, and conspecifics; however, these categories are not particularly useful clinically.[447] In general, fearfulness is correlated with high visual and auditory exploration.[154] Illness in puppies can impact social fears in later life.[394]

Of 258 cases at Texas A&M University over a 16-year period, 106 dogs were afraid of noise, including thunder; 29 dogs were afraid of multiple components in a storm; 127 were afraid of people or other dogs; 2 feared odors; 14 disliked certain surfaces; and 14 had a specific visual fear. Approximately half of the sensory-related fears are those associated with loud noises or thunderstorms; although under the right set of circumstances, any input to a dog's senses can cause fear.

Evidence exists that humans with fears or phobias have differences in neurophysiology. The locus caeruleus and its neurotransmitter norepinephrine are important in the genesis and expression of fear.[400] The locus caeruleus is the major noradrenergic nucleus in the human brain, with widespread connections, including some into the limbic system.[66,400] There is increased neuronal activity during anxiety and stress with an increased turnover of norepinephrine in areas of noradrenergic

innervation.[242] The amygdala is important for processing information about reinforcers and connects to higher cortical areas. A functioning forebrain is necessary to unlearn a fear.[340] Human patients with panic disorders have an increased sensitivity to pharmacologic stimulation and suppression of the locus caeruleus, suggesting abnormal neurotransmitter functions.[340,400] GABA and glutamate, acting on NMDA receptors, apparently help prevent excessive fear responses.[94] Epinephrine associated with the fear response indirectly causes a significant short-term increase in cognitive abilities.[66,242,340] Comparative studies between gun-shy and normal dogs showed that affected dogs had exaggerated startle responses, pronounced increases in heart rates, lack of curiosity, and fearful behavior toward people and objects.[161] These observations suggest that dogs as well as people may have inherent differences in neurophysiology.

Dogs can respond with a variety of fearful behaviors, from freezing in place, to flight or fight. In part, this is an individual response and in part it depends on the perceived intensity of the threat and the ability to escape. Reactivity can even arise owing to prenatal experiences, but more typically relate to genetics, amount of socialization, and previous learning. Treating a fear or phobia may be as simple as avoiding the fear-inducing stimuli. But treatment is more likely to involve a desensitization program, often with counterconditioning. The desensitization program uses the fearful stimulus but in such low amounts as not to provoke a fear-associated behavior. The amount of the stimulus is carefully increased and never allowed to occur spontaneously. It is extremely important that this controlled increase occur at such a slow rate as to never trigger any of the fearful responses.[168,438] This can be successful with a highly motivated owner, and the biggest change occurs during the first month.[249] The most common reason for failure of a desensitization program is that the owner does not have enough patience to properly administer it. Counterconditioning, usually with eating or playing, puts the dog in a mood incompatible with fear. While the dog is in this pleasant mood, the fearful stimulus is introduced in low doses, and the dog is rewarded for appropriate behavior. With repetition, the amount of stimulus can be gradually increased over a period of several days or weeks until the stimulus approaches that experienced naturally.

Drug therapy is receiving a great deal of attention in veterinary behavior because owners want an easy solution that does not involve a major time commitment on their part. No single drug or drug group is the complete answer to problems of fear. In newer and milder cases, drugs can be helpful, however. The Dog Appeasing Pheromone has been shown to reduce stress symptoms in dogs being trained, in veterinary hospitals, and in an animal shelter.[295,390,431] As stress levels increase, drugs also can be helpful in reducing a phobia to a fear, so that the animal will be more receptive to desensitization and counterconditioning. Reviews are mixed for drugs of all types, because they seem helpful in some individuals but not others. In humans, the benzodiazepines and buspirone are considered to have comparable efficacy working as anxiolytics in patients suffering problems with fear, even though the two types of drugs work differently.[400] In veterinary medicine, benzodiazepines work for some dogs,[103] and drugs that inhibit serotonin reuptake have successes, too.[341] Dogs that seem to have a chronic underlying anxiety may need both types of drugs concurrently. The dissociation effects of the benzodiazepines have the potential of blocking the learning process, but that is a desirable effect if used during an anxiety-provoking situation.

Spontaneous recovery from a fear-inducing stimulus can occur. Such a recovery is more likely for laboratory-induced fears than naturally occurring ones.[400] The disappearance of a fear is also more likely if the fear is a relatively new development and if there is a long time between the stimuli.[448]

Flooding techniques are generally not successful for fears, especially if the fear is severe.[442,447] Because flooding techniques are often inappropriately applied, or because the fear is too generalized or is associated with genetic factors, there is a real potential for escalating the severity of the problem rather than curing it with these techniques.[474]

### Generalized Anxiety Disorder

For some dogs, life is stressful. Generalized anxiety cases represent about 5.7% of canine cases seen in a behavior referral practice.[21] Signs of anxiety vary and are often missed by owners. Most people recognize trembling and cowering but miss lip licking and yawning.[311] Stressed dogs tend to raise one paw and show lowered body positions compared to nonstressed ones.[35] Pupils dilate. Heart rate increases, as does salivary cortisol. These dogs have blood cortisol levels significantly higher than non-anxious dogs.[39] In addition, anxious dogs tend to have lower blood and salivary immunoglobulin A (IgA) concentrations.[39] Although general activity decreases if escape is not possible, solitary housed dogs may actually begin repetitive movements like pacing, tail chasing, and flank sucking.[35] Their human counterparts describe chronic anxiety with restlessness, easy fatigue, poor concentration, and irritability.[374]

Treatment for generalized anxiety generally involves desensitization and counterconditioning if specific triggers are identified.[311] Chronically distressed dogs need long-term anxiolytic drug therapy using serotonergic agents too. At the same time owners can teach relaxation exercises in which the dog lies on its side for gentle stroking, and learns to do so on command. One study looked at the stress reaction of dogs to a novel stimulus after receiving human interaction or none, and half of each of those groups received a premium diet.[180] Plasma cortisol and adrenocorticotrophic hormone (ACTH) dropped significantly for dogs on the premium diet over time, but after the novel stimulus, it was the dogs that experienced human interactions that had a significantly low rise in cortisol and ACTH. Dopamine plasma levels may become a useful test for behavioral disorders.[327] Another blood test for prolactin levels has been looked at as an indicator of anxiety. Early work suggests that dogs with higher than normal levels might respond better to drugs that affect dopamine, whereas those with normal levels might do better with selected serotonin reuptake inhibitors.[350]

### Fear of Noise and Noise Phobias

Fears and phobias associated with noise are common in dogs and extremely varied in stimulus (Box 2-4).[293] Even puppies younger than 9 weeks of age can show sound-induced stress apart from separation distress.[93] Problems severe enough to cause

| BOX 2-4 | The top 15 noise fears in dogs |
|---|---|
| Thunderstorms | Wind |
| Fireworks | Beeping alarm systems |
| Vacuum cleaners | Screaming people |
| Guns | Foghorns |
| Motorcycle engines | Beeping microwaves |
| Car engines | Arguing voices |
| Backfiring engines | Hot air ballons |
| Airplanes | |

Data from reference 293.

owners to seek professional help occur in up to 20% of dogs, depending on the puppy's age, its location, and the type of noise.[40,69,438,448] Noise discomforts and fears, particularly those associated with thunder, usually develop over an extended period.[69,448,472] Sixty-one percent of dogs that are afraid of thunder developed that fear over time.[201] The rest of the noise fears are more likely to have an acute onset. They may be reinforced by owners' reactions and by chronic exposure. Because loud, sharp noises tend to produce defensive reactions,[63] single events can trigger fearful responses. If at one time firecrackers were tied to a dog's tail, the dog will usually remain very fearful of any loud, sharp noise.

Occasionally an owner will report that the dog has developed a skittish behavior, but they can not seem to pinpoint a trigger. Consider special noises such as those made by a smoke alarm when the battery gets weak. It can be intermittent enough at first that owners just do not pick up on it. There can be other concurrent problems as well as a fear of noise. About 87% of noise-phobic dogs had some degree of separation anxiety.[140,344] Dogs with separation anxiety had a 63% likelihood of also having a noise phobia and a 52% probability of thunderphobia.[344] Paw dominance, or rather the lack of a dominant paw, is related to noise phobias. Dogs without clear laterality are more likely to have a noise phobia.[44]

There is some evidence that severity and duration of severe fears may not be predictors of the success of the treatment.[151] It may be possible to keep the dog isolated from the specific noise if it is predictable. On July 4th and New Year's Eve, the dog may be fine if kept indoors, perhaps even in the basement, with the radio providing background noise. Other dogs with these reactions to specific loud noises can be successfully treated with behavior modification.[248] This involves an 8-week course of desensitization and counterconditioning and the use of the Dog Appeasing Pheromone. Sixty-six percent of owners reported moderate to great improvement and 74% were at least moderately pleased with the results.[248] Therefore drug therapy is not necessary if the owner is willing to devote some time and effort to modifying the behavior.

## Fear of Thunderstorms and Thunderphobia

A large percentage of dogs that are afraid of loud noises are afraid of thunderstorms. Although the onset tends to be gradual, it can be identified by owners while the dog is quite young. In one study, 42% of the dogs were showing thunderstorm phobia by 1 year of age.[274] That study also showed a tendency for dogs of herding breeds to be overrepresented. The most typical signs these dogs show are physical ones. Panting, pacing, and trembling each occur in 97% of affected dogs. Also, 90% remain with the owner, 86% hide, 72% salivate, 59% are destructive, and 55% vocalize.[86] Shaking, dilated pupils, salivation, escape, and elimination are typical of 68% of affected dogs.[274] Another 39% will hide.[274] In the presence of a fearful stimulus, a dog's cortisol levels will increase over 200% and then slowly recover.[101] If there are other dogs in the household, there is less reactivity and a more rapid recovery.[101]

If the animal is afraid only of the thunder, the problem can be treated like any other noise fear. Treatments for fear of thunder can be as simple as bringing a dog indoors if storms are threatening. The noise of a radio or television also may be preventive. Some dogs will show no signs of anxiety as long as they are surrounded by their owners' odors. Others may hide in a clothes closet or climb into a basket of dirty clothes. Security also may be found in a certain location, usually away from windows. One owner taught her dog to go to a bed area on command where it was very comfortable during normal times. If she could not be home when a storm came up, she would call home and give the "bed" command through her answering machine, and the dog would go to its safe area. Use of the Dog Appeasing Pheromone diffuser could be helpful in a situation like this too.[91] Ideally, it is best to learn about storm fears while the dog is still showing mild signs, because mildly affected dogs may be helped with anxiolytic drugs.[267] Questioning about early signs can be very important during yearly veterinary visits so therapy can be started before the problem escalates. In those cases, the use of a benzodiazepine, particularly alprazolam, can stop the escalation of the fear. The drug should be administered before the dog shows any signs, meaning at least an hour before a storm hits. When the dose is appropriate, there is no change in normal behavior so it is better that the owner give the dog the drug in anticipation of a storm than to not have it medicated to reconnect with the fearful stimulus. For more severe cases, acepromazine may need to be added. (Please note: acepromazine should not be used alone because it does nothing for the anxiety.) If acepromazine is added, it is started at 1/10 the normal sedative dose.[91] A special metallically lined cape, which is thought to reduce static electricity on the dog, has been recommended during thunderstorms. Approximately 71% of dogs in a small study seemed to show improvement while wearing the cape.[80]

When simple techniques are not effective or when dogs are more severely affected, treatment becomes more complicated. Severely affected dogs probably cannot be "cured," but intense therapy can help decrease the degree of fear or phobia. The various triggers need to be identified. Some dogs cue in on associated storm happenings, too, like lightning, wind, rain, barometric pressure changes, ionization, or odors.[373,401,448] Careful questioning of owners about their dogs' behaviors during rain only, thunder only, lightning but not thunder, windstorms, and other situations will help sort out the various fears. There is a 90% probability that a thunderphobic dog is also noise phobic and 76% probability that the noise phobic dog is also thunderphobic.[140,344] Using one trigger at a time, the owner can desensitize the dog to each that can be mimicked. Recordings of thunderstorms that produce the same behavioral response can be used for the initial desensitization process. Strobe lights might come next. Those types of changes that are harder to mimic make specific desensitization more difficult.

Of the affected dogs, 39% are considered to be fearful or reactive in temperament by their owners,[274] so maintaining them on a serotonergic drug like clomipramine or fluoxetine can be helpful too. Over 90% of storm phobic dogs will show improvement with a daily serotonergic drug and situational benzodiazepine desensitization program, and they will maintain that improvement for several months.[87] Both trazodone, an atypical antidepressant, and melatonin have also been used,[401] probably working best on milder cases. Desensitization and counterconditioning alone can be used successfully in mildly affected dogs.[438] These techniques are useful if the owner is willing to put in some effort, but they involve a lot of work and owners of mildly affected dogs would prefer to simply use medication.

The occurrence of an actual storm during a desensitization process can result in a loss of most of the real desensitization progress.[446,448] It may be necessary to tranquilize the dog just to get it through the storm. For this reason it is important to wait for thunderstorm season to be over and to use an intense program to achieve desensitization as quickly as is reasonable. Sessions should occur at least once daily and last 30 to 40 minutes each.[401,448] With this type of program, it could take the owner a few weeks of conscientious work for moderate fears to be abated in the dog and 1 to 1.5 months for more severe ones.[448] Once this retraining is completed, it may be necessary to repeat the procedure to different stimuli and in different locations.[442] If the dog does not experience a real storm in a reasonable amount of time, it may be necessary to reinforce the lessons with repetition.[448]

### Fear of Odors

Fear of an odor is unusual but does occur. When a furnace is first turned on in the fall, a smoky odor may cause the dog to react fearfully. In some cases, fear reaction to an odor is a one-time behavior. In other cases, dogs may associate an odor with other events and continue to show fear. For them, a desensitization and counterconditioning program can be useful if the problem odor can be identified.

## Genetic Makeup of Fears

Although fears and phobias can be caused by environmental events alone, evidence exists of a genetic component for some fears.* In one line of nervous Pointers, 80% of the puppies had personalities similar to those of their parents.[103,348] Experimentally, these dogs showed a stronger fear of humans than of objects, and habituation was more difficult than expected.[103] Signs become evident as early as 3 months of age and continually worsen until 12 to 36 months.[348] Oversensitivity to loud noises is reported to be homozygous recessive in some German Shepherds.[438] People with hunting and working dogs report that some lines seem to be "sound sensitive," also supporting the suggestion of the involvement of genetic composition.[348]

## Stress and Distress

A great deal of discussion takes place among behaviorists and psychologists as to what constitutes stress and distress. *Distress* generally has a negative connotation, whereas *stress* can have both positive and negative meanings. No specific definition of stress is available for several reasons. First, there is no specific biologic measure of stress.[297] Although numerous values, including cortisol levels and leukocyte counts, are studied, they represent only external parameters that often, but not always, parallel "stress levels." Second, no specific response is characteristic of all types of stress; considerable variability in biologic responses to the same stressor occurs among mdividuals.[297] Third, and this is probably the most complicating factor, no correlation has been proved between any type of stress and its impact on an animal's well-being.[297]

Dogs may respond to stress with reactions in the autonomic nervous system (ANS), changes in the neuroendocrine system, or changes in behavior.[297] The ANS reacts through the fight-or-flight mechanisms as dictated by the circumstances. Aggression in fear-biters is one example. The neuroendocrine system response can be helpful or potentially harmful, again depending on the circumstances. Release of beta-endorphins can induce an internal analgesia,[377] but the epinephrine and corticosteroids from adrenal origin can increase ventricular vulnerability[250] and alter both disease resistance and sex hormone levels.[297]

Behavior changes can be extremely variable. Stereotypic behaviors may represent one coping mechanism. These behaviors are not necessarily harmful,[297] although they are often viewed as undesirable. Because some stereotypies can be stopped by narcotic antagonists, it is reasonable to suppose that they may represent a neuroendocrine response. Development of extreme fears, submission, or aggression can accompany stress.

Veterinarians are acutely aware of stress-related behavior changes and frequently notice them in hospitalized patients undergoing various procedures.[71,251,451] Stress responses also are seen in sheltered dogs. Adopted dogs that had the highest cortisol levels preadoption ultimately had fewer behavior problems after adoption than did dogs with lower cortisol levels.[179] Psychogenic problems, such as those in Box 2-5, must be considered in differential diagnoses.[32,238] Psychogenic problems can be diagnosed only after ruling out medical conditions and other behavioral problems. Use of increased exercise, environmental manipulation, and behavior modification, perhaps with anxiolytic drug therapy, is usually needed to treat psychogenic problems.

## Aversive Conditioning

Coupling an aversive situation to the stimulus for a particular problem behavior will, over time, reduce the likelihood that the animal will perform that behavior. Aversive conditioning, then, affects

---

| BOX 2-5 | Psychogenic behavior problems |
| --- | --- |

Anorexia
Psychogenic alopecia
Psychogenic constipation
Psychogenic diarrhea
Psychogenic pain
Psychogenic polydipsia
Psychogenic vomiting
Seizures
Sympathy lameness

---

*References 30, 103, 226, 333, 348, 438.

the initiation of a behavior rather than punishing the animal after the behavior has started.[43] It depends on the dog learning through one or more senses, and success can be accomplished only by the dog enduring negative experiences. Creating a sensory aversion to things in the environment has been tried for a number of problem behaviors, from excessive grooming to destructive chewing, killing of livestock, and intake of dangerous substances.

*Taste aversion,* a possible treatment for oral behavior problems, is generally the most successful type of aversive conditioning, but there are times when *smell aversion* might be preferred. The learning concept in both types of aversive conditioning is that the dog learns from a negative experience with a taste or odor to back away from the next encounter.

For taste aversion, the dog should first be introduced to the odor of the taste repellent before the substance is put in its mouth. Substances that can be used are numerous and include acorn extracts, beta-chloroacetyl chloride, beta-mercaptopropionic acid, caffeine, capsaicin, L-carvone, L-naphthalene thiol, cayenne pepper, citronella oil, commercial bitter or hot flavors, horseradish extract, octaacetate, oleoresin, pepper sauce, pepperoni enhancers, petroleum jelly, quassia wood extract, quinine tonic, sucrose, triethylamine, and vanillamide.[192,199,244] A few milliliters of the substance are squirted into the dog's mouth after it smells the substance. The hoped for, very negative reaction is a wincing expression, a drawing back, and excessive salivation. The product can then be put on surfaces that the dog is to leave alone so that the dog's next encounter with the initial taste, or even just the odor, reminds the dog of the initial bad experience. Avoidance results. Occasionally, this lesson must be repeated as a reminder.

Smell aversion uses the same principle to instill a dislike of experiences associated with a particular odor. A spray can, aimed at a 90-degree angle from the dog's nose, creates an aversion to the hissing noise, the rapid movement of the can toward the dog, and the smell of the can's product. The odor can then be put on specific objects when the dog is not in the room to prevent extinguishing the effects of the odor. Fumes need to settle before the dog is allowed back into the room.

Capsaicin, a taste repellent, has been used to limit intake of ethylene glycol to sublethal amounts.[192] Emetics like lithium chloride have also been used to create an aversion, particularly in dogs that kill livestock and as a preventive against accidental poisonings.[62,192] Apomorphine, copper sulfate, and antimony potassium tartrate successfully cause emesis.[192] Controversy remains about whether long-term aversion really results from emetics because the vomiting usually occurs quite a while after the product and inappropriate substance are eaten. It is hoped that the negative experience of vomiting, in association with the taste of the inappropriate substance coming up again, creates a taste aversion.

## Shock Collars for Training

A word about electric-shock collars is probably appropriate, because they are a piece of equipment frustrated dog owners often inquire about. The remote control shock collar is most commonly used as a training aid and a form of punishment. A second type of shock collar is bark-activated. The latest use of electric shock for punishment is in association with an unseen perimeter fence. Various shock collars have been used by some trainers,[362,435] but they are seldom appropriate. They are even worse for the average dog owner because the owner does not have an extensive education about how to use them. The amount of punishment is too severe or inconsistent, depending on battery strength, shock-intensity setting, breed of dog, amount of hair on the dog, degree of direct skin contact, and presence of wet hair. Most important, the person controlling the switch may not understand the behavioral principles of learning, including the appropriate timing and application of the punishment.[165,317,454] Studies show that the use of a shock collar in training results in behaviors associated with stress, fear, and pain.[388] In addition, those same dogs quickly learn to associate the distress with the mere presence of the owner and with the commands even in the absence of a shock.[388] Shock is rarely an appropriate training tool, because it can cause major tissue damage (Fig. 2-12). Better alternatives exist.

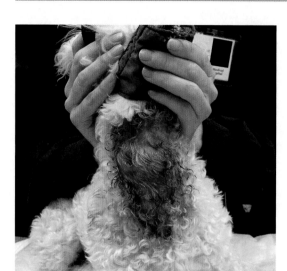

**Figure 2-12.** Shock collars can result in painful neck injuries.

## References

1. Adams B, Chan A, Callahan, et al: Use of a delayed non-matching to position task to model age-dependent cognitive decline in the dog. Behav Brain Res 2000; 109:47.
2. Adams DR, Weikamp MD: The canine vomeronasal organ. J Anat 1984; 138(4):771.
3. Adler LL, Adler HE: Ontogeny of observational learning in the dog *(Canis familiaris)*. Dev Psychobiol 1977; 10(3):267.
4. Ahl AS: The role of vibrissae in behavior: A status review. Vet Res Commun 1986; 10(4):245.
5. Ali MA, Klyne MA: Vision in Vertebrates. New York: Plenum Press, 1985.
6. Allen WF: Olfactory and trigeminal conditioned reflexes in dogs. Am J Physiol 1937; 118:532.
7. Amen DG: Attention, doctors. Newsweek (Feb. 26)2001:72.
8. American Psychiatric Association: Diagnostic and Statistical Manual of Mental Disorders, 3rd ed. Washington, DC: American Psychiatric Association, 1987.
9. Anastasi A, Fuller JL, Scott JP, et al: A factor analysis of the performance of dogs on certain learning tests. Zoologica 1955; 40(3):33.
10. Andersson B, Olsson K: Effects of bilateral amygdaloid lesions in nervous dogs. J Small Anim Pract 1965; 6:301.
11. Araujo JA, Landsberg G, Milgram NW, et al: A combination of acetyl-ʟ-carnitine and alpha lipoic acid improves learning, but not memory, in aged Beagle dogs. Am Coll Vet Behav/Am Vet Soc Anim Behav Scientific Session 2007:29.
12. Araujo JA, Milgram NW, Landsberg G, et al: A combination of acetyl-l-carnitine and alpha lipolic acid improves learning, but not memory, in aged Beagle dogs. In Landsberg G, Mattiello S, Mills D (eds): Proceedings of the 6th International Veterinary Behaviour Meeting and European College of Veterinary Behavioural Medicine-Companion Animals European Society of Veterinary Clinical Ethology. Brescia, Italy: Fondazione Iniziative Zooprofilattiche e Zootecniche, 2007, p. 66.
13. Arey LB, Bruesch SR, Castanares S: The relation between eyeball size and the number of optic nerve fibers in the dog. J Comp Neurol 1942; 76:417.
14. Arey LB, Gore M: The numerical relationship between the ganglion cells of the retina and the fibers in the optic nerve of the dog. J Comp Neurol 1942; 77:609.
15. Ashton EH, Eayrs JT, Moulton DG: Olfactory acuity in the dog. Nature 1957; 179:1069.
16. Bacon WE, Stanley WC: Effect of deprivation level in puppies on performance maintained by a passive person reinforcer. J Comp Physiol Psychol 1963; 56(4):783.
17. Bacon WE, Stanley WC: Avoidance learning in neonatal dogs. J Comp Physiol Psychol 1968; 71(3):448.
18. Bacon WE, Stanley WC: Reversal learning in neonatal dogs. J Comp Physiol Psychol 1970; 70(3):344.
19. Bain MJ, Hart BL, Cliff KD, et al: Predicting behavioral changes associated with age-related cognitive impairment in dogs. J Am Vet Med Assoc 2001; 218(11):1792.
20. Ballarini G: Animal psychodietetics. J Small Anim Pract 1990; 31:523.
21. Bamberger M, Houpt KA: Signalment factors, comorbidity, and trends in behavior diagnoses in dogs: 1,644 cases (1991-2001). J Am Vet Med Assoc 2006; 229(10):1591.
22. Barakat C: How well do horses hear? Equus 2004; 315:28.
23. Bareggi SR, Becker RE, Ginsburg BE, et al: Neurochemical investigation of an endogenous model of the "hyperkinetic syndrome" in a hybrid dog. Life Sci 1979; 24:481.
24. Bareggi SR, Becker RE, Ginsburg B, et al: Paradoxical effect of amphetamine in an endogenous model of the hyperkinetic syndrome in a hybrid dog: Correlation with amphetamine and p-hydroxyamphetamine blood levels. Psychopharmacology 1979; 62(3):217.
25. Bartlett M: Follow up: Puppy aptitude testing. AKC Gazette 1987; 104(5):64.
26. Bartoshuk LM: The functions of taste and olfaction. Ann N Y Acad Sci 1989; 575:353.
27. Bauer EB, Smuts BB: Cooperation and competition during dyadic play in domestic dogs. *Canis familiaris.* Anim Behav 2007; 73(3):489.
28. Baxter Jr LR: Neuroimaging studies of human anxiety disorders: Cutting paths of knowledge through the field of neurotic phenomena. In Bloom FE, Kupfer DJ (eds): Psychopharmacology: The Fourth Generation of Progress. New York: Raven Press Ltd, 1995, p. 1287.
29. Beaudet R, Chalifoux A, Dallaire A: Predictive value of activity level and behavioral evaluation on future dominance in puppies. Appl Anim Behav Sci 1994; 40(2-3):273.
30. Beaver BV: The genetics of canine behavior. Vet Med Small Anim Gin 1981; 76(10):1423.
31. Beaver BV: Somatosensory development in puppies. Vet Med Small Anim Clin 1982; 77(1):39.
32. Beaver BV: Psychosomatic behaviors in dogs and cats. Vet Med Small Anim Clin 1982; 77(11):1594.
33. Beaver BV: Feline Behavior: A Guide for Veterinarians. Philadelphia: Saunders, 2003.
34. Beaver BV: The Veterinarian's Encyclopedia of Animal Behavior. Ames: Iowa State University Press, 1994.

35. Beerda B, Schilder MBH, van Hoof JA, et al: Manifestations of chronic and acute stress in dogs. Appl Anim Behav Sci 1997; 52(3-4):307.

36. Begley S: How the brain rewires itself. Time 2007; 169(5):72.

37. Bekoff M: Social play and play-soliciting by infant canids. Am Zool 1974; 14:323.

38. Bekoff M, Hil HL, Mitton JB: Behavioral taxonomy in canids by discriminant function analyses. SCI 1975; 190:1223.

39. Berteselli GV, Servida F, Dall'Ara P, et al: Evaluation of immunological, stress and behavioural paramenters in dogs *(Canis familiaris)* with anxiety-related disorders. In Mills D, Levine E, Landsberg G, et al (eds): Current Issues and Research in Veterinary Behavioral Medicine. West Lafayette, IN: Purdue University Press, 2005, p. 18.

40. Blackshaw JK: Abnormal behaviour in dogs. Aust Vet J 1988; 65(12):393.

41. Blackshaw JK, Cook GE, Harding P, et al: Aversive responses of dogs to ultrasonic, sonic and flashing light units. Appl Anim Behav Sci 1990; 25(1-2):1.

42. Blackwell EJ, Twells C, Seawright A, et al: The relationship between training methods and the occurrence of behaviour problems in a population of domestic dogs. In Landsberg G, Mattiello S, Mills D (eds): Proceedings of the 6th International Veterinary Behaviour Meeting and European College of Veterinary Behavioural Medicine-Companion Animals European Society of Veterinary Clinical Ethology. Brescia, Italy: Fondazione Iniziative Zooprofilattiche e Zootecniche, 2007, p. 51.

43. Borchelt PL, Voith V: Punishment. Compend Contin Educ [Small Anim] 1985; 7(9):780.

44. Branson N: Landmark study: How does handedness affect behaviour? http://www.ava.com.au/news.php?action+show&news_id=246&c=0&PHPSESS1D=aoaflc08e5228f741ac86680a45439b8, 6/14/2007.

45. Bräuer J, Call J, Tomasello M: Visual perspective taking in dogs *(Canis familiaris)* in the presence of barriers. Appl Anim Behav Sci 2004; 88:299.

46. Breazile JE: Neurologic and behavioral development in the puppy. Vet Clin North Am 1978; 8(1):31.

47. Breitschwerdt EB, Breazile TE, Broadhurst JJ: Clinical and electroencephalographic findings associated with ten cases of suspected limbic epilepsy in the dog. J Am Anim Hosp Assoc 1979; 15(1):37.

48. Brisbin IL, Austad SN: The use of trained dogs to discriminate human scent: A reply. Anim Behav 1993; 46(1):191.

49. Brisbin Jr IL, Austad SN: Testing the individual odour theory of canine olfaction. Anim Behav 1991; 42:63.

50. Broderick PA, Blaha CD, Lane RF: In vivo electrochemical evidence for an enkephalinergic modulation underlying stereotyped behavior: Reversibility by naloxone. Brain Res 1983; 269:378.

51. Brown GL, Goodwin FK, Ballenger JC, et al: Aggression in humans correlates with cerebrospinal fluid amine metabolites. Psychiatry Res 1979; 1:131.

52. Burghardt Jr. WF: The use of prospective behavioral markers in prediction of later learning and performance in military working dogs. Newsl Am Vet Soc Anim Behav 1997; 19(2):9.

53. Burton M: The Sixth Sense of Animals. New York: Taplinger Publishing Co, 1972.

54. Cabib S, Puglisi-Allegra S, Oliverio A: Chronic stress enhances apomorphine-induced stereotyped behavior in mice: Involvement of endogenous opioids. Brain Res 1984; 298:138.

55. Campbell WE: A behavior test for puppy selection. Mod Vet Pract 1972; 53(12):29.

56. Campbell WE: Matching puppies and people. Gaines Dog Research Progress Spring 1973:2.

57. Campbell WE: Behavioral modification of hyperkinetic dogs. Mod Vet Pract 1973; 54(12):49.

58. Campbell WE: Canine hyperkinesis. Mod Vet Pract 1974; 55(4):313.

59. Campbell WE: Biologic clocks and canine neuroses. Mod Vet Pract 1974; 55(11):889.

60. Campbell WE: The when, how, and who of training. Mod Vet Pract 1975; 56(7):492.

61. Campbell WE: Behavior Problems in Dogs. Santa Barbara, CA: American Veterinary Publications, 1975.

62. Campbell WE: Fowl play. Mod Vet Pract 1977; 58(3):202.

63. Campbell WE: Conditioned global panic due to percussive sounds. Mod Vet Pract 1977; 58(11):963.

64. Campbell WE: Behavior Problems in Dogs, 2nd ed. Goleta, CA: American Veterinary Publications, 1992.

65. Cargill J, Hudson M: Temperament tests as puppy selection tools. Dog World April 1994:4049.

66. Casey R: Fear and stress. In Horwitz DF, Mills DS, Heath S (eds): BSAVA Manual of Canine and Feline Behavioural Medicine. Quedgeley, Gloucester, England: British Small Animal Veterinary Association, 2002, p. 144.

67. Cash WC, Blauch BS: Jaw snapping syndrome in eight dogs. J Am Vet Med Assoc 1979; 175(7):709.

68. Chapman B, Voith VL: Dog owners and their choice of a pet. American Veterinary Society of Animal Behavior meeting, Atlanta, July 20, 1986.

69. Chapman B, Voith VL: Geriatric behavior problems not always related to age. DVM 1987; 18(3):32.

70. Charles MS, Fuller JL: Developmental study of the electroencephalogram of the dog. EEG Clin Neurophysiol 1956; 8:645.

71. Chastain CB, Franklin RT, Ganjam VK, et al: Evaluation of the hypothalamic pituitary-adrenal axis in clinically stressed dogs. J Am Anim Hosp Assoc 1986; 22(4):435.

72. Coile DC, Pollitz CH, Smith JC: Behavioral determination of critical flicker fusion in dogs. Physiol Behav 1989; 45(6):1087.

73. Coon K: Dog Intelligence Test. Baton Rouge, LA: Dog Inc, 1977.

74. Corder RL, Latimer HB: The prenatal growth of the brain and of its parts and of the spinal cord in the dog. J Comp Neurol 1949; 90:193.

75. Coren S: The Intelligence of Dogs: Canine Consciousness and Capabilities. New York: The Free Press, 1994.

76. Cornwell AC, Fuller JL: Conditioned responses in young puppies. J Comp Physiol Psychol 1961; 54(1):13.

77. Corson SA: Corson EO'L: Philosophical and historical roots of Pavlovian psychobiology. In Corson SA, EO'L Corson (eds): Psychiatry and Psychology in the USSR. New York: Plenum Press, 1976, p. 19.

78. Corson SA, EO'L Corson, Arnold LE, et al: Interaction of psychopharmacologic and psychosocial therapy in behavior modification of animal models of violence and hyperkinesis. In Serban G (ed): Relevance of the Psychopathological Animal Model to the Human. New York: Plenum Press, 1975.

79. Corson SA, EO'L Corson, Arnold, LE et al: Animal models of violence and hyperkinesis: Interaction of psychopharmacologic and psychosocial therapy in behavior modification. In Serban G, Kling A (eds): Animal Models in Human Psychobiology. New York: Plenum Press, 1976, p. 111.

80. Cottam N, Dodman N, Critzer T: Use of a cape (The Storm Defender) in the treatment of canine *(Canis familiaris)* thunderstorm phobia. In Mills D, Levine E, Landsberg G, et al (eds): Current Issues and Research in Veterinary Behavioral Medicine. West Lafayette, IN: Purdue University Press, 2005, p. 165.

81. Craig DJ: Small-breed detector dog feasibility study. Report to Major General AP Iosue, USAF, Commander, AF Military Training Center, Lackland AFB, October 19, 1976.

82. Craig DJ: Personal communication, 1977.

83. Crighton GW: Thermal regulation in the newborn dog. Mod Vet Pract 1969; 50(2):35.

84. Crowell-Davis S: A case of psychomotor epilepsy responsive to environmental stimuli. American Veterinary Society of Animal Behavior meeting, Las Vegas, NV, July 22, 1985.

85. Crowell-Davis SL, Lappin M, Oliver JE: Stimulus-responsive psychomotor epilepsy in a Doberman Pinscher. J Am Anim Hosp Assoc 1989; 25:57.

86. Crowell-Davis SL, Seibert L, Sung W, et al: Treatment of storm phobia with a combination of clomipramine, alprazolam, and behavior modification: A prospective open trial. American Veterinary Society of Animal Behavior Meeting Proceedings 2001:5.

87. Crowell-Davis SL, Seibert LM, Sung W, et al: Use of clomipramine, alprazolam, and behavior modification for treatment of storm phobia in dogs. J Am Vet Med Assoc 2003; 222(6):744.

88. Cummings BJ, Head E, Ruehl W, et al: The canine as an animal model of human aging and dementia. Neurobiol Aging 1996; 17(2):259.

89. Cummings BJ, Su JH, Cotman CW, et al: Beta-amyloid accumulation in aged canine brain: A model of early plaque formation in Alzheimer's disease. Neurobiol Aging 1993; 14:547.

90. Cunningham JG, Farnbach GC: Inheritance and idiopathic canine epilepsy. J Am Anim Hosp Assoc 1988; 24:421.

91. Curtis TM: How I treat storm phobias. Am Vet Med Assoc Convention Proc 2007.

92. Dantzer R: Behavioral, physiological and functional aspects of sterotyped behavior: A review and a re-interpretation. J Anim Sci 1986; 62:1776.

93. Davis KL, Gurski JC, Scott JP: Interaction of separation distress with fear in infant dogs. Dev Psychobiol 1977; 10(3):203.

94. Davis M, Myers KM: The role of glutamate and gamma-aminobutyric acid in fear extinction: Clinical implications for exposure therapy. Biol Psychiatry 2002; 52:998.

95. Dehasse J: Intelligent activity for dogs as a tool in behavioural therapy. In Landsberg G, Mattiello S, Mills D (eds): Proceedings of the 6th International Veterinary Behaviour Meeting and European College of Veterinary Behavioural Medicine-Companion Animals European Society of Veterinary Clinical Ethology. Brescia, Italy: Fondazione Iniziative Zooprofilattiche e Zootecniche, 2007, p. 53.

96. Denenberg S, Landsberg G: Evaluation of the effect of Dog Appeasing Pheromones on the reduction of anxiety and fear in puppies during training. Am Coll Vet Behav/Am Vet Soc Anim Behav Scientific Session 2007:3.

97. Dodman NH, Knowles KE, Shuster L, et al: Behavioral changes associated with suspected complex partial seizures in bull terriers. J Am Vet Med Assoc 1996; 208(5):688.

98. Domínguez C, Ibíñez M, Biosca EY: Distribution of cases in a clinical ethology referral service in Spain. Proc Third International Cong Vet Behav Med 2001:158.

99. Dravid AR, Himwich WA, Davis JM: Some free amino acids in dog brain development. J Neurochem 1965; 12:901.

100. Dreschel NA: The effects of the immune system on behavior. AVSAB Annual Symposium on Anim Behav Res 2002 Meeting Proc:25.

101. Dreschel NA, Granger DA: Physiological and behavioral reactivity to stress in thunderstorm-phobic dogs and their caregivers. Appl Anim Behav Sci 2005; 95:153.

102. Dykman RA, Murphree OD, Ackerman PT: Litter patterns in the offspring of nervous and stable dogs. II. Autonomic and motor conditioning. J Nerv Ment Dis 1966; l41(4):419.

103. Dykman RA, Murphree OD, Reese WG: Familial anthropophobia in pointer dogs? Arch Gen Psychiatry 1979; 36:988.

104. Echteler SM, Fay RR, Popper AN: Structure of the mammalian cochlea. In Fay RR, Popper AN (eds): Comparative Hearing: Mammals. New York: Springer-Verlag, 1994, p. 134.

105. Educate owners in puppy selection. Small Anim Vet Report 1983; 1(5):78.

106. Elia J, Borcherding BG, Rapoport JL, et al: Methylphenidate and dextroamphetamine treatments of hyperactivity: Are there true nonresponders? Psychiatry Res 1991; 36:141.

107. Ernst M, Zametkin A: The interface of genetics, neuroimaging, and neurochemistry in attention-deficit hyperactivity disorder. In Bloom FE, Kupfer DJ (eds): Psychopharmacology: The Fourth Generation of Progress. New York: Raven Press Ltd, 1995, p. 1643.

108. Ewer RF: The Carnivores. Ithaca, NY: Cornell University Press, 1973.

109. Ezeh PI, Myers LJ: Functional visual acuity in the dog: Development and use of the refined optokinetic technique. Proc Am Coll Vet Internal Med Forum 1989:631.

110. Ezeh PI, Myers LJ, Cummins KA, et al: Utilizing an optokinetic device in assessing the functional visual acuity of the dog. Prog Vet Neurol 1990; 1(4):427.

111. Fagen R: Animal Play Behavior. New York: Oxford University Press, 1981.

112. Faraone SV, Biederman J, Spencer TJ, et al: Comparing the efficacy of medications for ADHD using meta-analysis. http://www.medscape.com/viewarticle/543952, 10/12/2006.

113. Fenner WR: Neurology of the geriatric patient. Vet Clin North Am [Small Anim Pract] 1988; 18(3):711.

114. Fernández-Teruel A, Giménez-Llort L, Escorihuela RM, et al: Early-life handling stimulation and environmental enrichment. Are some of their effects mediated by similar neural mechanisms? Pharmacol Biochem Behav 2002; 73:233.

115. Ferrell F: Tastebud morphology in the fetal and neonatal dog. Neurosci Biobehav Rev 1984; 8(2):175.

116. Ferrell F: Gustatory nerve response to sugars in neonatal puppies. Neurosci Biobehav Rev 1984; 8(2):185.

117. Filiatre JC, Millot JL, Eckerlin A: Behavioural variability of olfactory exploration of the pet dog in relation to human adults. Appl Anim Behav Sci 1991; 30(3-4):341.

118. Flood J, Smith GE, Morley JE: Modulation of memory processing by cholecystokinin: Dependence on the vagus nerve. SCI 1987; 236:832.

119. Fox MW: Conditioned reflexes and innate behaviour of the neonate dog. J Small Anim Pract 1963; 4(2):85.

120. Fox MW: Development and clinical significance of superficial reflexes in the dog. Vet Rec 1963; 75(14):378.

121. Fox MW: The postnatal growth of the canine brain and correlated anatomical and behavioral changes during neuro-ontogenesis. Growth 1964; 28:135.

122. Fox MW: The ontogeny of behaviour and neurologic responses in the dog. Anim Behav 1964; 12:301.

123. Fox MW: Canine Behavior. Springfield, IL: Charles C Thomas, 1965.

124. Fox MW: Brain-to-body relationships in ontogeny of canine brain. Experientia 1966; XXII:111.

125. Fox MW: Dog development, rearing and training: Practical applications of research findings. Southwest Vet 1966; 19:303.

126. Fox MW: Canine Pediatrics: Development, Neonatal and Congenital Diseases. Springfield, IL: Charles C Thomas, 1966.

127. Fox MW: Postnatal development of the EEG in the dog. II. Development of electrocortical activity. J Small Anim Pract 1967; 8:77.

128. Fox MW: Postnatal development of the EEG in the dog. III. Summary and discussion of development of canine EEG. J Small Anim Pract 1967; 8:109.

129. Fox MW: Neuronal development and ontogeny of evoked potentials in auditory and visual cortex of the dog. Electroenceph Clin Neurophysiol 1968; 24:213.

130. Fox MW: Overview and critique of stages and periods in canine development. Dev Psychobiol 1971; 4(1):37.

131. Fox MW: Psychopathology in man and lower animals. J Am Vet Med Assoc 1971; 159(1):66.

132. Fox MW: Integrative Development of Brain and Behavior in the Dog. Chicago: University of Chicago Press, 1971.

133. Fox MW: The Dog: Its Domestication and Behavior. New York: Garland STPM Press, 1978.

134. Fox MW, Bekoff M: The behaviour of dogs. In Hafez ESE (ed): The Behaviour of Domestic Animals, 3rd ed. Baltimore: Williams & Wilkins, 1975, p. 380.

135. Fox MW, Inman OR, Himwich WA: The postnatal development of neocortical neurons in the dog. J Comp Neurol 1966; 127:199.

136. Fox MW, Inman OR, Himwich WA: The postnatal development of the spinal cord of the dog. J Comp Neurol 1967; 130:233.

137. Fox MW, Spencer JW: Development of the delayed response in the dog. Anim Behav 1967; 15(1):162.

138. Fox MW, Spencer JW: Exploratory behavior in the dog: Experiential or age dependent? Dev Psychobiol 1969; 2(2):68.

139. Fox MW, Stelzner D: Behavioral effects of differential early experience in the dog. Anim Behav 1966; 14:273.

140. Frank D, Overall K, Dunham AE: Co-occurrence of noise and thunderstorm phobias and other anxieties. American Veterinary Society of Animal Behavior Proceedings 2000:7.

141. Frank H, Frank MG: Comparison of problem-solving performance in six-week-old wolves and dogs. Anim Behav 1982; 30:95.

142. Frazier LL, Brunjes PC: Unilateral odor deprivation: Early postnatal changes in olfactory bulb cell density and number. J Comp Neurol 1988; 269:355.

143. Fredericson E, Gurney N, Dubois E: The relationship between environmental temperature and behavior in neonatal puppies. J Comp Physiol Psychol 1956; 49:278.

144. Freedman DG: Constitutional and environmental interactions in rearing of four breeds of dogs. SCI 1958; 127:585.

145. Freedman DG: Some effects of early rearing on later obedience in dogs. Nord Vet Med 1965; 17:111.

146. Fuller JL: Experiential deprivation and later behavior. SCI 1967; 158:1645.

147. Fuller JL, Easler CA, Banks EM: Formation of conditioned avoidance responses in young puppies. Am J Physiol 1950; 160:462.

148. Fuller JL, Fox MW: The behaviour of dogs. In Hafez ESE (ed): The Behaviour of Domestic Animals, 2nd ed. Baltimore: Williams & Wilkins, 1969, p. 438.

149. Fuller JL, Rosvold HE, Pribram KH: The effect on affective and cognitive behavior in the dog of lesions of the pyriform-amygdala-hippocampal complex. J Comp Physiol Psychol 1957; 50:89.

150. Gaineldinov RR, Wetsel WC, Jones SR, et al: Role of serotonin in the paradoxical calming effect of psychostimulants on hyperactivity. SCI 1999; 283(5400):397.

151. Gandia Estellés M, Mills DS, Coleshaw PH, et al: A retrospective analysis of relationships with severity of signs of fear of fireworks and treatment outcome in 99 cases. In Mills D, Levine E, Landsberg G, et al (eds): Current Issues and Research in Veterinary Behavioral Medicine. West Lafayette, IN: Purdue University Press, 2005, p. 161.

152. Gazit I, Terkel J: Explosives detection by sniffer dogs following strenuous physical activity. Appl Anim Behav Sci 2003; 81(2):149.

153. Gazit I, Terkel J: Domination of olfaction over vision in explosives detection by dogs. Appl Anim Behav Sci 2003; 82(1):65.

154. Goddard ME, Beilharz RG: The relationship of fearfulness to, and the effects of, sex, age and experience on exploration and activity in dogs. Appl Anim Behav Sci 1984; 12(3):267.

155. Goddard ME, Beilharz RG: A factor analysis of fearfulness in potential guide dogs. Appl Anim Behav Sci 1984; 12:253.

156. Goddard ME, Beilharz RG: A multivariate analysis of the genetics of fearfulness in potential guide dogs. Behav Genet 1985; 15(1):69.

157. Goddard ME, Beilharz RG: Early prediction of adult behaviour in potential guide dogs. Appl Anim Behav Sci 1986; 15:247.

158. Gourevitch G: Directional hearing in terrestrial mammals. In Popper AN, Fay RR (eds): Comparative Studies of Hearing in Vertebrates. New York: Springer-Verlag, 1980, p. 357.

159. Graham L, Wells DL, Hepper PG: The influence of olfactory stimulation on the behaviour of dogs housed in a rescue shelter. Appl Anim Behav Sci 2005; 91:143.

160. Grillon C: Startle reactivity and anxiety disorders: Aversive conditioning, context, and neurobiology. Biol Psychiatry 2002; 52:958.
161. Gun-shy dogs. Vet Med 1944; 39:296.
162. Halász N: The Vertebrate Olfactory System. Budapest: Akadérniai Kiadó, 1990.
163. Halpern M: The organization and function of the vomeronasal system. Ann Rev Neurosci 1987; 10:325.
164. Hart BL: Gonadal androgen and sociosexual behavior of male mammals: A comparative analysis. Psychol Bull 1974; 81(7):383.
165. Hart BL: Acquired objectionable behavioral patterns: The role of reward and punishment. Canine Pract 1974; 1(3):5.
166. Hart BL: Brain disorders and abnormal behavior. Canine Pract 1977; 4(4):10.
167. Hart BL: Anthropomorphism: Two perspectives. Canine Pract 1978; 5(3):12.
168. Hart BL: Successive approximation: The key to behavioral therapy. Canine Pract 1978; 5(5):8.
169. Hart BL: Biological basis of the behavior of sick animals. Neurosci Biobehav Rev 1988; 12(2):123.
170. Hart BL: Effect of gonadectomy on subsequent development of age-related cognitive impairment in dogs. J Am Vet Med Assoc 2001; 219(1):51.
171. Hart BL, Ladewig J: Accelerated and enhanced testosterone secretion in juvenile male dogs following medial preoptic-anterior hypothalamic lesions. Neuroendocrinology 1980; 30:20.
172. Haug LI, Beaver BV, Longnecker MT: Comparison of dogs' reactions to four different head collars. Appl Anim Behav Sci 2002; 79:53.
173. Hawk HW, Conley HH, Kiddy CA: Estrus-related odors in milk detected by trained dogs. J Dairy Sci 1984; 67:392.
174. Head E, Mehta R, Hartley J, et al: Spatial learning and memory as a function of age in the dog. Behav Neurosci 1995; 109(5):851.
175. Hearing ability of animals. J Am Vet Med Assoc 1983; 183(2):211.
176. Heath S: Behaviour problems in the geriatric pet. In Horwitz DF, Mills DS, Heath S (eds): BSAVA Manual of Canine and Feline Behavioural Medicine. Quedgeley, Gloucester, England: British Small Animal Veterinary Association, 2002, p. 109.
177. Heffner HE: Hearing in large and small dogs: Absolute thresholds and size of the tympanic membrane. Behav Neuroscience 1983; 97(2):310.
178. Heffner HE: Auditory awareness. Appl Anim Behav Sci 1998; 57(3-4):259.
179. Hennessy MB: Human interaction and diet affect neuroendocrine stress responses and behavior of dogs in a public animal shelter. Am Vet Soc Anim Behav Proc 2001:1.
180. Hennessy MB, Voith VL, Hawke JL, et al: Effects of a program of human interaction and alterations in diet composition on activity of the hypothalamic-pituitary-adrenal axis in dogs housed in a public animal shelter. J Am Vet Med Assoc 2002; 221(1):65.
181. Hess EH: Sensory processes. In Waters RH, Rethlingshafer DA, Caldwell WE (eds): Principles of Comparative Psychology. New York: McGraw-Hill, 1960, p. 74.
182. Hewson CJ, Luescher UA, Parent JM, et al: Efficacy of clomipramine in the treatment of canine compulsive disorder. J Am Vet Med Assoc 1998; 213(12):1760.
183. Himwich HE, Fazekas JF: Comparative studies of the metabolism of the brain of infant and adult dogs. Am J Physiol 1941; 132:454.
184. Hoffman L, Kelley R, Waltz D: For smarter more trainable puppies: Effect of docosahexaenoic acid on puppy trainability. The Iams Co. ABSB #07356100, 2003.
185. Hollander E: Introduction. In Hollander E (ed): Obsessive-Compulsive-Related Disorders. Washington, DC: American Psychiatric Press Inc, 1993, p. 1.
186. Holliday TA, Cunningham JG, Gutnick MJ: Comparative clinical and electroencephalographic studies of canine epilepsy. Epilepsia 1970; 11:281.
187. Holloway CL: Loss of olfactory acuity in hunting animals. Auburn Vet 1961; 18(1):25.
188. Holy TE, Dulac C, Meister M: Responses of vomeronasal neurons to natural stimuli. SCI 2000; 289:1569.
189. Horwitz DF: Cognitive dysfunction in senior dogs. http://www.avma.org/conv/cv2002/cvnotes/CAn_CDS_hoD.asp, 7/3/2002.
190. Horwitz DF: Puppy development and welfare. http://www.avma.org/conv/cv2002/cvnotes/CAn_Ped_PDW_HoD.asp, 7/3/2002.
191. Horwitz D, Landsberg G, Luescher A, et al: Enriching the environment of our pets: Roundtable on the psychology of play and behavior modification. Vet Forum 2003; 20(1):46.
192. Houpt K, Zgoda JC, Stahlbaum CC: Use of taste repellents and emetics to prevent accidental poisoning of dogs. Am J Vet Res 1984; 45(8):1501.
193. Houpt KA, Davis PP, Hintz HF: Effect of peripheral anosmia on dogs trained as flavor validators. Am J Vet Res 1982; 43(5):841.
194. Houpt KA, Shepherd P, Hintz HF: Two methods for producing peripheral anosmia in dogs. Lab Anim Sci 1978; 28(2):173.
195. Hubrecht RC: A comparison of social and environmental enrichment methods for laboratory-housed dogs. Appl Anim Behav Sci 1993; 37(4):345.
196. Hughes A: The topography of vision in mammals of contrasting life style: Comparative optics and retinal organisation. In Crescitelli F (ed): The Visual System in Vertebrates. New York: Springer-Verlag, 1977, p. 613.
197. Hunthausen W: Identifying and treating behavior problems in geriatric dogs. Vet Med (Suppl) 1994; 89:688.
198. Hunthausen WL: Rule out medical etiologies first in geriatric behavior problems. DVM 1991; 22(7):24.
199. Hunthausen WL: The causes, treatment, and prevention of canine destructive chewing. Vet Med 1991; 86(10):1007.
200. Hyperkinesis and aggression. Lab Anim July-August 1974:38.
201. Iimura K, Mills DS, Levine E: An analysis of the relationship between the history of development of sensitivity to loud noises and behavioural signs in domestic dogs. In Landsberg G, Mattiello S, Mills D (eds): Proceedings of the 6th International Veterinary Behaviour Meeting and European College of Veterinary Behavioural Medicine-Companion Animals European Society of Veterinary Clinical Ethology. Brescia, Italy: Fondazione Iniziative Zooprofilattiche e Zootecniche, 2007, p. 70.
202. Ikeda-Douglas CJ, Zicker SC, Estrada J, et al: Prior experience, antioxidants, and mitochondrial co-factors improve cognitive dysfunction in aged beagles. Vet Therapeut 2004; 5:5.

203. Irimajiri M, Jay EE, Luescher AU, et al: Mild polycythemia in canine compulsive disorder. Proc Am Vet Soc Anim Behav meeting 2003:22.
204. Irimajiri M, Luescher AU: Effect of fluoxetine hydrochloride in treating canine compulsive disorder. In Mills D, Levine E, Landsberg G, et al (eds): Current Issues and Research in Veterinary Behavioral Medicine. West Lafayette, IN: Purdue University Press, 2005, p. 198.
205. Jacobs GH: Comparative Color Vision. New York: Academic Press, 1981.
206. Jacobs GH, Deegan JF, Crognale MA: Photopigments of dogs and foxes and their implications for canid vision. Vis Neurosci 1993; 10:173.
207. James WT: The geotropic reaction of newborn puppies. J Genet Psychol 1956; 89:127.
208. James WT: Preliminary observations on play behaviour in puppies. J Genet Psychol 1961; 98:273.
209. James WT, Cannon DJ: Conditioned avoiding responses in puppies. Am J Physiol 1952; 168:251.
210. Jeddi E: Contact comfort and behavioral thermoregulation. Physiol Behav 1970; 5(12):1487.
211. Jensen C, Ederstrom HE: Development of temperature regulation in the dog. Am J Physiol 1955; 183:340.
212. Jones AC, Gosing SD: Temperament and personality in dogs (Canis familiaris): A review and evaluation of past research. Appl Anim Behav Sci 2005; 95:1.
213. Jones RD: Use of thioridazine in the treatment of aberrant motor behavior in a dog. J Am Vet Med Assoc 1987; 191(1):89.
214. Kabat H: The greater resistance of very young animals to arrest of the brain circulation. Am J Physiol 1940; 130:588.
215. Kalmus H: The discrimination by the nose of the dog of individual human odours and in particular the odours of twins. Br J Anim Behav 1955; 3:25.
216. Kamerlang SG: Drugs and animal behavior. 138th Annual AVMA Convention Notes 2001. http://www.avma.org/noah/members/convention/conv01/notes/04050101.asp, 6/11/2001.
217. Kamin LJ: Traumatic avoidance learning: The effects of CS-US interval with a trace-conditioning procedure. J Comp Physiol Psychol 1954; 47:65.
218. Kaminski J, Call J, Fischer J: Word learning in a domestic dog: Evidence for "fast mapping." SCI June 11, 2004; 304:1682.
219. Kaulfuss P, Mills DS: Neophilia in domestic dogs (Canis familiaris). In Landsberg G, Mattiello S, Mills D (eds): Proceedings of the 6th International Veterinary Behaviour Meeting and European College of Veterinary Behavioural Medicine-Companion Animals European Society of Veterinary Clinical Ethology. Brescia, Italy: Fondazione Iniziative Zooprofilattiche e Zootecniche, 2007, p. 152.
220. Kay R, Palmer AC, Taylor PM: Hearing in the dog as assessed by auditory brainstem evoked potentials. Vet Rec 1984; 114:81.
221. Kelly K: The brainiest canines bark back. The Houston Post, April 3, 1994:E-7.
222. Khanna S: Carbamazepine in obsessive-compulsive disorder. Clin Neuropharmacol 1988; 11(5):478.
223. Kiddy CA, Mitchell DS, Hawk HW: Estrus-related odors in body fluids of dairy cows. J Dairy Sci 1984; 67:388.
224. King JE, Becker RF, Markee JE: Studies on olfactory discrimination in dogs: (3) Ability to detect human odour trace. Anim Behav 1964; XII(2-3):311.
225. Kirk DW: Domestic Security Dog. MS Thesis, College Station: Texas A&M University, 1976.
226. Klein E, Steinberg SA, Weiss SRB, et al: The relationship between genetic deafness and fear-related behaviors in nervous pointer dogs. Physiol Behav 1988; 43(3):307.
227. Knowles KE, Cash WC, Blanch BS: Auditory-evoked responses of dogs with different hearing abilities. Can J Vet Res 1988; 52(3):394.
228. Koch SA: Fly biters. J Am Vet Med Assoc 1980; 176(1):22.
229. Koch SA, Rubin LR: Distribution of cones in retina of the normal dog. Am J Vet Res 1972; 33(2):361.
230. Korsgaard S, Povlsen UJ, Randrup A: Effects of apomorphine and haloperidol on "spontaneous" stereotyped licking behavior in the Cebus monkey. Psychopharmacology 1985; 85:240.
231. Krestel D, Passe D, Smith JC, et al: Behavioral determination of olfactory thresholds to amylacetate in dogs. Neurosci Biobehav Rev 1984; 8(2):169.
232. Krushinskii LV, Fless DA: Strengthening of olfaction in police dogs. Pavlov J Higher Nerv Act 1959; 9:266.
233. Landsberg G: Products for preventing or controlling undesirable behavior. Vet Med 1994; 89(10):970.
234. Landsberg G: Behavior problems in the geriatric dog and cat. Friskies PetCare Symposium: Small Anim Behav Proc 1998:37.
235. Landsberg G: The summit on internal medicine. Part II: Behavior medicine. Vet Forum December 1998:47.
236. Landsberg G: Therapeutic options for cognitive decline in senior pets. J Am Anim Hosp Assoc 2006; 42(6):407.
237. Landsberg G, Araujo JA, Miolo A: Objective assessment of a proprietary neuroprotective nutraceutical on short-term memory of aged dogs. In Landsberg G, Mattiello S, Mills D (eds): Proceedings of the 6th International Veterinary Behaviour Meeting and European College of Veterinary Behavioural Medicine-Companion Animals European Society of Veterinary Clinical Ethology. Brescia, Italy: Fondazione Iniziative Zooprofilattiche e Zootecniche, 2007, p. 154.
238. Landsberg GM: Veterinarians as behavior consultants. Can Vet J 1990; 31:225.
239. Landsberg GM: The distribution of canine behavior cases at three behavior-referral practices. Vet Med 1991; 86(10):1011.
240. Landsberg GM: Clomipramine—Beyond separation anxiety. J Am Anim Hosp Assoc 2001; 37(4):313.
241. Landsberg GM: Senior pet anxiety disorders. Am Vet Med Assoc Conv Proc, July 2006.
242. Landsberg GM: Role of medical problems in the development of anxiety in pets. Am Vet Med Assoc Conv Proc, 2007.
243. Lawrence J, Bautista J, Hicks RA: Arousability and eye color: A test of Worthy's hypothesis. Percept Motor Skills 1994; 78(1):143.
244. Lehner PN, Krumm R, Cringan AT: Tests for olfactory repellents for coyotes and dogs. J Wildl Manage 1976; 40:145.
245. LeMoal M: Mesocorticolimbic dopaminergic neurons: Functional and regulatory roles. In Bloom FE, Kupfer DJ (eds): Psychopharmacology: The Fourth Generation of Progress. New York: Raven Press Ltd, 1995, p. 283.
246. Lessac MS, Solomon RL: Effects of early isolation on the later adaptive behavior of beagles: A methodological demonstration. Dev Psychol 1969; 1(1):14.

247. Leveque NW: Cognitive dysfunction in dogs, cats an Alzheimer's-like disease. J Am Vet Med Assoc 1988; 212(9):1351.

248. Levine ED, Mills DS: One year follow-up study on the efficacy of a treatment program for dogs with fear of firework noise. Am Coll Vet Behav/Am Vet Soc Anim Behav Scientific Session 2007:15.

249. Levine ED, Ramos D, Mills DS: The treatment of feara of fireworks in dogs *(Canis familiaris)*: A prospective study. In Mills D, Levine E, Landsberg G, et al (eds): Current Issues and Research in Veterinary Behavioral Medicine. West Lafayette, IN: Purdue University Press, 2005, p. 211.

250. Liang B, Verrier RL, Melman J, et al: Correlation between circulating catecholamine levels and ventricular vulnerability during psychological stress in conscious dogs. Proc Soc Exper BioI Med 1979; 161(3):266.

251. Light GS, Hardie EM, Young MS, et al: Pain and anxiety behaviors of dogs during intravenous catheterization after premedication with placebo, acepromazine, or oxymorphone. Appl Anim Behav Sci 1993; 37(4):331.

252. Lipman EA, Grassi JR: Comparative auditory sensitivity of man and dog. Am J Psychol 1942; 55:84.

253. Lit L, Crawford CA: Effects of training paradigms on search dog performance. Appl Anim Behav Sci 2006; 98:277.

254. Losier BJ, McGrath PJ, Klein RM: Error patterns on the continuous performance test in non-medicated and medicated samples of children with and without ADHD: A meta-analytic review. J Child Psychol Psychiatry 1996; 37(8):971.

255. Lott D, Hart BL, Verosub KL, et al: Is unusual animal behavior observed before earthquakes? Yes and no. DVM 1980; 11(3):65.

256. Luescher A: Compulsive behavior in companion animals. In Houpt KA (ed): Recent Advances in Companion Animal Behavior Problems, International Veterinary Information Service. www.ivis.org, 9/22/2000, p. 198.

257. Luescher UA: Conflict, stereotypic and compulsive behavior. American Veterinary Medical Association meeting, San Francisco, July 9, 1994.

258. Luescher UA: Compulsive behavior in dogs. Friskies PetCare Symposium: Small Animal Behavior Proceedings1998:9.

259. Luescher UA: Compulsive behavior in dogs. http://www.vetshow.com/friskies/comp.htm, 2/18/2000.

260. Luescher UA: Compulsive behaviour. In Horwitz DF, Mills DS, Heath S (eds): BSAVA Manual of Canine and Feline Behavioural Medicine. Quedgeley, Gloucester, England: British Small Animal Veterinary Association, 2002, p. 229.

261. Luescher UA: Diagnosis and management of compulsive disorders in dogs and cats. Vet Clin North Am [Small Anim Pract] 2003; 33(2):253.

262. Luescher UA, McKeown DB, Halip J: Stereotypic or obsessive-compulsive disorders in dogs and cats. Vet Clin North Am [Small Anim Pract] 1991; 21(2):401.

263. Luescher UA, Medlock T, Beck AM: The effects of training and environmental alterations on adoption success of shelter dogs. In Landsberg G, Mattiello S, Mills D (eds): Proceedings of the 6th International Veterinary Behaviour Meeting and European College of Veterinary Behavioural Medicine-Companion Animals European Society of Veterinary Clinical Ethology. Brescia, Italy: Fondazione Iniziative Zooprofilattiche e Zootecniche, 2007, p. 57.

264. MacKenzie SA, Oltenacu EAB, Leighton E: Heritability estimate for temperament scores in German shepherd dogs and its genetic correlation with hip dysplasia. Behav Genet 1985; 15(5):475.

265. Mackintosh NJ, Wilson B, Boakes RA: Differences in mechanisms of intelligence among vertebrates. Phil Trans Roy Soc Lond B 1985; 308:53.

266. Macphail EM: Vertebrate intelligence: The null hypothesis. Phil Trans Roy Soc Lond B 1985; 308:37.

267. Mandelker L: Clinical use of piperacetazine to modify behavior in dogs and cats: A practitioner's viewpoint. Vet Med Small Anim Clin 1979; 74(4):505.

268. Manteca X: Fly snapping syndrome in dogs. Vet Q 1994; 16(51):495.

269. Marlois N: Hyperactivity in dogs, a model for human pathology: Discrepancies between different approaches. Proc Third International Cong Vet Behav Med 2001:212.

270. Marr JN: Varying stimulation and imprinting in dogs. J Gen Psychol 1964; 104:351.

271. Mason GJ: Stereotypies: A critical review. Anim Behav 1991; 41:1015.

272. Mason MM, Scheflen AM: Senility in dogs. Cornell Vet 1953; 43:10.

273. Maurer BM, Dodman NH: Animal behavior case of the month. J Am Vet Med Assoc 2007; 231(4):536.

274. McCobb EC, Brown EA, Damiani K, et al: Thunderstorm phobia in dogs: An internet survey of 69 cases. J Am Anim Hosp Assoc 2001; 37(4):319.

275. McConnell PB: Acoustic structure and receiver response in domestic dogs. *Canis familiaris*. Anim Behav 1990; 39(5):897.

276. McCulloch M, Jezierski T, Broffman M, et al: Diagnostic accuracy of canine scent detection in early- and late-stage lung and breast cancers. Integrative Cancer Therapies 2006; 5(1):30.

277. McKeown DB, Luescher UA, Halip J: Stereotypies in companion animals and obsessive-compulsive disorders. Purina Specialty Review in Behavioral Problems in Small Animals 1992:30.

278. Meaney MJ, Aitken DH, van Berkel C, et al: Effect of neonatal handling on age-related impairments associated with the hippocampus. SCI 1988; 239:766.

279. Melzack R: The genesis of emotional behavior: An experimental study of the dog. J Comp Physiol Psycho I 1954; 47:166.

280. Melzack R, Scott TH: The effects of early experience on the response to pain. J Comp Physiol Psychol 1957; 50:155.

281. Messonnier S: Canine senile dementia: Does it exist? Texas Vet Med J 1991; 53(3):22.

282. Micaleff J, Blin O: Neurobiology and clinical pharmacology of obsessive-compulsive disorder. Clin Neuropharmacol 2001; 24(4):191.

283. Milgram NW, Head E, Cotman CW, et al: Age dependent cognitive dysfunction in canines: Dietary intervention. Proc Third International Cong Vet Behav Med, Wheathampstead, Herts, UK: Universities Federation for Animal Welfare, 2001, p. 53.

284. Milgram NW, Head E, Muggenburg B, et al: Landmark discrimination learning in the dog; effects of age, an antioxidant fortified food, and cognitive strategy. Neurosci Biobehav Rev 2002; 26:679.

285. Milgram NW, Head E, Weiner E, et al: Cognitive functions and aging in the dog: Acquisition of nonspatial visual tasks. Behav Neurosci 1994; 108(1):57.

286. Milgram NW, Head E, Zicker SC, et al: Long-term treatment with antioxidants and a program of behavioral enrichment reduces age-dependent impairment in discrimination and reversal learning in beagle dogs. Exp Gerontol 2004; 39:753.

287. Milgram NW, Ivy GO, Head E, et al: The effect of L-deprenyl on behavior, cognitive function, and biogenic amines in the dog. Neurochemical Res 1993; 18(12):1211.

288. Milgram NW, Siwak CT, Gruet P, et al: Oral administration of adrafinil improves discrimination learning in aged Beagle dogs. Pharmacol Biochem Beh 2000; 66(2):301.

289. Milgram NW, Zicker SC, Head EA, et al: Dietary enrichment counteracts age-associated cognitive dysfunction in canines. Neurobiol Aging 2002; 23:737.

290. Miller PE, Murphy CJ: Vision in dogs. J Am Vet Med Assoc 1995; 207(12):1623.

291. Millot JL, Filiatre JC, Eckerlin A, et al: Olfactory cues in the relations between children and their pet dogs. Appl Anim Behav Sci 1987; 19(1-2):189.

292. Mills DS: Welfare considerations relevant to the treatment of stereotypies in companion animals. Newsl Am Vet Soc Anim Behav 1997; 19(2):6.

293. Mills DS: Noise fears. E-mail correspondence to Am Vet Soc Anim Behav listserve, 6/15/2004.

294. Mills DS, Ledger RA: Oral selegiline hydrochloride improves attention in the dog to signals of reward during training. Proc Third International Cong Vet Behav Med, Wheathampstead, Herts, UK: Universities Federation for Animal Welfare, 2001, p. 200.

295. Mills DS, Ramos D, Estelles MG, et al: A triple blind placebo-controlled investigation into the assessment of the effect of Dog Appeasing Pheromone (DAP) on anxiety related behaviour of problem dogs in the veterinary clinic. Appl Anim Behav Sci 2006; 98:114.

296. Miolo A, Re G: Emerging role of polyphenols ginkgo biloba and resveratrol as neuroprotectors in brain aging of dogs and cats: A review. In Landsberg G, Mattiello S, Mills D (eds): Proceedings of the 6th International Veterinary Behaviour Meeting and European College of Veterinary Behavioural Medicine-Companion Animals European Society of Veterinary Clinical Ethology. Brescia, Italy: Fondazione Iniziative Zooprofilattiche e Zootecniche, 2007, p. 129.

297. Moberg GP: Problems in defining stress and distress in animals. J Am Vet Med Assoc 1987; 191(10):1207.

298. Moon BJ, Feigenbaum JJ, Carson PE, et al: The role of dopaminergic mechanisms in naloxone-induced inhibition of apomorphine-induced stereotyped behavior. Eur J Pharmacol 1980; 61:71.

299. Morgan JL, Coulter DB, Marshall AE, et al: Effects of neomycin on the waveform of auditory-evoked brain stem potentials in dogs. Am J Vet Res 1980; 41:1077.

300. Moulton DG: Factors influencing odor sensitivity in the dog. Air Force Office of Scientific Research, October 1972.

301. Moulton DG, Ashton EH, Eayrs JT: Studies in olfactory acuity. 4. Relative delectability of N-aliphatic acids by the dog. Anim Behav 1960; 8:117.

302. Muller G: Pseudo phobias in dogs. Proc Third International Cong Vet Behav Med, Wheathampstead, Herts, UK: Universities Federation for Animal Welfare, 2001, p.114.

303. Murphree OD, Dykman RA: Litter patterns in the offspring of nervous and stable dogs. I. Behavioral tests. J Nerv Ment Dis 1965; 141(3):321.

304. Myers LJ: Dysosmia of the dog in clinical veterinary medicine. Prog Vet Neurol 1990; 1(2):171.

305. Myers LJ: Use of innate behaviors to evaluate sensory function in the dog. Vet Clin North Am [Small Anim Pract] 1991; 21(2):389.

306. Myers LJ: Personal communication, October 18, 2006.

307. Myers LJ, Hanrahan LA, Swango L, et al: Anosmia associated with canine distemper. Am J Vet Res 1988; 49(8):1295.

308. Myers LJ, Nusbaum KE, Swango LJ, et al: Dysfunction of the sense of smell caused by canine parainfluenza virus infection in dogs. Am J Vet Res 1988; 49:188.

309. Myers LJ, Pugh R: Thresholds of the dog for detection of inhaled eugenol and benzaldehyde determined by electro-encephalographic and behavioral olfactometry. Am J Vet Res 1985; 46(11):2409.

310. Neer TM: Complex partial seizures (behavioral epilepsy). Texas Veterinary Medical Association Summer Seminar, Corpus Christi, August 6, 1995.

311. Neilson JC: The anxious animal. Wild West Veterinary Conference Veterinary Syllabus 2002:595.

312. Neilson JC: Fear of places or things. In Horwitz DF, Mills DS, Heath S (eds): BSAVA Manual of Canine and Feline Behavioural Medicine. Quedgeley, Gloucester, England: British Small Animal Veterinary Association, 2002, p. 173.

313. Neilson JC, Hart BL, Cliff KD, et al: Prevalence of behavioral changes associated with age-related cognitive impairment in dogs. J Am Vet Med Assoc 2001; 218(11):1787.

314. Neitz J, Geist T, Jacobs GH: Color vision in the dog. Vis Neurosci 1989; 3:119.

315. Newton JEO, Dykman RA, Chapin JL: The prediction of abnormal behavior from autonomic indices in dogs. J Nerv Ment Dis 1978; 166(9):635.

316. Newton JEO, Lucas LA: Differential heart-rate responses to person in nervous and normal Pointer dogs. Behav Genet 1982; 12(4):379.

317. Niebuhr BR, Nobbe DE: Shock collars. Canine Pract 1979; 6(1):4.

318. Nobbe DE, Niebuhr BR, Levinson M, et al: Use of time-out as punishment for aggressive behavior. Canine Pract 1978; 5(2):12.

319. Noonan GJ, Rand JS, Blackshaw JK, et al: Behavioural observations of puppies undergoing tail docking. Appl Anim Behav Sci 1996; 49(4):335.

320. Norris MP, Beaver BV: Application of behavior therapy techniques to the treatment of obesity in companion animals. J Am Vet Med Assoc 1993; 202(5):728.

321. Odom JV, Bromberg NM, Dawson WW: Canine visual acuity: Retinal and cortical field potentials evoked by pattern stimulation. Am J Physiol 1983; 245:R637.

322. O'Farrell V: Owner attitudes and dog behaviour problems. Appl Anim Behav Sci 1997; 52(3-4):205.

323. Ofri R, Dawson WW, Gelatt KN: Visual resolution in normal and glaucomatous dogs determined by pattern electroretinogram. Prog Vet Comp Ophthalmol 1993; 3(3):111.

324. Ogata N, Vandeloo J, Kikusui T, et al: Predicting the outcome of detector dog training based on their behaviour and genetic characteristics. In Landsberg G, Mattiello S, Mills D (eds): Proceedings of the 6th International Veterinary Behaviour Meeting and European College of Veterinary

Behavioural Medicine-Companion Animals European Society of Veterinary Clinical Ethology. Brescia, Italy: Fondazione Iniziative Zooprofilattiche e Zootecniche, 2007, p. 55.

325. Ogburn P, Crouse S, Martin F, et al: Comparison of behavioral and physiological responses of dogs wearing two different types of collars. Appl Anim Behav Sci 1998; 61(2):133.

326. Osella MC, Girardi C, Re G, et al: Evaluation of age-related cognitive impairment in pet dogs. In Landsberg G, Mattiello S, Mills D (eds): Proceedings of the 6th International Veterinary Behaviour Meeting and European College of Veterinary Behavioural Medicine-Companion Animals European Society of Veterinary Clinical Ethology. Brescia, Italy: Fondazione Iniziative Zooprofilattiche e Zootecniche, 2007, p. 64.

327. Osella MC, Odore R, Badino P, et al: Plasma dopamine neurophysiological correlates in anxious dogs. In Mills D, Levine E, Landsberg G, et al (eds): Current Issues and Research in Veterinary Behavioral Medicine. West Lafayette, IN: Purdue University Press, 2005, p. 274.

328. Osella MC, Re G, Badino P, et al: Phosphatidylserine: A novel nutraceutical weapon against brain aging in dogs and cats. In Landsberg G, Mattiello S, Mills D (eds): Proceedings of the 6th International Veterinary Behaviour Meeting and European College of Veterinary Behavioural Medicine-Companion Animals European Society of Veterinary Clinical Ethology. Brescia, Italy: Fondazione Iniziative Zooprofilattiche e Zootecniche, 2007, p. 161.

329. Osella MC, Re G, Odore R, et al: Canine cognitive dysfunction: Prevalence, clinical signs and treatment with a nutraceutical. In Mills D, Levine E, Landsberg G, et al (eds): Current Issues and Research in Veterinary Behavioral Medicine. West Lafayette, IN: Purdue University Press, 2005, p. 66.

330. Osthaus B, Lea SEG, Slater AM: Dogs *(Canis lupus familiaris)* fail to show understanding of means-end connection in a string-pulling task. Anim Cognition 2005; 8:37.

331. O'Sullivan G, Noshirvani H, Marks I, et al: Six-year follow-up after exposure and clomipramine therapy for obsessive-compulsive disorder. J Clin Psychiatry 1991; 52:150.

332. Overall K: Temperament testing and training: Do they prevent behavioral problems? Canine Pract 1994; 19(4):19.

333. Overall K: Combination of therapies could help shy Cairn Terrier; elderly owners at a loss. DVM 1995; 26(4):20S.

334. Overall K: Puppy temperament testing. APDT Newsl July/August 2000:16.

335. Overall KL: Preventing behavior problems: Early prevention and recognition in puppies and kittens. Purina Specialty Review: Behavioral Problems in Small Animals 1992:13.

336. Overall KL: Part 1: A rational approach: Recognition, diagnosis and management of obsessive-compulsive disorders. Canine Pract 1992; 17(2):40.

337. Overall KL: Part 2: A rational approach: Recognition, diagnosis and management of obsessive-compulsive disorders. Canine Pract 1992; 17(3):25.

338. Overall KL: Use of clomipramine to treat ritualistic stereotypic motor behavior in three dogs. J Am Vet Med Assoc 1994; 205(12):1733.

339. Overall KL: Understanding repetitive, stereotypic behaviors: Signs, history, diagnosis, and practical treatment. Talk at the American Veterinary Medical Association Convention, July 8, 1995.

340. Overall KL: Pharmacological treatment of fears and anxieties. Am Vet Med Assoc Convention Notes 1997:145.

341. Overall KL: Clinical Behavioral Medicine. St. Louis: Mosby, 1997.

342. Overall KL: The role of pharmacotherapy in treating dogs with dominance aggression. Vet Med 1999; 94(12):1049.

343. Overall KL: Early intervention and prevention of behavior problems. Step 1: The owner and pet must match. Vet Forum May 2001:42.

344. Overall KL: Noise phobias in dogs. In Horwitz DF, Mills DS, Heath S (eds): BSAVA Manual of Canine and Feline Behavioural Medicine. Quedgeley, Gloucester, England: British Small Animal Veterinary Association, 2002, p. 164.

345. Overall KL: Phenomenology, breed, age of onset, and outcome in dogs and cats with obsessive-compulsive disorder. Am Vet Soc Anim Behav Annual Symp Anim Behav Res Proc 2002:69.

346. Overall KL: Evaluation and management of behavioral conditions. http://www.ivis.org/special_books/braund/overall/chapter_frm.asp?LA=1, 9/17/2002.

347. Overall KL, Dunham AE: Clinical features and outcome in dogs and cats with obsessive-compulsive disorder: 126 cases (1989-2000). J Am Vet Med Assoc 2002; 221(10):1445.

348. Overall KL, Dunham AE: Behavioral responses to a physiologically provocative test for anxiety: Sentinel signs and concurrence with physiological changes. Proc AVSAB Annual Paper Presentations 2003:12.

349. Pageat P: Description, clinical, and histological validation of the A.R.C.A.D. score (evaluation of Age-Related Cognitive and Affective Disorders). Proc Third International Cong Vet Behav Med 2001:83.

350. Pageat P: Assessing prolactinaemia in anxious dogs *(Canis familiaris)*: Interest in diagnostic value and use in the selection of the most appropriate psychotropic drug. In Mills D, Levine E, Landsberg G, et al (eds): Current Issues and Research in Veterinary Behavioral Medicine. West Lafayette, IN: Purdue University Press, 2005, p. 155.

351. Parker AJ: Behavioral signs of organic disease. In Ettinger SJ (ed): Textbook of Veterinary Internal Medicine. Philadelphia: Saunders, 1989, p. 70.

352. Parker AJ: Behavioral changes of organic neurologic origin. Prog Vet Neurol 1990; 1(2):123.

353. Passe DH, Walker JC: Odor psychophysics in vertebrates. Neurosci Biobehav Rev 1985; 9:431.

354. Pauli AM, Bentley E, Diehl KA, et al: Effects of the application of neck pressure by a collar or harness on intraocular pressure in dogs. J Am Anim Hosp Assoc 2006; 42(3):207.

355. Perlson J: The Dog: An Historical, Psychological and Personality Study. New York: Vantage Press, 1968.

356. Perse T: Obsessive-compulsive disorder: A treatment review. J Clin Psychiatry 1988; 49(2):48.

357. Peterson EA, Heaton WC, Wruble SD: Levels of auditory response in fissiped carnivores. J Mammal 1969; 50(3):566.

358. Pfaffenberger CJ, Scott JP: The relationship between delayed socialization and trainability in guide dogs. J Genet Psychol 1959; 95:145.

359. Pi WP, Peng MT: Functional development of the central emetic mechanism in the puppy dog. Proc Soc Exper Biol Med 1971; 136(3):802.

360. Pickel D, Manucy GP, Walker DB, et al: Evidence for canine olfactory detection of melanoma. Appl Anim Behav Sci 2004; 89:107.

361. Pigott TA, Pato MT, Bernstein SE, et al: Controlled comparisons of clomipramine and fluoxetine in the treatment of obsessive-compulsive disorder. Arch Gen Psychiatry 1990; 47:926.

362. Polsky RH: Electronic shock collars: Are they worth the risks? J Am Anim Hosp Assoc 1994; 30(5):463.

363. Poncelet LC, Coppens AG, Meuris SI, et al: Maturation of the auditory system in clinically normal puppies as reflected by the brain stem auditory-evoked potential wave V latency-intensity curve and rerefaction-condensation differential potentials. Am J Vet Res 2000; 61(11):1343.

364. Pongrácz P, Miklósi Á, Vida V, et al: The pet dogs ability for learning from a human demonstrator in a detour task in independent from the breed and age. Appl Anim Behav Sci 2005; 90:309.

365. Pownall R, Crighton GW: Factors influencing body temperature in newborn dogs. Br Vet J 1977; 133:191.

366. Prince JH: Comparative Anatomy of the Eye. Springfield, IL: Charles C Thomas, 1956.

367. Prince JH, Diesem CD, Eglitis I, et al: Anatomy and Histology of the Eye and Orbit in Domestic Animals. Springfield, IL: Charles C Thomas, 1960.

368. Radinsky LB: Outlines of canid and felid brain evolution. Ann N Y Acad Sci 1969; 167(1):277.

369. Ramos-Remus C, González-Castañeda RE, González-Perez O, et al: Prednisone induces cognitive dysfunction, neuronal degeneration, and reactive gliosis in rats. J Investigative Med 2002; 50(6):458.

370. Rapoport JL, Buchsbaum MS, Weingartner H, et al: Dextroamphetamine. Its cognitive and behavioral effects in normal and hyperactive boys and normal men. Arch Gen Psychiatry 1980; 37(8):933.

371. Rapoport JL, Buchsbaum MS, Zahn TP, et al: Dextroamphetamine: Cognitive and behavior effects in normal prepubertal boys. SCI 1978; 199:565.

372. Rapoport JL, Ryland DH, Kriete M: Drug treatment of canine acral lick: An animal model of obsessive-compulsive disorder. Arch Gen Psychiatry 1992; 49:517.

373. Reed AB: Fear of thunderstorms, rain. Canine Pract 1977; 4(4):6.

374. Reisner IR: Diagnosis of canine generalized anxiety disorder and its short-term management with paroxetine. Proc Am College Vet Behavior Scientific Paper Session, 2003.

375. Roe DJ, Sales GD: Welfare implications of ultrasonic flea collars. Vet Rec 1992; 130(7):142.

376. Rooney NJ, Bradshaw JWS, Robinson IH: A comparison of dog-dog and dog-human play behaviour. Appl Anim Behav Sci 2000; 66(3):235.

377. Rossier J, French ED, Rivier C, et al: Foot-shock induced stress increases beta-endorphin levels in blood but not brain. Nature 1977; 270:618.

378. Rostain AL: Attention deficit disorders in children and adolescents. Pediatr Clin North Am 1991; 38(3):607.

379. Roudebush P, Zicker SC, Cotman CW, et al: Nutritional management of brain aging in dogs. J Am Vet Med Assoc 2005; 227(5):722.

380. Ruehl WW: Rationale to develop the investigational drug L-deprenyl for use in pet dogs. Am Vet Soc Anim Behav Newsl 1993; 15(1):4.

381. Ruehl WW: Treatment of geriatric behavior problems. Am Vet Med Assoc Convention Notes 1997:172.

382. Ruehl WW, Bruyett DS, DePaoli A, et al: Canine cognitive dysfunction as a model for human age-related cognitive decline, dementia and Alzheimer's disease: Clinical presentation, cognitive testing, pathology and response to L-deprenyl therapy. Prog Brain Res 1995; 106:217.

383. Ruehl WW, Bruyette DS, Entriken TL, et al: Adrenal axis dysregulation in geriatric dogs with cognitive dysfunction. J Vet Intern Med 1997:119.

384. Ruehl WW, DePaoli AC, Bruyette DS: L-Deprenyl for treatment of behavioral and cognitive problems in dogs: Preliminary report of an open-label trial. Appl Anim Behav Sci 1994; 39:191.

385. Ruehl WW, Hart BL: Canine cognitive dysfunction. In Dodman NH, Shuster L (eds): Pharmacology of Animal Behavior Disorders. Boston: Blackwell Science, 1998, p. 283.

386. Sadowski B: Intracranial self-stimulation patterns in dogs. Physiol Behav 1972; 8(2):189.

387. Sawyer DC: Pain control in small-animal patients. Appl Anim Behav Sci 1998; 59(1-3):135.

388. Schilder MBH, van der Borg JAM: Training dogs with help of the shock collar: Short and long term behavioural effects. Appl Anim Behav Sci 2004; 85:319.

389. Schoon GAA: Scent identification lineups by dogs (Canis familiaris): Experimental design and forensic application. Appl Anim Behav Sci 1996; 49(3):257.

390. Schroll S, Dehasse J, Palme R, et al: The use of the DAP collar to reduce stress during training of police dogs (Canis familiaris): A preliminary study. In Mills D, Levine E, Landsberg G, et al (eds): Current Issues and Research in Veterinary Behavioral Medicine. West Lafayette, IN: Purdue University Press, 2005, p. 31.

391. Scott JP: The effects of selection and domestication upon the behavior of the dog. J Natl Cancer Inst 1954; 15(3):739.

392. Scott JP: Critical periods in behavioral development. SCI 1962; 138(3544):949.

393. Scott JP, Fuller JL: Genetics and the Social Behavior of the Dog. Chicago: University of Chicago Press, 1965.

394. Serpell J, Jogoe JA: Early experience and the development of behaviour. In Serpell J (ed): The Domestic Dog: Its Evolution, Behaviour and Interactions with People. Cambridge, England: Cambridge University Press, 1995, p. 79.

395. Serpell JA, Hsu Y: Development and validation of a novel method for evaluating behavior and temperament in guide dogs. Appl Anim Behav Sci 2001; 72(4):347.

396. Settle RH, Sommerville BA, McCormick J, et al: Human scent matching using specially trained dogs. Anim Behav 1994; 48(6):1443.

397. Sherman SM, Wilson JR: Behavioral and morphological evidence for binocular competition in the postnatal development of the dog's visual system. J Comp Neurol 1975; 161:183.

398. Short CE: Fundamentals of pain perception in animals. Appl Anim Behav Sci 1998; 59(1-3):125.

399. Shull E: Personal communication. July 15, 2001.

400. Shull-Selcer EA, Stagg W: Advances in the understanding and treatment of noise phobias. Vet Clin North Am [Small Anim Pract] 1991; 21(2):353.

401. Simpson BS: Clinical treatment of thunderstorm phobia. http://www.avma.org/conv/cv2002/cvnotes/CAn_AnB_CTT_SiB.asp, 7/3/2002.

402. Simpson ST, Myers LJ: Dysosmia caused by encephalitis in a dog. J Am Vet Med Assoc 1987; 191(12):1593.

403. Sims MH, Shull-Selcer E: Electrodiagnostic evaluation of deafness in two English Setter littermates. J Am Vet Med Assoc 1985; 187(4):398.

404. Siwak CT, Gruet P, Woehrlé F, et al: Behavioral activating effects of adrafinil in aged canines. Pharmacol Biochem Behav 2000; 66(2):293.

405. Siwak CT, Gruet P, Woehrlé F, et al: Comparison of effects of adrafinil, propentofylline, and nicergoline on behavior in aged dogs. Am J Vet Res 2000; 61(11):1410.

406. Siwak CT, Tapp PD, Milgram NW: Age-associated changes in non-cognitive behaviours in a canine model of aging. Proc Third International Cong Vet Behav Med 2001:133.

407. Skoumalova A, Rofina J, Schwippelova Z, et al: The role of free radicles in canine counterpart of senile dementia of the Alzheimer type. Exper Gerontology 2003; 38(6):711.

408. Slabbert JM: Observational learning of an acquired maternal behaviour pattern by working dog pups: An alternative training method? Appl Anim Behav Sci 1997; 53(4):309.

409. Slabbert JM, Odendaal JSJ: Early prediction of adult police dog efficiency—a longitudinal study. Appl Anim Behav Sci 1999; 64(4):269.

410. Smith DA, Ralls K, Davenport B, et al: Canine assistants for conservationists. SCI 2001; 291:435.

411. Smythe RH: Vision in the Animal World. New York: St. Martin's Press, 1975.

412. Solanto MV: Neuropsychopharmacological mechanisms of stimulant drug action in attention-deficit hyperactivity disorder: A review and integration. Behav Brain Res 1998; 94(1):127.

413. Solomon RL, Kamin LJ, Wynne LC: Traumatic avoidance learning: The outcomes of several extinction procedures with dogs. In Hendersen RW (ed): Learning in Animals. Stroudsburg, PA: Hutchinson Ross Publishing Co, 1982, p. 221.

414. Sommerville BA, Green MA, Gee DJ: Using chromatography and a dog to identify some of the compounds in human sweat which are under genetic influence. In Macdonald DW, Müller-Schwarze D, Natynczuk SE (eds): Chemical Signals in Vertebrates 5. New York: Oxford University Press, 1990, p. 634.

415. Sommi RW, Crismon ML, Bowden CL: Fluoxetine: A serotonin-specific, second-generation antidepressant. Pharmacotherapy 1987; 7(1):1.

416. Spreat S, Spreat SR: Learning principles. Vet Clin North Am [Small Anim Pract] 1982; 12(4):593.

417. Stanley WC, Bacon WE, Fehr C: Discriminated instrumental learning in neonatal dogs. J Comp Physiol Psychol 1970; 70(3):335.

418. Stanley WC, Barrett JE, Bacon WE: Conditioning and extinction of avoidance and escape behavior in neonatal dogs. J Comp Physiol Psychol 1974; 87(1):163.

419. Stanley WC, Cornwell AC, Poggiani C, et al: Conditioning in the neonate puppy. J Comp Physiol Psychol 1963; 56(1):211.

420. Steen JB, Wilsson E: How do dogs determine the direction of tracks? Acta Physiol Scand 1990; 139:531.

421. Steiss JE, Wright JC, Storrs DP: Alterations in brain stem auditory evoked response threshold and latency-intensity curve associated with conductive hearing loss in dogs. Prog Vet Neurol 1990; 1(2):205.

422. Stoddart DM: The Ecology of Vertebrate Olfaction. New York: Chapman and Hall, 1980.

423. Stoddart DM: Olfaction in Mammals. New York: Academic Press, 1980.

424. Svartberg K: A comparison of behaviour in test and in everyday life: Evidence of three consistent boldness-related personality traits in dogs. Appl Anim Behav Sci 2005; 91:103.

425. Svartberg K, Tapper I, Temrin H, et al: Consistency of personality traits in dogs. Anim Behav 2005; 69(2):283.

426. Tancer ME, Stein MB, Bessette BB, et al: Behavioral effects of chronic imipramine treatment in genetically nervous pointer dogs. Physiol Behav 1990; 48(1):179.

427. Tapp PD, Siwak CT, Head E, et al: Sex differences in the effect of oestrogen on size discrimination learning and spatial memory. Proc Third International Cong Vet Behav Med, Wheathampstead, Herts, UK: Universities Federation for Animal Welfare, 2001, p. 136.

428. Tapp PD, Siwak CT, Head E, et al: Concept abstraction in the aging dog: Development of a protocol using successive discrimination and size concept tasks. Behav Brain Res 2004; 153:199.

429. Thesen A, Steen JB, Døving KB: Behaviour of dogs during olfactory tracking. J Exp Biol 1993; 180:247.

430. Tillung RH: Reward is suitable to achieve an obedient dog. Abstract, Master's Thesis, The Norwegian University of Life Sciences, August 21, 2006.

431. Tod E, Brander D, Waran N: Efficacy of dog appeasing pheromone in reducing stress and fear related behaviour in shelter dogs. Appl Anim Behav Sci 2005; 93:295.

432. Toner BS, Miller Jr DI: Olfactory discrimination of individual human odors using experienced tracking police workdogs. Anim Behav Consult Newsl 1993; 10(4):2.

433. Tonosaki K, Tucker D: Responsiveness of the olfactory receptor cells in dog to some odors. Comp Biochem Physiol 1985; 81(1):7.

434. Topál J, Miklósi Á, Csányi V: Dog-human relationship affects problem solving behavior in the dog. Anthrozoös 1997; 10(4):214.

435. Tortora DF: Understanding electronic dog training: Part 3. Canine Pract 1982; 9(4):8.

436. Towbin KE, Leckman JF: Attention deficit hyperactivity disorder in childhood and adolescence. In Klawans HL, Goetz CG, Tanner CM (eds): Textbook of Clinical Neuropharmacology and Therapeutics, 2nd ed. New York: Raven Press Ltd, 1992, p. 323.

437. Townsend RE, Johnson LC: Relation of frequency-analyzed EEG to monitoring behavior. Electroenceph Clin Neurophysiol 1979; 47(3):272.

438. Tuber DS, Hothersall D, Peters MF: Treatment of fears and phobias in dogs. Vet Clin North Am [Small Anim Pract] 1982; 12(4):607.

439. Tunturi AR: Audio frequency localization in the acoustic cortex of the dog. Am J Physiol 1944; 141:397.

440. Tunturi AR: Analysis of cortical auditory responses with the probability pulse. Am J Physiol 1955; 181:630.

441. Voith VL: Learning principles and behavioral problems. Mod Vet Pract 1979; 60(7):553.

442. Voith VL: Treatment of phobias. Mod Vet Pract 1979; 60(9):721.

443. Voith VL: Behavioural problems. In Chandler EA, Evans JM, Singleton WB, et al (eds): Canine Medicine and

Therapeutics. Oxford, England: Blackwell Scientific, 1979, p. 395.

444. Voith VL: Play: A form of hyperactivity and aggression. Mod Vet Pract 1980; 61(7):631.

445. Voith VL: Hyperactivity and hyperkinesis. Mod Vet Pract 1980; 61(9):787.

446. Voith VL: Behavioral disorders. In Ettinger S (ed): Textbook of Veterinary Internal Medicine. Philadelphia: Saunders, 1989, p. 227.

447. Voith VL, Borchelt P: Fears and phobias in companion animals. Compend Contin Educ 1985; 7(3):209.

448. Voith VL, Borchelt PL: Fear of Thunder and Other Loud Noises. Kankakee, IL: Veterinary Learning Systems, 1985.

449. Voith VL, Marder A: Overactivity. In Morgan R (ed): Handbook of Small Animal Practice. New York: Churchill Livingstone, 1988, p. 1036.

450. Volhard J, Fisher GT: Training Your Dog: The Step-by-Step Manual. New York: Howell Book House, 1983.

451. Vollmer PJ: Conditioned avoidance response to the veterinary clinic in dogs. Vet Med Small Anim Clin 1977; 72(11):1719.

452. Vollmer PJ: The new puppy. 2. Preventing problems through thoughtful selection. Vet Med Small Anim Clin 1978; 73(1):31.

453. Vollmer PJ: Puppy rearing. 9. Early stimulation. Vet Med Small Anim Clin 1979; 74(3):307.

454. Vollmer PJ: Electrical stimulation as an aid in training: Part 1. Vet Med Small Anim Clin 1979; 74(11):1598.

455. Volokhov AA: Comparative-physiological investigation of conditioned and unconditioned reflexes during ontogeny. Pavlov J Higher Nerv Act 1959; 9:49.

456. Walker AD: Taste preferences in the domestic dog and cat. Gaines Dog Research Progress Summer 1975:1.

457. Walls GL: The Vertebrate Eye and Its Adaptive Radiation. New York: Hafner Publishing Co, 1967.

458. Warden CJ: Animal intelligence. Sci Am 1951; 184:64.

459. Washburn MF: The Animal Mind, 3rd ed. New York: Macmillan Inc, 1926.

460. Wells DL: A review of environmental enrichment for kenneled dogs, *Canis familiaris*. Appl Anim Behav Sci 2004; 85:307.

461. Wells DL: Aromatherapy for travel-induced excitement in dogs. J Am Vet Med Assoc 2006; 229(6):964.

462. Wells DL, Hepper PG: Directional tracking in the domestic dog, *Canis familiaris*. Appl Anim Behav Sci 2003; 84(4):297.

463. Wells DL, Hepper PG: Prenatal olfactory learning in the domestic dog. Anim Behav 2006; 72(3):681.

464. Wiepkema PR: Developmental aspects of motivated behavior in domestic animals. J Anim Sci 1987; 65:1220.

465. Wilens TE, Biederman J, Spencer TJ, et al: Pharmacotherapy of adult attention deficit/hyperactivity disorder: A review. J Clin Psychopharmacol 1995; 15(4):270.

466. Williams GV, Goldman-Rakic PS: Modulation of memory fields by dopamine $D_1$ receptors in prefrontal cortex. Nature 1995; 376:572.

467. Wilson M, Warren JM, Abbott L: Infantile stimulation, activity, and learning by cats. Child Dev 1965; 36:843.

468. Wilsson E, Sundgren P-E: The use of a behaviour test for the selection of dogs for service and breeding, I: Method of testing and evaluating test results in the adult dog. Appl Anim Behav Sci 1997; 53(4):279.

469. Wilsson E: Sundren P-E: Behaviour test for eight-week old puppies—heritabilities of tested behaviour traits and its correspondence to later behaviour. Appl Anim Behav Sci 1998; 58(1-2):151.

470. Wiseman R, Smith M, Milton J: Can animals detect when their owners are returning home? An experimental test of the 'psychic pet' phenomenon. Brit J Psych 1198; 89(3):453.

471. Wright JC: The effects of differential rearing on exploratory behavior in puppies. Appl Anim Ethol 1983; 10:27.

472. Wright JG: Television with ultrasonic remote control and discomfort in dogs. Vet Rec 1973; 92(23):628.

473. Young CA: Verbal commands as discriminative stimuli in domestic dogs *(Canis familiaris)*. Appl Anim Behav Sci 1991; 32(1):75.

474. Young MS: Treatment of fear-induced aggression in dogs. Vet Clin North Am [Small Anim Pract] 1982; 12(4):645.

475. Zahn TP, Rapoport JL, Thompson CL: Autonomic and behavioral effects of dextroamphetamine and placebo in normal and hyperactive prepubertal boys. J Abnorm Child Psychol 1980; 8(2):145.

476. Zicker SC, Overall KL: Possible implications of oxidative stress in clinical veterinary medicine. Am Vet Soc Anim Behav Annual Symp Anim Behav Res Proc 2002:14.

477. Zohar J, Pato MT: Diagnostic considerations. In Pato MT, Zohar J (eds): Current Treatments of Obsessive-Compulsive Disorder. Washington, DC: American Psychiatric Press Inc, 1991, p. 1.

## Additional Readings

AAHA pet owner survey results. Trends Mag 1993; IX(2):32.

Adachi I, Kuwahata H, Fujita K: Dogs recall their owner's face upon hearing the owner's voice. Anim Cogn 2007; 10(1):17.

Animal vision research focuses on seeing colors: DVM 1986; 17(3):84.

Arata S, Kaneko F, Momozawa Y, et al: Search for temperament-associated genes in guide dogs. In Landsberg G, Mattiello S, Mills D (eds): Proceedings of the 6th International Veterinary Behaviour Meeting and European College of Veterinary Behavioural Medicine-Companion Animals European Society of Veterinary Clinical Ethology. Brescia, Italy: Fondazione Iniziative Zooprofilattiche e Zootecniche, 2007, p. 43.

Atkins DL., Dillon LS: Evolution of the cerebellum in the genus *Canis*. J Mammal 1971; 52:96.

A treatable medical condition in senior dogs. Vet Forum August 2000:44.

Beaver BV, Fischer M, Atkinson CE: Determination of favorite components of garbage by dogs. Appl Anim Behav Sci 1992; 34(1-2):129.

Becker F, Markee JE, King JE: Studies on olfactory acuity in dogs. (1) Discriminatory behaviour in problem box situations. Br J Anim Behav 1967; 5:94.

Berteselli GV, Michelazzi M: Use of l-theanine tablets (Anxitane) and behaviour modification for treatment of phobias in dogs: A preliminary study. In Landsberg G, Mattiello S, Mills D (eds): Proceedings of the 6th International Veterinary Behaviour Meeting and European College of Veterinary Behavioural Medicine-Companion Animals European Society of Veterinary Clinical Ethology. Brescia, Italy: Fondazione Iniziative Zooprofilattiche e Zootecniche, 2007, p. 185.

Blatt CM, Taylor CR, Habal MB: Thermal panting in dogs: The lateral nasal gland, a source of water for evaporative cooling. SCI 1972; 177:804.

Bolles RC: Species-specific defense reactions and avoidance learning. Psychol Rev 1970; 77(1):32.

Branis M, Burda H: Inner ear structure in the deaf and normally hearing Dalmatian dog. J Comp Pathol 1985; 95:295.

Breazile JE, Thompson WD: Motor cortex of the dog. Am J Vet Res 1967; 28(126):1483.

Brisbin Jr II L, Austad SN: Testing the individual odour theory of canine olfaction. Anim Behav 1991; 42:63.

Buchsbaum MS, Davis GC, Bunney Jr WE: Naloxone alters pain perception and somatosensory evoked potentials in normal subjects. Nature 1977; 270:620.

Cain WS: Testing olfaction in a clinical setting. Ear Nose Throat J 1989; 68:321.

Campbell WE: Correction of canine misbehavior. Mod Vet Pract 1973; 54(4):12.

Campbell WE: Social attraction: The ultimate tool for canine behavior control. Mod Vet Pract 1973; 54(5):73.

Campbell WE: Learning, behavior and health. Mod Vet Pract 1973; 54(9):87.

Campbell WE: Sympathy lameness, trauma, and the interpretive factor. Mod Vet Pract 1975; 56(1):45.

Campbell WE: Punishment—Valid teaching tool or dog owner's nemesis? Mod Vet Pract 1975; 56(3):207.

Canine geriatric behavior changes established. Vet Forum June 25, 1998:18.

Cannas S, Frank D, Minero M, et al: Puppy behaviours when left home alone. In Landsberg G, Mattiello S, Mills D (eds): Proceedings of the 6th International Veterinary Behaviour Meeting and European College of Veterinary Behavioural Medicine-Companion Animals European Society of Veterinary Clinical Ethology. Brescia, Italy: Fondazione Iniziative Zooprofilattiche e Zootecniche, 2007, p. 29.

Cassady JM: Avoidance and classical conditioning of leg flexion in dogs. Behav Brain Res 1996; 77:79.

Cattell RB, Korth B: The isolation of temperament dimensions in dogs. Behav Biol 1973; 9(1):15.

Cattet J, Etienne AS: Blindfolded dogs relocate a target through path integration. Anim Behav 2004; 68(1):203.

Chalifoux A, Dallaire A: Physiologic and behavioral evaluation of CO euthanasia of adult dogs. Am J Vet Res 1983; 44(12):2412.

Chaput RL, Kovacic RT, Fleming NL, et al: A discrimination problem for restrained beagles. Lab Anim Sci 1973; 23(5):707.

Coile DC, O'Keefe LP: Schematic eyes for domestic animals. Ophthalmic Physiol Opt 1988; 8:215.

Colgan P: Animal Motivation. New York: Chapman and Hall, 1989.

Cormarèche-Leydier M, Cabanac M: Dog behaviour as related to spinal cord temperature. Experientia 1976; 32(1):66.

Corson SA, Corson EO'L, Kirilcuk V: Individual differences in respiratory responses of dogs to psychologic stress and Anokhin's formulation of the functional system as a unit of biological adaptation. Int J Psychobiol 1970; 1(1):1.

Corson SA, Corson EO'L, Kirilcuk V, et al: Differential effects of amphetamines on clinically relevant dog models of hyperkinesis and stereotypy: Relevance to Huntington's chorea. In Barbeau A, Chase TN, Paulson GW (eds): Advances in Neurology, vol. 1. Huntington's Chorea. New York: Raven Press Ltd, 1973.

Crawford LM, Bowen JM: Thoracic compression reflex in the dog. Am J Vet Res 1968; 29(8):1625.

Davis GC, Buchsbaum MS, Naber D: Altered pain perception and cerebrospinal endorphins in psychiatric illness. Ann N Y Acad Sci 1982; 398:366.

Denenberg S, Landsberg GM, Gaultier E: Evaluation of DAP's effect on reduction of anxiety in puppies (*Canis familiaris*) as well as its usefulness in improving learning and socialization. In Mills D, Levine E, Landsberg G, et al (eds): Current Issues and Research in Veterinary Behavioral Medicine. West Lafayette, IN: Purdue University Press, 2005, p. 225.

Dodman NH: Animal behavior case of the month. J Am Vet Med Assoc 2004; 225(9):1339.

Doty RL, Brugger WE, Jurs PC, et al: Intranasal trigeminal stimulation from odorous volatiles: Psychometric responses from anosmic and normal humans. Physiol Behav 20(2):175.

Dramard V: Analysis of factors causing behavioral difficulties in three dogs destined to become dogs to assist the handicapped. Am Vet Soc Anim Behav Proc 2001:21.

Dramard V: Understanding and preventing sensory homeostasis problems in dogs or how to optimize the education of a companion dog. Am Vet Soc Anim Behav Proc 2001:22.

Ehrman RN, Overmier JB: Dissimilarity of mechanisms for evocation of escape and avoidance responding in dogs. Anim Learn Behav 1976; 4(3):347.

Eichelman Jr BS, Thoa NB: The aggressive monoamines. Biol Psychiatry 1973; 6(2):143.

Ezeh PI, Myers LJ, Hanrahan LA, et al: Preliminary studies on the effect of steroids on olfactory function of the dog. Chem Sens 1989; 14:698.

Firth AM, Haldane SL: Development of a scale to evaluate postoperative pain in dogs. J Am Vet Med Assoc 1999; 214(5):651.

Fogle B: The Dog's Mind. London: Pelham Books, 1970.

Fox MW: Canine behavior: A review article on the work of the Roscoe B. Jackson Memorial Laboratory. J Small Anim Pract (Suppl) 1963; 4:35.

Fox MW: The clinical significance of age differences in the effects of decerebration and spinal cord transection in the dog. J Small Anim Pract 1966; 7:91.

Fox MW: Behavioural and physiological aspects of cardiac development in the dog. J Small Anim Pract 1966; 7(4):321.

Fox MW: The development of learning and conditioned responses in the dog: Theoretical and practical implications. Can J Comp Med Vet Sci 1966; 30:282.

Fox MW: Postnatal development of the EEG of the dog. I. Introduction and EEG techniques. J Small Anim Pract 1967; 8:71.

Fox MW: Normal and abnormal behavioral development of the dog. In Kirk RW (ed): Current Veterinary Therapy, IV. Small Animal Practice. Philadelphia: Saunders, 1971, p. 506.

Fox MW: Inter-species interaction differences in play actions in canids. Appl Anim Ethol 1976; 2(2):181.

Fox MW, Spencer J: Exploratory behavior in the dog: Experiential or age dependent? Develop Psychobiol 1969; 2(2):68.

Fuller JL: Experiential deprivation and later behavior. SCI 1967; 158:1645.

Gallant DM, Bishop MP: Quide vs Mellaril in chronic schizophrenic patients. Curr Ther Res 1972; 14(1):10.

Getchell TV, Margolis FL, Getchell ML: Perireceptor and receptor events in vertebrate olfaction. Prog Neurobiol 1984; 23:317.

Glausiusz J: Scents and scents-ability. Discover 2007; 28(3):22.

Gorman ML, Trobridge BJ: The role of odor in the social lives of carnivores. In Gittleman JL (ed): Carnivore Behavior, Ecology and Evolution. Ithaca, NY: Cornell University Press, 1989, p. 57.

Griffin DR: Animal Minds. Chicago: University of Chicago Press, 1992.

Griffin RW, Beidler LM: Studies in canine olfaction, taste and feeding: A summing up and some comments on the academic-industrial relationship. Neurosci Biobehav Rev 1984; 8(2):261.

Hart BL: Three disturbing behavioral disorders in dogs: Idiopathic viciousness, hyperkinesis and flank sucking. Canine Pract 1977; 4(6):10.

Hart BL: Training dogs not to roam. Canine Pract 1980; 7(5):10.

Hetts S: Psychologic well-being: Conceptual issues, behavioral measures, and implications for dogs. Vet Clin North Am [Small Anim Pract] 1991; 21(2):369.

Hoskins JD: Natural aging can have direct and indirect effect on behavior. DVM February 2002:4S.

Hunthausen WL: Giving new puppy owners practical tips to curb unruly behavior can save lives. DVM 1990; 21:29.

Innes JRM: Canine hysteria. North Am Vet 1952; 33(12):862.

Jones AC, Josephs RA: Are we dog's best friend? Predicting canine cortisol response from human affiliative and punitive behaviors. In Mills D, Levine E, Landsberg G, et al (eds): Current Issues and Research in Veterinary Behavioral Medicine. West Lafayette, IN: Purdue University Press, 2005, p. 194.

Jones FN: An analysis of individual differences in olfactory thresholds. Am J Psychol 1957; 70:227.

Kent JM, Mathew SJ, Gorman JM: Molecular targets in the treatment of anxiety. Biol Psychiatry 2002; 52:1008.

King T, Hemsworth PH, Coleman GJ: Fear of novel and startling stimuli in domestic dogs. Appl Anim Behav Sci 2003; 82:45.

Kitchell RL: Taste perception and discrimination by the dog. Adv Vet Sci Comp Med 1978; 22:287.

Kliavina MP, Kobakova EM, Stelmakh LL, et al: Speed of formation of conditioned reflexes in dogs in the course of ontogenesis. Pavlov J Higher Nerv Act 1958; 8:859.

Koch RB, Gilliland Tl: Responses of $Na^+$-$K^+$ ATPase activities from dog olfactory tissue to selected odorants. Life Sci 1977; 20:1051.

Koolhaas JM, deBoer SF, Bohus B: Motivational systems or motivational states: Behavioral and physiological enidence. Appl Anim Behav Sci 1997; 53(1-2):131.

Lane JG: Ototoxicity in the dog and cat. Vet Rec 1985; 117(July):94.

Lashley KS: Experimental analysis of instinctive behavior. Psychol Rev 1938; 45(6):445.

Lem M: Animal behavior case of the month. J Am Vet Med Assoc 2006; 229(8):1254.

Lester D: Body build and temperament in dogs. Perceptual and Motor Skills 1983; 56:590.

Mackenzie SA, Oltenacu EAB, Houpt KA: Canine behavioral genetics—A review. Appl Anim Behav Sci 1986; 15(4):365.

Marshall DA, Doty RL: Taste responses of dogs to ethylene glycol, propylene glycol, and ethylene glycol-based antifreeze. J Am Vet Med Assoc 1990; 197(12):1599.

Marx J: How stimulant drugs may calm hyperactivity. SCI 1999; 283(5400):306.

Mason B: What's your dog thinking? http://sciencenow. sciencemag.org/cgi/content/full/2005/808/2, 8/23/2005.

McCutcheon PD: Stress, that insidious, intriguing element interwoven into every element of health in the animals we are entrusted to treat. Calif Vet 1980; 34(5):22.

McKinley S, Young RJ: The efficacy of the model-rival method when compared with operant conditioning for training domestic dogs to perform a retrieval-selection task. Appl Anim Behav Sci 2003; 81(4):357.

McMillan FD: Emotional pain management. Vet Med 2002; 97(11):822.

Meaney MJ, Stewart J, Beatty WW: Sex differences in social play: The socialization of sex roles. Adv Study Behav 1985; 15:1.

Millichamp NJ, Arden GB: Transretinal mass receptor potentials recorded from the canine retina in vitro. Am J Vet Res 1989; 50(10):1710.

Mills DS.: Using learning theory in animal behavior therapy practice. Vet Clin North Am [Small Anim Pract] 1997; 27(3):617.

Mills DS, Ledger RA: Oral selegiline hydrochloride improves attention in the dog to signals of reward during training. Proc Third International Cong Vet Behav Med 2001:200.

Monks of New Skete: The Art of Raising a Puppy. Boston: Little, Brown and Co, 1991.

Murphy JA: Describing categories of temperament in potential guide dogs for the blind. Appl Anim Behav Sci 1998; 58(1-2):163.

Myers LJ, Boddie R, May K: Electrophysiolcgical and innate behavioral responses of the dog to intravenous application of sweet compounds. Ann N Y Acad Sci 1987; 510:519.

Myers LJ, Nash R, Elledge HS: Electroolfactography: A technique with potential for diagnosis of anosmia in the dog. Am J Vet Res 1984; 45(11):2296.

Myles S: Trainers and chokers: How dog trainers affect behavior problems in dogs. Vet Clin North Am [Small Anim Pract] 1991; 21(2):239.

Nicol JAC: Tapeta lucida of vertebrates. In Enoch JM, Tobey Jr FL (eds): Vertebrate Photoreceptor Optics. New York: Springer-Verlag, 1981, p. 401.

Nicolaïdis S: A hormone-based characterization and taxonomy of stress: Possible usefulness in management. Metabolism 2002; 51(6, Suppl 1):31.

Ogata N, Takeuchi Y, Kikusui T, et al: Objective measurement of fear-associated learning in dogs *(Canis familiaris)*. In Mills D, Levine E, Landsberg G, et al (eds): Current Issues and Research in Veterinary Behavioral Medicine. West Lafayette, IN: Purdue University Press, 2005, p. 48.

Osella MC, Girardi C, Re G, et al: Behavioural and physiological evaluation of age-related cognitive impairment in pet dogs. In Landsberg G, Mattiello S, Mills D (eds): Proceedings of the 6th International Veterinary Behaviour Meeting and European College of Veterinary Behavioural Medicine-Companion Animals European Society of Veterinary Clinical Ethology. Brescia, Italy: Fondazione Iniziative Zooprofilattiche e Zootecniche, 2007, p. 100.

Overall KL: Part 3: A rational approach: Recognition, diagnosis and management of obsessive-compulsive disorders. Canine Pract 1992; 17(4):39.

Overall KL: Reluctance to collar could be result of abuse; desensitizing puppy can help. DVM 1995; 26(12):8S.

Overall KL, Arnold SE, Milgram NW: Assessment of olfactory function: An integrated approach to assess cognition in dogs. In Mills D, Levine E, Landsberg G, et al (eds): Current Issues and Research in Veterinary Behavioral Medicine. West Lafayette, IN: Purdue University Press, 2005, p. 298.

Overall KL, Dyer D, Dunham AE, et al: Hereditary fear, panic, and anxiety in dogs *(Canis familiaris)*. In Mills D, Levine E, Landsberg G, et al (eds): Current Issues and Research in Veterinary Behavioral Medicine. West Lafayette, IN: Purdue University Press, 2005, p. 221.

Pageat P: Description, clinical, and histological validation of the A.R.C.A.D. score (evaluation of age-related cognitive and affective disorders). Proc Third International Cong Vet Behav Med 2001:83.

Palestrini C, Previde EP, Spiezio C, et al: Heart rate and behavioural responses of dogs in the Ainsworth's Strange Situation: A pilot study. Appl Anim Behav Sci 2005; 94:75.

Pierantoni L, Verga M: Behavioural consequences of premature maternal separation and of a lack of stimulation during the socialization period in dogs. In Landsberg G, Mattiello S, Mills D (eds): Proceedings of the 6th International Veterinary Behaviour Meeting and European College of Veterinary Behavioural Medicine-Companion Animals European Society of Veterinary Clinical Ethology. Brescia, Italy: Fondazione Iniziative Zooprofilattiche e Zootecniche, 2007, p. 102.

Polley DD: Shaping puppy personalities. Vet Forum February 1994: 22.

Pryor P: Animal behavior case of the month. J Am Vet Med Assoc 2003; 223(6):790.

Rader RD, Stevens CM: Telemetered renal responses in dogs during detection of explosives. Biotelemetry 1975; 2(5):265.

Range F, Viranyl Z, Huber L: Selective imitation in domestic dogs. Current Biol 2007; 17(10):868.

Reuterwal C, Ryman N: An estimate of the magnitude of additive genetic variation of some mental characters in Alsatian dogs. Heredity 1973; 73:277.

Riedel J, Buttelmann D, Call J, et al: Domestic dogs *(Canis familiaris)* use a physical marker to locate hidden food. Anim Cogn 2006; 9(1):27.

Rogerson J: Canine fears and phobias: A regime for treatment without recourse to drugs. Appl Anim Behav Sci 1997; 52(3-4):291.

Romanes GJ: Dog-General intelligence. In Henderson RW (ed): Learning in Animals. Stroudsburg, PA: Hutchinson Ross Publishing Co, 1982, p. 24.

Rosenthal M: Remembrance of things past. Vet Forum Fall 2006:14.

Roundtable on canine cognitive dysfunction, Part 2: Treatment. Vet Forum March 29, 1999:56.

Royce JR: A factorial study of emotionality in the dog. Psychol Monogr 1955; 69(22):1.

Russell ES: Playing with a dog. Q Rev Biol 1936; 11(1):1.

Salazar I, Rueda A, Cifuentes M: A contribution to the knowledge of the organum vomeronasale in the dog. Anat Histol Embryol 1982; 11(4):366.

Schmidt-Morand D: Vision in the animal kingdom. Vet Int 1992; 4(1):3.

Seksel K: Behavior problems in the senior dog. http://www.avma.org/conv/cv2002/cvnotes/CAn_AnB_BPS_SeK.asp, 7/3/2002.

Serpell JA: The influence of inheritance and environment on canine behavior: Myth and fact. J Small Anim Pract 1987; 28(11):949.

Shepherd WT: Tests on adaptive intelligence in dogs and cats, as compared with adaptive intelligence in rhesus monkeys. Am J Psychol 1915; 26:211.

Shively JN, Epling GP, Jensen R: Fine structure of the canine eye: Retina. Am J Vet Res 1970; 31:1339.

Sims MH, Moore RE: Auditory-evoked response in the clinically normal dog: Early latency components. Am J Vet Res 1984; 45(0):2019.

Siracusa C, Manteca X, Cerón JJ, et al: Perioperative stress in dogs: Neuroendocrine and immune responses. In Landsberg G, Mattiello S, Mills D (eds): Proceedings of the 6th International Veterinary Behaviour Meeting and European College of Veterinary Behavioural Medicine-Companion Animals European Society of Veterinary Clinical Ethology. Brescia, Italy: Fondazione Iniziative Zooprofilattiche e Zootecniche, 2007, p. 159.

Sommerville BA, Settle RH, Darling FM, et al: The use of trained dogs to discriminate human scent. Anim Behav 1993; 46(1):189.

Stiles E, Palestrini C, Beauchamp G, et al: A placebo-controlled double-blind comparative study on the effects of dextroamphetamine on motor activity, cardiac frequency, and behaviour in beagles. In Landsberg G, Malliello S, Mills D (eds): Proceedings of the 6th International Veterinary Behaviorists Meeting & European College of Veterinary Behavioural Medicine-Companion Animal European Society of Veterinary Clinical Ethology. Brescia, Italy: Fondazione Iniziative Zooprofilattiche e Zootecniche, 2007, p. 49.

Terenius L, Wahlström A, Lindström L, et al: Increased CSF levels of endorphins in chronic psychosis. Neurosci Lett 1976; 3:157.

The brain on the wane: Roundtable on canine cognitive dysfunction. Part 1: Incidence and diagnosis. Vet Forum July 25, 1998:54.

Tokuriki M, Matsunami K, Uzuka Y: Relative effects of xylazine-atropine, xylazine-atropine-ketamine, and xylazine-atropine-pentobarbital combinations and fine-course effects of the latter two combinations on brainstem auditory-evoked potentials in dogs. Am J Vet Res 1990; 51(1):97.

Tortora DF: Understanding electronic dog training: Part 1. Canine Pract 1982; 9(2):17.

Tortora DF: Understanding electronic dog training: Part 2. Canine Pract 1982; 9(3):31.

Triana E, Pasnak R: Object permanence in cats and dogs. Anim Learn Behav 1981; 9(1):135.

Tunturi AR: Masking of cortical responses in middle ectosylvian auditory area of the dog. Am J Physiol 1956; 184:321.

Voith VL: Fear-induced aggressive behavior. Canine Pract 1976; 3(5):14.

Voith VL: Multiple approaches to treating behavior problems. Mod Vet Pract 1979; 60(8):651.

Voith VL: Play behavior interpreted as aggression or hyperactivity: Case histories. Mod Vet Pract 1980; 61(8):707.

Voith VL, Borchelt PL: Introduction to animal behavior therapy. Vet Clin North Am [Small Anim Pract] 1982; 12(4):565.

Voith VL, Borchelt PL: Fear of thunder and other loud noises. Vet Tech 1985; 6(4):189.

Vollmer PJ: The new puppy: Preventing problems through thoughtful selection. Vet Med Small Anim Clin 1977; 72(2):1823.

Vollmer PJ: Electrical stimulation. 2. Bark-training collars. Vet Med Small Anim Clin 1979; 80(12):1737.

Vollmer PJ: Electrical stimulation. 3. Conclusion. Vet Med Small Anim Clin 1980; 75(1):57.

Walker DB, Walker JC, Cavnar PJ, et al: Naturalistic quantification of canine olfactory sensitivity. Appl Anim Behav Sci 2006; 97:241.

Walker R, Fisher J, Neville P: The treatment of phobias in the dog. Appl Anim Behav Sci 1997; 52(3-4):275.

Ward C, Smuts BB: Quantity-based judgements in the domestic dog *(Canis lupus familiaris)*. Anim Cogn 2007; 10(1):71.

Watkins LR, Mayer DJ: Organization of endogenous opiate and nonopiate pain control systems. SCI 1982; 216:1185.

Wiesel TN, Gilbert CD: Morphological basis of visual cortical function. Q J Exp Physiol 1983; 68:525.

Wiseman-Orr ML, Nolan AM, Reid J, et al: Development of a questionnaire to measure the effects of chronic pain on health-related quality of life in dogs. Am J Vet Res 2004; 65(8):1077.

Wysocki CJ, Wellington JL, Beauchamp GK: Access of urinary nonvolatiles to the mammalian vomeronasal organ. SCI 1980; 207:781.

Young D: Nerve Cells and Animal Behavior. New York: Cambridge University Press, 1989.

# Canine Communicative Behavior

When humans think of communication, we usually think of the verbal form. For dogs, however, vocal communications are the least significant; body signals and odors are primary. The types of information transmitted also differ between the two species. Language allows specific messages. Without language, the messages are more general in nature, usually reflecting an emotional state.[52] Because people use language to communicate with dogs, and because dogs understand generalities in vocal communication, it is important to be consistent in word and voice quality when giving commands.[20] Many times the dog actually picks up on a body language message rather than a verbal one.

General messages can be given by dogs via vocal or silent communications, and mixed messages can be expressed as well.[54] The agonistic message system includes six types of messages: territorial defense, advertisement, submission, defensive threat, offensive threat, dominance, and readiness to fight.[107] The sexual message system includes five types of messages: male advertisement, female advertisement, courtship, synchronization and suppression, and copulatory signals.[107] The most general category includes those messages commonly used in day-to-day routines: play, affiliation, assembly, identity, familiarization, solicitation, alarm, distress, and satisfaction.[107] Even the youngest dogs give and receive messages. The neonatal message system includes infant distress, infant identity, infant affiliation, infant satisfaction, neonatal contact, maternal assembly, maternal identity, and maternal alarm.[107]

## VOCAL COMMUNICATION

The dog has a variety of sounds for communication. Unlike its wolf relative, which uses only four to nine types of vocalizations,[46] the dog is significantly more vocal, almost to the point of hypertrophic barking.[30,44] This characteristic has been equated with paedomorphosis associated with the selective breeding of domestication. Excessive barking is considered a juvenile behavior.[32]

Puppies develop the vocal patterns of adult dogs gradually. A newborn puppy starts with three calls, two for distress and one for nondistress situations.[17,54,107] Distress vocalizations—whines and yelps—have an et-epimeletic function to reunite the neonate and the bitch.[48,56,117] The use of whines and yelps tends to increase, peaking at 7 to 9 days after birth, and they gradually decrease over the next 3 weeks.[48] Use of the nonprotest grunt, mew, and clicking sounds is associated with relief of stress or relief of discomfort, contact with the bitch or littermates, and warmth.[16,31] These sounds peak at 4 to 9 days and then gradually decrease until they are gone by 5 weeks of age.[17,48] Around 4 weeks of age, the more adult-like phase of vocal communication begins, with some structural changes occurring after that.[107]

Distress vocalizations in young puppies have been well studied. They are characterized as a rapid series of whines and yelps occurring at rates that can exceed 100 per minute in 3-week-old puppies during situations of obvious discomfort.[36,117] This frequency decreases with experience from repetition, but situational and genetic variations occur.

As puppies mature, they develop a larger repertoire of vocalizations. These can be described by acoustic signs,[133] situational arousal, or type of sound. The later is described here.

### Bark

Barking starts abruptly between 2 and 4 weeks of age,[17,36,48,54,107] with most puppies showing a response as if they are startled by their first bark. Initially, barking occurs in a play-soliciting context

| TABLE 3-1 | Vocalization patterns of adult and neoadult dogs | | | | | | | | | | | |
|---|---|---|---|---|---|---|---|---|---|---|---|---|
| | Bark | Groan | Growl | Grunt | Hiss | Howl | Mew/ Click | Pant | Puffing | Scream | Tooth snap | Whine/ Whimper | Yelp |
| Alarm | A | | A | | | | | | | | | | |
| Care Seeking | A | | | A | | | | | | | | NA | N |
| Contact Seeking | A | | | | | A | | | | | | NA | A |
| Defense | A | | A | | | | | | A | | A | A | A |
| Distress | A | A | A | | | | | | | NA | | NA | N |
| Distress Relief | | | | N | | | N | | | | | | |
| Greeting | A | | A | A | | A | | | | | | A | A |
| Group Vocalization | A | | A | | | A | | | | | | A | |
| Play Solicitation | A | | | | | | | A | | | A | A | A |
| Predatory-Related | A | | | | | | | | | A | | | |
| Submission | | | A | | A | A | | | A | | | A | A |
| Threat/ Warning | A | | A | | | | | | | | A | | |

Data from references 17, 35, 54, 56, 67, 92, 142.
*A*, Adult dogs; *N*, Neonatal dogs; *NA*, Neonatal and adult dogs.

and is not associated with serious aggression until after 8 weeks of age, when puppies will respond to their dam's growl.[17] Aggressive barks by puppies generally do not occur before 12 weeks.[17] By the fourth month, the aggressive bark is more marked in defense of food and toward strange dogs, probably more as an announcement of presence rather than a warning.[17]

Different pitches indicate different situations, with the higher tones more for greetings and play and lower tones for threats. Because barks can carry a number of different messages, it is easier to put them into context when the dog's body language can also be observed.[17] Barks are most commonly associated with greeting, play solicitation, alarm, hunting, tracking, herding, vocal alerting, defense, threat, care seeking, distress, contact seeking, and group vocalization (Table 3-1).* Disturbances are

associated with a harsh, low-frequency, unmodulated characteristic.[95,143,144] It is longer in duration and has a more rapid repetition than barks for other reasons. Without knowing the context, 70% of people can identify this harsh bark as a bark of disturbance.[143,144] They can also recognize barks from other general situations by general acoustic patterns.[95,98,110,111] Owners who are around their dogs more are better at recognizing the tone of bark and the situation that prompts it. Certain breeds or lines pass on an inherited tendency to bark more often, but individuals can also learn to bark excessively through rewards.[67] In contrast, wolf cubs bark a lot, but adult wolves do so only for alarm, threat, protest, while hunting and during pair behavior.[118] Their barks are brief and infrequent.

Tone quality varies within a barking episode, and more than one message can be conveyed at a time.[32] In general, barking is characterized as complex, wide-banded, segmented bursts of sound of 200 to 6000 Hz, with a mean of 650 Hz.[17,32,54]

*References 31, 35, 54, 56, 67, 92, 142.

These bursts last 0.2 second each,[17] and they tend to be cyclic. The frequency of barks during an event ranges from one single bark to a continuous series. One Beagle barked 907 times in 10 minutes.[32] In contrast, only 2.5% of the vocalizations of captive wolves were barks.[32]

Quantifying the frequency and duration of barking episodes is important to differentiate normal from abnormal. On average, dogs bark 3.1 (0 to 8) times in 24 hours when owners are home.[47] Each episode lasts 50.9 (1 to 302) seconds for a total of 198 (0 to 430) seconds spent barking in that 24-hour period.[47]

Over two thirds of dogs in various urban habitats in one study barked during the night. Half of those barking dogs had five or more bouts of barking during the 8-hour period.[1] When asleep, dogs apparently remain more alert to alarm barking than to other stimuli, even though the other types of stimuli might be of more significance to the owner.[2] Individual dogs living in a group are more likely to bark than single individuals.[2]

## Cough

Obviously coughing is usually associated with tracheobronchial irritations, but it occasionally can have a communication function. As in human communication, coughing-like sounds can be used by canids as a threat or warning.[31] They can also be heard in defensive situations.

## Groan

A groan is an acute distress call that has been described as sounding like a saw cutting wood or a snore.[17] The fundamental pitch is 250 to 450 Hz, with the main harmonics at 500 to 700 Hz.[17] The spectrogram shows a segmented rate of 125 per second, a duration of 0.06 second and a frequency of 15 per second.[17]

## Growl

Whereas dog owners usually associate growling with an aggressive behavior of defense, warning, or threat, it usually is more complex than that (see Table 3-1). For example, growling can occur as a greeting, perhaps to reinforce dominance relationships.[54] Play bouts between dogs or between dogs

and humans may contain play growls in addition to the more traditional signals of play.

Growling usually occurs first during puppy play fights at approximately 24 days of age.[17] At that time the fundamental pitch is 150 to 450 Hz, with poor harmonics to 3000 Hz.[17] By 9 weeks, the fundamental play growls are more segmented, and the fundamental pitch is 150 to 300 Hz, with no harmonics.[17] In adult dogs, it is difficult to define a fundamental pitch any longer; however, the energy level associated with growling remains.[17,56] The pattern is noncyclic.[56] Spectrograms of growls in various contexts show similar patterns regardless of the initiating factors.[17]

## Grunt

Newborn puppies grunt as a nonprotest sound for greeting, care seeking, or contact.[16,31,56] Initially, the sound starts between 250 and 1500 Hz,[54] lasting 0.2 second at a rate of two grunts per second.[16,17] The frequency and rate increase slightly by the second day. By 6 weeks, the sonogram pattern shows segmentation and a shorter duration.[17] In adults, grunts are usually associated with the animal being stroked or held by its owner.[17] Then the fundamental frequencies are 85 to 200 Hz.[31]

## Hiss

The hiss is a mechanical sound of air being forced through the nose.[17] It has been suggested that the hiss is a primitive predecessor of threat sounds.[17]

## Howl

The howl is a canine vocalization that can both fascinate and annoy humans. In wolves, the howl is used by isolated individuals, perhaps as a long-distance vocalization.[80,134,135] Members of a pack may join in a chorus of howls as a group vocalization.[43] It has been shown that, for wolves at least, there are seasonal fluctuations in the number of howls. The number of elicited howls remains relatively constant over time, but the increase in spontaneous howls by pack members during the wolf's breeding season correlates to the increase in frequency of howling by the alpha male.[81] Thus, group howling may be a show of pack affinity, a display of strength, or a spontaneous vocalization. It can also be used as a warning and a show of group power toward strangers approaching a pack. A perimeter wolf will howl when it becomes aware of a stranger approaching.[127] This howl gets the attention of the others in the pack, and all join in unison to stop the stranger's advance.[127] The closer the approach of the stranger, the deeper the pitch is of the howling, and the more harmonically unrelated frequency sidebands are added.[64]

In the modern dog, these wolf traits associated with howling may still be expressed. Contrary to popular opinion, dogs are probably not howling as the result of a noise hurting their ears. As described in Chapter 2, their hearing is not that much different from a human's hearing. Instead, the pet dog that howls to the wailing siren may be responding to an approaching "stranger," and the one that sings with its owner's voice or musical instrument may be joining in the vocalization of others in its pack.

The harmonics of a howl are in the range of 400 to 2000 Hz for the fundamental frequency and 1200 to 2900 Hz for the dominant one.[31,54] The lower frequencies are more prominent,[56] and they are used most in situations in which a greater threat or warning is needed.[64] The duration of a howl is greater than 1.0 second, and there are few variations of frequency during the howl.[56] Although a howl may be repeated, it is not considered cyclic.[56] In wolves, the voice quality is unique enough that individuals can be identified by their howl alone.[64, 135]

## Mew/Click

The mew or click sound is made by distressed neonates when they are in pain or seek maternal or littermate contacts.[31,56] These are short, wide-banded, cyclic sounds with moderate frequency variation.[56]

## Moan

A moan can be heard occasionally in conjunction with situations of apparent pleasure. As an example, when the inside of the ear is rubbed by the owner, the dog may moan as it tilts its head.

## Pant

Noises of panting are not vocalizations of the larynx but rather of air movements of the oropharynx. In canine communication, they are associated with play solicitation.[56]

## Puffing

Puffing can be described as the lowest-intensity aggressive vocalization,[17] and its origin is mechanical rather than from the vocal folds. The sound results when air is forced through a slightly opened mouth. The lip folds can be seen to move.[17]

## Scream

The scream is used as a vocalization by both puppies and adults when they are distressed, in pain, or showing submission.[31,56] Characteristically, these sounds are of great intensity and are wide banded, noncyclic, and long in duration.[56] Great frequency variations exist, with a fundamental frequency of 1200 to 2700 Hz and a pitch of dominant frequency of 1800 to 3200 Hz.[31,54]

## Sneeze

The sneeze is used by some dogs when excited and when soliciting play.

## Tooth Snap

Another mechanical sound coming from the mouth is the tooth snap, made by teeth hitting each other as the jaw rapidly closes. The sound has been associated with play solicitation, defense, and threat behaviors.[31,54]

## Whine/Whimper

Whines and whimpers can be associated with a number of different events, so they have a number of meanings, but they mainly signify distress.[16,17] Situations that appear to provoke whines and whimpers can include care seeking, contact seeking, defense, distress, greeting, group vocalizations, pain, play solicitation, and submission.[31,56] In newborns the pitch varies from 500 Hz to 1500 Hz, and the average duration is 1 second.[16,17] The usual frequencies associated with the whine or whimper in older dogs are cyclic, ranging between 500 Hz and 3400 Hz. Clear harmonics exist at 1000-cycle intervals, and the duration decreases.[16,17,54,56] The distress vocalizations in puppies as young as 8 days can exceed 100 per minute but average about 20 per minute in unfamiliar environments.[129]

One variation, the sex whine, is a vocalization of intact male dogs associated with a male being near a copulating pair, refused by or separated from an estrous female, or near a whelping bitch.[17] The frequency for the sex whine ranges from 3250 Hz to 4200 Hz, with no harmonics.[17]

### Yawn

The yawn is often accompanied by an "aaaa . . ." sound that increases in pitch. These behaviors are associated with stress and anxiety, not with boredom or sleepiness as happens in people.

### Yelp

The yelp begins to develop with the whine at 14 to 20 days of age.[17,54] Initially, the combination will start at 1300 Hz, then drop to 800 Hz, with a duration of 0.2 to 0.3 second.[17] From this will develop the more abrupt, bark-like yelps, with harmonics extending to 6000 Hz.[17] True yelps first occur at 20 to 24 days of age.[17] Yelps are associated with greetings and play solicitation, as well as with distress, pain, submission, contact seeking, and defense.[54]

Tone quality of yelps can cause different responses in other dogs. Short notes, especially of higher frequency, are more likely to increase motor activity levels than are long, low-frequency notes.[88,89] Inhibitory signals tend to be prolonged and descending single notes.[89]

Vocalizations can occur alone, simultaneously with other vocalizations, or successively in various combinations. The pairs of vocalizations that occur simultaneously include the whine-bark, bark-scream, growl-whine, and bark-growl.[31] Combinations that occur sequentially vary from the mew-grunt in puppies to whine-bark, whine-growl, whine-pant, bark-growl, growl-scream, and howl-bark in adults.[31]

Mutism is also possible in dogs. Experimentally, a mute can be created by bilateral destruction of the central gray matter beneath the superior colliculus.[126]

## POSTURAL COMMUNICATION

Canids use a wide variety of genetically programmed body postures to communicate,[68] and they are adept at reading subtle changes. Owners may think that their moods are sensed by their dogs without recognizing that their pets are actually reacting to specific human behavior. The "guilty" look of submission, for example, is more likely the dog's response to the owner's increased dominant postures than to remembering that it defecated in the house several hours earlier. Experimentally this ability of dogs to interpret, react to, and even rely on human gestures has been confirmed in a number of different ways.* The responses are also dependent on a moving image as compared to only a voice.[109]

Postural signals generally carry distance-reducing, distance-increasing, or ambivalent messages. These are not equivalent to a submissive or dominant dog because they can be used by any dog under specific circumstances. Each type of message tends to start with more subtle signals and progressively becomes more obvious. Sometimes, however, stages are skipped or mixed.

### Distance-Reducing (Submissive) Signals

Body signs that tend to decrease a threat or encourage an approach are classified as distance-reducing, or submissive, signals. Showing submission helps stop or attenuate aggression or punishment by a more dominant dog,[68] and puppies quickly learn the usefulness of these signals as appeasement gestures.[124] It represents an effort by a lower ranking animal to attain a harmonic social integration and assumes that the higher ranking individual will respond appropriately.[30,121] This type of communication can be broadly divided into three categories: passive submission, active submission, and play.[9,12,52]

#### Passive Submission

The body signals of passive submission are derived from postures the young adopt when being cleaned by their mother.[121] These signals range from the very subtle to the very extreme.[52] At the subtle end of the scale is the simplest of responses—that of avoiding direct eye contact. Progressively more

---

*References 21, 22, 37, 45, 57, 62, 63, 93, 94, 96, 116, 128, 131, 136.

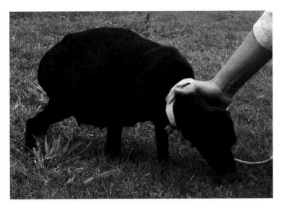

**Figure 3-1.** The lowered head, neck, ears, and tail of submission.

obvious signs may follow in any order. The dog will tend to lower the ears back against the neck, and the head will be lowered as the neck is lowered and extended forward or twisted sideways (Fig. 3-1). The lowered ears, head, and neck for submission must be carefully interpreted to be consistent with other body signs because of the similarity with signals used by aggressive dogs. The tongue can flick in and out, or the more dominant animal may be licked in greeting.[56,125] A submissive grin, with its horizontal retraction of the lips, may be observed.[56] If the submissive dog is touched, it will hold completely still.

The tail is held lower, often between the legs, as an indicator of fear or submission. It may be wagged there (Table 3-2). Tail wagging has been equated with a human's smile and can be used as an index of emotionality.[78] Motion in the tail should be viewed cautiously though. The flagging of dominance, while stiffer, more upright, and more rigid, is still easily confused with the wagging of submission. One study indicated that the tail swings farther to the right in the presence of a person and to the left for an unfamiliar dog.[113] Wolves wag their tails in much the same way as dogs. The limber tail indicates a friendly, possibly submissive message.[82] This is almost always true if the wolf's tail is wagged in a circle.[82] Domestication has increased the tendency of the dog to use a tail wag.[32,78] Dogs do differ from wolves in other ways, however. Overall their visual communicative repertoire is less complex, their facial displays more limited, and signals can vary by breed.[125]

The general aim of distance-reducing signals is to decrease any sign of threat, so the dog will gradually crouch into a lower position, perhaps raising a front paw (Fig. 3-2).[48,56] A raised paw can also signal a defensive warding-off reaction or a play-soliciting behavior.[56] The submissive dog may actually lie down (Fig. 3-3). It may then even roll over to expose the abdomen. Because the abdomen is the only body part not protected by bone, attack of it by a more dominant animal could be fatal. As a result, rolling over is an extremely submissive posture. In addition, the dog may urinate in submission. Some dogs will roll over onto their backs and present their abdomens to solicit "tummy rubs." This is a submissive posture but one soliciting interactions. The difference is generally easily distinguished from the submissive message alone because the one's seeking interactions will have their eyes wide open and be looking at the person from whom they want attention.

It is important to note that submissive postures are often associated with fear. In addition to the tendency to shrink in size, dogs may also tremble, freeze in place, or run away. There are physiologic changes of stress that can include increased salivary cortisol levels.[13]

A few dogs that are passively submissive will show the "mimic grin" facial expression (Fig. 3-4).[9] The expression is easily confused with an aggressive one because of the bared teeth, but with the mimic grin, all other body signals indicate submission. Although some authors feel the mimic grin is a learned behavior,[52] it is most likely an inherited submissive behavior, as it is common in certain bloodlines in both purebred and mixed-ancestry dogs. The "pleasure face," or "grin,"[124] is another facial expression that does not carry a threat.[52] This expression includes lips that are pulled back horizontally a little from normal, ears that are lowered, and eyelids that are half-closed (Fig. 3-5). A dog is most likely to show the pleasure face when it is scratching or rolling over odiferous things.

## Active Submission

Individual dogs use active submission significantly more often than passive submission. This behavior pattern is derived from the puppy's initial begging for milk and food, olfactory investigation, and receiving

**TABLE 3-2**    The relationship of a dog's tail position to activities

| | Over back | Vertical | Slightly vertical | Lowered | Between legs |
|---|---|---|---|---|---|
| Aggressive Approach | X | X | | | |
| Ambivalent Approach | X | X | X | X | |
| Defensive Threat | | | | | X |
| Elimination Postures | X | | | | |
| Fear-Induced | | | | X | X |
| Fighting | X | X | | | |
| Greeting | X | X | | | |
| Investigative Approach | X | X | | | |
| Isolation | X | X | X | X | |
| Locomotion | | | | | |
|   Walk | X | X | X | X | |
|   Trot | X | X | X | X | |
|   Upright trot | X | X | X | | |
|   Canter | | X | X | | |
|   Gallop | | X | X | | |
|   Leaping | | | | | |
| Orient to Object | X | X | X | | |
| Pain | | | | X | X |
| Sex Behavior | | | | | |
|   Courtship by males | X | X | X | | |
|   Estrous females | X | X | X | | |
|   Sexual approach—males | X | X | | | |
|   Sexual approach—females | X | X | X | | |
| Sickness | | | | X | X |
| Standing | | | | X | |
| Stress-Induced | X | X | | | |
| Submission | | | | X | X |
| Tactile Stimulation | X | X | X | X | |

Data from reference 78.

anogenital licking from the mother.[30,78,121] The most distinguishing characteristic of active submission is the approach of the dog to a person or other dog. The approach is usually accompanied initially by the head and tail held high as the dog bounds forward. Tail wagging is common when a dog greets a social peer or superior.[78] Once the dog has reached its goal, it will show one or more signs of passive submission: diverted eyes, lowered head, immobile response to touch, submissive urination. Shortly after acknowledgment, the dog may bound around again.

The "greeting grin" is associated with active submission (Fig. 3-6).[9, 52] This facial expression resembles a human smile, with the corners of the mouth pulled back.[52] It is seen only in human-dog interactions, not in dog-dog ones.[53]

## Play

Play is another series of postures used in friendly, nonconfrontational interactions by dogs. In puppies, the behaviors mimic adult behaviors in fragmented forms. The various components of fighting,

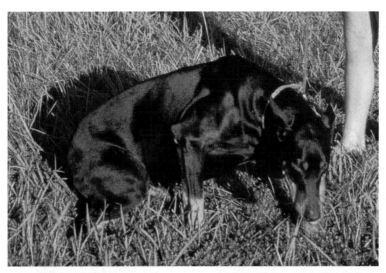

**Figure 3-2.** Crouching is another one of the body postures of submission. (From reference 9. Used with permission of Veterinary Medicine Publishing Group.)

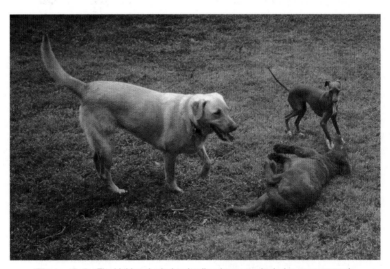

**Figure 3-3.** The highly submissive dog lies down as submissive ones approach.

sexual, and predatory behaviors are shown out of context and in incomplete sequences.

Adult dogs maintain specific postures for play solicitation. The front-end-lowered rear-end-up position of play intention posture, called the play bow, is well recognized (Fig. 3-7).[9] It is significant that adult dogs use a specific posture associated with play intention to be sure that the context that follows is not confused with other intentions, such

as aggression.[14,124] This play bow is usually followed after approximately one third of a second by a quick return to a standing position[14] and then by some jumping around the intended playmate. Play activity involves rapid and exaggerated movements.[125] This behavior is first used at about 23 days of age.[14] The posture is rarely used outside the context of play, but occasionally there is a dog that solicits play with the play bow and then attacks.[69]

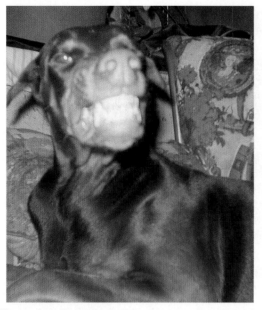

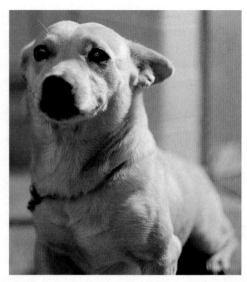

**Figure 3-6.** The greeting grin. (From reference 9. Used with permission of Veterinary Medicine Publishing Group.)

**Figure 3-4.** The mimic grin. Notice the ears are lowered, and the dog is avoiding direct eye contact.

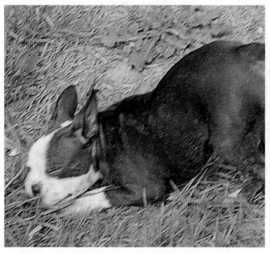

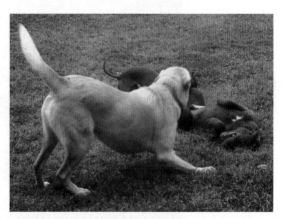

**Figure 3-7.** Play solicitation with the lowered chest and raised hindquarters is called the play bow.

**Figure 3-5.** The pleasure face.

A raised forepaw can be a play-solicitation gesture.[56,125] The context in which it is displayed is important to its interpretation. Other play solicitation behaviors include open mouth panting, running off while looking back, and exaggerated loping (leaping) approaches.[19,87]

Humans can also use canine postures to solicit playful interactions with a dog. A play bow posture and a "lunge" often result in play, including an increase in play bout frequency and mean duration.[115,116] Adding play vocalizations increases both even more.[115]

The "play face" expression is an intensification of the greeting grin.[52, 56] The ears are erect and forward, anatomy permitting, and panting may occur. At the same time, the tail is often high and wagging while the front is in the play bow.[52]

## Distance-Increasing (Agonistic, Aggressive, Dominant) Signals

Body postures that appear to increase the size of an individual by optical illusion are meant to convey a "go away" message. As with submissive postures, signals intended to increase a dog's threat come on a graduated scale and diverge in opposite directions. Although submission involves a reduction in size and use of a soft whine, a threat involves increasing body size and a loud vocalization.[125] The tendency is for displays to begin as subtle messages and increase if necessary; however, a dog can mix signals in any order of presentation.[10,125]

Nine behaviors have been described as agonistic signals observed in wolves.[51,58] These include the growl, displacement (moving the opponent away), standing over, inhibited bite, standing erect, body wrestling, aggressive gape, bared teeth (snarl), and stare. These are also behaviors seen in dogs, but not in all breeds of dogs. Breeds that are physically, and perhaps evolutionarily, closer to wolves show more of the behaviors, whereas breeds more physically dissimilar show progressively fewer of the signals.[58] Behavioral paedomorphism parallels physical paedomorphism.[58]

Direct eye contact, with eyelids wide open—the stare—is the most subtle of threats but one generally recognized among dogs. Its use effectively settles disputes between most dogs, minimizing the need for escalation of the confrontation and reducing the potential for life-threatening injuries. The mouth shows the next signals when the lips are pulled back at the corners and eventually retracted vertically into a snarl (bared teeth) (Fig. 3-8).[56] The aggressive gape also shows teeth, but adds a partially open mouth.[51] The head, neck, and ears are elevated during the initial phases of distance-increasing communication, but as the threat becomes more intense, they may be lowered.[52] This is to protect the throat and ear pinnas during an actual attack. This lowered position can resemble the posture of passive submission, but each leads to a very different next step.

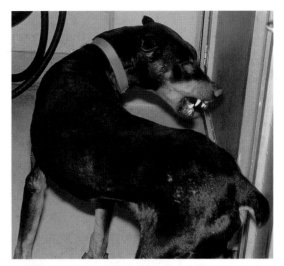

**Figure 3-8.** The retracted lips and stare typical of a snarl.

The dog will create the illusion of increasing size. First the weight is shifted forward to indicate a strong position. Then the legs and toes are stiffened (standing erect) to maximize what length is there. Piloerection of the hairs over the shoulders and rump also creates a deceptive sudden increase in height, especially in dogs with longer hair (Fig. 3-9). These postures are used for threat aversion, indicating high arousal, not necessarily dominance.[124] Dogs showing fear tend to have hair raised in two areas—over the shoulders and over the rump—whereas a dominant dog has it raised all the way down its back.[101] The tail is held vertically or arched over the back, where it can be flagged in either a slow, deliberate motion or a rapid motion in which it is almost vibrating back and forth (see Table 3-2).[10,52] The relative height of the tail gives a good indication of the level of confidence of the dog[78] and of the relative dominance between individual dogs (Fig. 3-10). Confusion about the meaning of a vertical tail can result because this is also a behavior of excitement.[52]

At any stage of posturing to create a distance-increasing message, a male dog may go over to an object to urinate on it, perhaps even scraping the ground afterward. During this time, however, the stare, piloerection, and other distance-increasing signs are maintained.[52]

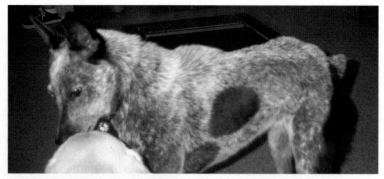

**Figure 3-9.** Piloerection of hair over the shoulders and rump.

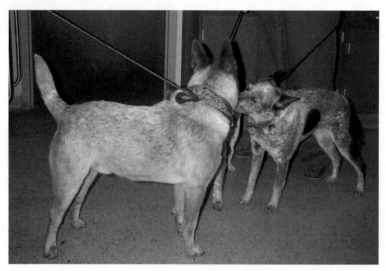

**Figure 3-10.** Two Blue Heelers show a facial-lingual approach, one with a vertical tail and the other with a tucked tail.

Ultimately, the distance-increasing signals can escalate until they approach an actual attack.[52] The dog may show an inhibited bite (bite-intention movement or snap) as a warning or threat.[52] Biting into the victim and holding on, with or without the head shake, is the primary method of fighting, and the ultimate position in the fight is to achieve a firm grip on the ventral neck (Fig. 3-11). This neck-grip position is used in fights between dogs and for bringing down prey.

Another behavior that can be shown is the displacement of the opponent. The physical presence or approach of a more dominant dog can result in the submissive one moving away. It is common for

owners to miss the subtle but intense displacement interactions.

A dominant dog may show other behaviors to a less dominant one to reinforce their relationship but these are not necessarily intended to make the lower ranking dog leave. A higher ranking dog may rest its head or stand with its forelimbs on the neck or shoulders of a lower ranking one (Fig. 3-12). It may also grasp the muzzle or head of the more submissive dog in its mouth using an inhibited bite.[30] When two dogs are interacting, the degree of distance-reducing signs shown by the submissive dog varies with the degree of threat shown by the more dominant one. The primary purpose of

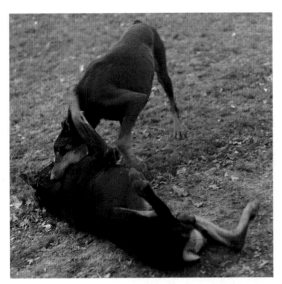

**Figure 3-11.** A ritualized neck grip during a fight between two Doberman Pinschers.

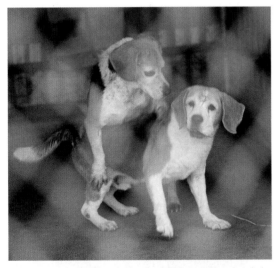

**Figure 3-12.** Social mounting by a higher ranking dog during a disturbance in the kennel area of male Beagles.

this variation evolved from wolves' behavior that was designed to inhibit fights-to-the-death by animals that are especially skilled at killing. Dogs used in fighting have been selected to have less reliance on threat displays so there is less warning of an impending attack.[125] They also have a tendency to bite and hold their prey.[125]

## Ambivalent Signals

Ambivalent signals are a normal part of communicative behavior. They are frequently seen in wolves too.[43] Signals are often mixed, with a dominant wolf showing submissive behavior and low-ranking ones showing an occasional agonistic posture, like bared teeth. The animals can quickly flip between messages too.

Dogs can show this mix of signals as part of normal intraspecies communication or they can show the mixed signals arising from internal conflict.[52] As an example, a small dog that generally likes people may be fearful of an extremely large person or of a person who approaches it when there is no escape. The head may be up and eyes staring while the rest of the body is lowered to the ground or the tail is held between the legs and wagged (Fig. 3-13), or the dog may be staring while it is backing away (Fig. 3-14). These postures of frontal threat with rearend retreat may suddenly reverse, so that the eyes are diverted but the hair over the rump is elevated and the tail becomes vertical.

Because of the internal conflict of these dogs, it is safest to read the worse end. Mixed signals are the classic indication of a fear-biter. Although aggression does not always occur, it is best to assume that it might. To read these dogs more accurately, or any other dog being approached, a person should use the "Captain, may I?" approach. By slowly shifting your weight forward, you are essentially asking permission to move forward. As long as the dog shifts its weight back, drops its tail, and shows other distance-reducing signs, the person can slowly continue toward the dog.[52] If, however, the dog's weight shifts forward and distance-increasing signs become more intense, increased caution is appropriate.

Other, less obvious behaviors may also indicate a conflict. Although licking is generally considered a submissive behavior, a licking motion, where the tongue curls back to touch the nose, shows ambivalence.[56] Yawning or stretching before an active approach may also convey this message.[56]

## Active Defense

Dogs can show a behavior that has both aggressive and submissive elements, called the active-defense behavior. The body signals include bared teeth,

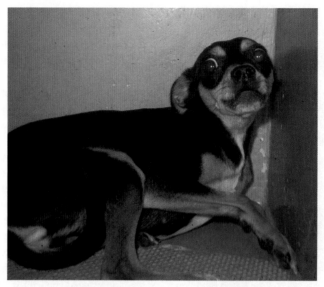

**Figure 3-13.** A classic fear-biter body posture.

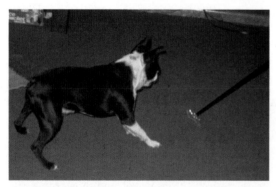

**Figure 3-14.** An ambivalent body posture in which the front end is facing the stick as the dog stares at it, but the weight is shifted backward.

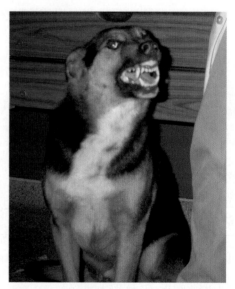

**Figure 3-15.** Active defense signals (toward camera holder) of bared teeth and growling interspersed with flicking the tongue and looking toward the owner.

piloerection, pupillary dilation, licking or protruding of the tongue between the teeth, and a turning away of the head to avoid eye contact (Fig. 3-15).[49]

## Confusing Signals

Because of anatomic features, the body language of certain dogs can be very difficult to read.[52] It has even been suggested that dogs have become less reliant on body language than are wolves, with olfactory signals being increasingly important.[19] Tails are quite variable. Some are docked very short,

so on a Pembroke Welsh Corgi, for example, the whole rear end has to move for the wagging to be obvious. Doberman Pinschers and Rottweilers are difficult to read because they have short tails and because it is hard to evaluate their dark eyes for a stare. It is also difficult to try to read the eyes and tail at the same time. Boston Terriers have the short, screw tail that can be wagged but does not move vertically very much. Curly-tailed breeds like Basenjis and Norwegian Elkhounds can uncurl the tail in extreme cases, but the tail's height does not directly correlate with the distance-increasing message for the rest of the dog. Chow Chows not only have the curly tail, but their hair coat appears to be in constant piloerection. The combination of confusing signs decreases the available signals that can be studied to predict aggression.

Hairy faces complicate interpretation, because it is difficult to see the eyes, and lifted lips may go unnoticed. For this reason, the aggressive nature of some Old English Sheepdogs has been particularly difficult to predict. Hair draped over the eyes can favor aggression in a dog with that tendency, because it is less likely to see well. This not only makes some dogs more reactive if bothered, but they do not convey the more subtle signals.

Large, pendulous lips and ears are anatomic features that make a dog's body language difficult to read. The weight makes the lips and ears difficult to move, so facial expressions do not change much between distance-reducing and -increasing situations. Saint Bernards, Bassett Hounds, and Bloodhounds are example breeds.

Geriatric animals may have difficulty showing appropriate signals because of painful conditions. Also, dogs that have medical problems, like a broken tail that has healed in a permanent downward direction, may not be able to signal appropriately and complicate the interdog communication.

## COMMUNICATION BY SCENTS

Scents are commonly used by animals to communicate information between individuals. In dogs we automatically think of urine marking, but odors are used other ways too. Scent marking has been defined as urinating, defecating, or rubbing certain body areas while oriented toward specific objects. The behavior is elicited by familiar landmarks, novel objects, or certain odors; it occurs frequently and is repeated on the same object.[79,85] Scent-marking behavior can be used to mark a particular object, territory, individual, or

| TABLE 3-3 | Contexts and types of scent marks used by wolves | | | |
|---|---|---|---|---|
| | Raised-leg urination | Squatting urination | Defecation | Ground-scraping |
| Agonistic | 2 | 3 | 4 | 4 |
| Assertive | 8 | 4 | 2 | 9 |
| Disturbed | 1 | 1 | 2 | 1 |
| Friendly | 0 | 11 | 0 | 0 |
| Sexual | 5 | 5 | 1 | 7 |

Data from reference 108.

self.[12] In dogs, scent marking occurs through two primary methods: anal sac secretions and urine. Other scents, like those of feces, saliva, sebaceous gland secretions, and those released by earth scraping also can be used for communications. In view of the significance of olfaction to dogs, as discussed in Chapter 2, it is reasonable to expect that a dog could obtain a great deal of information from a scent mark.

The purpose of scent marking and the type of mark used for each situation may vary (Table 3-3). The behavior may have originally been performed to familiarize and reassure an animal when it entered a strange area. Over time, it also became useful in bringing sexual partners together, possessing a territory, and maintaining a territory.[56,79,108] Mammals typically mark more frequently when they are intolerant of or dominant to other members of their own species.[60,114] Scent marking can also occur when an animal is motivated toward aggression and is likely to attack.[114] If the attack does occur, the marking animal is more likely to win the fight.[114] Stimuli that affect scent marking are extremely variable. In general, however, they fall into two categories.[79] One group includes objects that are familiar and conspicuous, as would be the case with wolves marking prominent rock formations or bushes. For dogs, this could be a fence corner, light pole, or fire hydrant. The second group of stimuli can be described as novel things, such as objects with such odors as urine from a new dog or novel visual objects, including the occasional suitcase.

### Anal Sac Secretions

Veterinarians typically think of anal sac secretions as being odiferous substances to be carefully avoided when manually expressing the impacted sac of a dog presented for scooting. In most dogs, however, these secretions are routinely expressed during the first and last part of defecation.[6,85] Evacuation without defecation is rare in dogs,[6] but it can occur in distress. Experimentally, anal sac contents cause other adult dogs to recoil and show apparent apprehension.[38]

In a Greyhound-sized dog, each anal sac holds 1.0 to 1.5 ml of material.[6] When the sac is full, some of its contents will be squirted up to 4 feet from the body as defecation starts.[6,104] The remaining material is passed intermittently during defecation for up to 80 hours.[6,85] Anal sac secretions are similar for both males and females.[39,85,112]

The secretion is composed mostly of short-chain aliphatic acids and trimethylamine.[3,85,112] Also present in smaller amounts are ethanol, acetic acid, isobutanol, propionic acid, 2- and 3-methylbutanol, isobutyric acid, η-butyric acid, 2-methylbutyric acid, isovaleric acid, *n*-valeric acid, 4-methylvaleric acid, 2-methylvaleric acid, and 2-piperdone.[60,85,112] Marked individual differences exist in the secretion's properties, and dogs may have some control over composition, at least of the lipid and aqueous pH.[18] Estrus increases the concentrations of $C_2$ to $C_5$ aliphatic acids, acetone, and trimethylamine.[104] Modification can also occur from microorganisms within the sac and from interaction with environmental factors.[18] The potential exists that anal sac problems could change the chemical composition of anal sac materials enough that previously friendly dogs act aggressively toward the one with the problem.[104]

## Urine Marking

Dogs use urine to mark, with males significantly more likely to do so than females. Like anal sac secretions, urine contains a number of different chemicals that may contribute to its unique scents. Odorants that have been identified include isopent-3-enyl methyl sulphide, 2-phenylethyl methyl sulphide, 4-heptanone, 6-methylhept-5-en-2-one, benzaldehyde, acetophenone, and 2-methylquinoline.[60] In addition, a variety of steroids could also be important to dogs.[60] Dogs can remember specific individual urine-scent signals.[18]

Marks associated with urine are more important to males, but both sexes tend to urinate in locations that other dogs have previously used,[5,125] sometimes immediately after one.[19] In wolves, packs tend to overmark the urine of a lone wolf but not the other way around, suggesting that urine marks a territory or home range.[19] Males will mark at least twice as often as females, especially just after they meet another dog or see another dog urinate.[73,85] Females, on the other hand, seldom or never mark in the presence of a strange dog.[55] Experimentally, males mark an average of once every 1.6 minutes, compared with once every 4.7 minutes for females.[85] Of the urine marks in one study, more than 70% were made by males,[85] and male dogs marked over the urine of a female dog 30 of 36 times.[55] Sometimes a male will urinate over the urine mark of another male that had covered over female urine.[55] Urine marks are frequently made by male dogs over the marks of other dogs, especially within the first 2 hours after they are encountered.[66] When put in a pen previously occupied by other dogs, adult males urine marked 24.6 times in the first 2 hours versus only two to five times in any other 2-hour segments.[66] Castration does not change the rate of this marking behavior.[66]

Wolves leave scent marks at regular intervals along their established trails, especially at the junction of different trails and along the edges of their territory.[60,108] Along the territorial boundaries, urine marks are much higher in number than within the territory.[60] However, wolves will repeatedly overmark scent-posts within their home range that were left by strangers.[125] Dogs can use any urinary posture in scent marking, although the raised-leg posture typical of males is most commonly used by them. This posture is thought to elevate the mark to nose height. It also facilitates dispersal of the odor by the wind, increases the evaporating surface, and minimizes the chances of its being covered by snow or washed away by rain.[108]

## Feces Marking

For wolves, feces marks are left at trail junctions and the borders of the home range.[125] In contrast, dogs do not commonly use feces odors for marking, although they are interested in the odors of the feces left by other dogs. Individual dogs may mark objects with feces, and when they do, the handstand position is the one usually used. The dog backs up to a tree or post, smearing the feces onto the object as it defecates. This behavior places the odor closer to nose level for other dogs to find.

## Scent Rubbing

In wolves, and probably in dogs, scent rubbing is most likely to occur for odors that are not commonly encountered, familiar odors that deviate from the norm, or scents that are strongly attractive or aversive.[119] The behavior actually starts as a rubbing in the material by lowering the front half of the body and rubbing both sides of the neck and head over the odor.[79] The dog may then roll over completely onto its back and wiggle in a back-and-forth pattern. A "pleasure face" is typical during this behavior (see Fig. 3-5).[50] On vertical objects with scent marks, the dog rubs its head, body, and neck against the odor mark.[79]

Although it is impossible to know the actual reasons for scent rubbing, five theories have been proposed. In certain instances, the rubbing-rolling behavior may be used to camouflage or cover the dog with a particular scent.[80,84] Rolling, then, would be somewhat similar to humans putting on perfume or aftershave lotion, although obviously the aesthetics of scent selection differ between the two species. A second possible reason for scent rubbing is for the dog to add its scent to another object.[80,84] A third theory is that the behavior is used to facilitate long-term memory of that scent.[119] The fourth theory is to provide an olfactory identity to the animal's pack.[84] It is common in wolf packs for all members to rub the same scent spot. Lastly, it has been suggested that scent rubbing is to take on environmental information to share with pack-mates at a later time.[84]

## Scratching the Ground

After urinating or defecating, a dog will occasionally scratch the ground with its feet, sending clumps of leaves and earth flying backward. Dog owners have been known to speculate that the behavior is the canine equivalent of the cats covering behavior, but it probably is not. Dogs cannot be taught to use a litterbox nor to consistently cover feces. In addition, this ground scratching action is rarely sufficient

to cover the excreta. The behavior is probably intended to leave a visual marker of fresh gouges in the soil and an additional olfactory one of the scent of fresh earth and pheromones from the feet. In wolves, the behavior is increasingly seen with the arousal associated with a stranger.[125] In dogs, ground scratching occurs more often when a dog is in a new location, there is competition between male dogs, or strangers have intruded.[104]

## Odors of Estrus

It is commonly observed that male dogs are particularly interested in the odors of estrous bitches. The chemical methyl *p*-hydroxybenzoate has been identified as the main component of estrous vaginal secretions.[59,60] Sex differences exist in preferred odors of dogs. Sexually experienced males are more attracted to urine and vaginal secretions from estrous females than from diestrous ones,[40,41] and they spend more time investigating female dog urine than either vaginal or anal sac secretions.[40] All males prefer female urine and feces to those of other males.[41] Anal sac secretions from estrous females also have been reported to elicit excitement in males,[38] but later studies indicate that there is really no difference in the amount of attraction to estrous versus diestrous anal sac secretions.[40]

## Pheromones

The role pheromones play in communication between dogs is hard for people to appreciate because we cannot smell them. Many can appreciate that there may be a fear pheromone emitted by very distressed people that results in protective aggression by their dogs. In contrast, pheromones are associated with normal activities too. The primary pheromone-secreting glands in the dog are the labial, auricular, perianal, genital (vulvar or preputial), interdigital (pedal), and mammary complexes of sebaceous glands.[104] Most of the information apparently enters via the vomeronasal organ.

The labial and auricular glands are related to social status with higher ranking dogs "smelling" the lower ranking dog. Interdigital glands are used in marking territory and to produce alarm pheromones.[104] For dogs, the circumanal glands and those of the anal sacs are the most important of the perianal complex. The circumanal glands convey social information that must be of significant importance to males, because they increase in size over the years. Methyl dihydroxybenzoate secretion from the vulvar areas of an estrous bitch is highly attractive to male dogs.[104] Mammary pheromones of a nursing bitch have been synthesized commercially and are marketed as a calming product called the Dog Appeasing Pheromone (DAP).

## COMMUNICATIVE BEHAVIOR PROBLEMS

### Excessive Vocalization

Dogs that bark too much represent a large group of problem dogs. Excessive barking is one of the top five behavior problems,[24,26] constituting between 6.0% and 35% of all owner complaints to behaviorists.* In geriatric dogs that have developed behavior problems, slightly over one fourth were presented for the problem of excessive vocalization.[29] It is interesting to note that although certain breeds are commonly thought of as being barkers, client complaints about barking are usually for dogs not among those breeds. An above-average proportion of barking complaints has come from people who have Beagles, Cocker Spaniels, Collies, Dachshunds, Dalmations, Miniature Schnauzers, Shetland Sheepdogs, Silky Terriers, and Yorkshire Terriers.[23,25]

Genetic predisposition certainly is not the cause of all barking. Early experience can reinforce barking so that it is continued at a greater than normal rate.[122] If barking is reinforced, such as when the owner gives attention to the barking dog, the dog quickly learns how to get attention. Fearful dogs might also bark to deter a closer approach. Distress barking is frequently associated with separation anxiety too.

The current environment can trigger excessive barking.[122] Dogs that are overly excited or in mental or physical distress will bark. The other situation that is often not well appreciated is the lack of mental stimulation, or "boredom." If there is nothing to

do, and especially if the dog is somewhat genetically programmed to bark anyway, barking becomes the default behavior.

Thus, there are many reasons for barking. In some cases, the behavior is perfectly normal, but the owner is not in a mood to tolerate it. True excessive vocalization has been associated with infection, hormonal or metabolic disease, too much or too little environmental stimuli, attention seeking, hyperactivity or hyperkinesis, anxiety (including separation anxiety), stereotypies, and obsessive-compulsive disorders.[91,102,103] It is also a common problem in older puppies and adult dogs adopted from animal shelters,[140] although in these dogs, the problem tends to decrease significantly after a few months.[86] Of the various sounds a dog makes, barking is the least appreciated.

Why is the dog that barks excessively a problem? In addition to the obvious answer of its keeping an owner awake, noise-level measurements and complaints registered provide some insight. Noise levels at a distance of 2 meters (m) from a barking dog are over 100 decibels (db)—the loudness of a jackhammer.[123] At 10 m from the dog, noise levels are still 80 db.[123] Even in an adjoining room, the levels can be 70 to 85 db.[123] If the dog is outside but near a bedroom window, the level is still around 68 db, and even with the window closed in an air-conditioned house, the noise level from the outside dog is approximately 55 db.[123] Compared with an acceptable noise level below 40 db, even 55 db is too loud.[42] In addition, the randomness of barking, the timing of its occurrences, the frequency of its occurrences, the quality of its sound, its interference with human sleep, and the human inability to control its noise all contribute to its irritative effect.[4]

Of complaints received at the Los Angeles Society for the Prevention of Cruelty to Animals, which averages 2200 per year, most were related to being awakened at night by barking.[123] Efforts to control the problem by passing ordinances and laws appeal only to those being bothered. Owners typically bring the problem to the veterinarian's attention when the dog's barking has been keeping them awake or when neighbors' complaints have led to intervention by some law-enforcement agency.

---

*References 15, 27, 28, 72, 75, 76, 83.

In the first case, the owners are highly motivated to correct the problem. In the latter, they usually want a simple solution that requires minimal effort,[11] as is reflected in the increased number of requests to "debark" a dog when a new city ordinance is passed.

Barking is also a welfare problem in animal shelters and dog kennels, neither of which tends to consider noise abatement in their designs. Peak noise levels frequently exceed 100 db and could be as high as 125 db.[33,120]

Puppies are known to bark or whine when they first go to a new home. There is less vocalization if the puppy sleeps with another dog,[132] although, that is often not possible. Puppies from breeds developed to be gun dogs tend to vocalize more nights than those of other breeds.[132] The duration of this "crying" can be decreased in half by using the DAP nearby.[132]

Young dogs may show barking tendencies before 6 months of age and are often set off by environmental stimuli. The barking of other dogs triggers 38.1% of the barking episodes, sirens 12.7%, garbage trucks 6.3%, buses 6.3%, and children playing 4.8%.[4] Owners may reinforce the barking behavior as well, through increased attention or praise.[24,92,138] It is important to emphasize to new puppy owners not to encourage barking for a feeling of increased security. Protectiveness is an instinctive behavior, as discussed in Chapter 4, and is not related to barking tendencies.

For dogs that bark when the owner is home, a number of options can be tried to stop the problem. The first is extinction. Because most barking is triggered by an outside stimulus, such as another dog barking or a nearby noise, ignoring the behavior may help it stop on its own. The idea is to avoid accidental reinforcement through owner attention. If the dog has learned to expect attention, even negative attention, extinction of the behavior can take longer. At first, the dog will try barking louder or longer, but it will eventually learn that the rules have changed. The duration of barking bouts will then decrease. This process, of course, can mean there will be some long, sleepless nights for the owner. Neighbors might not appreciate this choice, either, if the dog normally stays near their window.

Punishing the dog for barking is another treatment option. It is one, however, that requires some very careful consideration to be sure that the dog does not interpret the act as reinforcing the behavior instead. Yelling does not work, because the presence of the owner sends the wrong message.[67] Punishment, not the owner's presence, should be associated with the act of barking, and every episode of barking must be punished.[67] Remote punishment can be used. The owner can place a garden hose with a pistol-grip sprayer near the bedroom window, then grab it when the barking starts and blast the dog with a water spray, never interacting with the dog. Balloons on a pulley clothesline can be popped on a nail placed above the dog's kennel.

An antibarking muzzle significantly reduces barking levels without affecting indices of stress, such as salivary cortisol.[34] This might be an option when owners do not interact with the dog, such as during the night or while gone during the day. Dogs show submissive behaviors like the lowered head and tail and they are less active.[34] Because owners view these as signs of depression, they are not likely to want to use the equipment when they can observe the dog.

Antibark collars are another treatment option. There are three basic types. The first is a bark-activated collar that repeatedly makes a clicking noise or other sound that can serve as a punishment to some dogs.[12,141] Bark-activated collars also are made that spray a citronella mist as a punishment. Electronic shock collars come in models that are bark activated or remotely triggered. In the latter case, the owner must trigger the shock each and every time the dog barks and as soon as the barking starts. Appropriate operation of the remotely controlled shock collar is a real problem. All three of the bark-activated collars punish each occurrence of barking. They seem to work because of the element of surprise.[8] Many dogs quickly learn to tell when the collar is around their neck and when it is not, so intermittent use may prolong the best response.[139] These collars also can be set off by other things besides the barks of the target dog. Close-up barking by other dogs or hitting the collar against a piece of furniture may accidentally set off the collar, confusing the wearer about cause and effect.

Of the three types of collars, external factors could be the most serious problem with the shock collars. In addition, shock collars are the most difficult to adjust to be sure the degree of punishment is consistent and not too severe for the individual dog.[11,67] Comparative studies of shock, high-frequency, and citronella collars with and without the actual citronella odor found the citronella-containing spray collar resulted in a 77.8% to 88.9% decrease in the frequency, intensity, and duration of barking, whereas 59% improved with a scentless spray collar, 50% responded to the high-frequency collar, and 25% to 44.4% of the dogs responded as well to shock collars.[76,97,118] About 20% of a control group improved without treatment.[97] Overall owner satisfaction was 88.9% for the citronella collar compared with 50% for the shock collar.[76] With the spray collars, 67.7% of dogs continued to bark but at reduced levels, even after the removal of the spray but with retention of the collar.[8]

If specific stimuli can be identified that trigger barking, it may be possible to use counterconditioning or desensitization to stop the excessive reaction.[67,92,137] As an example, teaching the dog to sit quietly during a stimulus that causes barking requires persistence, but it can be accomplished.[138]

Three fourths of the problem dogs bark during the day, and the majority of those are kept outdoors.[106] These generate more complaints to authorities because it disturbs the neighborhood. The motivation to stop the barking results from potential legal action, not because the owner is actually being disturbed. It is the neighbor who suffers through the problem. There is a device on the market that emits a very loud noise in response to barking that might be helpful for the neighbor to use, but some dogs become afraid to go back into the yard.[71] Because owners are less motivated to stop this behavior, as it does not bother them,[11] understanding specific stimuli can be helpful when the owners are forced to do something. Dogs that bark when the owner is not home usually do not get reinforcement through attention, although there may be some type of internal reward involved. The owner can videotape the dog's behavior to identify exactly what the dog is doing. If barking is accompanied by panting, salivation, restlessness, and excessive activity, the pet may be experiencing separation anxiety, which is a more extensive problem (see Chapter 4).[90]

Owners who are very emotional toward the dog either immediately before they leave or as soon as they return can cause the dog to become overly excited. Barking would be one way the dog could express this excitement. Minimal attention should be given for approximately 30 minutes before leaving so there is not a high level of excitement that needs to be dissipated when the door closes. When returning home, the owner should barely acknowledge the dog until some other activity is begun, like taking the dog outside, changing clothes, or starting supper. The signal for active attention then becomes the specific activity rather than a certain time, and the dog is less likely to become anxious as the time of the owner's reappearance approaches.

Remote punishment, as through the use of bark-activated collars, may be the best option for dogs that bark when the owner is away, provided that separation anxiety or other anxiety-related causes of barking have been ruled out.[99] This option requires the least work on the part of the owner, but it does not address the barking stimulus. Surgical devocalization is generally not a good long-term solution. Unless the vocal folds are sutured against the laryngeal wall, scar tissue will grow back across the remnants, and the dog will regain a hoarse-sounding voice.

Puppy classes are becoming popular options for new owners, but by the time there are more than five puppies together, there is a significant increase in the number and loudness of vocalizations.[61] The DAP used during the sessions results in more appeasing, quieter interactions.[61]

Older dogs may start barking without any of the usual precipitating stimuli. It is necessary to consider medically related problems, such as deafness or brain disease.[28,74,105] This barking may be caused by a lack of auditory feedback, but it may also be the result of separation anxiety.[28] Decreased sensory capabilities that accompany aging can leave the dog feeling more isolated or less able to function in the minimal light of night. For some dogs, leaving a hall light on is sufficient to stop the barking. Others may be showing the behavior as the result of aging changes on certain brain centers. Canine cognitive dysfunction is currently being studied, and selegiline and other current treatments are discussed in Chapter 2.

Excessive vocalizations have also been described as stereotypies and obsessive-compulsive disorders.[91,93] If there is a rhythmic bark or a persistent, high-priority need to bark or growl, these syndromes may be suspected. Until specific patterns are understood at the neurotransmitter level, a drug trial of a narcotic antagonist or drug to increase serotonin levels at the synapse level might be tried.

## Excessive Submission

Most people are not particularly good at reading body language except for the obvious display of the dog that wiggles all over in its excitement to see them.[7] Nor do people consider what postural message they may be sending a dog as it approaches. Timid dogs, especially young ones, have a tendency to show submissive behaviors that are more excessive than dictated by the situation. If the owner becomes upset or tries to discipline the dog, matters only get worse, especially when submissive urination is involved. Whereas the number of dogs referred to a behavior practice for problems of submission may represent only 2.4% of the caseload according to one study,[83] practitioners who routinely ask about behavior problems find the numbers much larger.

For the excessively submissive dog, treatment plans are generally built around two concepts. First, punishment is not appropriate, and second, the best overall approach is to decrease the perception of approaching dominance. Many times the extremely submissive dog will try hiding or will show submissive urination, neither of which pleases the owner. The owner becomes angry and punishes the dog for not coming when called or for urinating in the house. The person's presence becomes more threatening instead of less so, and the dog increases its submissive response or avoidance to the maximum extent. Eventually, the perception of threat can become so great that a warning fear-bite may occur as an attempt to stop the progression of events.

As puppies grow, most develop increasing amounts of self confidence, so that by 6 to 12 months of age, the extremes of submissive behavior have faded, provided the owner did not escalate dominant interactions with the dog. For submissive puppies, owners should carefully evaluate those situations most likely to precipitate the shy response and look for ways to decrease the threats they present. Certain human postures are more helpful than others with these dogs. Avoid direct or prolonged eye contact. Instead, look to the side and watch the dog with your peripheral vision, or use long, deliberate blinks to make obvious breaks in eye contact. Decreasing one's apparent size uses the same type of message a dog would use. Crouching down instead of bending over, and turning sideways instead of straight on, decreases the threat. Encouraging the dog to approach with a high-pitched, happy-sounding voice is less threatening than grabbing for the dog or yelling at it.

Fear-biters are more difficult to work with because of the possibility of injury. Owners often do not recognize the submissive component in the behavior of a fear-biter, only the aggressive. A fine line exists between effectively dealing with these dogs and overreacting in punishment. Fear-induced aggression will be discussed along with the other types of aggression in Chapter 4.

## Urine Marking

Urine marking is a male sexually dimorphic behavior, meaning it can be occasionally shown by females. As such, problems with this behavior tend to occur in socially dominant, male dogs[73] and are at least partially responsive to elimination of testosterone. Castration of male dogs that urine marked in their homes was helpful in approximately 50% of the dogs.[70,137] For dogs older than 2 years of age, 78% show an improvement by decreased amounts of urine marking of at least 50% after castration, and 39% had an improvement of 90% to 100%.[100] Responses varied from a rapid decrease in this problem in 30% of the cases to a more gradual reduction in 20% and no change in 50%.[70] Age at the time of castration, and therefore previous learning, was not related to the eventual success or failure of castration for this problem.[70] In some practices, apparently, the success of castration for urine marking in the home is much greater.[130,137] It is also important to differentiate marking in the home versus marking in a scent-enriched environment, because castration does not seem to decrease the frequency of the latter.[65]

Because progestins also decrease levels of serum testosterone, they have been used successfully for controlling male sexually dimorphic behaviors. Initially, the use of megestrol acetate improved the behavior in 74% of urine-marking male dogs.[77] Over time, however, many relapsed, so that after 3 months, less than half of those that initially responded were still improved.[77] Because urine marking is used to mark objects within a territory and the boundaries of the territory, dogs that start marking manifest an apparent psychological need to do so. If the problem is relatively new and the dog is caught in the act, stern, prompt punishment, either directly from the owner or remotely triggered, may be sufficient to stop the marking. For the occasional offender, it may be possible to anticipate the problem and take preventive measures. For example, the dog that marks chairs where house guests sit may be calmed by putting a towel with the owner's or dog's scent on the chair for a few days. Restricting the dog's fun times so that they occur only when the new baby is nearby or involved can stop a dog from marking baby toys and baby furniture.

## References

1. Adams GJ, Johnson KG: Sleep-wake cycles and other nighttime behaviours of the domestic dog, *Canis familiaris.* Appl Anim Behav Sci 1993; 36:233.
2. Adams GJ, Johnson KG: Behavioural responses to barking and other auditory stimuli during night-time sleeping and waking in the domestic dog *(Canis familiaris).* Appl Anim Behav Sci 1994; 39:151.
3. Albone ES: Mammalian Semiochemistry: The Investigation of Chemical Signals Between Mammals. New York: John Wiley & Sons Inc, 1984.
4. Alvord LS: Annoyance factors for common neighborhood stationary noise. J Acous Soc Am 1988; 84(2):780.
5. Anisko J: Communication by chemical signals in canidae. In Doty RL (ed): Mammalian Olfaction, Reproductive Processes and Behavior. New York: Academic Press, 1976, p. 283.
6. Ashdown RR: Symposium on canine recto-anal disorders. 1. Clinical anatomy. J Small Anim Pract 1968; 9(7):315.
7. AVMA Animal Welfare Forum: Human-canine interactions. J Am Vet Med Assoc 1997; 210(8):1121.
8. Beaudet R: Comparing the effectiveness of citronella with unscented odours in the anit-barking spray collar. Proc Third International Cong Vet Behav Med 2001:190.
9. Beaver BV: Friendly communication by the dog. Vet Med Small Anim Clin 1981; 76(5):647.
10. Beaver BV: Distance-increasing postures of dogs. Vet Med Small Anim Clin 1982; 77(7):1023.
11. Beaver BV: Therapy of behavior problems. In Kirk RW (ed): Current Veterinary Therapy VIII: Small Animal Practice. Philadelphia: Saunders, 1983, p. 58.
12. Beaver BV: The Veterinarian's Encyclopedia of Animal Behavior. Ames: Iowa State University Press, 1994.
13. Beerda B, Schilder MBH, van Hooff JARAM, et al: Behavioural, saliva, cortisol, and heart rate responses to different types of stimuli in dogs. Appl Anim Beh Sci 1998; 58 (3-4):365.
14. Bekoff M: Social communication in canids: Evidence for the evolution of a stereotyped mammalian display. SCI 1977; 197:1097.
15. Blackshaw JK: Abnormal behavior in dogs. Aust Vet J 1988; 65:393.
16. Bleicher N: Behavior of the bitch during parturition. J Am Vet Med Assoc 1962; 140:1076.
17. Bleicher N: Physical and behavioral analysis of dog vocalizations. Am J Vet Res 1963; 24(100):415.
18. Bradshaw JWS, Natynczuk SE, Macdonald DW: Potential for applications of anal sac volatiles from domestic dogs. In Macdonald DW, Müller-Schwarze D, Natynczuk SE (eds): Chemical Signals in Vertebrates 5. New York: Oxford University Press, 1990, p. 640.
19. Bradshaw JWS, Nott HMR: Social and communication behaviour of companion dogs. In Serpell J (ed): The Domestic Dog: Its Evolution, Behaviour and Interactions with People. Cambridge, England: Cambridge University Press, 1995, p. 115.
20. Braem MD, Mills D: How does additional verbal information influence a dog's obedience to a command? In Landsberg G, Mattiello S, Mills D (eds): Proceedings of the 6th International Veterinary Behaviour Meeting & European College of Veterinary Behavioural Medicine-Companion Animals European Society of Veterinary Clinical Ethology. Brescia, Italy: Fondazione Iniziative Zooprofilattiche e Zootecniche, 2007, p. 144.
21. Bräuer J, Kaminski J, Riedel J, et al: Making inferences about the location of hidden food: Social dog, causal ape. J Comp Psychol 2006; 120(1):38.
22. Call J, Bräuer J, Kaminski J, et al: Domestic dogs *(Canis familiaris)* are sensitive to the attentional state of humans. J Comp Psychol 2003; 117(3):257.
23. Campbell WE: Which dog breeds develop what behavioral problems? Mod Vet Pract 1972; 53:31.
24. Campbell WE: Excessive barking. Mod Vet Pract 1973; 54:73.
25. Campbell WE: Which dog breeds develop what behavior problems? Mod Vet Pract 1974; 55(3):229.
26. Campbell WE: Effects of training, feeding regimens, isolation and physical environment on canine behavior. Mod Vet Pract 1986; 67:239.
27. Chapman B, Voith V: Dog owners and their choice of a pet. American Veterinary Society of Animal Behavior meeting, Atlanta, July 20, 1986.
28. Chapman B, Voith VL: Geriatric behavior problems not always related to age. DVM 1987; 18(3):32.
29. Chapman BL, Voith VL: Behavioral problems in old dogs: 26 cases (1984-1987). J Am Vet Med Assoc 1990; 196(6):944.

30. Clutton-Brock J: Domesticated Animals from Early Times. Austin: University of Texas Press, 1981.

31. Cohen JA, Fox MW: Vocalizations of wild canids and possible effects of domestication. Behav Processes 1976; 1:77.

32. Coppinger R, Feinstein M: 'Hark! Hark! The dogs do bark…' and bark and bark. Smithsonian 1991; 2l(10):119.

33. Coppola CL, Enns RM, Grandin T: Noise in the animal shelter environment: Building design and the effects of daily noise exposure. J Appl Anim Welfare Sci 9(1): http://www.psyeta.org/jaawa/abv9n1.shtml, 9/29/2006.

34. Cronin GM, Hemsworth PH, Barnett JL, et al: An antibarking muzzle for dogs and its short-term effects on behaviour and saliva cortisol concentrations. Appl Anim Behav Sci 2003; 83:215.

35. Daniels TJ, Dekoff M: Spatial and temporal resource use by feral and abandoned dogs. Ethology 1989; 81:300.

36. DeGhett VJ, Stewart JM, Scott JP: Habituation of distress vocalization response of puppies of different dog breeds in constant and varying environments. Am Zool 1970; 10:294.

37. Does your dog understand you? http://www.vetscite.org/publish/items/002027//index.html, 1/19/2005.

38. Donovan CA: Some clinical observations on sexual attraction and deterrence in dogs and cattle. Vet Med Small Anim Clin 1967; 62:1047.

39. Doty RL, Dunbar I: Color, odor, consistency, and secretion rate of anal sac secretions from male, female, and early-androgenized female beagles. Am J Vet Res 1974; 35(5):729.

40. Doty RL, Dunbar I: Attraction of beagles to conspecific urine, vaginal and anal sac secretion odors. Physiol Behav 1974; 12(5):825.

41. Dunbar IF: Olfactory preferences in dogs: The response of male and female beagles to conspecific odors. Behav Biol 1977; 20:471.

42. Eldred KMck: Demographics of noise pollution with respect to potential hearing loss. In Henderson D, Hamernik RP, Dosanjh DS, et al (eds): Effects of Noise on Hearing. New York: Raven Press, 1976, p. 21.

43. Fatjó JF, Mets M, Braus B, et al: Aggression in wolves (*Canis lupus*): Ambivalent behaviour as a model for comparable behaviour in dogs (*Canis familiaris*). In Mills D, Levine E, Landsberg G, et al (eds): Current Issues and Research in Veterinary Behavioral Medicine. West Lafayette, IN: Purdue University Press, 2005, p. 98.

44. Feddersen-Petersen D: Social behavior of wolves and dogs. Voorjaarsdagem, Amsterdam, Netherlands: April 22, 1994.

45. Feddersen-Petersen D: Some interactive aspects between dogs and their owners: Are there reciprocal influences between both inter- and intraspecific communication? Appl Anim Behav Sci 1994; 40(1):78.

46. Field R: A perspective on syntactics of wolf vocalizations. In Klinghammer E (ed): The Behavior and Ecology of Wolves. New York: Garland STPM Press, 1979, p. 182.

47. Flint EL: The tragedy of a quick-fix approach to canine behaviour problems: A New Zealand perspective. In Mills D, Levine E, Landsberg G, et al (eds): Current Issues and Research in Veterinary Behavioral Medicine. West Lafayette, IN: Purdue University Press, 2005, p. 255.

48. Fox MW: Canine Behavior. Springfield, IL: Charles C Thomas, 1965.

49. Fox MW: The anatomy of aggression and its ritualization in Canidae: A developmental and comparative study. Behavior 1969; 35:242.

50. Fox MW: Ontogeny of prey-killing behavior in Canidae. Behavior 1969; 35:259.

51. Fox MW: A comparative study of the development of facial expressions in canids; wolf, coyote and foxes. Behavior 1970; 36:49.

52. Fox MW: Understanding Your Dog. New York: Coward, McCann and Geoghegan Inc, 1972.

53. Fox MW: Inter-species interaction differences in play actions in canids. Appl Anim Ethol 1976; 2(2):181.

54. Fox MW: The Dog: Its Domestication and Behavior. New York: Garland STPM Press, 1978.

55. Fox MW, Beck AM, Blackman E: Behavior and ecology of a small group of urban dogs (*Canis familiaris*). Appl Anim Ethol 1975; 1(2):119.

56. Fox MW, Cohen JA: Canid communication. In Sebeok TA (ed): How Animals Communicate. Bloomington: Indiana University Press, 1977, p. 728.

57. Fukuzawa M, Mills DS, Cooper JJ: More than just a word: Non-semantic command variables affect obedience in the domestic dog (*Canis familiaris*). Appl Anim Behav Sci 2005; 91:129.

58. Goodwin D, Bradshaw JWS, Wickens SM: Paedomorphosis affects agonistic visual signals of domestic dogs. Anim Behav 1997; 53(2):297.

59. Goodwin M, Gooding KM, Regnier F: Sex pheromone in the dog. SCI 1979; 203:559.

60. Gorman ML, Trowbridge BJ: The role of odor in the social lives of carnivores. In Gittleman JL (ed): Carnivore Behavior, Ecology and Evolution. Ithaca, NY: Comstock Publishing Associates, 1989, p. 57.

61. Graham D, Mills DS, Bailey G: Evaluation of the effect of temporary exposure to synthetic dog appeasing pheromone (DAP) on levels of arousal in puppy classes. In Landsberg G, Mattiello S, Mills D (eds): Proceedings of the 6th International Veterinary Behaviour Meeting and European College of Veterinary Behavioural Medicine—Companion Animals European Society of Veterinary Clinical Ethology. Brescia, Italy: Fondazione Iniziative Zooprofilattiche e Zootecniche, 2007, p.133.

62. Hare B, Brown M, Williamson C, et al: The domestication of social cognition in dogs. Science 2002; 298(5598):1634.

63. Hare B, Tomasello M: Domestic dogs (*Canis familiaris*) use human and conspecific social cues to locate hidden food. J Comp Psychol 1999; 113(2):173.

64. Harrington FH: Aggressive howling in wolves. Anim Behav 1987; 35(1):7.

65. Hart BL: Effect of castration on urine marking. J Am Vet Med Assoc 1974; 164(2):140.

66. Hart BL: Environmental and hormonal influences on urine marking behavior in the adult male dog. Behav Biol 1974; 11:167.

67. Hart BL: Problems with the barking dog. Canine Pract 1978; 5(1):8.

68. Hart BL: Anthropomorphism: Two perspectives. Canine Pract 1978; 5(3):12.

69. Haug L: Personal communication, 3/16/2005.

70. Hopkins SG, Schubert TA, Hart BL: Castration of adult male dogs: Effects on roaming, aggression, urine marking, and mounting. J Am Vet Med Assoc 1976; 168(12):1108.

71. Houpt K: Good neighbor barker breaker, DACVB Listserve, 3/13/2007.

72. Houpt KA: Disruption of the human-companion animal bond: Aggressive behavior in dogs. In Katcher AH, Beck AM (eds): New Perspectives on Our Lives with Companion Animals. Philadelphia: University of Pennsylvania Press, 1983, p. 197.

73. Houpt KA: Companion animal behavior: A review of dog and cat behavior in the field, the laboratory, and the clinic. Cornell Vet 1985; 75:248.

74. Houpt KA, Beaver B: Behavioral problems of geriatric dogs and cats. Vet Clin North Am [Small Anim Pract] 1981; 114:643.

75. Hunthausen W: Identifying and treating behavior problems in geriatric dogs. Vet Med (Suppl) 1994; 89:688.

76. Juarbe-Diaz SV, Houpt KA: Comparison of two antibarking collars for treatment of nuisance barking. J Am Anim Hosp Assoc 1996; 32(3):231.

77. Joby R: The control of undesirable behaviour in male dogs using megestrol acetate. J Small Anim Pract 1984; 25:567.

78. Kiley-Worthington M: The tail movements of ungulates, canids and felids with particular reference to their causation and function as displays. Behavior 1976; LVI(1-2):69.

79. Kleiman D: Scent marking in the Canidae. Symposia Zool Soc Lond 1966; 18:167.

80. Kleiman DG, Eisenberg JF: Comparisons of canid and felid social systems from an evolutionary perspective. Anim Behav 1973; 21:637.

81. Klinghammer E, Laidlaw L: Analysis of 23 months of daily howl records in a captive grey wolf pack *(Canis lupus)*. In Klinghammer E (ed): The Behavior and Ecology of Wolves. New York: Garland STPM Press, 1979, p. 153.

82. Lambert CA: Wolf tail wag. E-mail communication, 9/26/2003.

83. Landsberg GM: The distribution of canine behavior cases at three behavior referral practices. Vet Med 1991; 86(10):1011.

84. Lindsay S: Eau-de-Canide? E-mail communication, 3/13/1998.

85. Macdonald DW: The carnivores: Order Carnivore. In Brown RE, Macdonald DW (eds): Social Odours in Mammals, vol. 2. Oxford, England: Clarendon Press, 1985, p. 619.

86. Marder A, Engel J: Behavior problems after adoption. AVSAB Annual Symposium on Anim Behav Res 2002 Meeting Proc 2002:6.

87. Mason B: What's your dog thinking? http://sciencenow. sciencemag.org/cgi/content/full/2005/808/2, 8/23/2005.

88. McConnell PB: Acoustic structure and receiver response in domestic dogs. *Canis familiaris.* Anim Behav 1990; 39:897.

89. McConnell PB, Baylis JR: Interspecific communication in cooperative herding: Acoustic and visual signals from human shepherds and herding dogs. Z Tierpsychol 1985; 67:302.

90. McCrave EA: Diagnostic criteria for separation anxiety in the dog. Vet Clin North Am [Small Anim Pract] 1991; 21(2):247.

91. McKeown DB, Luescher UA, Halip J: Stereotypies in companion animals and obsessive compulsive disorder. Purina Specialty Review in Behavioral Problems, 1992:30.

92. Meeham SK: When a bark is as bad as a bite. J Am Vet Med Assoc 1995; 207(6):682.

93. Miklósi Á, Kubinyi E, Topál J, et al: A simple reason for a big difference: Wolves do not look back at humans, but dogs do. Current Biol 2003; 13(9):763.

94. Miklósi Á, Pongrácz P, Lakatos G, et al: A comparative study of the use of visual communicative signals in interactions between dogs *(Canis familiaris)* and humans and cats *(Felis catus)* and humans. J Comp Psychol 2005; 119(2):179.

95. Miklósi Á, Pongrácz P, Molnár CS: On the communicative nature of barking. In Mills D, Levine E, Landsberg G, et al (eds): Current Issues and Research in Veterinary Behavioral Medicine. West Lafayette, IN: Purdue University Press, 2005, p. 58.

96. Miklósi Á, Soproni K: A comparative analysis of animal's understanding of the human pointing gesture. Anim Cogn 2006; 9(2):81.

97. Moffat K, Landsberg G: Effectiveness and comparison of both a citronella and scentless spray bark collar for the control of barking in a veterinary hospital setting. Am Vet Soc Anim Behav Proc 2001:7.

98. Molnár C, Pongrácz P, Dóka A, et al: Can humans discriminate between dogs on the basis of the acoustic parameters of barks? Behav Processes 2006; 73(1):76.

99. Neilson JC: Unruly and annoying behaviors in dogs and cats. http://www.avma.org/conv/cv2002/cvnotes/CAn_AnB_UAB_NeJ.asp, 7/3/2002.

100. Neilson JC, Eckstein RA, Hart BL: Effects of castration on problem behaviors in male dogs with reference to age and duration of behavior. J Am Vet Med Assoc 1997; 211(2):180.

101. Overall K: Neurochemistry of anxiety and aggression. Western Vet Conf Proc 2000.

102. Overall KL: Part 3: A rational approach: Recognition, diagnosis and management of obsessive compulsive disorders. Canine Pract 1992; 17(4):39.

103. Overall KL, Dunham AE: Clinical features and outcome in dogs and cats with obsessive-compulsive disorder: 126 cases (1989-2000). J Am Vet Med Assoc 2002; 221(10):1445.

104. Pageat P, Gaultier E: Current research in canine and feline pheromones. Vet Clin North Am [Small Anim Pract] 2003; 33(2):187.

105. Parker AJ: Behavioral changes of organic neurologic origin. Prog Vet Neurol 1990; 1(2):123.

106. Perry GA, Seksel K: A survey of barking dogs in southeast Queensland, Australia. In Mills D, Levine E, Landsberg G, et al (eds): Current Issues and Research in Veterinary Behavioral Medicine. West Lafayette, IN: Purdue University Press, 2005, p. 60.

107. Peters G, Wozencraft WC: Acoustic communication by fissiped carnivores. In Gittleman JL (ed): Carnivore Behavior, Ecology and Evolution. Ithaca, NY: Comstock Publishing Associates, 1989, p. 14.

108. Peters RP, Mech LD: Scent-marking in wolves. Am Sci 1975; 63:628.

109. Pongrácz P, Miklósi Á, Dóka A, et al: Successful application of video-projected human images for signalling to dogs. Ethology 2003; 109(10):809.

110. Pongrácz P, Molnár C, Miklósi Á: Acoustic parameters of dog barks carry emotional information for humans. Appl Anim Behav Sci 2006; 100:228.

111. Pongrácz P, Molnár C, Miklósi, et al: Human listeners are able to classify dog *(Canis familiaris)* barks recorded in different situations. J Comp Psychol 2005; 119(2):136.

112. Preti G, Muetterties EL, Furman JM, et al: Volatile constituents of dog *(Canis familiaris)* and coyote *(Canis latrans)* anal sacs. J Chem Ecol 1976; 2(2):177.

113. Quaranta A, Siniscalchi M, Vallortigara G: Asymmetric tail-wagging responses by dogs to different emotive stimuli. Curr Biol 2007; 17(6):R199.

114. Ralls K: Mammalian scent marking. SCI 1971; 171:443.

115. Rooney NJ, Bradshaw JWS, Robinson IH: The importance of play signals during dog-human games. Proc Third International Cong Vet Behav Med 2001:43.

116. Rooney NJ, Bradshaw JWS, Robinson IH: Do dogs respond to play signals given by humans? Anim Behav 2001; 61(4):715.

117. Ross S, Scott JP, Cherrier M, et al: Effects of restraint and isolation on yelping in puppies. Anim Behav 1960; 8:1.

118. Rudolph JK, Myers LJ: Is the bark worse than the bite? Vet Forum 2004; 21(3):26.

119. Ryon J, Fentress JC, Harrington FH, et al: Scent rubbing in wolves *(Canis lupus)*: The effect of novelty. Can J Zool 1986; 64:573.

120. Sales G, Hubrecht R, Peyvandi A, et al: Noise in dog kenneling: Is barking a welfare problem for dogs? Appl Anim Behav Sci 1997; 52(3-4):321.

121. Schenkel R: Submission: Its features and functions in the wolf and dog. Am Zool 1967; 7:319.

122. Seksel K: The problem of barking. Proc 75th Jubilee New Zealand Vet Assoc, Vet Continuing Edu, Massey Univ Pub No. 185 1998.

123. Senn CL, Lewin JD: Barking dogs as an environmental problem. J Am Vet Med Assoc 1975; 166(1l):1065.

124. Shepherd K: Development of behaviour, social behaviour and communication in dogs. In Horwitz DF, Mills DS, Heath S (eds): BSAVA Manual of Canine and Feline Behavioural Medicine. Quedgeley, Gloucester, England: Brit Small Anim Vet Assoc, 2002, p.8.

125. Simpson BS: Canine communication. Vet Clin North Am [Small Anim Pract] 1997; 27(3):445.

126. Skultety FM: Experimental mutism in dogs. Arch Neurol 1962; 6:235.

127. Smythe RH: Animals Habits. The Things Animals Do. Springfield, IL: Charles C Thomas, 1962.

128. Soproni K, Miklósi Á, Topál J, et al: Dogs' *(Canis familiaris)* responsiveness to human pointing gestures. J Comp Psychol 2002; 116(1):27.

129. Stewart JM, DeGhett VJ, Scott JP: Age of onset of puppies' distress vocalizations in strange and familiar situations. Am Zool 1970; 10:293.

130. Stuart J: Castration and "urine marking" in dogs. J Am Vet Med Assoc 1973; 163(9):1014.

131. Szetei V, Miklósi Á, Topál J, et al: When dogs seem to lose their nose: An investigation on the use of visual and olfactory cues in communicative context between dog and owner. Appl Anim Behav Sci 2003; 83(2):141.

132. Taylor K, Mills DS: The control of puppy *(Canis familiaris)* disturbance of owners at night. In Mills D, Levine E, Landsberg G, et al (eds): Current Issues and Research in Veterinary Behavioral Medicine. West Lafayette, IN: Purdue University Press, 2005, p. 27.

133. Tembrock G: Canid vocalizations. Behav Processes 1976; 1:57.

134. Theberge JB, Falls JB: Howling as a means of communication in wolves. Am Zool 1967; 7:331.

135. Tooze ZJ, Harrington FH, Fentress JC: Individually distinct vocalizations in timber wolves, *Canis lupus*. Anim Behav 1990; 40(4):723.

136. Virányi Z, Topál J, Gácsi M, et al.: Dogs respond appropriately to cues of humans' attentional focus. Behav Processes 2004; 66(2):161.

137. Voith VL: Behavioral disorders. In Ettinger S (ed): Textbook of Veterinary Internal Medicine. Philadelphia: Saunders, 1989, p. 227.

138. Voith VL, Marder AR: Canine behavioral disorders: Excessive vocalization. In Morgan R (ed): Handbook of Small Animal Practice. New York: Churchill Livingstone, 1988, p. 1035.

139. Wells DL: The effectiveness of a citronella spray collar in reducing certain forms of barking in dogs. Appl Anim Behav Sci 2001; 73(4):299.

140. Wells DL, Hepper PG: Prevalence of behaviour problems reported by owners of dogs purchased from an animal rescue shelter. Appl Anim Behav Sci 2000; 69(1):55.

141. Willis J: Behavior modification of excessive noise in a young Basenji. Psychol Rep 1972; 31:525.

142. Yeon SC: The vocal communication of canines. J Vet Beh 2007; 2(4):141.

143. Yin S: Barking in dogs: Communication or noise? AVSAB Annual Symp Anim Behav Res 2002 Meeting Proc 2002:5.

144. Yin S, McCowan B: Barking in domestic dogs: Context specificity and individual identification. Anim Behav 2004; 68(2):343.

## Additional Readings

Antelyes J: The Antelyes touch: Funny faces? Mod Vet Pract 1976; 57(11):963.

Ashdown RR, Lea T: Explaining Basenji barklessness. J Am Vet Med Assoc 1980; 177(11):1154.

Bamberger M, Houpt KA: Signalment factors, comorbidity, and trends in behavior diagnoses in dogs: 1,644 cases (1991-2001). J Am Vet Med Assoc 2006; 229(10):1591.

Burnett AS: Behavior modification for barking. Mod Vet Pract 1985; 66(12):1012.

Campbell W: Branding and aggression (territory). Mod Vet Pract 1975; 56(12):849.

Campbell WE: Between pets and people: The communications gap. Mod Vet Pract 1977; 58(6):549.

Coppinger R, Zuccotti J: Kennel enrichment: Exercise and socialization of dogs. J Appl Anim Welfare Sci 1999; 2(4):281.

Coren S: The Intelligence of Dogs: Canine Consciousness and Capabilities. New York: The Free Press; 1994.

Dehasse J, Schroll S: The influence of the experimenter's expectancy in the results of the assessment of appeasing pheromones in stress of police dogs *(Canis familiaris)* during training. In Mills D, Levine E, Landsberg G, et al (eds): Current Issues and Research in Veterinary Behavioral Medicine. West Lafayette, IN: Purdue University Press, 2005, p. 23.

Donovan CA: Canine anal glands and chemical signals (pheromones). J Am Vet Med Assoc 1969; 155(12): 1995.

Gácsi M, Miklósi Á, Varga O, et al: Are readers of our face readers of our minds? Dogs *(Canis familiaris)* show situation-dependent recognition of human's attention. Anim Cogn 2004; 7(3):144.

Gese EM, Ruff RL: Scent-marking by coyotes, *Canis latrans*: The influence of social and ecological factors. Anim Behav 1998; 54(5):1155.

Hemmer H: Domestication: The Decline of Environmental Appreciation. New York: Cambridge University Press, 1990.

Juarbe-Diaz SV: Assessment and treatment of excessive barking in the domestic dog. Vet Clin North Am [Small Anim Pract] 1997; 27(3):515.

Kaminski J, Call J, Fischer J: Word learning in a domestic dog: Evidence for "Fast Mapping." Sci 2004; 304(5677):1682.

Laven-Butler RD: Evaluating the effectiveness of the Aboistop as a treatment for excessive vocalizing in the dog. International Society for Applied Ethology meeting abstracts, part 1, June 23, 1996.

Lewin JD: Barking dog noise in veterinary hospitals. J Am Anim Hosp Assoc 1974; 10(2):183.

Matthews SL: Elimination barking as an attention-getting device. Canine Pract 1984; 11(1):6.

Mills DS, Fukuzawa M, Cooper JJ: The effect of emotional content of verbal commands on the response of dogs *(Canis familiaris)*. In Mills D, Levine E, Landsberg G, et al (eds): Current Issues and Research in Veterinary Behavioral Medicine. West Lafayette, IN: Purdue University Press, 2005, p. 217.

Montagna W, Parks HF: A histochemical study of the glands of the anal sac of the dog. Anat Rec 1948; 100:297.

Moore RA: Behavioral vices in dogs: Educates owners. Mod Vet Pract 1985; 66(12):1010.

Neilson JC: The anxious animal. Wild West Vet Conf Vet Syllabus 2002:595.

Osella MC, Bergamasco L, Cost F: Use of a synthetic analogue of dog-appeasing pheromone in sheltered dogs after adoption. In Mills D, Levine E, Landsberg G, et al (eds): Current Issues and Research in Veterinary Behavioral Medicine. West Lafayette, IN: Purdue University Press, 2005, p. 270.

Psychologist develops anti-aggression training: DVM 1983; 14(10):55.

Romanes GJ: Dog-General intelligence. In Hendersen RW (ed): Learning in Animals. Stroudsburg, PA: Hutchinson Ross Publishing Co, 1982, p. 24.

Tripp R: Control barking in the veterinary kennel. Vet Pract News 2000; 12(9):34.

Virányi Z, Topál J, Miklósi Á, et al.: A nonverbal test of knowledge attribution: A comparative study on dogs and children. Anim Cogn 2006; 9(1):13.

Voith VL, Borchelt PL: Diagnosis and treatment of dominance aggression in dogs. Vet Clin North Am [Small Anim Pract] 1982; 12(4):655.

Vollmer PJ: Puppy rearing-6: Vocalizing. Vet Med Small Anim Clin 1978; 73:1519.

Vollmer PJ: Electrical stimulation-2: Bark-training collars. Vet Med Small Anim Clin 1979; 80(12):1737.

# CHAPTER 4

# Canine Social Behavior

Dogs are a social species, like humans. During the selective breeding process, some modifications were made to the group structure. As a result, many of the interactions and problem behaviors of dogs are associated with intercanid relations. From sexual behavior to predatory behavior, from urine marking to mutual grooming, the subtleties for much of the canine daily life are based on social relationships. To complicate this process, humans are accepted as group members, bringing in the factor of interspecies interactions.

Social behaviors start at birth and become more intricate as a puppy gets older. Social learning passes through the stages of socialization, development of dominant-subordinate relationships, behavioral maturation, and group interactions.

The largest and most complete study of the social interactions of the dog was headed by J.P. Scott and J.L. Fuller at Bar Harbour, Maine. These findings were published in a number of scientific articles cited throughout this chapter and in the classic text, *Genetics and the Social Behavior of the Dog*.[290] Any serious student of dog behavior is encouraged to read this text.

## SOCIALIZATION AND OTHER CRITICAL PERIODS

The hypothesis that a specific experience will lead to different behavioral results at different periods during the development of an animal is the one on which the existence of *critical periods* is based.[292] The concept of critical periods (also called *sensitive periods*) means that certain important events must happen in specific time periods or else that learning opportunity is lost.[32] It would be expected that one of these critical periods occurs when new social relationships can be easily developed and another when memory becomes consistent.[292] Using these

types of landmarks, social behavior for dogs has been divided into four time periods: neonatal, transition, socialization, and juvenile.

The *neonatal period* covers the first 2 weeks of life, from birth until the eyes and ears open.* Because of the immature physical and neurologic state of the puppy at this age, behavior is restricted to infantile patterns—mainly sleeping and nursing. Only a lack of tactile input from the dam or littermates causes a neonatal puppy to become active.[165]

The *transition period* is a short time frame starting when the eyes and ears open and during which the locomotor skills change from a crawl to a walk.[20,105,284,292] It is a time of rapid neurologic and physical development, when puppies first begin to respond to environmental stimuli.[298] This is usually the time that puppies become mobile enough to start leaving the nest box, first notice others, and start eating semisolid foods.

*Socialization* is the third critical period for a young puppy, It probably is the single most important time in the dog's life relative to social interaction.[32] This period begins at 3 weeks of age, when the puppy becomes capable of seeking nonmaternal social interaction, and it lasts until infantile behavior patterns end and environmental interactions become more attractive than social ones—about 12 weeks of age.† A lot of other things happen during this time relative to the maturation of physical, neurologic, and behavioral features. Motor skills mature to allow active interaction and reaction. The nervous system approaches adult-like patterns, and stable learning begins. Evidence exists that events during the socialization period may be critical for other effects, such as attachment to

---

*References 20, 105, 197, 223, 284, 292, 298.
†References 20, 105, 223, 288, 290, 292.

particular places,[286] formation of basic food habits,[286] development of agile motor skills,[97] and reaction to isolation.[97]

Because the socialization period is so significant, it is important to understand the various types of learning that go on during that time. Rapid brain development and maturation, along with myelination of the spinal cord parallel the social significance of this period.[298] The most significant lesson that should occur during this time period is species identification. By raising puppies in solitary isolation, paired isolation, around cats, or around people and then testing at various intervals, investigators have learned much about the importance of puppies being with other dogs and with people. At 3 to 5 weeks of age, puppies will actively approach people who are either familiar or strangers.[116,117,197] Eventually puppies will develop an attachment to their owner and approach them in preference to a stranger. In contrast, well-socialized wolf cubs do not show approach differences between known individuals and strangers.[310] Five to 8 weeks is considered to be the optimum time to socialize puppies.[288] Shortly thereafter, avoidance of strangers begins and slowly escalates until it peaks at 12 to 14 weeks of age.[106,116,117] This progressive avoidance helps protect the youngster from predators,[106,197] but it can also prevent normal relationships with humans.[116]

Although there are breed differences in responses,[121,290] puppies that are completely isolated from humans until 14 weeks of age are never comfortable around people.[117] They act unapproachable, like a wild wolf,* usually attempting to avoid interactions and acting fearful if escape is not possible.[104,106] If raised only around humans or cats for 14 weeks (no other dogs), the puppy tends to avoid its own species both socially and sexually.[104,108,112,122,123] A hand-reared puppy is more apt to show inappropriate social behaviors toward other dogs, from aggression to avoidance (Fig. 4-1).[223]

At the other extreme, in wolves and dogs, the adult that was not socialized to people as a cub or puppy can nevertheless be socialized to a few

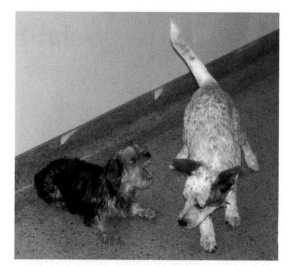

**Figure 4-1.** The Yorkshire Terrier was not raised around other dogs and now shows aggression even to puppies.

individual humans with very careful handling.[108] The period between puppyhood and adulthood when socialization apparently cannot occur may be related to the increased physical and emotional development that can finally be overcome as an adult.[108]

Puppies isolated in cages from 8 weeks to 6 months of age, or kept in kennels beyond 14 weeks of age, showed a generalized fear of different environments.[108,218,288] Those kept in relatively bland surroundings showed behavior aberrations in new, more complex environments.[108,119] This *institutionalization syndrome,* or *kennelosis,* is expressed as a lack of interest in exploring a new environment; the puppy will withdraw into the transport crate and show timidity or other inappropriate responses to strangers.[108,218,223] It is only comfortable in its original environment.[288] Even the inclusion of toys, especially rawhides, in the puppy environment is of some enrichment to help prevent this.[159] If this isolation also includes social isolation, significant changes occur in behavior and in brain chemistry.[4] Although there are genetic differences, the general reaction after social isolation is one of withdrawal from social activities. Glutamic acid, glutamine, gamma-aminobutyric acid (GABA), and aspartic acid levels in the superior colliculi, thalamus-hypothalamus, and caudate nucleus are

---

*References 104, 106, 108, 116, 117, 337

significantly different between puppies raised in isolation and their littermate controls.[4]

The actual amount of contact needed for socialization to another species is probably quite brief, and it can be influenced by outside factors. Studies suggest a minimum of 2 minutes per week is sufficient.[288] Food rewards are not necessary for socialization, nor does punishment inhibit it; however, hunger and its gratification will speed up the process.[284] Emotional stress associated with separation begins at 3 weeks,[288] then strong emotional experiences, such as occur when the puppy is separated from its mother and littermates in a strange location, will also speed up socialization toward human handlers.[284] This natural separation at weaning coincides with the barking and whining of isolation, which peaks by 6 to 7 weeks.[223,284]

Isolation and restraint significantly increase the amount of distress vocalization a puppy uses, but the addition of a companion can reduce the distress vocalization by 50% to 60%.[96,277] Because this age also happens to be a common one for new puppies to go to new homes, socialization to people may actually be facilitated. New owners, however, should be advised to not overreact to whining episodes. The experience of distress in general will be sufficient for socialization, and response to the vocalizations could reward the undesired behavior.

An interesting study was done on the effects of punishment at different times during socialization.[106,111] Puppies raised with normal human contact were divided into three groups that were tested at either 5 to 6 weeks, 8 to 9 weeks, or 12 to 13 weeks of age. Each group was first tested for the approach response to humans. If the puppies did approach, they were given a mild electric shock. The puppies of age 5 to 6 weeks who actively approached the human ran away when shocked. When retested a few weeks later, these same puppies actively approached again as if they had no memory of the first episode. The puppies of age 8 to 9 weeks that approached the human also retreated from the shock. When these puppies were later retested, though, they would not approach the person. The oldest group, those of age 12 to 13 weeks, continued to approach the human even though they received the shock.

These were three different reactions at three different ages. Stable learning does not start until approximately 8 weeks of age. Therefore, the young puppies of age 5 to 6 weeks first showed the typical active approach to humans and, when retested, showed no memory of the early traumatic experience. This result would be consistent with a new pet puppy actively approaching a resident cat, getting clawed on the nose, but returning to pester the cat again.

Because of the start of stable learning at around 8 weeks, the puppies of age 8 to 9 weeks remembered the trauma and chose to avoid a similar situation. Traumatic episodes (trauma from the puppy's perspective) can desocialize a dog. A discharge of static electricity, a toe accidentally stepped on, or a painful vaccination may be sufficient for the puppy to become cautious of an individual or a similar group of individuals.

The older puppies of age 12 to 13 weeks had been socialized, and their continued approach indicated a strong emotional attachment toward humans. As is the case in interactions with children, the puppies may have felt safer by being close than by running away. For example, a dog may follow a child leaving home on a bicycle, even though the dog is not supposed to leave the property. The child then gets off the bicycle and hits or throws stones at the dog, yelling for it to go home. The dog responds by lying down next to the child instead of running home, so the frustrated child has to ride the bicycle home and tie up the dog before starting out again.

Separation of 6-week-old puppies from their mother, as would occur during weaning, has been shown to have a negative effect on their well being for the next 6 weeks.[302] Parameters affected include higher susceptibility to disease and mortality.[302] Separation from the dam either at 6 weeks or 12 weeks did not affect socialization to humans if daily human contact was received.[302]

Not everything happening during the socialization period relates strictly to social behavior. Fear of strange objects begins at 7 weeks and peaks at 14 weeks.[288] When puppies are introduced to new environments, it is important that owners allow appropriate time and positive situations as the puppy learns that the new object poses no threat.

The fourth and last of a puppy's critical periods is the *juvenile period,* which extends from approximately 12 weeks until sexual maturity.[20,197,290,292] The lessons of socialization will need occasional reinforcement during the juvenile period and afterward, or they can be forgotten within 6 months.[122] If the original learning did not occur, the dog will be socially handicapped throughout the remainder of its life.[104,338] Environmental exploration increases during the juvenile period, and if the puppy has not been around people, it will show avoidance of them. The basic learning capacity is fully developed, and the speed for conditional learning begins to slow, perhaps because of the interference of previous learning.[197]

Other critical periods occur related to specific events, although specifics for these periods are less well understood. One critical period occurs for mothers to learn to identify their newborn as their own. Another coincides with sexual maturity, when dogs learn territorial boundaries.[284]

## SOCIAL (REACTIVE) DISTANCES

It is generally true for any social species that individuals will spend a considerable amount of time in proximity with their own kind. To maintain a social unit, most intercanine interactions must be friendly and of a cooperative nature, that is, *allelomimetic.* Dogs in a pack spend 43% to 85% of their time within 50 feet of each other.[122] By becoming the equivalent of a pack member, the dog owner must consider this social need. Of course, it is often impractical for a person to spend 10 to 20 hours a day with the dog, and most dogs can adjust to less time together if maintained on a fairly regular schedule. The reaction of the dog to other species and individuals depends on socialization, environmental context, physiologic state, "mood," intensity of stimulation, and early learning.[32]

### Home Range

The *home range* of a dog is the farthest distance from home that it would normally travel.[32] It usually consists of a dense core area, with farther distances used less often.[41,166] The dog turned out each morning will typically have a pattern of travel around the neighborhood. Although an unusual scent trail may cause an occasional deviation, it generally will not affect the normal home range.

In the wild, the size of a home range is influenced by the availability of food.[166] For wolves the size of the home range is correlated with metabolic needs and in proportion to the amount of meat in the diet.[127] Plentiful amounts and reliable sources of food tend to be associated with smaller home ranges, as in urban areas where home ranges vary from 0.01 to 61.0 hectares (ha) (0.02 to 150.7 acres).* Dogs in rural areas tend to have larger home ranges of 444 to 1050 ha (1100 to 2600 acres).[109,153,294] These figures correspond to home-range information for free-ranging dogs as well.[125,240,241]

The size of a home range also may show seasonal variations, with those of winter being approximately half as large as those of summer.[79,241] Seasonal variations are not, however, always observed.[80] The size of a home range correlates to neither the dog's size nor sex, and the home ranges of owned dogs are not significantly smaller than those of unowned dogs.[79] Abandoned dogs usually remain very near a food source, so their home range averages 0.02 ha (0.049 acres) in size.[80]

The distance of a daily excursion varies from 500 to 8200 m (0.3 to 5.1 miles) for a pack of owned dogs to 10,000 m (6 miles) for feral dog packs.[108,109,125,294] This movement occurs at approximately equal distances in all directions from the core.[278] Activity is primarily in the cool periods of the day, so the pack-group dogs are most active at night and early morning, especially from 8 PM to 11 PM in the evening and 5 AM to 8 AM in the morning.[80,294] Urban dogs are most active when humans are the least—that is, early morning and late in the day[109,278]—or at times when people typically turn the dogs out of their homes, like 7 AM and 5 PM.[41,103] Feral dogs are seasonally more active when the weather is cool.[125]

### Territory

In general terms, a *territory* is the part of the home range that is actively defended.[32,103,166] This defense can be by aggressive encounters, vocalization,

---

*References 41, 103, 108, 109, 155, 278.

or threat displays.[166] It is also a space where the boundaries are marked to create olfactory fences. For dogs, the most important area is usually near the core of the home range, where a dog spends most of its time. Barriers like chain link fences can artificially limit the size of both the territory and home range.[278]

Many, but not all, dogs are very protective of their territory. The intensity of a dog's threat will increase as an intruder moves closer toward its territory and toward the center of its territory. When a stranger first approaches a territorial boundary, the dog responds with a high-pitched, rapid bark. If the intruder enters the territory, the pitch lowers and the dog's body language becomes more threatening. As the stranger goes deeper into the territory, the bark may turn to a growl, and the growl may give way to an attack.

The dog is somewhat ambivalent about how aggressively it should defend the edges of a territory, in essence having to weigh the importance of holding the space against the potential for being hurt. But the closer to the center of the territory an intruder approaches, the greater is the shift in importance toward holding the space. For this reason, dogs are often very aggressive in defending small territories such as cars. If the opportunity is available, the average dog territory will consist of 2 ha (4.9 acres), with a 0.65 ha (0.6 acre) core area in which the dog has its favorite resting spots and spends approximately 60% of its time.

Other types of territories can exist. Aggression at a food bowl may occasionally represent the protection of a feeding territory, although it may also be associated with food-protection aggression. Breeding locations, nest sites, and sleeping locations can all be territories defended by a dog.

## Distances When Approached

When a dog is approached by a member of a species to which it is poorly socialized, the dog will first become aware of the stranger when it reaches the *perceptive distance*.[32] It may show no visible acknowledgment of this awareness, it may look toward the approaching individual, or it may actually walk a short distance toward the intruder. In this latter case, the actual distance the dog walks forward is the *approach distance*.[32] If the intruder continues to come toward the dog, a point will be reached at which the discomfort is so great that the dog will flee. The distance at which this escape behavior happens is the *flight distance*.[32,107] The distance the dog runs away from the potential danger is the *withdrawal distance*.[32] In many cases, the dog will then stop, reassess the situation, and leave the area at a somewhat slower pace. If for some reason the dog was unaware of the intruder's approach or was unable to flee, the dog will attack as the stranger reaches the animal's *critical distance*.[32,107] This type of attack usually has the characteristics of fear biting, but the wounds inflicted can be quite serious.

If the approaching individual is recognized by the dog, the aforementioned distances do not apply. Instead, they are replaced by individual, social, and submissive distances. Close associates are allowed within a space immediately surrounding the dog, the *individual* or *personal distance*.[32,107] This is the space in which veterinarians must work. If the dog is uncomfortable with a person entering that space, it will try to move away, putting the person into the more remote *social distance*.[32] If the dog is comfortable with the person's approach, it may show submissive behaviors as the person gets to its *submissive distance*.[32]

## SOCIAL ORGANIZATION

How dogs interact with one another is influenced by many factors: proximity, dominant-subordinate relationships, and species-specific interrelations. Interactions between dogs can result in social facilitation and competition for food,[293, 316] especially when that food is highly palatable.[74] Wolf behavior and that of feral, untamed, or genetically selected dog populations can provide insight into the behavior of the pet dog. Puppies born to free-ranging bitches have a high mortality rate—68% by 4 months of age.[241] When old enough, the surviving offspring tend to disperse, especially males. The mean distance they go from their birth place is just under 2 km.[241]

### Social Orders

Dominant-subordinate relations ultimately promote group harmony and a decreased incidence of agonistic interactions. Disputes can be settled through the use of subtle threats instead of more serious aggression. When puppies are raised together, they can establish their dominance hierarchy over food or play without inflicting serious injury.[122] Older dogs depend mainly on the language of body positions, with occasional aggressive bouts needed for dominant-personality individuals. Social ranks are generally thought of as having a stair-step order, with each individual a step below the more dominant one above it. This linear A over B over C ranking generally holds true in dogs, although certain positions can be shared by two individuals, and occasionally there can even be a triangular relationship such as A over B over C over A.[32,122]

The social hierarchy will be established by 15 weeks of age in 88% of the puppies.[290,291] Dominant puppies control access to the food bowl and other favorite resources. Once the dominant-subordinate relationships are established, there is a reduction in the number of fights and in the seriousness of the play fights.[98,290] Instead, the group members play more often and interact more in general. Siblings recognize and prefer one another to other puppies.[143] This group may even attack or mock-attack strangers,[290] and if raised around members of only one breed, they may direct their attentions more toward the recognized breed of dog.

Once dogs establish a social order, they tend to retain that order, but a few changes can occur over time. After 11 weeks of age, there can be marked differences in hierarchy based on breeds.[243] Some breeds tend to maintain positions once they have been established. Others have a deterioration of rank so that all the puppies again become equals. The most clear-cut differences seem to be in the tendencies for males to be dominant over most females, especially female littermates.* Litter size, physical size, and relative dominance of the bitch can also influence dominance.† In trials between Terriers and Beagles, terriers are dominant. They control food availability and, as adults, sire all the puppies.[164] It is also interesting to note that if given a choice for social interaction, both breeds will choose to be with a Beagle as opposed to a terrier.[164] Puppies that are introduced to older dogs typically come in at the bottom of the social order.

In discussions about dog social ranks, there is a tendency to compare it to wolves. Although lessons can be learned by doing this, it is important to be careful not to expect exact duplication. For example, group members are almost all related individuals of different ages. Also, wolves live in packs in which there is a dominance ranking for males and a separate one for females. There is a well-defined alpha wolf that is not only the leader, but also a decision maker, intervening to settle disputes.[108] The highest ranking male and highest ranking female are usually the only two that can successfully mate.[108] It is also noted that for both the male and female social orders, the highest ranking individuals are well defined, but it becomes harder to identify hierarchical positions as you get further from the top.[51] For dogs, we have put them as individuals in a human "pack" with different social rules, surgically neutered the dogs so hormonal influences of social behaviors are removed, and mixed sexes within the "pack." Dogs do not signal like wolves, complicating interactions even more.[51] Few dogs try to assume an alpha position and readily yield that role to humans. Instead of needing the "put in your place" handling advocated by some trainers, dogs seek a pack leader figure.

Relative dominance is usually tested by giving two dogs access to one bone (Fig. 4-2). The dog that gets possession is considered the higher ranking dog. Adult dogs rarely take bones from young puppies, but by 7 months of age a puppy will always lose its bone to an adult male dog and will lose it 54% of the time to an adult female.[93] Between male and female adults, males will gain possession of the bone 2.5 times more often than females. If possession is shared, the male usually has the largest end.[93]

Once established, the interdog hierarchy may remain stable for several years with only minor fluctuations occurring, by breed, as mentioned earlier, or during estrus.[18,93,285] If dogs are also studied during interactions with other dogs, it is possible in some cases to find differences between the results of dominance tests with bones and those with

---

*References 18, 19, 93, 107, 243, 291.
†References 93, 105, 107, 140, 164, 291.

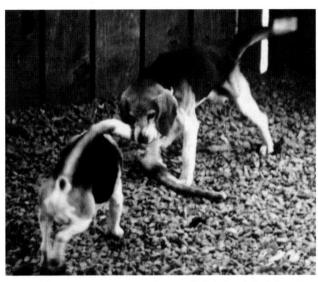

**Figure 4-2.** Testing relative dominance of two dogs with access to food (oxtail). Note the relative tail position and the placement of the paw on the food as a sign of possession by the lower ranking dog. (From Ian Dunbar, Center for Applied Animal Behavior, used with permission.)

social interactions. This result points to more than one type of dominance: dominance can be competitive or social.[342] Maintaining possession of a bone, then, is unrelated to physical size.[18] If food is not a strong motivator, an individual may not appear very dominant and yet actually be fairly high ranking socially. A direct correlation has been made between exploratory behavior and competitive dominance.[343]

If puppies are raised around humans, humans will usually be viewed as dominant.[105] Humans are viewed as dominant in part because of their relatively greater size and age. Certain individuals, especially from some breeds, are less likely to accept this rank as automatic. Firm but gentle guidance during puppyhood may be necessary to establish a human as the pack leader. Care must be used to ensure that the appropriate lessons are learned but that excessive force is not exerted.

A dominant wolf may pin a subordinate to the ground by the neck.[285] Although it has been reported not to be part of the 71 behavior patterns that dogs share with wolves,[285] this behavior does occasionally occur in dogs, but more in play than serious altercations (see Chapter 3, Fig. 3-11). Despite its popularity with a few dog trainers, the

*alpha-roll technique,* in which the human pins the adult dog or puppy down on its back, even growling near its neck, is excessive and not appropriate, because it is not a common dog behavior. It can result in a very dominant dog becoming more aggressive or any dog showing aggression because of fear. The dog is also likely to develop a distrust of the person. The individual attempting such a move can be injured by teeth or claws from the fearful dog and may even misinterpret the fear reaction to mean the dog is acting "like an alpha."

## Feral versus Domestic Dogs

Pack behaviors vary somewhat between feral dogs and their domestic relatives, whether the domestic dogs are stray or just loose (free ranging). The term *feral* is most appropriately applied to a group of animals that have been together long enough that their innate behaviors, physiology, or anatomy have changed from the original domesticated version. True feral populations are generally low, perhaps 2.5% of the free-ranging population.[183] Most feral individuals are solitary scavengers that participate in a pack for only brief periods under a rigid hierarchy.[108,109,125] When feral dogs do pack together, the pack has up to 10 members,[125,171,294] consisting of two males and six to eight females.[125] A feral dog pack typically lasts only 1 to 2.5 weeks and has a large dog as its leader.[125] When a new pack is formed, the lead dog barks loudly until a sufficient number of other feral dogs join.

Canine specializations to accommodate the hunting of large herbivores have developed in parallel with pack-hunting techniques.[171] Peripheral dogs may follow this group, but they are not allowed to share any kill. During their travels, the feral dogs will frequently stop to test dominance, but a definite order can be identified, both during travel and when eating. Aggression is rare, with avoidance preferred.[41,79] If aggression does occur, dogs unfamiliar with each other are 5 to 15 times more likely to be involved than familiar ones.[79]

Cases have been recorded in which members of a feral pack suddenly turn on and kill a weak member.[125] This type of behavior has also been seen in domestic dogs. It has happened in at least two research colonies of geriatric Beagles and in occasional household environments. Because people have not been around to see the actual attacks, precipitating factors are unknown.

Feral dogs can be tamed individually but, like a wild animal, they usually become very aggressive when forced to interact with humans.[294] As might be expected, feral dogs have a greater flight distance, are more elusive when being followed, are not active in the morning between 6:30 and 9:00, and systematically forage for food.

Stray dogs are unowned animals that tend to show remarkable plasticity in pack behavior, leading to group stability.[103] The density of stray dogs reflects this plasticity, varying from 127 dogs to 1304 dogs per square kilometer.[103] Stray-dog packs tend to be a little smaller than feral packs and have two to three times as many males as females.[79,103,125]

Free-ranging (loose but owned) dogs tend to be solitary, but approximately 60% of their dog interactions develop into temporary groups of two to five dogs.[41,125,183,278] Whereas strays are wary and tend to retreat from humans, free-ranging dogs are more likely to show aggression or bark at humans.[278] As many as 60% of these free-ranging dogs are wearing collars.[278] Strays have larger flight distances than free-ranging dogs.

## Social Maturity

Evolution of canine behavior resulted in sophisticated pack hunting techniques and with them, a group structure based on long-term affiliations.[171] Domestication of the wolf to the dog has resulted in other changes, just as Belgaev's experimental domestication of foxes did.[38,73] Comparisons between identically raised wolf cubs and Malamute puppies suggest that differences can be attributed to the genetic selection for prolongation of juvenile behaviors and morphologic characteristics.[115] Changes associated with domestication have resulted in canids that can read human communicative signals.[131] On the negative side, it has also been blamed for the breakdown in ritualized aggression,[115] perhaps resulting in the inability of many dog owners to know exactly what to expect in certain situations.

Although dog behavior is similar to wolf behavior, it is not the same, and a wolf may or may not recognize various components of a dog's behavior.[51,115] Cubs have approximately 100 facial expressions by 18 weeks of age; puppies have significantly fewer.[101] Play and social behaviors also differ. Whereas cubs show an increase in both social and solitary play during their first year, the young dog reaches a maximum of play at around 6 months and then decreases.[101] In one study, Poodle puppies showed little interaction with the adult males that were part of the group until the females' first estrus. By comparison, wolf cubs had frequent, nonstressful encounters with adults.[101] This difference may have a bearing on the tendency toward unstable social orders in dogs.[101] It has been shown that there are considerable differences in social affinity among nonestrous females, each showing an individual pattern of preference.[18] It has also been suggested that the interactions between the puppies and bitch facilitate the appearance of submission and affect later trainability.[340]

As a social species, dogs develop certain behavior patterns that allow safe interaction among individuals, and these patterns change as dogs age. As with the young of most species, the physical properties of the puppy tend to inhibit aggression by adults. This fact holds true even when the puppy's playful interactions take on an added play-fighting

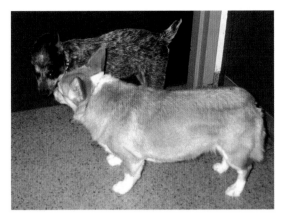

**Figure 4-3.** The facial-lingual approach for canine greeting.

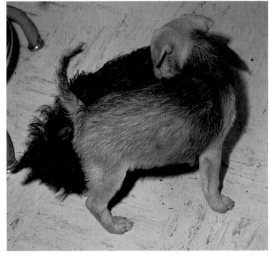

**Figure 4-5.** The anogenital approach for canine greeting.

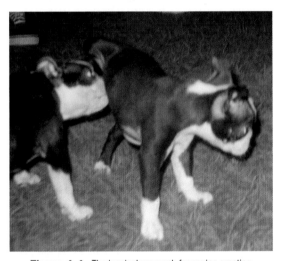

**Figure 4-4.** The inguinal approach for canine greeting.

component by 5 weeks of age.[122] By 6 weeks of age, the puppy shows most of the species-specific patterns, including the facial-lingual greeting response, the inguinal approach, and the anogenital approach (Figs. 4-3, 4-4, and 4-5).[38,122] At 9 weeks, the pup's behavior repertoire includes submissive postures, et-epimeletic (care soliciting), forelimb raising, licking, and investigation-initiated rear-limb raising.[122] Social maturity is reached much later, usually at 12 to 24 months of age, approximately twice the age of sexual maturity. It may occasionally be as late as 36 months in very large breeds.[218]

Responses of a dog to being petted indicate the extent to which the dog is able to include humans as a member of its pack. It would correspond with mutual grooming between dogs. Simple tactile contact can dramatically lower the dog's heart rate, blood pressure, respiratory rate, aortic blood flow, and coronary artery blood flow.[188] Responses can also vary somewhat depending on the sex of the dog and the person involved. Female dogs show little reluctance to approach unfamiliar people regardless of gender. Male dogs are much less likely to approach unfamiliar men.[187] Most dogs solicit petting from their owner but few really are relaxed when an owner tries to hug them.

## Social Cognition

Social cognition is the derivation of social information from the observation between group members.[274] In many ways it puts observational learning in the social context. Although social cognition has been extensively studied in primates, only recently has it been investigated in dogs. An observer dog will interact first and/or more rapidly with the winner of a play bout than with the loser.[274] If the social context was a contest over a resource instead of a play bout, the observer dog is less likely to seek interaction with either winner or loser.[274] Dogs have been shown also to be able to learn from human demonstrations, not just that from other dogs,[254,255] but verbal attention-getting may be an important aspect of that success.[256]

# SPECIAL HUMAN-CANINE SITUATIONS

The long history of dogs and humans was discussed in Chapter 1. It is the social characteristics of dogs that have allowed this to come about. This interspecies social interaction has some unique situations that are worthy of separate discussion.

## Moving to a New Home

There is no question that moving to a new home, while exciting, is stressful to people. All the disruptions in schedules and human interactions make it stressful for dogs too. Almost 50% of dogs will show signs of distress, including 23% that show excessive vocalization, 15% will have changes in urination or defecation patterns, and 13% will overgroom.[295] About 20% of dogs may escape from the new home,[295] turning the move into a tragedy.

A few precautions can minimize the dog's stress. Owners should try to keep the pet's schedule as close to normal as possible. That includes social interactions as well as meals. Exercise helps reduce stress and can be helpful to both the owner and the animal. Getting the dog gradually used to being in a crate or exercise pen long before the move will mean it has a familiar place to be after the move. In addition the owner can put in a clothing item, like a dirty tee shirt, that has a lot of owner odor on it, as an olfactory reassurance. The pheromone diffusers may also be helpful.

Pets that move or travel should be microchipped, and that microchip needs to be registered with the parent company nationally. Contact information should be changed right away and should include the phone number of a friend or relative in a different geographic location, in case of a significant disaster like a hurricane.

## Rehoming of a Dog

Unfortunately in the United States, it is common for a dog to go to a new home after it has grown up. It could be a dog adopted from a shelter, one that was returned to a breeder because of unacceptable conformation, or one given to another family for personal reasons. It is obvious that the dog shows the distress of abandonment and adjustment for a few weeks or longer. The dog is certainly capable of building a quality relationship with the new owner, but the abandonment does affect the dog.[258,296] They play less with people, are more attentive to people, and tend to be more restless when separated from their owners.[258]

## Working Dogs

Dogs have been used by humans for many tasks. In fact, many of the modern breeds resulted from selective breeding for a specific task. Retrievers are still used to bring in downed birds and Border Collies still work sheep. Some dogs guard businesses and property.[3] Dogs also are used for tasks that are newer, like catching criminals, finding lost or trapped people, guiding the blind, alerting a deaf owner to certain noise-related events, and assisting severely handicapped people. A number of scientific studies are beginning to evaluate the success of the various uses of dogs and look for ways to make them even more effective.

## New Babies and Small Children

Dogs and babies are often part of the same household and it is important that they get along together. The most extreme case of positive interaction between the two was reported by witnesses of the event in Kenya. A young mother had abandoned her newborn and it was retrieved by a dog and carried to be with her puppies.[341] In the United States, the baby-dog interaction is more likely to be negative without special considerations.

Bringing a new baby into a home that previously did not have children can cause a lot of tensions for a dog. This single event results in major changes to the dog's routine and social interactions. There are lots of visitors in and out, fewer interactions with the owner, less predictable interactions, loud crying noises, and strange smells. To the dog it might be as if an alien invaded its space. Owners, however, may not recognize the disruptions that occur for the dog because they are so distracted with the new family member. The dog's resulting behaviors, like urine marking and attention seeking, are inappropriately handled.[32] The dog may be punished and is often banned from interactions with the owners when the baby is present. If the dog is not socialized to infants, it may even show threatening behaviors in the presence of the infant. Severe discipline may suppress a dog's aggression toward a child when the adult is present, but it is often not inhibited when the adult is gone.[322] There are better ways to introduce dogs to babies.

The best time to begin minimizing the impact of the newest family member is several months before the arrival. Obedience training gives owners better verbal control and a higher comfort level in their ability to handle situations when baby and dog interact.[161,327] The dog should gradually be put on a schedule of feeding, exercise, and reduced attention that can be continued after the baby comes.[32,161] Owners can also incorporate fun interactions with the dog in the baby's room, rather than making the room off-limits.[32] The sounds and smells of new babies can be introduced by audiotape recordings and used items of baby clothing borrowed from friends before the newest member arrives.[32,161]

When the family comes home from the hospital, the adults should greet the dog as they usually do, alternating who holds the baby as necessary. This will allow the mother to interact with the dog, who is excited enough simply by her return.[161,327] The dog will be curious about the baby, so after the dog has settled down, it should be introduced to the new family member. This is more so it can smell the baby rather than see it up close, so a little distance is desirable. Protection of the infant is important, of course, so using a leash is appropriate and a muzzle is appropriate if there is any concern.[161,327] This should not be confused with jealousy, nor should it be punished.[161,327] At this time, there are also likely to be many visitors. Because both the dog and family members are already stressed by all the recent changes, caution needs to be used to protect guests.

To help the dog adjust to the newest family member, positive owner interactions with the dog should occur primarily when the baby is also present, so that the dog comes to associate good things with the presence of the new infant.[32,138,161,323,327] The dog can even be asked to "sit," "down," or do a trick, with the baby seeming to give the food reward with "help" from the parent. All too often owners want to ban the dog from the baby's room

and use punishment when the dog seeks attention, thus setting up an ever-increasing series of negative interactions.

**The most important consideration with any small child and dog is to never allow the two together unsupervised.** Not every dog will accept a new baby, even with the best preparation. Certain situations dictate caution. A greater likelihood for problems exists if the dog has had little or no contact with babies,[161] has already shown aggression to other babies, is aggressive to adults, or has a history of predatory aggression toward small animals.[326] Owners should be particularly alert to the possibility of problems when the baby cries, crawls, and begins to walk. Protective barriers are a must.[40] The cries of a newborn baby can be very upsetting to certain dogs. They may hide in some distant corner of the house, or they may respond by pacing back and forth between the baby and owner.[32] A parent may incorrectly interpret this pacing as protective behavior when in reality the behavior is the dog's comfort-seeking attempt. If the source of the irritating noise does not stop, a stressed dog may eventually attack.

The other two times of special concern are when the baby begins to crawl and later when it begins to walk. At these times, the dog finds it more difficult to escape the approaching child and may bite as a warning.[32] Unfortunately, young children can hurt dogs by pulling tails, grabbing a handful of hair, or losing their balance and falling on the dog. Dogs usually try to withdraw from these types of situations if possible,[205] but when that is not possible, they may react defensively.

Dogs also want quiet time away from the two-legged pest. The dog goes off by itself but the child seeks it out. It may try to move away again or it may begin to show other signs. When trying to communicate this "leave-me-alone" message, the dog can become irritable, but the child is not able to understand the nonverbal message. These situations can be particularly dangerous for small children because they are at face level with a dog. In cases where the dog is unable to get peace from a busy child, parents should remove the child or dog from the vicinity or strictly shield the child from interactions with the dog.[32]

## Veterinarians

Veterinary clinics can be stressful places for dogs because no matter how many times the dog comes, there is almost always a painful or stressful experience. In some cases, it is the strange environment that causes stress. In others, it is many unfamiliar people or animals.[336] The dog may get a thermometer placed in its anus, be put on a slippery table, stuck with needles, have tender ears swabbed, and get pills poked down its throat—all for a pat on the head or a so-so food treat. Sixty percent of dogs coming into a veterinary clinic for routine examinations show submissive apprehension.[303] Another 18% are fear-biters or potential fear-biters, and 5% show active defensive tendencies.[303] All types of breeds have shown aggression to veterinarians, and not necessarily in proportion to their distribution in the population.[190] Only 17% are relaxed and easy to approach.[303]

Problems at the veterinary clinic can be caused in part by negative experiences during the socialization period, particularly if they happened as stable learning was beginning. It is during this time that puppies are getting vaccinations and fecal exams frequently. There are several ways to help minimize the likelihood of the visit being negative. By spending the first few minutes interacting with the puppy or dog in a positive way, the veterinarian allows the animal to get comfortable with the new person and environment. Small pieces of a highly palatable food treat help create a positive first impression. If this happens routinely, many dogs will eventually walk right up to the veterinarian and put their nose in the treat pocket. Shy dogs take a little more effort. In addition to the treats and soft voice tones, it may be necessary to avoid direct eye contact. When it is time to actually do a procedure, such as getting the weight, obtaining a fecal sample, or vaccinating, distracting the puppy or dog with spreadable cheese can make the procedures go unnoticed (Fig. 4-6). Then, time spent by the veterinarian to end each visit on an upbeat interaction is probably time well spent in regard to future visits.

## Dog Heroes

Of special note in human-canine interactions are the numerous times dogs have been helpful, even lifesaving, to humans. The best of the best may

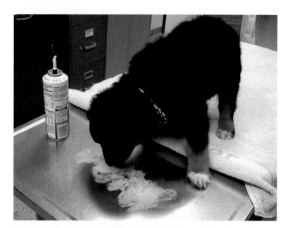

**Figure 4-6.**  Cheese or other treats that can be licked can be used as a distracter during puppy vaccinations.

even be honored with special awards. Dog heroes have saved people from drowning and from burning buildings. They have prevented harm from cars, blizzards, burglars, other dogs, and dangerous animals. They have sheltered the lost and injured and sought help for injured humans and other dogs. These heartwarming stories occur because special dogs use their social behavior to the fullest degree. In almost all cases, the dog is reacting to a member of its extended pack in trouble or is showing territorial protection.[32,107] Except for toy breeds, which retain puppy characteristics, and terriers, which tend toward independent behaviors, most dogs will instinctively protect their owners if they respect the owner as a higher ranking pack member.[32,63] Terriers tend to be territorially protective instead.

Occasionally, owners try to set up situations to see if their dog will come to the rescue. This generally is not recommended because innocent people can be hurt in the process, or owners can be disappointed when they do not see the desired response. Rarely is it possible to set up a lifelike scenario that includes the true reactions of fear. Owners tend to confuse territorial protection with owner protection, so a dog that may lick a burglar could still be very protective if the owner were threatened.

## Human-Dog Play

Social play between puppies, and to a lesser extent between adult dogs, provides social interaction, an opportunity to learn new skills, and physical toning. Play with humans is characteristically and motivationally different than play with another dog.[275] A dog that plays with other dogs will still play as much with its owner as does a dog without a canine play partner. This indicates the types of play are motivationally different. Dogs are also capable of responding to play signals from humans, especially the play bows and lunges.[276] Dogs are also less likely to possess toys than to present a toy when playing with the owner.[275] In interdog play, they tend to keep the toy for themselves.

## AGGRESSION

Aggression is a threat of harmful behavior directed toward an individual.[32] It is a normal behavior between dogs and is commonly seen in free-ranging dogs. Their interactions occur between dog packs 69% of the time and within them the remaining 31%.[240] Dominance hierarchies are established among all adults of a pack via aggressive encounters, with juvenile males showing the highest levels of submission and adult females showing the highest levels of aggression.[240,247] Dog packs have a linear dominance hierarchy, with 56% of the aggressive bouts initiated by the dominant male or female.[240] The number of agonistic episodes varies considerably by season, sex, and age.[240]

There is a relationship between defeat (subordination) and the neural mechanisms involved in regulating adrenocorticotrophic hormone (ACTH), thyroid-stimulating hormone (TSH), and luteinizing hormone (LH) secretion in males.[52] This serves as one example of the relationship between behavior and the neuroendocrine system. In several animal species, including wild dogs, the most dominant female has the highest cortisol levels,[207] suggesting the chronic stress of "life at the top." As a result, the life span of this alpha dog is shorter,[207] and it may affect other aspects of life, including reproduction. Other researchers have suggested that alpha males of various species have higher testosterone levels, but specific information is not available for dogs.

Aggression represents a normal expression of distance-increasing vocal and postural communication between dogs. Often, however, it is reported as a problem because of the fear it elicits,

a misunderstanding of its message, or injuries that have resulted. Aggression can also occur in excess of the acceptable limits for normal behavior.

Clinically, aggression means that one or more of the distance-increasing behaviors was expressed in an agonistic way as the dog asserted itself at the expense of someone else.[321] Careful history taking is essential to assess fully the situation in which the behavior was shown and how it was expressed. Additional information may be obtained from a physical examination and laboratory test data. Only then can the specific type of aggression be determined and appropriately treated. Normal agonistic behaviors have been described as being related to eating, reproduction, and hazard-avoidance activities.[74] Their expression as aggression varies by quality, frequency, and sequencing because of the environmental context, as well as the dog's genetic and developmental history.[74] The number of functional diagnoses is usually larger and contextual but ranges from 2 to 20.* Applied behaviorists tend to use the most extensive lists of differential diagnoses. Because it has been helpful to use the broadest grouping, the discussion here recognizes 15 major categories, with several subcategories (Box 4-1).

Before any discussion can take place about the types of canine aggression, their diagnostic criteria, and treatment protocols, it is worthwhile to assess overall outcomes relative to public safety. Many factors contribute to the success or failure of a treatment program:

1. Competence of veterinarian gathering the information
2. Client's ability to predict the triggering circumstances
3. Accuracy of client's observations
4. Owner expectations
5. Environmental factors
6. Dog's health
7. Hormonal status of dog
8. Previous learning by dog
9. Degree of owner commitment
10. Accuracy of diagnosis

---

*References 24, 26, 27, 95, 133, 134, 194, 224-226, 307, 319, 321, 328, 335, 345.

| BOX 4-1 | Functional classifications of canine aggression |
|---|---|

Dominance
   Dominance over humans
      Alpha personality
      Mismatched dog-to-owner personality
      Dog never learned proper rank
   Dominance over another dog
      Owner sides with lower-ranking dog
      Lower-ranking dog tries to climb the ranks
      Dominant dog enforces position
      Shared dominance rank
Fear-induced
Idiopathic
Intrasexual
   Interfemale
   Intermale
Learned
   Purposely taught
   Unconsciously taught by owner
Material-protective
   Food-protective
Maternal (parental)
Medical
   Epilepsy
   Hepatoencephalopathy
   Hormone imbalance
      Pseudocyesis
   Hydrocephalus
   Hyperthyroid
   Hypothyroid
   Irritable
   Mental lapse
Owner-protective
Pain-induced
Play
Predatory
Redirected
Sex-related
Territorial/protective

11. Appropriateness of therapeutic plan
12. Ability of owner to follow therapeutic plan
13. Susceptibility of dog to drug therapy

The first concern when dealing with canine aggression must be for human safety. Handling an aggressive dog makes the veterinary staff particularly vulnerable to dog bites. Proper restraint, whether physical or chemical, is a must.[272] Gauze, leather, wire, cloth, and plastic muzzles can be very important tools. Catch (rabies) poles, double leashes, and swing gates or doors may also be necessary, if only until a drug has time to become effective. Sometimes it is possible that the dog will allow the owner to safely put on a collar without showing any aggression. When this is the case, they can slip a collar on and then slip a big loop made by the leash passing back through the ring of the collar over the dog's nose. The veterinarian can then tighten the leash and thus create a makeshift head halter (Fig. 4-7).

Even with safety as the primary concern, every veterinarian realizes that "euthanasia" is not the first word to utter to certain owners, especially if they have clearly stated they are unwilling to consider it. For some aggressive cases, the appropriate recommendation is nevertheless euthanasia.[257] For others, there may be therapeutic options. Because the client may stop listening if given an ultimatum, it is important to discuss various options and all ramifications leaving euthanasia as the last one discussed.[229] Topics for discussion include risk to family, anticipated age-related or physical changes in the dog that may improve or worsen its condition, owner liability for the dog's aggressive acts in regard to state and local laws, owners' commitment to facilitating change, prognosis for improvement, current level of fear of the dog in each family member, degree of attachment to the dog of each family member, and severity of the aggression problem.[229,334]

Just as there are multiple types of aggression, there are also many different treatment protocols, usually based on the specific cause. Unpredictable and severe manifestations of the aggression make treatment more difficult, as do certain family characteristics and the overall complexity of the situation.[160] Even though everyone wants the magic pill to stop aggression, drug therapy may be of no value,[315] or it may actually make it worse, as in the case of an anxiolytic that removes the fear that has kept the aggression to a minimum.[210]

It is important that owners understand there is no way to guarantee a successful outcome or that the dog will never bite again.[227,318,328,335] Biologic systems are not completely predictable, and not all environmental influences can be controlled. In addition, an aggressive reaction can still be triggered by a very different stimulus. A food protective dog can learn to not guard its food, but it is

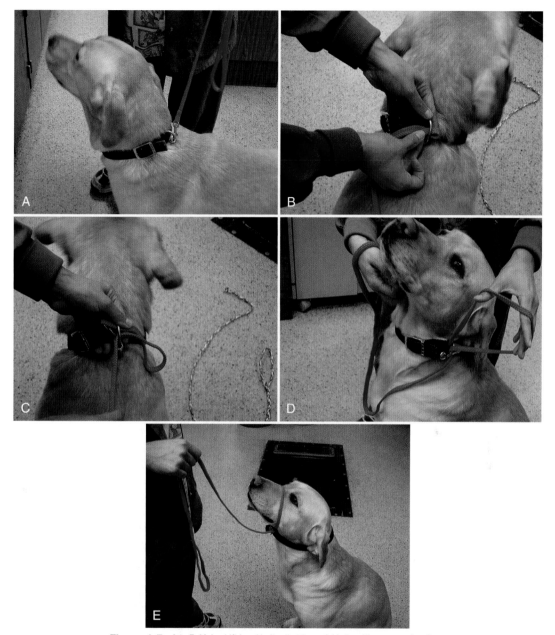

**Figure 4-7.** A to E, Makeshift head halter that is useful in handling aggressive dogs.

still likely to bite if someone steps on its tail. Successful treatment is usually defined by the owner as completely eliminating the problem or at least significantly reducing the frequency and intensity of the aggressive episodes. For veterinary behaviorists, the overall success rate for aggression cases is probably between 50% and 75% for fair-to-good improvement.[154,172,224]

Although any dog has the ability to show aggression, certain variables have been identified that influence its development (Box 4-2). Approximately 10% of dogs surrendered to animal shelters are

| BOX 4-2 | Variables influencing development of canine aggression |
| --- | --- |

| Dog variables | Owner variables |
| --- | --- |
| Age | Attachment to dog |
| Age of onset | Attitude toward behavior |
| Breed/hereditary | Commitment to change |
| background | Compliance with |
| Duration of problem | therapeutic program |
| Early experience | Confidence in therapeutic |
| Frequency of occurrence | program |
| Health | Experience with dogs |
| Other problems | |
| Predictability | |
| Presence of other dogs | |
| Previous training | |
| Severity of display | |
| Sex/reproductive status | |
| Sizes | |

Data from references 227, 253.

there because of aggression.[195] Unfortunately, it is difficult to truly evaluate the dog's personality in a shelter, but most places do try to use some type of temperament test. Many dogs are successfully placed and typically take 2 to 3 months to adjust in their new home. Then to the dismay of all concerned, the adjustment period gives way to their real nature and there is a marked increase in aggression toward strangers.[192]

The incidence of aggression as a behavior problem varies depending on the stage being examined. Aggression is not frequently mentioned as a problem by the average dog owner, but if actually asked about any undesirable behavior, 18% complain about aggression.[30] On the other hand, aggression represents a high percentage of cases seen by veterinary behaviorists—that is, anywhere from 20% to 66% of the cases,* with most being directed toward people.[15] Another 5% to 18% of all cases are fights between dogs.[203] Intact male dogs are significantly more likely to be involved in problems with aggression, although sex differences are apparent in some types of aggression. Figures for aggression show that intact male dogs account for over half of

*References 24, 26, 27, 95, 133, 134, 194, 224-226, 307, 319, 321, 328, 335, 345.

all bites,[202,345] but fights between dogs are more apt to be female against females.[203] More than 86% of biting dogs have an owner, and almost 56% are restrained at the time of the bite.[202]

As would be expected, dogs presented to a behaviorist for aggression are usually males.[15] Overall 52% of biting dogs are intact males, 16% are castrated males, 16% are intact females, and 16% are spayed females.[24,26,27,154,344] The mean age at which aggression appears as a behavior problem is generally between 2 and 3 years old—young adults—but it can occur in geriatric dogs as well as in puppies.[24,26,344] Neither the age of the dog nor the duration of the aggression has value for predicting whether castration will be beneficial.[214] The correlation between several factors has been reported as a multidimensional grouping.[128] Dogs that bite are more likely to show other oral behaviors, like excessive chewing on objects or excessive barking.[129] Biting dogs also are more likely to have a history of pruritic skin disease,[129] illness as a puppy,[296] or getting its first vaccination as an older puppy.[296]

Dogs bite a significant number of people each year, and as long as people and dogs coexist, this problem will continue. Although the actual incidence of dog bites within a population may vary, there is no question that dog bites remain a significant public health problem worldwide.[309] It is not in the scope of this book to thoroughly address the problem of dogs biting people, but a few words are in order. Even with mandatory reporting of all injuries from dogs, the actual number of dog bites will be underreported, because owners bitten by their own dogs seldom report minor confrontations that do not require medical attention.[12] Thus, any data about the actual number of bites that occur each year are purely speculative and probably on the low side.[48,312,346] The American Veterinary Medical Association took an important multidisciplinary first step in addressing this issue with the 1996 Animal Welfare Forum.[1]

When dogs bite people, they may be using one of the many types of aggression to be described. An appropriate diagnosis is necessary to help the dog. It should also be mentioned that a dog that fights with other dogs will not automatically aggress toward people. The type of victim and type of aggression can vary. A few generalizations can be made about the dogs that inflict the most injury to people: The dogs are more likely to be young adult, intact males; large in size; and known by the victim.* The victim is most likely a boy younger than 10 years of age who receives injuries to one or more limbs.[130,168] Of bites to children, 26% occur as a dog guards a resource such as food or a toy, but 18% happen during apparently benign interactions.[271]

The actual bite rate is probably in proportion to the general age and breed distribution of dogs in a community.[344] Almost every breed has been represented in statistics on aggressive dogs, although reports suggest that mixed-breed dogs have either a higher or lower than expected frequency of aggression problems.[24,27,55,154] Unless breed incidence of the problem is compared with the actual population as a whole in that community at that time, the numbers may represent only popular breeds, popular large breeds, dogs owned by certain irresponsible types of owners, types of dogs that the media highlight, or the breeds that tend to be owned by cautious owners wanting a watchdog. Lawmakers must be extremely careful to have valid data on bites and dog populations before considering any type of breed-specific or dangerous dog legislation.[35,273,279,281]

The victims of canine aggression can be other dogs, humans (adults, children, strangers, or owners), cats, horses, or other animals. In most cases, the expression of one type of aggression toward one category of victim does not mean the dog is predisposed to different types of aggression or to other victims. However, dogs presented for aggression are frequently diagnosed with more than one type of aggression. Dogs that aggress toward other dogs are frequently said to be showing dominance aggression.[203] In reality, they could be showing any of a number of other types of aggression instead. It is important to consider several differentials for interdog aggression.

The incidence of canine aggression toward humans is unknown, but estimates indicate between 4 and 5 million people are bitten each year, with 800,000 requiring medical care, and 6000 being hospitalized.[36,126,202] Studies estimate almost half of all children age 18 years old or younger have been bitten.[34,168] Of those cases in which owners sought help from a veterinarian for any behavior problem, approximately 40% wanted help with aggressive dogs.[27] In 54% to 67% of these aggression cases, the aggression was directed toward people. In the remaining one third, the aggression was directed toward other animals.[24,27,42] The incidence of aggressive animal interactions resulting in admittance to a veterinary hospital for treatment is also significant. Approximately 10% of traumatic injury cases are associated with these interactions.[174] Animal control workers are 500 times more likely to be bitten by a dog than is the general population, and 92% to 97% of veterinarians also have had this happen.[89,206] Unfortunately, only 37% of biting dogs displayed traits usually associated with the problem or had given enough warning to warrant a muzzle.[89]

Even the dog's owner does not do a good job of knowing the dog's signals.[75] Aggression can exist for months to years before the owner actually recognizes that there is a problem. They usually miss a dog's stare warning, justify a growl, or blame themselves for a snap. They only remember 51% of the aggressive signals their dog displayed, and only 10% were interpreted in the context they had learned about.[75] A fearful dog's signals of aggression tend to be masked and so are harder to read.[75] It may take a serious bite before the owner realizes there is a problem. This makes it very important to ask specific questions during yearly exams to be sure there really is no problem.

A classification scheme can be used to identify the level of injuries that occurred[91]:

0 = growl/snap/stare, but no contact
1 = snap touches skin/clothing but not injury to victim
2 = snap/bite leaving a red mark/bruise/torn clothing
3 = single bite with puncture/large bruise/slash
4 = multiple bites on the same occasion with punctures/bruising/slashes
5 = disfiguring bite that removed a chunk of flesh or multiple severe bites on the same occasion
6 = bite resulting in death of the victim

*References 12, 28, 47, 69, 130, 154, 181, 189, 208, 344.

When a dog shows aggression, it is usually very accurate with the severity intended. A nip was intended to be a warning and does not represent a serious bite that missed its target. Only those trained to recognize the subtle warning signs and who have taken safety precautions might escape the full brunt of a bite. And even for them, the precautions do not always work. The end result of the aggression, especially in categories 3 to 6, is emotionally and medically draining. It is difficult to measure the mental toll, but the damage is expensive in terms of medical costs—over $170 million a year.[238] It is also expensive in terms of workers' compensation claims, currently over $10,000,000 per year.[259] Homeowners liability insurance claims total over $1 billion,[1,36] and another $25,000,000 is lost in ancillary costs, such as torn clothes and lost income.[238]

In certain situations, the genetic makeup of the dog influences its aggressive response. For example, various breeds have the ability to be trained easily as a guard dog, and this ability has been refined over many generations of selective breeding.[22,37,133,283,290] This can also affect how they respond to human body language. For example, Belgian Shepherds shift from friendly to threatening as the human does, but retrievers are more likely to retain their friendly attitudes.[314] This does not make dogs like Belgian Shepherds generally more aggressive, but it allows individuals to be more easily trained for guarding than dogs of other breeds. Genetics can also be associated with problem dogs. The English Springer Spaniel has a higher than expected incidence of severe dominance aggression (see Rage Syndrome, below).[156,264,270] In the United Kingdom, the English Cocker Spaniel, Doberman Pinscher, Saint Bernard, German Shepherd, Bernese Mountain Dog, and Golden Retriever breeds have been reported to have similar behaviors.* The terms *Springer rage* and *Cocker rage* have been tagged to problem dogs; however, other popular breeds are also known to develop similar problems.

Genetics can play a role in the development of aggression in other ways too. In some cases, the trait of dominance aggression can be traced back to a show dog whose success in the show ring made it a popular sire. The "presence" that helps the dog stand out may be related to confident, dominant dogs. Indiscriminate breeding to produce lots of puppies of a popular breed such as a Chow Chow, German Shepherd, Dalmatian, Saint Bernard, or Jack Russell Terrier concentrates only on physical appearance, not on temperament. In addition to the association of dominance aggression in English Springer Spaniels, other breeds have a genetic tendency toward aggression within certain bloodlines or colors.[156] German Shepherds are more likely to show fear-induced aggression. Yellow and chocolate Labrador Retrievers tend to be more aggressive than black ones, and in the United Kingdom, red Cocker Spaniels are more likely to be aggressive than black ones.

Diet, previous history, and location are other factors that can be related to aggression. A tendency for an increased amount of aggression can arise when dogs go from an unrestricted to a restricted diet (aggression can decrease in the reverse type of feeding program).[77,78,86] Protein levels in a diet can also affect aggression. Dominant aggressive dogs fed high-protein diets are more aggressive.[158] Territorial aggression decreases on a low-protein diet with added tryptophan. Because other proteins are better able to cross the blood-brain barrier, it makes sense that less tryptophan would be able to cross when protein levels are high. Tryptophan is a precursor of serotonin (tryptophan → tryptophan hydroxylase → 5-hydroxytryptophan → 5-hydroxytryptamine = serotonin) and this is the "feel good" neurotransmitter.[158] New owners of dogs adopted from animal shelters underreport aggression.[192] Location can be significant in that dogs tend to show more aggression in small spaces, including a veterinary examination room. It may be possible to eliminate this particular problem by having the veterinarian in the room before the dog is brought in. Changing the stimuli is another technique, such as examining the dog in the waiting room or having a different veterinarian perform the exam.[328]

Dog to dog aggression is the second most common aggressor-to-victim form seen. Unique differences between the aggressor and victim have been identified (Table 4-1).[273]

Unfortunately, these differences are not so unique as to be predictable. It would be desirable

---

*References 94, 137, 155, 209, 250, 251.

| TABLE 4-1 | Characteristics of dogs involved in interdog aggression | | |
|---|---|---|---|
| | Aggressors | Victims | General |
| Sex of dog | >70% intact male | >70% intact male | — |
| Source of dog | 62% from breeder | 40% from breeder | — |
| Time off leash daily | 52% | 35% | — |
| Fights occur off leash | — | — | 52% both off leash; 30.1% aggressor free, victim on leash |
| Previous attacks on dogs | 65% | — | — |
| Grew up with another dog | 7.3% | — | — |
| Both dogs previously fought each other | — | — | 31% |

Data from reference 273.

to have a test to predict future aggression, but none currently exists. Recent attempts indicate researchers are hopeful[244,249]; however, various types of aggression have different motivating factors. It would be nice to have a test to quickly and accurately diagnose those dogs most likely to show aggression in the future. There are lots of behavior tests to measure or predict many different behaviors. The problem is that they have not been validated. The Dutch have been working on a test to identify aggressive dogs so that they are not allowed to breed,[216] and they are close to one that is validated, at least under certain situations. Environmental factors play such a big role in so many forms of aggression that a comprehensive evaluation is not very likely.

## The Brain and Aggression

A number of brain areas have been implicated in aggression. These have been best studied in rodents and cats (see *Feline Behavior: A Guide for Veterinarians*).[25] Limited success with various neuropharmacologic agents has renewed interest in both the anatomic brain and the neurotransmitters as keys to understanding aggressive behavior. At the simplest level, there are two forms of aggression based on responses: nonaffective (predatory) and affective. *Nonaffective (predatory) aggression* is triggered by moving prey, involves minimal mood changes, has a hypothalamic origin, and uses acetylcholine as the neurotransmitter. *Affective aggression* is associated with a marked mood change, has autonomic activation, involves the frontal cortex or amygdala, and may involve serotoninergic,

catecholaminergic, cholinergic, and/or GABA neurotransmitter systems.[87]

The affective type of aggression has identifiable body language that is typically associated with an aggressive dog. This body language includes what have been called warning signs. Nonaffective (predatory) aggression is not associated with those signs. The dog may just attack. The attack of predation is the classic form of nonaffective aggression. Although some believe that this two-type classification is adequate for treatment purposes, the clinical impression is that this view is too simplistic.

Others define three types of aggression: predatory, irritable, and spontaneous.[95] *Predatory aggression,* according to this definition in rats at least, is facilitated by *p*-chlorophenylalanine with concurrent serotonin depletion.[95] *Irritable aggression* is caused by variations in norepinephrine levels and metabolism of dopamine and other enzymes.[95] *Spontaneous aggression,* which probably includes several more specific types of aggression, appears to be related to increased levels of dopamine metabolism or stimulation of dopamine receptors.[95] Chronically stressed rats tend to remain more aggressive several weeks after apparent clinical recovery. In those rats, brain levels of tyrosine hydroxylase remain high in the hypothalamus, and norepinephrine levels are higher than expected.[95]

Certain brain areas have been associated with aggression in dogs. Removal of the septal areas or ventromedial hypothalamus results in an increase in aggression or irritability.[136] Stimulation of the amygdala, diencephalon, periaqueductal gray, tectum, or reticular regions can result in aggression.[319] Fear and defensive responses occur when the dorsal area of the amygdaloid nucleus is stimulated,[319] so bilateral destruction of the amygdaloid nuclei may or may not be used to treat aggression—primarily fear-induced aggression.[7,319] Stimulation of part of the hypothalamus, the so-called aggressiveness center, results in an attack or ingestion of food.[14] This region is normally controlled by the *aggressive inhibition center* in the anterolateral hypothalamus, so lesions of the inhibition center can also result in increased aggression.[14] Other areas that inhibit aggression have been isolated in the amygdala (corpus amygdaloideum) and frontal lobes in the cortex.[14]

At the neurotransmitter level, there is a great deal of ongoing research in several species. Monoamine oxidase A (MAOA) deficiencies have been associated with aggression in humans and mice.[65] This enzyme normally degrades serotonin and norepinephrine. Acetylcholine and androgenic hormones activate the aggressiveness center of the hypothalamus, whereas serotonin tends to inhibit it.[27] The presence of long repeats in dopamine $D_4$ receptors has been correlated with dominance aggression in one breed.[156] It is also known that melatonin and dopamine share a common biochemical pathway,[156] which could be related to the association of aggression with certain colors. Ideally, a site of origin could be identified and specifically targeted for surgical or pharmacologic intervention. Electroconvulsive therapy is an example of a treatment that would not target specific locations.[260] Advanced research should lead to drugs that are not only neurotransmitter specific but site specific for various nuclei. An example of advances in research includes the development of a gene-deficient knockout mouse that lacks a-calcium-calmodulin kinase II. Also, homozygous and heterozygous mice have a well-defined syndrome that includes a reduction in fear and an increase in defensive aggression. In these mice, serotonin release in the dorsal raphe is reduced.[68] As new research continues, indications are that it will become increasingly important to identify specific categories of aggression to pick the correct pharmacologic therapy.[95]

## Dominance (Competitive, Status-Related) Aggression

In dogs, aggression is the behavior problem that is most likely to result in an owner's seeking professional help. In behavior referral practices, the incidence of aggression is variable, but up to 59% of those cases are eventually diagnosed as dominance aggression.* Dominance aggression, then, represents 19% to 34% of all problem behavior cases.[66,68,225]

The concept of dominance aggression has undergone a lot of discussion lately because of some general misunderstandings. Dominance is a relative social ranking between two individuals (dog to dog or dog to human) in a particular situation; thus, the other terms of "competitive" and "status-related" aggression. The lower ranking individual would yield to the higher ranking one to avoid escalating a conflict or a fight.[202] There are different types of dominance, such as social dominance, sexual dominance, food dominance, and resource dominance, so aggression can be seen in different contexts. There are times when the aggression occurs without relevance to the wider social structure, such as a dog that is very protective of a bone, showing dominance aggression toward someone it would never aggress to in any other setting. Some behaviorists have chosen to call dominance aggression either competitive or status-related aggression instead. For the purposes of this book, dominance aggression is used to describe those situations when a dog challenges another dog or person because it views itself as having a higher social rank at the time of the aggressive act. Situational aggression without social context is reflected in other types of aggression, such as food-protective aggression or territorial aggression. It is also important to recognize that there is a very close connection between dominance and fear aggression. A dog challenging a person may change into a fear mode without the person noticing the body language or contextual shift. When both types of aggression coexist in the same incidence, it might appropriately be called *conflict aggression*.[213]

---

*References 24, 26, 27, 43, 46, 49, 224.

A statistical look at dogs with dominance aggression presents an interesting picture. Between 65% and 90% of the dominant-aggressive dogs are males, and of those males, more than 90% are intact at the time of presentation.[26,27,46,185,225] It is also common for the dog to have been sexually intact when the problems first started and castration tried therapeutically, but unsuccessfully, to treat the dominance aggression. Purebred dogs also appear to be overrepresented, with 82% to 87% of dominant-aggressive dogs being purebreds.[49,185,334] Dogs that were ill as puppies are also overrepresented in dominance aggression statistics.[296]

Dominance aggression can occur in puppies as young as 6 weeks, because this is when littermates establish their hierarchy, usually over food. This aggression between puppies, however, is normal and not correlated to how any puppy will relate to people, either as a puppy or as an adult dog.[49,290] The young puppy that growls and snaps at an owner over food or handling should be put through the antiaggressive puppy-training procedures discussed later so that the owner will become the leader and not a threat. Dominance aggression toward people may not become obvious until some time between sexual maturity (6 to 12 months) and behavioral maturity (18 to 36 months).* This behavior is not controlled by hormones, but the presence of testosterone or lack of estrogen may exacerbate the amount of aggression shown.[217,230,247] The spayed females that are more likely to show increased aggression are those that were already showing signs as puppies.[142,217]

## Dominance Over People

Dominance aggression can be toward a person or toward another dog. When dominance aggression is directed toward humans, it can be one of three different types. The first, fortunately, is rare, but it is the most dangerous. A few dogs have a dominant personality in the extreme—an alpha personality. As puppies, they tend to be "pushy," as if questioning authority. As they get older, they gradually stop obeying commands, first from strangers and then

from various family members. Finally there is one, usually a man, that has some remaining control over the dog, and that too is now being challenged. By the time the owner, usually a person with a very dominant personality, seeks help, it is obvious that the dog is increasingly challenging the owner's authority. Even brief eye contact by a stranger will result in an aggressive advance by this kind of dog. This dog will pass a stranger with a stiff-legged walk and vertical tail, while staring at the person as if to provoke eye contact. If given a "sit" command by a stranger, this dog responds very slowly, even for a very prized treat. The second time the stranger gives the command, the dog is very apt to walk away.

The second type of situation in which dominance aggression is likely to occur toward a person is when there is a significant mismatch in personalities of the owner and the dog. If the owner has a timid personality and the dog is a fairly dominant type, problems are almost guaranteed. A fairly dominant dog can be an excellent pet for an owner with a dominant personality, but not for a person who is very mild and subdued. Yet, matching of personalities between a young puppy and its future owner is difficult to impossible to do. We are lucky that things go right between random matches of canine and human personalities as often as they do.

The third category of canine dominance aggression toward humans is that occurring in a dog that never learned it was not the dominant member. The social nature of most dogs, except perhaps terriers, demands a social order. Shared positions of equal status were never a part of their ancestral social scheme. If no top individual is obvious, the dog may take the role for itself. Some owners raise their dogs permissively, letting them do whatever they want and perhaps inadvertently rewarding the dominant signals. The dog gradually determines the day to day rules of the interactions. The problem may not become apparent until circumstances make it necessary to put restraints on the dog.

Presenting complaints for dominance aggression toward people will vary, but they usually center around the dog's control over what is happening in the home. In all three types of dominance aggression toward humans, the owners may complain of an acute onset, because from their perspective there

---

*References 26, 49, 219, 225, 230, 265, 266, 267.

was no problem until the dog actually bit. Before the actual bite, the behaviors were rationalized to be "natural."[325] These owners subconsciously alter their lives to avoid confrontation. Some owners, though, do recognize the more gradual escalation of aggression that typifies this problem. The gradual assumption of the top dominant position by a dog may begin with its growling, snapping, or "grumbling" when it is disturbed during sleep; the owner reaches over its head to attach a leash; or the owner cannot restrain the dog, medicate it, or handle its feet.[230] The dog may physically block access to areas from the owners, stiffen and "talk back" if forced to move, or constantly seek owner interaction.[230] They may be described as "pushy." The number of aggressive bouts increases over time, as does the number of circumstances in which the dog seeks control. It can get to the point that the owners are afraid to sit on a piece of furniture if the dog is present and may even be prevented from sleeping in their own bed. Complicating this picture is the likelihood that the owner misreads the intent of the dog. Controlling access may be viewed as "protective" and putting feet on the owner's shoulders viewed as "hugging."

The diagnosis of dominance aggression usually requires three or more situations that predictably result in aggression, not just a single event (Box 4-3). These situations tend to involve physical manipulation, discipline, or guarding of limited resources like food or resting areas.[49,132,185,235] A typical history will reveal a gradually escalating problem, although it may be necessary to ask probing questions to find the earlier signs. For example, the dog did not want the owner to take food away or brush its coat, so it growled, and the owner backed away. Over time, a dog like this will gradually assume authority over an increasing number of things. Whereas the first confrontation is often over the food bowl, other things will become significant, such as a toy, a stolen "prize," a chair, a resting place, or the owner's bed. Owners often deal with food-bowl aggression by waiting until the dog finishes its meal before picking up the bowl. Only when there is a threat to a small child does this issue become significant.

Aggression over food alone is not diagnostic of dominance aggression. The total picture of

| BOX 4-3 | Events that may be associated with dominance aggression |
|---|---|

Body slamming against people
Disturbing dog during its rest or sleep results in aggression
Escalating aggression upon receiving physical correction
Failing to yield right-of-way to people
Acting aggressive when given a command
Acting aggressive when being groomed or having feet handled
Leaning over the owner
Making eye contact (the stare)
Posing a minimal problem to groomer or veterinarian but being aggressive just to certain family members
Acting aggressive when being picked up or restrained
Placing forepaws on owner's shoulders or back
Protecting food
Protecting toys or stolen objects
Pushing dog off a bed or sofa results in aggression
Reaching for the door results in aggression
Spontaneously growling
Threatening a person stepping over its body
"Talking back" to verbal corrections
Acting aggressive when touched or hugged

Data from references 49, 76, 133, 178, 225, 263, 268, 325, 328, 331.

dominance aggression will include some of the following features: Toys have been taken away when the dog was not around and then not given back so as to avoid the aggression associated with the toys. Guarded "prizes" have been ignored until they are abandoned for the same reason. Bribery with a food treat has taught the owner how to respond to the dog's goal. If the dog is on the owner's lap, the person will not move or stand up until the dog decides to leave. If the dog happens to be lying on a stair step or in front of the bathroom door, the owner will find either an alternate way around or wait until the dog moves away rather than disturb the animal. Owners have learned that stepping over the dog, trying to make it move, or accidentally touching it can result in serious injury. Over time, the dog may bite if disturbed on the owner's bed. Some of these dogs begin to challenge the owner's attempt to get into bed. The owner may try tossing a favorite food treat off the bed and then diving into the bed while the dog chases its treat. This becomes a game for the dog, and many can get the treat and still beat the owner onto the bed. A few owners have actually given up and slept on the floor rather than confront the dog. In spite of working their lives around what seems to displease the dog, these owners are not likely to seek professional help until the dog growls or bites them severely when it is disturbed.

The severity of the aggressive behavior tends to escalate over time. The first sign of a problem for many dogs may be food-bowl protection. It is important to note that not all dominant dogs are food-bowl protective, and not all food-bowl protective dogs will develop dominance problems. It depends on the relative importance of food to the individual. Behavioral maturity occurs at an age approximately twice that of sexual maturity, generally 18 to 36 months, and the subtleties of dominance aggression will slowly progress until they become obvious to the owner around this time. Although the initial history may say that the problem started when the dog was 15 months of age, careful questioning will reveal that less obvious but historically significant events were occurring for many months before that.

Prevention of dominance aggression is better than trying to stop the problem once it has started. Quality time spent with new puppy owners is a bargain in the long run for the veterinarian. Unfortunately, many dogs are presented after the problem is well developed. There are two basic ways these cases can be handled, but before any course of therapy is initiated, owners must be educated about some important concepts. For dominance aggression, there are usually no magic cures. The treatment goals must first and foremost ensure the owner's safety. It is important to avoid the types of situations that provoke the aggression.[202,231,232] This list includes several "do nots":

1. Do not allow access to things that can trigger the aggression.
2. Do not abruptly reach for the dog; have it sit first.
3. Do not disturb the sleeping dog; have it come instead.
4. Do not give food or attention if solicited; have the dog respond to a command to earn the reward.
5. Do not permit the dog on furniture, including the bed; have it remain on the floor at a lower level.
6. Do not play aggressively, including games of tug; have it remain calm.
7. Do not feed the dog food from the table; feed the dog only in its own dish.
8. Do not physically punish the dog; use a simple "*No*" and withdraw attention.
9. Do not allow access to visitors; access to people must be highly controlled.

Then the program will include finding ways to gradually teach the dog not to show aggression in situations that used to elicit problems. Finally, it is not likely that all problematic interactions can be prevented,[335] so the dog should be made to assume a submissive role in all situations where a dominant-subordinate interaction is likely to occur.[49,326,331] The behaviors of "sit," "down," and "rollover" are examples. These commands are not just to have the dogs show the physical response, but also, over time, to learn to relax too.[232] It is suggested that the owner give voice signals, not hand signals.[232] A hand movement might be interpreted as a threat by the dog.

Neutering the intact dog is a common recommendation, but it probably will not make a significant difference. Only about 30% of male dogs show an improvement of 50+% after castration for any type of aggression.[142] For a few young dogs that show dominance aggression, castration can make a dramatic difference. Surgery, then, should be recommended as the first treatment. Testosterone is thought to facilitate the development of dominance aggression, but once the behavior is established, the hormone is no longer needed to maintain it. Plasma testosterone and LH levels were similar for dominant and subordinate male dogs, so regulation is not hierarchy-dependent.[173] If castration helps somewhat, great! If it does not work, then at least it has removed this dog from the breeding population and prevented any genetic components of the behavior from being passed on. For this same reason, an ovariohysterectomy is recommended for intact bitches, even though the amount of aggression may increase as a result of the surgery in some.[76,142]

Owners need to be educated about what a normal social order is for a dog and how humans are to fit into that order. Owners must also understand the time and effort commitment they will need to make. The process of reversing a dominance order can be very stressful and, even if successfully accomplished, will require a lifelong effort to maintain. A combined approach of castration, behavior modification, and drug therapy is generally the most successful.*

A hot topic in regard to preventing the development of dominance aggression or treating it is the *alpha-roll technique*. Any sign of aggression is met with an immediate rolling of the dog onto its back and holding it in that position until the aggressive behavior stops. The theory sounds logical until you consider the possible consequences and realize that it is more apt to cause aggression from fear than prevent aggression from dominance. To roll the dog over, the owner must have a direct, confrontational interaction with the dog. That could easily result in escalated aggression, with the owner being bitten and even with the dog winning the interaction. It is better to avoid situations in which confrontation would typically occur and then gradually teach the dog that the human is in control. Pain as a punishment also escalates aggression, with some owners being seriously injured.[6]

The treatment for switching dominance begins with the premise that "nothing in life is free." [178,202,326,331] The dog must earn food, attention, and a chance to play its favorite games.[76,317,327] Instead of being fed specific meals, the dog must earn the daily meal allotment in small increments, and the commands used are for simple, basic, obedience behaviors that are also submissive ones, such as "sit" and "down." The concept is to reward submissive, never dominant, behaviors.[179] If the dog does not obey a command or if it begs for food or attention, it is ignored, not rewarded. When the owner is ready, a specific command is given, like "sit." As has already been discussed in Chapter 2, timing of the reward is extremely important and should be emphasized in discussions of treatments.

If the dog has not previously learned the "sit" command, the owner can gradually shape the behavior by moving the piece of food from in front of the dog's face to slightly above and behind the back of the head while repeating the command. This forces the dog toward a sitting position, and partial correct motion can then be rewarded. Each lesson demands a position closer to the correct sitting one until it is achieved. Similarly, "down" can be taught from the sit position by lowering the piece of food and then gradually working it forward on the ground. As these lessons are learned, the dog is then to be gradually expected to show a more relaxed nature.[232] The tense dominance postures become more relaxed as the dog comes to recognize the owner as its leader.

At the same time the reward system is being started, other major changes must occur. The owner should avoid any situations that trigger an aggressive or antagonistic episode to ensure that the dog does not have any opportunity to reinforce its dominance. The dog should no longer be permitted on furniture, including the bed. This ensures that the dog remains on a lower level than the owner, and it avoids situations that might provoke aggression. The dog can drag a leash from its head halter or collar to give the owner a way to enforce an "off" command without risking a bite. It may even be necessary to shut the dog out of the bedroom. Although this is difficult for some owners to do, they must be prepared to enforce the new rules. The reward technique works best if the amount of dominance shown by the dog is minimal. With extreme cases of dominance aggression, the technique seems to be less effective.

A second technique to reduce a dog's dominance position is a more authoritative approach, in which controlled confrontations teach the dog the new boundaries. Again, the owner must be advised to avoid any situation that is likely to provoke aggressive behavior except as specifically set up. From the beginning, the dog will wear a collar and drag a leash at all times. This will allow the owners to get control of the dog while remaining far from its teeth. Any type of collar can be used. The head halter (collar) with an adjustable nose piece that can be left on the dog tends to work best. If choke collars

---

*References 49, 179, 185, 326, 328, 331, 335.

are used, they should not be abused. Painful correction or hanging the dog until it passes out are excessive and inappropriate. Instead of the intended lesson, the pain associated with stern handling of a choke chain usually creates more fear. The dog fights harder, panics, and physically injures itself or the owner.[219]

Once the dog is fitted to drag a leash from its collar, preferably a head halter, the owner can have physical control without being endangered.[213] Then they should avoid all aggression-provoking situations except one. Carefully set the dog up to a guaranteed loss. For example, for the dog that guards its toys, the owner chooses the dog's least favorite. The dog, while wearing its head halter with attached leash, is near its toy. The owner can call the dog away from the toy and then reward a "come" and "sit-stay" with a favorite food treat after picking up the toy. If the dog growls, rushes to the toy, grabs at the toy, or grabs at the person, the owner gives a quick, firm jerk on the leash and firmly says "No." The process is repeated several times with the least favorite toy until the owner can pick up the toy from beside the dog without any reaction by the dog. The process is then repeated with a slightly more prized toy and repeated progressively to the favorite toy.

Desensitization is added to the program for other things as well.[233] If the dog shows aggression when a hand goes over its head, as an example, the program begins with someone standing away from the dog. They bend one arm at the elbow, palm down, and make slow back/forth and left/right motions. The goal with each session is that the dog shows no reaction and remains relaxed. Very gradually the hand gets closer to the dog's head until it can be touched. It is important for the handler to identify increased tension in the dog, without keeping a tight leash to send the wrong signal.

If the dog guards a favorite location, like a chair, a similar process is used. Allow controlled access to the chair only while the dog has the head halter and leash. When the "come" command is met with a growl, the owner is ready with a firm "No," while briskly pulling the dog off the chair by the leash. Once the dog is off, the owner can then give another command, like "sit," so as to reward a correct response.

Pharmacologic intervention can be a useful addition to treatment of certain cases of aggression toward humans. In laboratory animals and primates, the level of serotonin in cerebrospinal fluid (CSF) is lowest in the most dominant-aggressive animals.[265] It is also low in a subgroup of relatively young men with personality disorders, but the serotonin-aggression hypothesis in humans has not been unequivocally confirmed.[311] In dogs showing dominance aggression, the urine serotonin levels are significantly lower than in dogs presented for other behavior problems,[265] and there is a significant reuptake of serotonin$_{2A}$ in all cortical areas of the brain,[245] with lower amounts of the serotonin metabolite 5-hydroxyindoleactic acid (5-HIAA) in the CSF.[266] In a subset of dogs that attack without warning, CSF levels of 5-HIAA are lower than for dogs that just growl.[266] Unfortunately there is no correlation between serotonin levels in the CSF and blood plasma.[204] Research indicates that drugs that enhance brain serotonin levels, particularly the tricyclic antidepressants and selective serotonin reuptake inhibitors, may decrease the amount of dominance aggression shown.[85,234] But recent studies of amitriptyline and clomipramine have shown that the tricyclic antidepressants may actually be no better than placebos.[315,339] Using a serotonin-enhancing drug does not change a dominant personality, but it may reduce the aggression in susceptible dogs. If there is also a fear component, use of these drugs is contraindicated, because they may reduce the fearful inhibitions before the serotonin levels increase.

Dietary changes can have an effect in dominance aggression. Problem dogs on high-protein diets may return to normal if the protein level is reduced to a more normal level of 20% to 22%. They may also respond if tryptophan is added to their high-protein diet.[82] Because tryptophan is important for the formation of serotonin and is the least competitive of the amino acids, a high-protein diet may actually result in lower tryptophan levels. Adding it would result in serotonin increases.

Progestins also have been recommended for dominance aggression.[42,76,167,331,335] The results, however, are inconsistent, and the newer serotoninergic drugs are replacing progestins. Lithium carbonate has been tried in dominance aggression, but more studies are needed before its potential will be properly understood.[262]

Changing the dog's position in the family social order can be a very trying experience for some owners, because the firmness needed to obtain and maintain control may not be a natural character trait for that person. It may be necessary to retain some level of discipline over the dog forever if the dog's relative personality is quite dominant,[218] and some people are uncomfortable with that prospect. There is approximately 80% compliance with avoiding triggering situations and 70% compliance with affection control.[305] Therefore, it is important to tell owners at the beginning that there may come a time when they no longer want to maintain their new personality just to keep the dog's behavior in line. That may be the time when it is better for all considered to get the dog out of the home. This result should not be considered a failure by the owner; it is simply the outcome of a mismatch of personalities. Long term, 93% of the dogs in one study remained in the home regardless of the degree of owner compliance.[305]

Some dominant dogs will need to be euthanized for the sake of the safety of those who live in the same household. This option must be considered whenever the owners no longer trust the dog, they are actually afraid of it, or there are people at special risk in the home, such as a baby or small child. Dogs that are most likely to be euthanized are those whose aggression is (1) unpredictable or (2) severe in response to benign challenges.[266,268,269] Other factors that have been documented to play a major part in the owner's decision for euthanasia include a history of multiple bite attacks, a dog weighing more than 40 lb, an abrupt escalation of intensity, a history of dominance challenges,[100,266,268] and a history of aggression for longer than 1 year. The request for euthanasia is generally honored, because these dogs would often be a problem in other homes[49,331] and would expose the new owners to significant liability.

### Dominance Over Other Dogs

Not all fights between dogs are related to dominance or social ranking. For those that are, they tend to fall into one of three types.[280] The first type is severe and ends with the subordinate fleeing or dying. More commonly, canids fight in a ritualized way over some privilege, and the submissive postures of the lower ranking animal eventually terminate the aggression. In the third situation, minor conflicts within a group involve growls and snaps. They are usually settled by the submissive behaviors of the lowest ranking dog. Of these fights between dogs, 57% are between females, 13% are between males, and 30% are between a male and a female.[102] The younger dog initiates the fight almost 90% of the time.[102] Although owner attention and general excitement are common triggers, more than one third of the cases had a serious fight when no person was present.[102] A poor prognosis should be given if the aggressive interactions occur at least once a week.[102]

Dominance aggression can affect the interactions between dogs in five ways. First, this type of aggression between dogs is common when the owner interferes by giving an unintended message. The typical history is one in which the owner complains that the dogs fight "all the time" and there is a concern that one might kill the other. When the owner is gone, however, the dogs stay together and there is never any indication of blood, saliva, or injuries when the owner returns home. Aggression is really occurring only in the presence of the owner. The higher ranking dog may approach when the Number 2 dog is being petted or groomed. Number 1 stares at Number 2 to displace it from the owner so that Number 1 can get the attention. This is allowable under "dog law." When Number 2 does not see the subtle threat or does not acknowledge it, Number 1 escalates the threat to a low growl—also allowable under "dog law." The owner, not appreciating the growl, admonishes Number 1. Number 2 wins and quickly learns that whenever the owner is present, it can get favored attention. When the owner is not present, Number 2 respects the higher-ranking dog. As the old cliché goes, the owner has a tendency to "side with the underdog."

Treatment for this first type of dominance aggression is generally straightforward and successful. First, it may be necessary to educate the owner about canine social orders and that living as "equals" is not natural.[212] Although the owners want their dogs to be equals, the dogs may not view their relationship in the same way. It is important to first determine which is the highest ranking dog, because it will be necessary to reinforce the social rank. Ideally, when the Number 1 dog approaches and shows any indication of wanting to displace the Number 2 dog, the owner should also reinforce the displacement.[135] Many owners are uncomfortable doing this, so an alternative plan can accomplish the same goal. Whenever aggression is likely to occur between the dogs, the owner can walk away. This way neither dog's behavior is reinforced, and the encounter is defused before it gets out of hand. The prognosis is poor if the problem has been going on for a long time, involves fights leading to injuries, or if the occurrence is not predictable to the owner.[203]

A second type of interdog dominance aggression occurs when a lower ranking dog tries to become a higher ranking one. This attempt at change can be related to several events, many of which cannot be predicted or prevented. Early handling of littermates in which one receives a lot more attention than the other can result in aggression between the two dogs that is carried over into competitive situations at a later age.[289] The relative size, age, sex, breeds, and personalities of the two dogs are usually significant, too. As an obvious example, an intact male Jack Russell Terrier approaching behavioral maturity would be highly likely to challenge the dominant position of a 14-year-old spayed female Bassett Hound. In many cases, the change in ranking would be unnoticed by the owner, because social orders are relatively insignificant to most Bassetts. If the Jack Russell lived with an 8-year-old castrated male Boston Terrier, the resulting aggression would be more obvious. What might not be so obvious, however, is that the Boston Terrier is handicapped in its ability to hold its top-ranking position by physical displays. Its tail cannot be elevated, and piloerection is insignificant. The Jack Russell might incorrectly read the Boston Terrier's body language as somewhat ambivalent, and the challenge would continue. A younger dog can also grow to be larger than the older dog, as would happen in a household with a young Chow Chow male that is growing up with a miniature Poodle, and then challenge the older dog.[145,149,212]

Aggressive episodes between dogs can happen at any time regardless of whether the owner is present. Aggression between housemates is similar to dominance aggression between wolves.[299] It occurs more often between same-sex pairs, is more likely to be started by the younger dog, and is started more often by the newest dog introduced into the home.[299] Often the first episodes are triggered over access to an important resource, such as food.[145]

Treatment for dominance aggression associated with a lower ranking dog trying to become dominant to a higher ranking one requires careful determination of which dog is higher ranking and consideration of which dog should be. Sometimes the owner has a preference for which dog should be the higher ranking dog. At other times physical frailty in the higher ranking dog means a change might be the safest situation. In a changeover, controlled interactions between the dogs are important, so they must be kept separate except during the sessions.[221] With both dogs on long leashes, the owner takes them to a fairly neutral location, such as a nearby park or the front yard. The dog which is to become the lower ranking one is put on a "down-stay" command as the dog to become higher ranking walks by on a "heel" command. This passing first occurs at a distance, but the interdog distance is decreased with subsequent passes, as both dogs accept the dominant-subordinate situation imposed on them. Gradually the sessions are moved closer to home, with the final ones being in the location where most of the aggressive encounters previously occurred.

The dogs can learn to repress aggressive behavior in the presence of the owners, but they do not always transfer those lessons to times when the owners are not present. Therefore, it is safest to keep the dogs separate when they cannot be supervised. Owners are often willing to try some behavior modification, but they may tire of how the dogs' behaviors affect their lives. Getting one of the dogs out of that environment is the best long-term solution for many owners. This solution should be mentioned as one option when talking about treatments, so if the owners do decide to get rid of one dog, they understand it is an acceptable option and do not have to feel like failures as dog owners.

A common sequela to a lower ranking dog obtaining a higher rank is that the amount of aggression does not decrease. This aggression also can appear to be excessive for the situation in which it is shown. The old dog readily relinquishes its top position and now responds to the young dog's growls by rolling over on its back in a very submissive posture. The young dog, though, aggressively attacks the submissive dog, inflicting serious injury. The reason why submissive postures fail to defuse the situation is unknown. In some cases, the new top dog may be so worked up before the submissive posture is assumed that it takes a while for it to settle down. At other times, it appears as if the new top dog has learned to focus in on a particular target, and even though the signals have changed, the target remains the same. It is also possible that domestication has reduced the significance of submissive postures in dogs. In this situation, separating the dogs is the only sure way to prevent injury. The serotonin-enhancing drugs offer promise for these extreme cases.

A third type of dominance aggression between dogs occurs when a dominant dog enforces its dominance position relative to another. A higher ranking dog may challenge a lower ranking pack member for a favored possession or location. If highly excited or stressed, the top dog may show aggression to a lower ranking pack member and it, in turn, will redirect aggression to an even lower ranking dog, passing on the blows to the "ego."[246] A subtle glance, a positioning over, or low-throat mutterings are subtle indicators of this kind of aggression. These interactions are usually not problematic unless the lower ranking dog becomes unable to respond. Blindness and osteoarthritis are examples of physical ailments that could slow an appropriate response, causing problems between dogs that had previously gotten along very well.

The fourth situation of interdog dominance aggression involves shared dominance positions between dogs. Two dogs can share a single ranking in a dominance hierarchy, and this relationship can be further complicated by owners who raise their dogs to be equal. In each situation, there must be a new decision about which dog gets first access. The dogs tend to show a lot of aggression toward each other, but there usually is no clear winner. The presence of food may be more likely to trigger aggression by one; disturbed sleep may be more serious to the other. The dogs can be helped to settle on a definite rank by means of the techniques just described, putting the dog that is to be the lower ranking one on a down-stay as the other is walked past.

General treatment considerations discussed for dominance aggression toward people also apply when the target is another dog. It is important to take precautions for human safety because injuries obtained when breaking up a dog fight can be very serious. A multifaceted approach is recommended for interdog dominance aggression. Castration is recommended for intact males, and drug therapy with serotonin-enhancing drugs can be used. The dogs should be separated for 3 to 5 days, then reintroduced in a neutral location while reinforcing previous social ranks.[132] Behavior modification teaches the dogs the long-term social interactions that will ultimately be important to successfully keeping both dogs in the same household. Surgical treatment by prefrontal lobotomy has been successful for dogs that had been aggressive toward other dogs. It has not been used for a long time and at best should be considered only a salvage procedure at this time.[5]

The fifth type of interdog dominance aggression is fence fighting. This behavior may have elements of intermale and/or territorial aggression too. Fence fighting is also seen in pen-housed wild canids where it tends to be ritualized. In a study of wolves, a fence was found to be the equivalent of having a 15-foot horizontal boundary between wolves.[175] The presence of the barrier may increase confidence to display that normally would need a space between individuals in a natural setting.

## Drug-Related (Drug-Induced) Aggression

Although not common, aggressive reactions have been reported to be associated with a number of drugs and probably for various reasons.[297,304] Several years ago, the use of a product containing fentanyl and droperidol in guard dog breeds, such as German Shepherds, was associated with aggression

15% of the times used.[201] Reasons for the reaction are unknown, but fentanyl remains associated with occasional bouts of aggression. Ketamine has been associated with aggressive behavior, especially in cats, and typically after the sedation wore off. Humans describe hallucinations while under the drug's influence, so perhaps this was happening in animals too. This problem does not seem to occur if ketamine is used in combination with other drugs, like diazepam. Medetomidine, related drugs like detomidine, and xylazine have had associated aggressive reactions reported anecdotally.[196] These may be associated with arousal, fear, or pain. The current recommendation to minimize the possibility of this reaction is to use these drugs in combination with other drugs, such as opioids. Yohimbine-associated aggression has also been noted.[196]

## Fear-Induced (Defensive) Aggression

Fear is a feeling of distress or uneasiness caused by the proximity of a particular object or individual.[32] Objects that precipitate fear in a dog can be diverse, but many are related to social encounters. A more dominant dog or person can elicit a fearful response from a dog, as can a child rapidly approaching while maintaining eye contact, or even an owner who inadvertently causes pain while pulling a dog out from under a bed where it took a stolen "prize." Dogs that were raised in benign environments that also lacked social stimuli are more fearful of new places and people than those from enriched experiences.[8,202] In a fearful situation, an animal may respond by avoiding the situation through flight or hiding, or it may confront the situation with an extreme response, such as a very submissive body posture, or it may show aggression as a defensive behavior.[29,132,134,317] The classic fear-biter seen by veterinarians is the small dog that has been put in the top cage where its view of the approaching person is an entranceway framing only a head with staring eyes. If the person approaches such a fear-biter and fails to read the dog's signals or if he or she blocks its retreat, the dog may bite out of fear.

Fear biting is the second most common form of aggression problem in dogs reported to behaviorists, making up between 6% and 23% of aggressive

cases.* It is also a behavior that tends to occur at a rate somewhat higher than expected in females, both intact and neutered.[46,247] Castration does not reduce the incidence of fear-induced aggression in affected males.[144,267] Generalized anxiety can increase the likelihood that a dog will become fearful and show this or other types of aggression.[267] It is important to differentiate an anxious dog, where specific stimuli are unclear, from a fearful dog that is reacting to a specific threatening stimulus. Fear biting is a very common type of aggression to veterinary staff, so safety precautions can be helpful.[206]

A fear-biter shows ambivalent body language—that is, mixed signals. It often stares as a distance-increasing sign, but the rear quarters are lowered as a submissive sign. Occasionally, the dog will suddenly divert eye contact but elevate its tail, and the hair over its hips will rise. The safest advice is to read the worst end. This kind of dog is usually fine with people, except when a unique situation is fear inducing for it.

The tendency for an individual dog to bite out of fear can be related to one of three situations. In some cases, the tendency for fear biting is passed directly from one generation to the next genetically.[31,105] A second mode of inheritance can occur when a very timid dog is bred to a very dominant dog, with some of the puppies getting the worst of both parents. In the third situation of fear biting, extreme environmental factors precipitate fear.

Both fear and aggression are very difficult to extinguish with operant conditioning,[74] so treatments for fear-biters are quite variable. They depend on the environment of the dog, triggering factors, the frequency of occurrence of fear biting, and the presence or absence of genetic factors. For a dog that is hiding under a chair, table, or bed and threatening those who approach, the owner must decide whether the need to get the dog is great enough to warrant a potential confrontation. If the answer is yes, a food bribe may be successful so that a confrontation is not necessary. But use of the food reward increases the likelihood of the event happening again. Pulling the dog out from its hiding

---

*References 24, 26, 27, 43, 46, 66, 224, 225.

place may cause pain, or at least it may involve an excessive threat posture and stare from the owner as a negative experience for the dog. The next time a similar situation occurs, the dog will be fearful of being hurt or threatened again. Using dominance is appropriate for controlling a dog's responses, but the amount necessary should be just enough to achieve the desired results. In excess, dominant behaviors are more likely to cause a fearful response. To complicate things even more, a dominant dog can quickly shift into a fearful mode, and the person approaching may not notice the subtle changes that occur.

Treatment for fear-induced aggressive dogs involves minimizing those situations that are most apt to induce fear. When that is not possible, a desensitization program may be helpful. Gradually the dog is introduced to increasing intensities of specific stimuli it fears. As an example, the dog that is afraid of people can learn to "sit-stay" for a special reward, such as a food treat or a ball-playing session. Once the dog learns what is expected, with the owner giving the reward, a familiar person whom the dog accepts can work on the same lesson. Gradually, less familiar people should work with the dog as it slowly learns to associate the fun with the presence of people. It is important that there be no negative experiences with strangers while this training occurs and that each step not be rushed. The owner should also decrease his or her amount of interaction with the dog when not involved in a training session, to increase the reward value of social interaction that occurs during the training sessions.

Fear-biting dogs in veterinary hospitals can present special challenges. First slow down to think through options, to read the animal's body language carefully, and to give the dog some time to adjust too. Muzzles, Elizabethan collars, and head halters can be successful tools to try before having to bring out the snares and drugs. In another common scenario, the veterinarian learns a dog is a fear-biter only after putting it in a top cage. A few other techniques may be helpful. As the threat to the dog comes from the facial approach, backing into the cage significantly decreases the degree of threat (Fig. 4-8). If the dog has been upset by unsuccessful attempts to get it out of the cage, it is advisable to wear heavy gloves. If, however, the dog is known to be a fear-biter from previous experience but is not currently upset, the heavy gloves are usually not necessary. As the dog will be against the back of the cage, removing it is a simple matter of sliding an arm around the animal and picking it up. Once a fear-biter has been picked up, it is usually not a problem to handle. Fear-biters in lower cages or in runs are usually accepting of human interaction once they have a leash on. It may take some patience and "pseudo-lasso" work to get the leash on, but it is usually not necessary to get overly assertive with these dogs. A long leash can be left on the dog identified as a fear-biter and tied to the outside of the cage or run to simplify procedures the next time the animal needs to be brought out of the cage.

Experimentally, surgical amygdalectomies have been effective in eliminating fear biting.[320] Another surgical procedure, castration, is not effective in reducing the incidence of fear biting. Surgery has never become popular in fear-induced aggression, but as the neurotransmitters are becoming more understood, drug therapy is gaining acceptance. Drug therapy can help those dogs that are extremely fearful of most things. For this, the selective serotonin reuptake inhibitors are used. Amitriptyline has not proven useful.[315] If specific events trigger the fearful behavior, benzodiazepines may be helpful.

## Idiopathic Aggression

In spite of careful history taking, detailed descriptions by owners, and extensive laboratory or special testing, a small percent of aggression cases will probably remain undiagnosed. Some of these may represent complicated interactions of multiple kinds of aggression, some may be due to inaccurate information in the history, and others may be due to factors that are yet to be identified. Regardless, a category for idiopathic aggression will probably always exist. Currently it serves as a catch-all for the apparently unprovoked, unpredictable, and unexplainable serious attacks that do not fit other diagnostic criteria.[134,137,226,313] If brain lesions cause these serious attacks, studies show the presence of bilateral lesions if they are destructive in nature, or perhaps a single focus if the lesions are only irritative.[321]

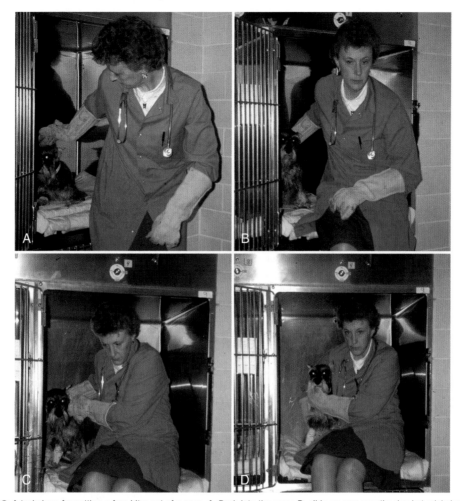

**Figure 4-8** A technique for getting a fear biter out of a cage. **A**, Back into the cage; **B**, slide an arm over the dog but minimize eye contact; **C**, secure the dog with both arms; **D**, pick the dog up and remove it from the cage.

## Intrasexual Aggression

Certain acts of aggression between dogs of the same sex appear to be driven only by the fact that they are the same sex.

### Intermale Aggression

Intermale aggression is the most common form of this intrasexual aggression. Many intact males have an instinctive tendency to fight any other intact male. This trait is common in terriers and guarding types of dogs like German Shepherds, Doberman Pinschers, and Rottweilers. The mere sight of another dog that looks, smells, and acts male is enough to trigger an attack. Intermale aggression is relatively common, accounting for 5.4% to 12.5% of aggressive cases.[24,27,43] In a survey of almost 400 owners of intact male dogs in Britain, 30% indicated their dogs fought with other male dogs.[320,328]

Intermale aggression is a male sexually dimorphic behavior. As such, it is most likely to be shown by intact males, then castrated males, neutered females, and least likely by intact females.[46] The behavior is apparently testosterone-dependent, at least for a while. Learning may result in the behavior continuing, even after castration, making the problem one of control, not cure. When unfamiliar dogs come together, 79% of them (usually male) would fight in 75% of the encounters.[202] Castration of intact males will eliminate aggression toward other male dogs in approximately 60% of the dogs[144] and more if both dogs are castrated.[334] For approximately half the cases that do not respond to castration, progestin therapy may reduce or eliminate the undesired behavior,[133,141,320] but the advantage of long-term use must be carefully weighed against potential side effects. Environmental factors that can contribute to the problem, like the presence of a bitch in estrus or a taunting but inaccessible male dog, should be avoided. If the two aggressive male dogs live in the same home, it will probably be necessary to find another home for one of them or keep them separated. Positive reinforcement and counterconditioning can be used to teach a dog to stay near the owner and relax in the presence of another male dog, but fighting may occur without such supervision.[220,321,328,335]

Terriers have a stronger tendency than most types of dogs to develop intrasexual aggression.[107] Puppies may need to be separated into pairs as early as 9 weeks of age because of coordinated attacks on the most submissive animal.[71,122] By choosing those individuals with the greatest tendency to show this aggression, fighting dogs have been developed. These dogs tend to be so interdog aggressive that the sex of the intended victim is ignored.[71] They also have a high pain tolerance.

When dogs fight, the most important consideration has to be prevention of human injuries while trying to separate the dogs. The dog seldom recognizes who is grabbing at it or trying to restrain it, so redirected aggression is common. To break up a fight, a person should not reach into the action, but rather should throw something over the dogs, like a blanket or water, to distract them.[220] Pulling on the dog's collar during a fight can cause the dog to actually lean into the fight more.[220] Prevention of a fight is easier and safer than separating dogs during a fight.

### Interfemale Aggression

Interfemale aggression is much less common than intermale aggression, and it is more difficult to treat because hormonal manipulation does not work. An ovariohysterectomy or progestin therapy will not eliminate the problem unless the aggressive episodes are associated with the estrous cycle.[328,335] Estrogen does lower the threshold for aggression.[72] In addition, aggression can be associated with pseudopregnancy, as discussed later. Owners can try behavior modification to control the dogs in their presence,[328,335] or they can keep the dogs physically separate. In the long term, however, many owners find it necessary to place one of the dogs in a new home.

### Learned Aggression

Learned aggression occurs in two forms: it can be purposely or unconsciously taught. In the first case, dogs are trained to show aggression. In the second, their owners unwittingly reinforce aggressive behavior.

#### Purposely Taught Aggression

Certain dogs are easily trained to show aggression—purposely taught aggression. Many breeds that can be trained this way were originally developed to protect livestock or property. German Shepherds, Belgian Malinois, Doberman Pinschers, and Rottweilers are a few of the breeds that can easily be trained to show aggression on command. Fortunately for veterinarians, most owners of working guard dogs know how to handle the animal, and these dogs willingly allow their owners to restrain them. A problem can occur when the dog owner teaches the dog to be aggressive for protection purposes or when the owner attempts to demonstrate a macho character through the dog. These owners seldom have adequate control over their dogs, and without that control, they own a potentially dangerous animal. Such owners need to realize the possible consequences of having such a dog, including their legal obligations in regard to public safety.

#### Unconsciously Taught Aggression

Another problem dog is the dog that has learned to be aggressive without the owner realizing it—unconsciously taught aggression. This learning can happen whenever aggressive behavior is reinforced. As an example, an owner crawls under the bed to pull a fear-biter out, but the dog anticipates the painful pull and the dominant stare. The dog growls, and the owner withdraws. The result is negative reinforcement of an aggressive behavior. The dog may transfer this learning to control other situations.

As another example, a dog can learn to be aggressive at the front door because of an owner who has some safety concerns. The dog is taken to the door each time the doorbell rings, and it starts barking. The owner verbally reassures the dog that everything is all right, but the voice tones and petting actually reinforce the barking behavior. The bark threat escalates to a growl with the same reinforcement. Eventually the dog lunges at visitors. The situation is now one in which the dog is behaving as if it feels responsible *for* the owners rather than *to* the owners.[58] The presenting complaint in this case is that the dog shows aggression at guests. Upon being told that the behavior can be stopped, owners often confess that they really would like the behavior to continue toward strangers, just not toward friends.

Unconsciously taught aggression represents between 2.2% and 4.2% of aggression cases.[24,27] To change the behavior, it is important to identify possible complicating factors. For the owners who are afraid of their neighborhood—and have communicated that fear to their dogs—actual crime statistics may help them understand they have less to fear than they thought. For the fearful dog that steals "prize" tissues from the garbage, ignoring it or putting the garbage out of reach can defuse potential confrontations. The veterinarian needs to identify how the owner has been reinforcing the undesired behavior, so that reinforcement can be stopped. The behavior can be eliminated either by no longer reinforcing it (extinction), punishing it, applying counterconditioning, or using a combination of techniques.[321]

A dog may also learn to show aggression toward an oncoming person or dog during a walk for other reasons, such as fear resulting from poor socialization or for anticipated pain. The owner tightens up on the leash, which sends an "alert" message to the dog. Over time the owner begins to tighten the leash at the sight of someone approaching and the dog gradually learns to increase its aggressive signals in response to the owner's concerns. The owner has unconsciously reinforced the exact behavior they do not want.

Counterconditioning can be used to treat these cases.[152] The dog is fitted with a head halter and in a series of controlled situations, introduced to the triggering stimulus when it is so far away as to not provoke any reaction. The dog is also taught a "watch me" behavior so its attention can be focused on the owner on command. Very gradually over many trials, the triggering stimulus comes closer, but never so that the aggressive behavior reoccurs.

## Material-Protective Aggression

Some dogs become very protective of specific objects like a ball or toy, rawhide chew, or stolen "prize" like a facial tissue taken from the bathroom garbage can. The dog may even present the object to the owner but become aggressive if the owner reaches to take it away.[226] Guarding of objects, with material-protective aggression, can start as early as the fourth or fifth week of life.[122] The behavior can take on a play quality, because each success has its own internal reward.[32] It can also be associated with dominance-related situations.[46] Owners often reward the behavior by chasing the dog or using a tasty food bribe to get the protected object away. The dog may learn that aggressive guarding causes the owner or another animal to back away, leading eventually to an increase in aggression and a shift in its focus from protection to dominance. Up to 17% of the complaints about aggression are related to material protection.[46]

To treat the problem of material-protective aggression, the owner needs to be proactive. The easiest approach is to throw away all toys that the dog covets. If the "prize" comes from the garbage, the owner should prevent access to the garbage can by putting it in a cupboard or on top of a counter or by closing off the room where it is located. Bribery with a food treat or removal by excessive force should be avoided unless the "prize" is potentially dangerous to the dog. Bribery rewards the behavior and increases the likelihood it will occur again. Excessive force can trigger aggression from fear or pain.

It is possible to teach a dog to give up its toy or "prize." The lesson is best taught with young puppies by taking the toy away from the puppy at the end of each session with it. For the older dog, the lesson starts by using the least favorite toy.

The owner should control each session by having the dog in a collar or head halter and on leash. The specific toy is given to the dog, and after a short period, the owner ends the session by taking the toy away. Before taking it away, the owner or a second person who has the leash should put the dog on a "sit" or "down" command for a food or praise reward. At the same time, with careful control of the dog so that it cannot reach the owner's hand, the toy is picked up. If the dog will sit quietly, it is rewarded. Then the lesson is repeated several times, and more favored toys are gradually introduced into the lessons.

## Food-Protective Aggression

Food-protective aggression tends to be most pronounced for the tastier foods.[226] A few dogs are very protective of food, yet show no other types of aggression. In other dogs, food-protective aggression may be a sign of other problems, especially dominance aggression. Owners must be careful in dealing with this type of dog, because it is easier to escalate the problem than to solve it. Because it is an evolutionary behavior, protection of a food source is difficult to eliminate.[226]

Very young puppies should learn that growling or snapping at a person picking up their food means they do not get it back for several minutes, whereas passive behavior is rewarded by its immediate return. An older dog that guards its food can inflict injury, so the approach to treatment needs to be more subtle. One approach is for the owner to just feed the dog its meal and leave. In this way, confrontation never happens. This approach is generally acceptable in an adults-only household when a dog eats its meal in a short amount of time. When small children are around, especially if the dog nibbles food throughout the day, there will be a confrontation at some time. One technique uses counterconditioning to teach the dog that it is the presence of the owner that results in food.[335] In one variation, the owner puts down the empty food dish, makes the dog sit, and then dispenses a small amount of food reward. The owner stands by the dish as the dog eats the few pieces of dry food. If the dog growls, snaps, or does not eat, it does not receive any of the food until the next trial. If the

dog eats without aggression, the owner puts in a few more pieces of food. This is repeated frequently throughout the day until the amount normally fed is reached. Bad manners mean the dog might be hungry, but this lesson rarely takes long to learn.

In another variation, the dog is fed a very small meal of untasty food. At the very beginning, the owner approaches as close as possible without eliciting a growl. (If a growl occurs before the owner stops, he or she should stop and stand still rather than retreating. The next time the owner should not advance as far.) As the dog nears the end of its tiny meal, the owner can toss individual pieces of a more palatable food into the bowl one at a time. This feeding routine is repeated three or four times a day, but appropriate caloric intake during the day should not exceed normal. On successive days, the owner moves slightly closer to the dish, with the eventual goal of being able to place food directly in the bowl. Any aggressive behavior results in an immediate cessation of feeding, and the owner walks away. For both variations, all family members should work with the dog so that the dog can generalize that people around the food bowl bring good things.

Another technique can be used, but it depends on the person holding the leash to be observant and not excessive in their response. By using a collar or head halter and long leash, two people can teach the older dog to control its aggression around food. One person holds the leash to control the dog. The second person puts the food down. After the dog has taken a few bites, the second person reaches for the dog's dish. If the dog shows no aggression as the food bowl is being picked up, the bowl is returned immediately. If any aggression is shown, the dog is pulled away and firmly told "No" at the same instant. The second person removes the food bowl as soon as it is safe to do so, and the food is not returned until the next training session. The process is repeated several times, using small meals of a minimally palatable food. As the dog learns the new expectations, small portions of the regular food can be added to the less palatable food until the regular food is eventually all that is fed. This technique does not change the motive for protective aggression; it just teaches restraint around certain individuals.

## Maternal (Parental) Aggression

After whelping, bitches show a strong protective behavior toward their young and may show aggression without a threat display.[32,132] This behavior is related to the post-parturient hormonal state and to the physical presence of young puppies, not necessarily their own.[132] Over the next several weeks, the intensity of the aggressive reaction decreases. Punishment is not useful for maternal aggression. If the puppies must be stressed, their cries will trigger the behavior, so situational management is dependent on keeping the puppies separated from their mother until the interaction is complete. While handling the puppies, keep the puppy between the bitch and the person because she is less apt to run over her own puppy to get to the person. Nonfamily members should avoid the bitch for the few weeks of highest protective tendencies.[45] When avoidance is undesirable or not possible, counterconditioning with food may be possible.[321,328]

## Medically Related Aggression

Not only can aggressive behavior be associated with the "not acting right" complaints typical of fever, gastrointestinal upset, and other common problems in veterinary medicine, there are also deeper relationships with medical conditions expressed as behavioral signs only. Changes in behavior can occur in dogs with infectious and acquired conditions. A large number of medical conditions are related to aggression.[237] They can be as obvious as rabies and tumors. They can also be associated with less understood problems like hepatoencephalopathy and cardiac problems.[186] There are, however, a number of classic medical problems that may be presented as behavior problems and lack the more typical signs of the medical condition. Diagnostic work-ups can be straightforward, or special procedures may be necessary. A complete blood count, blood chemistry, urinalysis, and thyroid profile are minimal. Magnetic resonance imaging (MRI) or computed tomography (CT) may be helpful when brain disease is suspected. Sometimes, though, only an electroencephalogram (EEG) may be abnormal.[39]

## Hormone Imbalance Aggression

Aggression related to a hormone imbalance can occur in the bitch. In some cases, an intact female becomes aggressive during her first estrus. The obvious solution is to remove the ovaries. If surgical treatment is not an option, the owner will need to find ways to prevent interactions that precipitate aggression until estrus is over. A neutered female may also show periods of aggression that occur in a cyclic nature—approximately every 6 months—with the periods lasting a few weeks. This timing is about the same as for an estrous cycle. Hormonal assays for estrogen levels do not indicate elevated amounts of the hormone, but the body cycles in other ways too. Whereas ovarian cycles tend to predominate the biologic rhythms, more subtle ones may become noticeable after the ovaries are removed.

One of the unusual types of aggression associated with hormonal imbalance is that which some bitches will show during pseudopregnancy (pseudocyesis). In the nonpregnant bitch, the corpora lutea of estrus lasts approximately 2 months. Progesterone from the corpora lutea can produce behavioral signs typical of pregnancy and whelping even in the nonpregnant state. The restlessness, nesting, and even aggression will disappear as the progesterone levels return to those typical of anestrus. Although clients may pressure the veterinarian to stop the unwanted signs of pseudopregnancy, it is best to let the behaviors gradually return to normal and then remove the ovaries to prevent their return with the next cycle.[335] Use of progestins will give temporary relief of signs, but the drugs are actually just bringing the hormonal state closer to that of early metestrus, and signs will return as the hormone level decreases again. A prolactin antagonist, cabergoline, has been used successfully in Europe.[72] Drugs like the phenothiazines and butyrophenones that inhibit or antagonize dopamine should be avoided at this time, because they are likely to enhance the pseudopregnancy.[319,328,335]

## Hydrocephalus

Hydrocephalus is a medical condition that can be manifested only as aggression. This condition accounts for 0.8% of aggressive behaviors.[24] Hydrocephalus should be high on a list of differential diagnoses for any aggressive dog weighing less than 10 lb, regardless of whether the dog has an open fontanelle. Because clinical signs of hydrocephalus depend on which areas of the brain are affected most by the increased pressure, abnormal behavior, including aggression, is often a sign of the condition. Historically, many of the aggressive dogs with hydrocephalus are also reported to be "stubborn" and not completely housetrained. Whether these secondary signs are associated with the hydrocephalus or are the exaggerated retention of juvenile characteristics is uncertain. Clinical evidence from necropsies done on aggressive dogs suggests that hydrocephalus is not restricted to the little dogs. Several larger dogs, including Bull Terriers, Saint Bernards, and Rottweilers, have been found to have varying degrees of the condition. Many of these breeds also have a tendency toward a more spherical-shaped skull. Continued investigation will give a better understanding of the role hydrocephalus plays in the aggressive problems in larger dogs.

### Hyperthyroidism

Hyperthyroidism is uncommon in dogs, but when it does occur, aggression can be the primary presenting complaint. This fact was discovered when thyroid screening became part of a minimum database for screening aggressive dogs. Although hypothyroidism is relatively common, an occasional case of hyperthyroidism can be identified as well. Treatment depends on the cause, so an additional medical work-up is indicated.

### Hypothyroidism

Hypothyroidism can manifest itself as a behavior change of seizures, altered mental state, extreme shyness, or aggression.[10,84,215] Hypothyroid aggression has a distinctly different presentation than other more classic forms of hypothyroidism, and it represents 1.7% of the aggressive behaviors.[24,261] Affected dogs rarely show other signs typical of hypothyroidism, such as associated alopecia. In fact, the dog may actually have a beautiful, show-quality coat. No lethargy or weight gain is demonstrated, either. The typical presentation for hypothyroid aggression is a grumpy dog. It may sleep on the bed but occasionally not want to share the sofa with the owner. When going through a door with the owner, one time the dog may be fine but the next time it may snap.

Hypothyroidism is an overdiagnosed condition in veterinary medicine, because so many things can influence thyroid levels, from time of day to drug therapy. Stress, by its effects on glucocorticoid levels, influences behavior and affects the hypothalamic-pituitary-adrenal axis.[17] Other behavior changes, including hyperness, separation anxiety, and noise phobias, may also be associated with hypothyroidism.[10] For all these reasons, the thyroid status should be evaluated as part of a behavioral work-up, but all results must be carefully evaluated.

Onset of hypothyroid aggression is usually gradual, and episodes that trigger the aggression are inconsistent. Usually the dogs are middle-aged adults, but hypothyroidism can occur in younger dogs, too. Consequently, the condition is easy to confuse with dominance aggression. For this reason, testing for hypothyroidism is an appropriate part of a minimum database for aggression cases. Thyroid-replacement therapy brings marked improvement in the dog's behavior without the need for other drug therapy or behavior modification. Coexisting problems will need separate treatments.[99] Occasional monitoring of thyroid levels helps identify dogs that need adjustment of their dosages.

### Irritable Aggression

Dogs that suffer from various medical conditions may show aggression more readily than physically healthy dogs, especially if they really just want to be left alone but are not. Irritable aggression is implicated in approximately 7% of aggression cases.[24,26,27] This kind of aggression can be understood by us humans; when people are suffering from a headache or toothache, they become less tolerant of things that normally would not bother them, like a child screaming in a restaurant or a driver suddenly cutting them off in traffic. Dogs with hot spots, fleas, hip dysplasia, discospondylosis, progressive retina atrophy, or a number of other conditions would certainly be candidates for irritable aggression. Geriatric dogs are highly likely to have a reason for this type of behavior.[157] Treatment means finding a way to eliminate or temper the underlying cause. Flea control has taken giant steps forward within the last few years. When orthopedic problems are not correctable with surgery, the use of pain relievers and environmental management that gives the dog a quiet and child-free safety zone may be necessary.

### Mental-Lapse Aggression

Up to 5% of aggressive dogs show a mental-lapse type of aggression that is quite unusual.[24] The affected dog, usually from a currently popular breed, will show aggression to those it used to like, usually without warning. It may back the owner into a room and aggressively keep him or her there for several hours. Even though that episode may end, the dog is likely to continue to show aggression almost continuously thereafter.

The dog with mental-lapse aggression does not show brief periods of aggression interspersed with long periods of normalcy, nor does it contain the development typical of dominance. The onset is sudden and serious. The diagnosis is confirmed by an EEG done under anesthesia.[21] The atypical pattern is a low-voltage, fast-activity one. Whether this EEG pattern was present before the onset of the aggression or resulted in it is not known. The pattern, however, is more common in wild animals, suggesting a potential for serious consequences. The animal may become the equivalent of a wild animal, with no fear of humans. For the owner's safety, euthanasia is the option of choice.

In a general veterinary practice, it is difficult to diagnose mental-lapse aggression, and neurologists are tending not to do EEGs anymore, so referrals to a neurologist still may not result in a firm diagnosis. Mental-lapse aggression can also be misdiagnosed as a severe form of dominance aggression. When the aggression is as severe as this usually is, regardless of cause, it is better to err on the side of human safety and euthanize the dog.

### Owner-Protective Aggression

Some people get dogs for protection or unconsciously want them to be protective. The result can be a dog that is overprotective. Formally trained dogs are the least overprotective, and untrained ones are the most.[61] Dogs that learn to show aggression—the recipients of purposely taught aggression—are discussed earlier in this chapter. Most dogs are instinctively protective of their owners when they perceive a serious threat. A few dogs become overly protective and will react to any approach of the owner by another person, even for a handshake or hug. These dogs constitute approximately 3.4% to 4.2% of aggression problems.[24,27] The instinctive nature of the protective behavior brings with it an internal reward for successfully driving the approacher away. Punishment is rarely successful because of this internal reward, but a desensitization-counterconditioning program can teach the dog it will be rewarded for another behavior. Some owners still need reassurance that the dog will protect them if the animal perceives danger.

The lesson starts with two people the dog gets along with approaching each other. The dog is told to "sit-stay" while the people shake hands. The dog is given a highly favored reward like food or ball play for appropriate behavior only at the end of the handshake and a release word like "okay." This is repeated several times. In the next set of lessons, the owner shakes hands with a nonfamily member but close friend whom the dog likes. The owner gives the "sit-stay" command, and the friend engages in the food reward/play bout after the dog responds correctly. In following sessions, the dog becomes accustomed to successively less well-known visitors but has learned that the release word will bring a reward from the visitors.

### Pain-Induced Aggression

When a dog is hurt, it may respond aggressively toward the source of the pain or something nearby.[155,317] Even the anticipation of pain because of previous experience can cause the same reaction.[202,252] This pain-induced aggression is the primary problem in approximately 2% to 3% of referred aggression cases[24,46,88]; however, it occurs much more often than that. This can become a significant problem in geriatric dogs, as it may be associated with osteoarthritis or even dental disease.[149] Because pain-induced aggression is a common problem when small children are around, dog-child interactions should always be supervised—a foot gets stepped on, an ear is pulled, an eye is poked, or a handful of hair is used to pull a toddler up to its wobbly feet.

For adults that trigger pain, the end result is usually a brief, warning nip. Unfortunately for a small child at the same height as the dog, even a nip can result in serious injury. When there is a significant dominance difference and the dog outranks the person, the severity of the bite could be way out of proportion to the intensity of the initial situation. As an example, an accidental touch by a foot under a kitchen table usually just displaces the dog, but a dog like this could respond with dominance and pain-induced aggression using a bite that is bad enough to result in the loss of a toenail. Careful history-taking may reveal that other components of dominance aggression are also present.

Some dogs, such as hounds and terriers, are very pain tolerant. Others react to the mildest of stimuli. The only way to prevent pain-induced aggression is to prevent pain.[321,328,335] If the dog bit because it was stepped on by the owner while getting up to go to the bathroom in the middle of the night, the owner could be advised to keep the dog out of the bedroom, crate the dog, or use a night-light so both the dog and owner can be seen.

## Play Aggression

Play in young dogs consists of segments of behavior that are parts of adult behaviors. Play allows the youngster to develop appropriate motor skills, release excess energy, interact with peers, and practice patterns that when put in context at a later time would be necessary for survival in the wild. From the first growls at 4 to 5 weeks,[122] to snarling and baring of teeth, to the attack and bite, the puppy can perfect its techniques. Mock attacks are perfected on littermates, and the playful bites on floppy ears teach jaw pressure. The amount of pressure it takes to make a littermate yelp and withdraw teaches how much is needed to inflict pain.

Two situations can occur in which humans are affected by play aggression. The first is when the puppy learns jaw pressure by practicing on the owner's hand, especially likely to occur when a littermate's ear is not available. Allowing biting during play and permitting rough play teach the puppy that those behaviors are acceptable and that a great deal of jaw pressure is necessary to inflict pain. Instead, the owner should remove his or her hand as soon as the puppy's mouth touches it and then distract the youngster to change the focus of attention.

The second interaction of humans with canine play aggression occurs when play escalates to what the owner is convinced is serious aggression. This situation is reported in 2.25% to 3.3% of aggressive-behavior problem cases.[24,27] It is important for the owner to avoid overreacting, which could cause the play to be replaced by fear. Because play aggression is a normal behavior, punishment is not appropriate.[328] Instead, the play should be redirected toward acceptable objects, or the person can move away from the puppy.[335] Play aggression can be minimized through encouraging lots of exercise, avoiding rough play, and making the dog earn human attention.[228]

## Predatory Aggression

Predation is a normal behavior in a carnivore, so it should be expected in dogs. The form it takes is variable because of generations of selective breeding. In general, predatory behavior includes an alert, usually by sight or sound; a stalk; an attack; a kill; and an eating series. Using the cat as a model, we know that each step in behavior requires a different level of excitement before it will occur.[25] Dogs bred to work livestock, such as the Border Collie, Welsh Corgi, and Blue Heeler, have a strong tendency to chase and bark at things that move. Their tendency to progress to attack the object is usually arrested. Predatory drives are strong and have their own internal reward. As an indication of how strong the internal reward is, half the dogs hit while chasing a car will chase again. The movement of an object, such as a running cat, triggers prey chasing, and if the prey is caught, the dog may then progress to the attack. Between 2.5% and 12.5% of complaints about aggression involve predatory aggression.[24,43] If the object chased is small enough, or if the attacker injures a vulnerable body part like a jugular vein, serious to fatal consequences can result.

In rat models of predatory aggression, lesions of the olfactory bulb facilitate the behavior, but those in the amygdala abolish it.[95] Enhanced serotonin levels may be inhibitive, and high cholinergic levels induce predation.[95]

Rapid movement of any object away from the dog tends to trigger the predatory chase response. If the chase is successful, predatory aggression follows. To avoid that response, two strategies have developed in prey animals. The first is to not move. Cats flatten down to the ground if a tall object is not close by to climb. Rabbits freeze. Similarly, children should be taught to "stand like a tree" or "lie like a log." Without the chase, the dog often loses interest. They may sniff the object or child, but quickly move on to new interests. The second strategy works well with the average dog that chases for the inward reward the chase brings. If the prey suddenly becomes the chaser, the carnivore acts confused and stops running. Deer, rabbits, and other prey species will occasionally stop running and turn on the chaser. A jogger who stops and turns on the dog that tries to chase ruins the dog's internal reward and within a few days will be left alone by that dog. Counterconditioning and strong punishment are other techniques that can be tried,[321,328,335] but their success has been limited.

Predatory aggression can be directed toward livestock species, and one or more uncontrolled dogs can do a lot of damage. Owners are usually reluctant to believe that their lovable family pet could kill or maim a sheep, calf, or pony, so they are seldom cooperative in controlling an ongoing problem. Once livestock chasing starts, the internal reward for the behavior makes it difficult to stop. The dog that barks and bounds after the intended victim is generally less dangerous than the one that silently stalks.[226] Vocalizing was not part of the evolutionary pattern that allowed a successful hunt. A number of remedies have been tried to control predatory aggression toward livestock. Carcasses have been laced with materials to induce vomiting—the Garcia effect.[328,335] Dead prey has been tied around the neck of the dog or tied in its mouth even until the carcass rots away. Ultrasonic noise and remote punishment also have been tried. Overall, however, the end results are not very satisfying. If they work, they usually work only when the owner is present.[335]

The only successful treatment of predatory chasing and aggression, including livestock chasing, is prevention, that is, to confine the dog so there is no access to the prey.[23,32,328] Related behaviors are discussed in relation to behaviors of eating and locomotion.

## Rage Syndrome

The rage syndrome has typically been associated with English Springer Spaniels and called *Springer rage*. In reality, the same type of aggression has been associated with other breeds too, such as the Bernese Mountain Dog[334] and the Cocker Spaniel (*Cocker rage*). For both English Springer Spaniels and English Cocker Spaniels, a large number (30% and 24%, respectively) showed aggression with attempts to remove food or bones (a form of protective aggression).[270] They also had a high incidence of dominance aggression.[270] The incidence of all types of aggression was higher in the English Springer Spaniel breed than would normally be expected for a hunting dog, and certain traits associated with owner-directed aggression have been identified.[266,270] They include males, then neutered males, then females; show lines; at least 4 years of age; less responsive to obedience cues; acquired from a hobby breeder; and the presence of a specific kennel and a specific sire in a four-generation pedigree. The tendency to label any type of aggression shown by an English Springer Spaniel as Springer rage is unfair to the breed. The term more accurately is used to describe extremely severe, difficult to predict, aggressive episodes that are disproportionate to the stimulus and which historically are really an excessive form of dominance aggression. The dog lacks inhibition so there are multiple bites per episode and there is a prolonged post-exposure arousal period.[266] This explosive type of dominance aggression shown by a rather large dog makes it particularly dangerous to those around them. In some cases the dog might be expressing mental-lapse aggression, but their brain waves have not been studied.

There is a report of a dog dying from myocardial necrosis following a particularly severe bout of aggression.[248] It is speculated that the release of catecholamines during the aggression may have caused the damage and death.

## Redirected Aggression

Redirected aggression is quite common in dogs and represents about 5% of the problem cases with aggression.[24,27,88] In this type of aggression, the dog becomes very excited, as when a neighbor dog runs along the fence, someone walks past the front picture window, or another dog provokes an aggressive response. At that point, if the dog is prevented from directing its aggression at the cause of the emotional arousal, it may redirect its aggression toward a nearby person or animal. People have been severely bitten while trying to hold two dogs apart that had been fighting, not because the dog meant to bite the people, but because it was trying to break the restraint keeping it from getting at the other dog again. Many times the dog is so focused on the target animal that it fails to recognize the person or animal who is the recipient of its redirected aggression. Prevention of the causative situations is the best approach to this problem.[335] For example, when a large dog gets very excited running the yard fence with the dog in the neighboring yard, it may do serious body damage to a small canine yardmate. Several approaches could be taken, such as keeping the small dog inside if the large dog is outside, or putting the dogs outside only when the neighbor dog is not in the yard. Another solution is to put another fence down the middle of the yard so the dogs are separated from the neighbor dog by a buffer zone.

## Sex-Related Aggression

During mating, male dogs may use an inhibited bite, the nape bite, on the skin of the shoulder area of the bitch. This is normal and represents one type of sex-related aggression in dogs, but it is not always understood by dog owners.[32] Another form of sex-related aggression can be shown by the female toward a male with an apparently undesirable mating style or by an anestrous female toward a male attempting to mount. The normal and abnormal behaviors are more thoroughly discussed under male and female sexual behaviors.

## Territorial-Protective Aggression

Some dogs have a strong instinctive tendency to protect their territory from intruders. Territorial-protective aggression may be demonstrated by these dogs. The behavior occurs regardless of whether the owner is present, and it begins to show about the time of behavioral maturity.[267] In general, territorial defense is strongest near the center of the territory and gradually gets weaker as the distance from the center increases. The actual degree of defense will vary. It may be a warning bark, especially if the intruder is farther from the center, or just a bite without any vocalization at all. Territorial aggression is infrequent in feral dogs.[80] Small or crowded territories, as in a car or on a bed, are more strongly defended than large ones.[107]

There is a relationship between the age when a puppy was first vaccinated and its tendency to show territorial aggression later. The older it was when first vaccinated, the more likely it will show the territorial behavior.[296] Diet may also affect territorial aggression. Dogs on a high-protein diet show a higher amount of territorial aggression, and those on a low-protein diet show significantly less.[86] Supplementing a low-protein diet with tryptophan also may help lower the incidence.[82,83]

Territorial-protective aggression has its own internal reward when the approacher is successfully driven off. These dogs, then, should not be expected to distinguish friend from foe.[328] Because of the reward inherent in territorial-protective behavior, it is difficult to eliminate. Castration has no effect.[144,328] If the owner successfully teaches the dog not to be so protective, the lesson is usually remembered only when the owner is present.[335] Problems occur when the territorial protection occurs out of proper context, as happens in 5% to 29% of aggression cases.[24,26,27,43,88]

The safest method of handling the territorial dog is to not allow it to be in a patrolling mode uusupervised.[321] One successful treatment for territorially protective dogs is to teach them that visitors are to be looked forward to—that is, through counterconditioning.[321] The owner must be careful not to reinforce the undesired behavior by picking the dog up or "scolding" it with a soft, reassuring voice. The dog can be taught not to be reactive at the doorbell by means of a sit-for-a-reward lesson. The goal is for the dog to learn it will get a command and reward when the doorbell rings if it acts appropriately. The owner should leave a collar and leash on the dog so that the lesson can be reinforced if the doorbell rings unexpectedly. The lesson begins with the dog learning to "sit" on command near the front door. After it does this well, a second family member will ring the bell. Without opening the door, the owner gives the dog a "sit" command and rewards the sit response. The dog is gradually expected to sit quietly for longer periods after the ringing of the bell. Eventually, when the dog will sit quietly at the door after several lessons, the owner opens the door, and a family member walks in to reward the good behavior with a special food treat. When that lesson is perfected, the people who are recruited to ring the bell and give the food treat become gradually less familiar to the dog. The dog's quiet, sitting response should continue. The dog is learning to expect good things from people coming in and gradually comes to look forward to people coming over. A special treat jar can even be located outside the front door, so anyone coming in can reward the good behavior. It is very important during this several-week period of training that no one else rings the bell. It may take a sign outside sending them to another door or a phone call before arrival to alert the owner.

## Aggression When Waking Up

The problem of a sudden, explosive aggression shown by a dog when it is awakened will be discussed in Chapter 9. Because the trigger is predictable, the owner should always call to a sleeping dog, having it come to them, rather than touching the dog. This means the dog should not be allowed to sleep on the bed and must be in an area where small children cannot inadvertently wander over.

## Drug Therapy for Cases of Aggression

The use of psychotherapeutic drugs for dogs showing aggression must be evaluated on a case-by-case basis. Certainly, if the dog has a medical condition, such as hypothyroid aggression, drug treatment is indicated. When generalized anxiety contributes to

the ease of triggering aggression, drug therapy is indicated. There are special considerations that must be made, however. If a fearful dog's aggression is being held in check, removing the fear component may allow the increased expression of aggression. Another consideration is the owner's commitment to make a change. Many owners want a simple answer to a complex problem and would rather give one or two pills a day than have to modify the environment and work on behavior modification. It is safer to make the owner show a several-week commitment to making a difference first and to then add drug therapy to improve results already shown.

It is important to remember there is no drug labeled for use in cases of aggression. This means owners must understand no drug is going to "cure" aggression. Potentially too, any drug can disinhibit a dog's control over aggression, making it even more aggressive. This has been associated with the benzodiazepines[53] and also has been reported with other classes of drugs.[267]

## Antiaggressive Puppy Training

Nonaggressive or antiaggressive puppy training teaches tolerance to a puppy, and it teaches the owner to become a leader rather than a master. The easiest lessons for young puppies are the submissive behaviors of "sit," "down" and "come."[151] Play aggression that is unchanneled or actually encouraged may ultimately result in a dog that is too rough. Biting and protective aggression are problems caused by inappropriate training or lack of training.[92,182] Early interaction is the answer for prevention of aggressive behavior, especially for the assertive, pushy puppy. Lessons can be started with newly weaned puppies, and veterinarians should advise owners to start training as soon as they detect a potential problem.

Puppies should not be allowed to bite an owner's hand.[57,107] Playful interactions among littermates, even as early as 3 to 4 weeks of age, teach how hard to bite to inflict pain.[33,147,151] When owners tolerate play bites because they are "cute," the puppy learns to bite hard, because the behavior is reinforced.[298] A littermate would yelp and stop the play when the bite became painful, but people do not. The puppy uses the situation to learn acceptable behaviors. Because the puppy behavior is a normal one, punishment for biting is inappropriate. Owners need to stop the interaction as soon as mouthing occurs and either ignore the puppy, divert its attention, or leave the area.

A behavior shown by Greyhounds has them nibbling on the owner in an abbreviated bite. The behavior, called "nitting," is probably related to mutual grooming.[169]

The food bowl is another area where early lessons can be very helpful in preventing dominance and protective aggressions.[90,92] Young puppies should readily allow the owner to pick up its food. The puppy should learn to wait before the food bowl is put down—no patience, no food. The bowl will only contain a small amount of food so that the lesson can be repeated often.[147] For the puppy that aggressively guards its food, the owner works through it by placing the empty bowl in place. The owner then literally puts one piece of kibble in the bowl if there is no growling or snapping, then adds another and another. If aggression occurs, the food is not put into the bowl and the owner leaves for a minute or two before trying again. Treats such as rawhides and toys can present similar problems, so teaching the puppy not to growl or bite when a hand gets near the prize is important. It can be learned while the dog is on a leash, with one person having the dog sit while the other picks up the prize and gives it back to the dog if the dog is good. When small children are in the family, the "no bite" lesson is particularly important because children have a habit of trying to take things from dogs. Lessons to teach acceptance should be started even before there is a problem. If the dog is particularly bad about guarding a type of treat or toy, the owner should stop providing that particular item altogether.

Puppies also need to tolerate other lessons that will facilitate handling them as adults. Dorsal recumbency while being held gently by the sternum is one. Others include submission to cleaning of the ear canals, trimming of the toenails, grooming, and wearing a collar and leash. If these actions are not tolerated or result in growling or biting, the owner should continue their actions persistently, until the puppy's behavior is no longer aggressive. The action should then be repeated frequently in subsequent days until aggression is no longer elicited.[62]

Games played with a puppy are extremely important in shaping its future behavior. Only those behaviors acceptable in an adult dog should be considered acceptable in a puppy. The owner must always be able to control access to a toy, so the puppy is never to win a game of tug-of-war. Toys should be given to the puppy at the start of play and physically taken away before the puppy is through playing. Owners should never chase the dog to get a toy—"chase me" should not be allowed to become a game. Instead, the environment should be managed by an enclosure or leash to ensure that the owner controls the situation. Rambunctious play should be with a toy rather than with the owner's arms or legs.[223] If the puppy actively solicits play, the owner can ignore it, walk away, or let the puppy drag a leash attached to a head halter for physical control. Owners should encourage puppies to exercise to relieve excess energy, but not because the puppy solicits it. Obviously there needs to be limits, but puppies need an acceptable outlet for their energy. As an adult, a rambunctious dog may go from a "thinking" mode into an "emotional" mode if play gets out of control. It is important for owners to learn how quickly this happens in their puppy so they can prevent it as the dog gets older.

Encouragement and reward for following the owner should also be practiced to help the puppy see the human as a leader figure.[56,63] Rewards should be given for obeying a specific command, not just for being a cute, fuzzy, carbon-based life form. Rewards can be food tidbits and petting, which may be interpreted as a social grooming of a subordinate by a higher ranking pack member.[56] Although the attention span of puppies is short, they are capable of learning simple lessons in obedience. Learning to sit and lie down on command will reinforce the leadership of the owner. Shaking hands, licking, and rolling over by the dog are submissive behaviors that also reinforce the owner's higher social position.[90] For puppies, food rewards and tactile interactions are usually more significant than praise[200]; however, combinations should be used to teach the puppies that a correct response will be rewarded.

# SOCIAL BEHAVIOR PROBLEMS

Owners generally seek help faster for those behavior problems that are potentially dangerous or cause the most disruption to their daily lives. Aggressive behaviors require attention, but other social behavior problems do, too. In owner surveys, socially disruptive behaviors were common complaints. These included behaviors like begging for food, jumping on furniture, jumping on people, running away, disobeying, and acting unruly. Almost 90% of owners admitted that their dogs needed training.[191] Overall, problems with social behaviors make up about 30% of complaints,[2,30] with aggression being the most common. Of problems in which help was sought from a behaviorist, social disruptions made up less than 5%.[27]

## Problems from Early Experience

Dogs that as adults are to interact with humans need contact with them as puppies. When that contact does not occur or is greatly restricted, undesirable behaviors can result. Learning about people is important for a puppy. In much the same way, it is important for the puppy to be exposed to an enriched, extended environment. Genetic traits also have been shown to affect a dog's relationship to humans regardless of socialization.[211] Although the actual incidence of problem behaviors resulting from genetic traits is not known, the possibility of a genetic influence must be considered when young puppies of good backgrounds continue to show the tendency to avoid people. The outcomes when various elements are present or absent are summarized in Table 4-2.

The most significant of the possible problems is termed *isolation syndrome*. This syndrome consists of deficits in the ability of a dog to form appropriate social relationships with people or occasionally with other dogs.[32,287] Bizarre behaviors and learning deficits also can occur when the dog is placed in an environment for which it had no early preparation.[287] In the most typical cases, a puppy is taken into a very quiet home with one or two adult humans. It grows up there without interaction with other dogs, human guests, or trips to other locations. The problem may then be revealed when the

| | TABLE 4-2 | Impact of various environments on puppies' socialization | | |
|---|---|---|---|

| People | Dogs | Physical environment | Outcome |
|---|---|---|---|
| Present | Present | Enriched | Normal |
| Present | Present | Restricted | Kennelosis |
| Present | Absent | Enriched | Confident in strange situations |
| Present | Absent | Restricted | Socially unresponsive to dogs |
| Absent | Present | Enriched | "Wild" dog |
| Absent | Present | Restricted | Isolation syndrome |
| Absent | Absent | Enriched | Unknown |
| Absent | Absent | Restricted | Hyper behavior; inappropriate approach response; isolation syndrome |

Data from references 32, 140, 197, 287.

humans have a large party or take the dog on a trip. It tries to hide from all the commotion or else it becomes aggressive, especially if approached by a stranger.

Because the isolation syndrome results from how the puppy was raised during a sensitive period, the missed opportunity cannot be corrected. Treatment for this problem really starts with owner awareness of why the dog behaves as it does. Although the dog can learn to accept an occasional new individual with gradual, friendly interactions, it should never be expected to do well with most people, especially in strange locations. Opiates and chlorpromazine have produced short-term improvement but are not helpful for long-term rehabilitation.[120,242] The kindest way to manage a dog with isolation syndrome is to put it in a back room or yard when guests visit in order to minimize social contact.[32]

*Kennelosis* (kennel dog syndrome; kennel-shy) is a behavior problem related to the isolation syndrome. The condition is a developmental response to an environmental deficit.[74] Dogs with kennelosis have had socially reduced input and limited environmental experiences, as tends to occur with kennel-raised dogs. When the dog is taken from its normal home, it shows signs of distress and deficits in trainability.[32,287] The coping response might be irritable aggression, anorexia, housesoiling, or hiding.[32] Some strains of dogs seem to be more sensitive to the development of kennelosis or show a greater variation of responses to a kennel environment, suggesting polygenetic predispositions.[74]

Once identified, this problem is best managed by minimizing the dog's contact with other environments, especially those quite different from its typical one. It is possible to teach the dog to accept a new location, such as a crate, if the lessons are taught slowly and the new locations are associated with only pleasant experiences. Familiar odors, like an old dog blanket or owner-handled towel, can also help the dog feel comfortable. These give familiarity to a new location. Short-term travel away from the home environment may be facilitated with use of a benzodiazepine drug.

The development of the isolation syndrome and kennelosis has been well studied. It seems that the approach and contact responses are the significant events,[120] as there is no difference in response of laboratory-raised versus home-raised dogs to similar environmental deprivation or deficits of physical contact. Some recovery from complete social isolation can occur up to approximately 8 weeks of age, but this capability decreases as the puppy gets older.[54] Early stress, before 5 weeks of age, such as to cold, noise, flashing lights, and other forms of environmental manipulation, speeds up maturation of the brain, as shown on the EEG, and increases problem-solving ability. This early stress also increases the size of the adrenal glands and raises the heart rate.[108] Puppies subjected to early stress are significantly more resistant to later stresses.[104,108] Even interacting with a human a day before being put into a novel environment results in more exploration and less fear.[110] The interplay of genetic type, environmental richness, and specific learning experiences produces wide individual variability in degrees of adjustment.[118]

In the United States, puppies are commonly weaned from the bitch at around 6 weeks of age, occasionally even earlier. No advantage exists in choosing this time for socialization as compared with an older age.[302] Some evidence even points to increased mortality in pet dogs that were weaned early.[302]

When an owner fails to take a leadership role, uses severe or excessive punishment, rationalizes every canine behavior as acceptable, is inconsistent in expectations, or unconsciously rewards undesirable actions, the dog can develop some very unusual behaviors.[13,81] The small dog that is picked up whenever it whimpers learns that whimpering is socially rewarded and soon is carried everywhere. Another dog might lick an owner's legs excessively, but the person accepts the behavior by rationalizing the dog needs the salt from the skin.[59] The most common problems reported by dog trainers are related to owners not knowing how to choose the right dog for their personality, how to socialize or bond with the puppy, or how to train the growing dog, because they lack an understanding of the time, energy, and responsibility needed.[191]

Dogs that were ill as puppies are overrepresented in data on dominance aggression, aggression toward strangers, fear of strangers, fear of children, and separation-related barking.[296] In part this could reflect poor socialization opportunities, but other things may be involved too.

## Separation Anxiety

Why some dogs develop separation anxiety and others do not is unclear. When young puppies are separated from their mother, they use distress vocalizations as a technique to reunite them. Puppies also tend to be quite vocal when first left alone at night in their new human home. If this behavior is not rewarded, the puppy adapts. Some dogs apparently become sensitized to social isolation or never have the early experience of being left alone.[186,301] Dogs that have no obedience training nor daily planned interactions with the owners are much more likely to have separation anxiety.[70] Strays may have had a similar problem before they were abandoned by their previous owner, or perhaps the experience of abandonment predisposes them to forming strong attachments.[332] Other causes have been speculated on as well.[301] There may be an inherited predisposition; a learned component, such as a site-specific factor; an environmental influence, such as a recent move; or a pathologic hyperattachment as a developmental anomaly.

The presenting complaint(s) for a dog with separation anxiety can be quite varied, so the veterinarian must consider several differential diagnoses. Included in the list of major presenting signs are one or more of the following: inappropriate urination, inappropriate defecation, excessive vocalization, destructive chewing, and/or digging. Other signs may occur, including excessive salivation, fearful behavior, trembling, vomiting, diarrhea, excessive licking, self-mutilation, overactive greetings, excessive attention seeking, and aggression at departures.* Because these dogs are close to normal when the owners are home, the behaviors are often described as being done for "spite" or in "anger." [199,332] Some dogs, though, will show the same signs if they are prevented from getting physically close to the owner, even though the owner is home, or if they are left with other people or animals.[146,199,331]

When the owner is home, many of these dogs have a hyperattachment to the owner.[9] They are excessively attentive, following the owner everywhere, being constantly underfoot, leaning on the owner, always wanting to be held, or becoming anorexic if the owner is not physically present.[199] The significant manifestations of separation anxiety usually begin within 5 to 30 minutes after the owner leaves,[100,150,332] although some dogs anticipate the departure and show signs consistent with an increased restlessness or clinginess even before that time. The behavioral expression of separation anxiety may continue all day until the owner returns, or the dog may recover and relax sooner.[332] The dog may even show signs for quite a while, return to normal to eat a previously left treat, and then resume the anxious behavior.[113] The degree of the problem is underappreciated because the owner finds only the end result—a feces-covered or drool-covered dog in a crate or a destroyed object, such as a door frame.

Dogs with separation anxiety are similar in signalment to the general dog population with other behavior problems.[332,333] The presenting problem also can have many differential causes.[146,236] One third are of mixed breeds, and two thirds are males.[9,333] There may be no difference by age,[332] or the dogs may be older than 1.5 years.[9] In geriatric dogs, the incidence of separation anxiety increases to include 29% to 50% of dogs.[146] A significant difference is seen in regard to the source of the pet. Dogs with separation anxiety are three times more likely to have come from an animal shelter than are dogs with other problems (87% versus 26%).[11,146,333] They are also more likely to have been a stray—about 30% of rehomed dogs show separation anxiety.[44] These dogs are more likely to have a noise phobia, show territorial aggression, have fear aggression toward strangers, or have dominance aggression.[16]

When owned dogs develop separation anxiety, there is often a history of a major change in the amount of time the owner and dog are together. Such a change can occur when an owner who had been at home all day takes an outside job. An extended illness or period of unemployment followed by a return to work can be associated with the beginning of this problem, as can a move or other dramatic change in the owner's schedule.[199]

The diagnosis of separation anxiety can be established after careful history-taking, and it will usually include two or more signs (Box 4-4). Some may be very subtle. Laboratory tests, such as a urinalysis and urine culture, may be necessary to rule out medical problems. Video recordings made of the dog after the owner leaves can be particularly useful to determine the true extent of the problem and to help rule out other causes of the same signs. These recordings can also provide strong motivation for owners to work to help the dog.[114] If an owner cannot make a video, they should at least try to get an audiotape. Once separation anxiety is diagnosed, an appropriate therapeutic protocol can be developed for the individual dog.

Therapy requires both an understanding and dedicated owner. Punishment is not appropriate for this or other fearful behavior,[322] although, as patience runs out, the temptation to punish is strong. In all cases, it is necessary to have the dog remain calm. Predeparture anxiety is the first part

---

*References 9, 148, 150, 199, 282, 332.

| BOX 4-4 | Differential diagnoses or behavioral problems confused with or related to separation anxiety |
|---|---|

Aggression (various types)
Attention-seeking behavior
"Boredom"
    Lack of exercise
    Poor environmental stimulation
Destructive behaviors
    Barrier frustration
    Destructive chewing
    Digging
    Raiding garbage pails
Excessive grooming
Excess vocalization
    Barking
    Howling
    Whining
Housesoiling
    Defecation
    Urination
Obsessive compulsive disorder
Psychogenic diarrhea
Psychogenic vomiting
Self-mutilation

Data from references 153, 186, 193.

to deal with if it is part of the problem. The owner will need to identify specific cues that trigger the anxiety. Jingling the car keys, picking up a briefcase, and putting on makeup are some common examples. When specific cues are identified, either they should be eliminated from typical preparture events, or the dog can be desensitized to them. Desensitization occurs by repeatedly doing them at times when the owner is not leaving. The owner can walk around the house jingling the keys. When the morning shower triggers the behavior, the owner can take the shower in the evening instead. Eventually cues will lose significance. The owner also needs to avoid emotional actions or excitement related to departures or homecomings.

In a mild case of separation anxiety, simple techniques can be tried first. If the dog is focused on things with the owner's scent, like shoes, bed, or dirty clothes, leaving the dog with a "security blanket" may be sufficient. After the owner sleeps with the blanket, towel, or other piece of cloth, that scent-rich item is left by the dog's bed or the area where the dog tends to focus its attention. Voices from a radio, television, or owner-recorded audiotape can comfort some animals. The owner can also rotate high-value toys and pick them up when arriving home. These can include food-stuffed hollow rubber items. If the high-value toy is given to the dog about 15 minutes before leaving, the dog has time to get engrossed in the item.[308]

Drug therapy may help mild cases, but it is usually not the magic cure for severe cases.[331] Most antianxiety drugs can be used, but what works for one dog may not work for another. Veterinary-approved forms of clomipramine and fluoxetine are available and have proved helpful, particularly when used with a behavior modification program.* It takes a few weeks for their effects to be helpful, so owners must be cautioned not to expect instant results. Amitriptyline, which is a tricyclic antidepressant like clomipramine, can be the exception, because its anxiolytic properties can almost immediately affect some dogs.[332] This is probably related to its antihistamine properties. The serotonergic component also takes several weeks to have an effect, and it tends not to be as strong as with the other two drugs mentioned. Dog Appeasing Pheromone (DAP) can be another adjunct to therapy to improve the overall success rate.[124,150,184,239] When a DAP diffuser is used with some behavior modification, it can be just as effective as clomipramine with the same behavior modification. About three fourths of the dogs with separation anxiety show either improvement or resolution.[239] Benzodiazepine drugs have some success in dogs and are most useful before the others have had a chance to build up serotonin levels.[184] Benzodiazepines are occasionally associated with a paradoxic reaction.[331] Progestins are another group of drugs that have been used, but long-term therapy is associated with a number of medical problems. The barbiturates and phenothiazines also have been tried. If drug therapy is going to be tried, preliminary blood work is advised to be sure there are no complicating conditions.

Dogs that have come from a shelter into a new home are stressed and may show separation anxiety

---

*References 150, 170, 176, 177, 222, 300, 301.

even if they never did before. These dogs will often improve gradually as they adjust to their new homes. Therapy is appropriate, but it is hard to determine if the improvement is the result of gradual adjustment to the new home or to the therapy the dog has received.

Systematic desensitization is the best way for owners to work with dogs affected with separation anxiety, regardless of whether drug therapy is used as well. Because the retraining time may take a few weeks of concentrated effort, it is ideal if owners can carve out some time to spend addressing this problem. Until that block of time is available, owners will have to look at alternative ways to cope. Confining the dog to a crate or kennel is not a good short-term or long-term solution. These dogs can be so frantic that they destroy the crate or severely injure their mouth or paws trying to get out. Alternatives include having a friend or pet-sitter stay with the dog, taking the dog to work, or boarding the dog.

The techniques of systematic desensitization for separation anxiety are designed to get the dog used to the owner's absence gradually. As was previously mentioned, predeparture cues are dissociated from actual leaving events. Owners will start the desensitization program too.

Step 1: The owner should find an activity that the dog can focus on with great intensity for a prolonged period. Most dogs will pay attention to a food reward. They can easily be distracted by cream cheese, peanut butter, or processed cheese spreads. Because these can be quickly consumed, efforts must be taken to prolong their attraction to the dog. Chew-toys shaped like dumbbells, those with flexible ridges, and those with holes in the center allow foods to be stuffed into or spread on them and then frozen so the dog really has to work to get the rewards. For some dogs, a rawhide chew is appropriate; others may be interested in small pieces of cheese, wieners, or semimoist treats. Unfortunately they tend not to last as long, making it more difficult to do the desensitization program. Initially, these are given to the dog when the owner is present.

Step 2: The owner should designate a "safe spot," such as a throw rug, blanket, or open crate—if the dog has not had a bad experience with one already. If there has been a negative experience, a different crate could be used instead.[330]

Step 3: With the dog resting on the "safe spot" and the owner sitting on a chair next to the dog, the owner gives the dog the "treat," which has a small amount of food on it. The owner does not move while the dog eats the food. Then there is a break. This is repeated several times before moving on to the next step.

Step 4: The owner repeats the sitting next to the dog and giving the dog the "treat." This time as the dog eats the treat, the owner will stand up for a short time and then sit down. This step is repeated several times with the goal that the dog continues to focus only on the "treat" and never gets up to come to the owner.

Step 5: The owner repeats all of Step 4, but this time the owner will stand up, take one step forward, one step back, and sit down. With this and all subsequent steps, the dog should never show anxiety with the owner's movement, and it should not get up to go to the owner. If this happens the owner has not made sufficient repetitions of the preceding step.

Step 6: In this step the owner repeats Step 5 but takes two steps forward and back. This gradual increase in distance from the chair continues until the owner can move around the room without the dog paying attention. In subsequent steps, the owner will exit the room for 1 second and come right back in. This also is repeated with small incremental increases in time spent out of the room without the dog seeking the owner out. The time out of the room is gradually increased, and eventually the owner will exit the home.

In all cases, it is *extremely* important that the person reappear in the room before the dog starts looking for him or her or showing any signs of distress. Teaching the dog to accept the first 30 minutes requires the longest training time, but by the time the dog is comfortable for 90 minutes, it will probably be fine for 3 to 4 hours.[331] Because too rapid an increase in the length of separation can escalate the severity of the problem, it is important for the owners to have patience and work slowly. Departures can then be varied in length to reinforce these early lessons. Owners can be gone for long, then short, then medium lengths of time after the dog is used to longer periods alone. Owners also can leave with and without a briefcase, jingling or not jingling keys, with and without the sound of the car engine (the car can be parked down the block), and dressed in either casual or business attire.

Taking time off from work to retrain a dog with separation anxiety is a luxury many owners cannot afford. The normal departure should not vary from that associated with the separation anxiety while the new program is being learned, so it will be necessary to take the pet to doggy daycare, visit a friend, or find another alternative. Success will depend on the dog learning a new protocol in which separation is not significant.

Other cues can be incorporated into the start of the training sessions to help differentiate them from work-time departures, such as key words and actions like turning on a radio. Owners will need to be very careful to make clear distinctions in their actions to differentiate clearly between the training sessions and the old-fashioned, problem-plagued departures. Only after the dog is well grounded in acceptable departure behavior and can be left alone for several hours should the owner replace the old way with the new.

Most owners are glad they made the effort to try to help their pet, yet only 46% report an overall success rate of 80% to 100%.[333] None of the dogs for whom treatment is started get worse.[333] The overall rate of improvement is 62% to 84%.[301,306] If left untreated, however, 54% get worse or remain unchanged.[301,333] Another 36% of the problem dogs left untreated are described as being 80% to 100% better.[301] The more treatment is needed, the less likely the program is to be followed. Significantly fewer dogs improved or were cured if the owners were given more than five instructions.[306] The owners tended to comply with instructions that took little time, avoided punishment, added a chew toy, and increased exercise.[306] Interestingly, many owners were not willing to uncouple departure cues.[306]

## Attention-Seeking Behaviors

Because of their social nature, dogs seek social interactions. Initially, the whines and distress vocalizations of a distressed puppy call the bitch back. Puppies in new homes may try the same behavior. Older dogs can learn that they will get attention for showing a specific behavior, like making eye contact, nudging, or pawing the person.[50] The most typical behavior used to seek attention from the owner as expressed to a veterinarian is sympathy lameness, even though unruly behaviors, like jumping up in greeting, are much more common. A dog can be a very convincing actor. Other symptoms may vary from vomiting or diarrhea to anorexia or constipation, from asthma-like wheezing to pseudoseizures or realistic paralysis.[139] The reward for showing the behavior is usually an owner's attention, even if it is negative.

Diagnosing an attention-seeking behavior can be difficult. First, obvious medical causes must be ruled out, and the process of elimination will narrow the list of differential diagnoses. Careful history-taking may prompt the owner to recall that the behavior occurs mainly with one person and the dog is being ignored.[50] Owners may admit to giving large amounts of attention to the dogs for the behavior problem.[93] Video recording the dog's behavior in the owner's absence can be revealing. From personal observation, the owner may pick up on the fact that the lame leg is not always the same one, or the dog may forget to limp at times, or the behavior became normal in a unique, attention-distracting situation.

Treatment usually has to take into account the owner's attachment to the dog. First, the owner must be convinced that there really is no medical problem and that the clever little dog is playing a game. The best approach is one of totally ignoring the undesirable behavior and rewarding a desired one, such as a response to a specific command. Punishment can be used to disrupt the problem behavior and speed up the treatment, but most owners do not want to use this technique or cannot do it correctly. Inattention or walking away from the dog when the behavior starts is appropriate. But it is important to build in times where the dog can be rewarded for the proper response to commands and given play sessions with the owner.[50] When this type of program is started, the problem may initially get worse because the dog tries what it knows has worked in the past. Gradually the behavior is extinguished as the new rules are learned.

Punishment, if properly done, can be used for some attention-seeking behaviors. For dogs that jump up in greeting, walking into them as if to push them over can be used if they will not obey a "sit" command. Tightly squeezing a front paw, immediately using a nail trimmer, stepping on toes, or kneeing the dog in the chest have also been suggested,[60,198] but these teach the dog to avoid letting people touch the feet or to jump on the person from the side instead. If the dog is squirted with a spray of water each and every time it jumps up on a person, the behavior will stop, provided the dog finds the squirt to be undesirable. In all cases, however, it is important to have a routine, and positive interaction between the dog and owner as well. Punishment of sympathy lameness, fear, or anorexia is not appropriate.

## Social Problems in Older Dogs

Behavior problems associated with aging are not significantly different from those seen in younger dogs, but there is a shift in incidence.[163] Separation anxiety and associated behaviors are the most common in older dogs.[64,67,163] Major changes in schedules, environment, social interactions, or physical health can be fear inducing or stressful enough to result in problem behaviors, including those of separation anxiety or aggression.[163] Generally, there tends to be a normal decrease in social interactions with age. When problems occur, they are often associated with the introduction of a new puppy or challenges by a younger dog for the higher dominance position.[162,163] As medical problems are also common in geriatric dogs, it is important to rule out sources of pain or decreased sensory perception as causative or complicating factors.

## References

1. AVMA animal welfare forum: Human-canine interactions. J Am Vet Med Assoc 1997; 210(8):1121.
2. AAHA pet owner survey results. Trends Mag 1993; lX(2):3233.
3. Adams GJ, Johnson KG: Guard dogs: Sleep, work and behavioural responses to people and other stimuli. Appl Anim Behav Sci 1995; 46(1-2):103.
4. Agrawal HC, Fox MW, Himwich WA: Neurochemical and behavioral effects of isolation rearing in the dog. Life Sci 1967; 6:71.
5. Allen BD, Cummings JF, DeLahunta A: The effects of prefrontal lobotomy on aggressive behavior in dogs. Cornell Vet 1974; 64:201.
6. Alnot-Perronin M: Inappropriate use of pain as punishment in canine aggression toward household members. In Mills D, Levine E, Landsberg G, et al (eds): Current Issues and Research in Veterinary Behavioral Medicine. West Lafayette, IN: Purdue University Press, 2005, p. 232.
7. Andersson B, Olsson K: Effects of bilateral amygdaloid lesions in nervous dogs. J Small Anim Pract 1965; 6:301.
8. Appleby D, Bradshaw JWS: The relationship between canine aggression and avoidance behaviour and early experience. Proc Third International Cong Vet Behav Med 2001:23.
9. Appleby D, Pluijmakers J: Separation anxiety in dogs: The function of homeostasis in its development and treatment. Vet Clin North Am [Small Anim Pract] 2003; 33(2):321.
10. Aronson LP, Dodds WJ: The effect of hypothyroid function on canine behavior. In Mills D, Levine E, Landsberg G, et al (eds): Current Issues and Research in Veterinary Behavioral Medicine. West Lafayette, IN: Purdue University Press, 2005, p. 131.
11. Association of Pet Behaviour Counsellors: Annual review of cases 2000. http://www.apbc.org.uk/2000/report.htm, 4/9/2001.
12. August JR: Dog and cat bites. J Am Vet Med Assoc 1988; 193(11):1394.
13. Bacon WE, Stanley WC: Effect of deprivation level in puppies on performance maintained by a passive person reinforcer. J Comp Physiol Psychol 1963; 56(4):783.
14. Ballarini G: Animal psychodietetics. J Small Anim Pract 1990; 31:523.
15. Bamberger M, Houpt KA: Trends in canine and feline behavioral diagnoses: 1991-2001. In Mills D, Levine E, Landsberg G, et al (eds): Current Issues and Research in Veterinary Behavioral Medicine. West Lafayette, IN: Purdue University Press, 2005, p. 168.
16. Bamberger M, Houpt KA: Signalment factors, comorbidity, and trends in behavior diagnoses in dogs: 1,644 cases (1991-2001). J Am Vet Med Assoc 2006; 229(10):1591.
17. Barlow TA, Bradshaw JWS, Casey RA: Hypothyroidism and behavioural change in the domestic dog *Canis familiaris*. Proc Third Internatl Cong Vet Behav Med 2001:130.
18. Beach FA: Coital behaviour in dogs. VIII. Social affinity, dominance and sexual preference in the bitch. Behaviour 1970; 36:13.
19. Beach FA, Buehler MG, Dunbar IF: Competitive behavior in male, female, and pseudohermaphroditic female dogs. J Comp Physiol Psychol 1982; 96(6):855.
20. Beaver BG: Puppy socialization and behavioral development. Southwestern Vet 1973; 26(Winter):133.
21. Beaver BV: Mental lapse aggression syndrome. J Am Anim Hosp Assoc 1980; 16(6):937.
22. Beaver BV: The genetics of canine behavior. Vet Med Small Anim Clin 1981; 76(10):1423.
23. Beaver BV: Why dogs chase cars. Vet Med Small Anim Clin 1982; 77(8):1178.

24. Beaver BV: Clinical classification of canine aggression. Appl Anim Ethol 1983; 10(1-2):35.
25. Beaver BV: Feline Behavior: A Guide for Veterinarians. Philadelphia: Saunders, 2002.
26. Beaver BV: Canine aggression. Appl Anim Behav Sci 1993; 37(1):8.
27. Beaver BV: Profiles of dogs presented for aggression. J Am Anim Hosp Assoc 1993; 29:564.
28. Beaver BV: Review of court cases involving canine aggression. Appl Anim Behav Sci 1994; 39:183.
29. Beaver BV: Fear biting in dogs. The Friskies Symposium on Behavior 1994:1.
30. Beaver BV: Owner complaints about canine behavior. J Am Vet Med Assoc 1994; 204(12):1953.
31. Beaver BV: Fear biting in dogs. Vet Int 1994; 4:36.
32. Beaver BV: The Veterinarian's Encyclopedia of Animal Behavior. Ames: Iowa State University Press, 1994.
33. Beaver BV: Behavior development and behavioral disorders. In Hoskins JD (ed): Veterinary Pediatrics: Dogs and Cats from Birth to Six Months of Age, 2nd ed. Philadelphia: Saunders, 1995, p. 23.
34. Beaver BV: Human-canine interactions: A summary of perspectives. J Am Vet Med Assoc 1997; 210(8):1148.
35. Beaver BV: Pit bull bans: In opposition to the Ontario law. Convention Proceedings of the American Veterinary Medical Association 2006.
36. Beaver BV, Baker MD, Gloster RC, et al: A community approach to dog bite prevention. J Am Vet Med Assoc 2001; 218(11):1732.
37. Bekoff M, Hill HL, Mitton JB: Behavioral taxonomy in canids by discriminant function analyses. SCI 1975; 190:1223.
38. Belyaev DK: Destabilizing selection as a factor in domestication. J Heredity 1979; 70:301.
39. Bergamasco L, Osella MC, Capogreco G, et al: Electroencephalographic findings in aggressive dogs. In Landsberg G, Mattiello S, Mills D (eds): Proceedings of the 6th International Veterinary Behaviour Meeting & European College of Veterinary Behavioural Medicine-Companion Animals European Society of Veterinary Clinical Ethology. Brescia, Italy: Fondazione Iniziative Zooprofilattiche e Zootecniche, 2007, p. 127.
40. Bergman L: Ensuring a behaviorally healthy pet-child relationship. Vet Med 2006; 10:670.
41. Berman M, Dunbar I: The social behaviour of free-ranging suburban dogs. Appl Anim Ethol 1983; (100-2):5.
42. Blackshaw JK: Abnormal behaviour in dogs. Aust Vet J 1988; 65(12):393.
43. Blackshaw JK: An overview of types of aggressive behavior in dogs and methods of treatment. Appl Anim Behav Sci 1991; 30:351.
44. Blackwell E, Casey RA, Bradshaw JWS: The prevention of separation-related behaviour problems in dogs re-homed from rescue centres. In Mills D, Levine E, Landsberg G, et al (eds): Current Issues and Research in Veterinary Behavioral Medicine. West Lafayette, IN: Purdue University Press, 2005, p. 236.
45. Bleicher N: Behavior of the bitch during parturition. J Am Vet Med Assoc 1962; 140(10):1076.
46. Borchelt PL: Aggressive behavior of dogs kept as companion animals: Classification and influence of sex, reproductive status and breed. Appl Anim Ethol 1983; 10(1-2):45.
47. Borchelt PL, Lockwood R, Beck AM, et al: Attacks by packs of dogs involving predation on human beings. Pub Health Rept 1983; 98(1):57.
48. Borchelt PL, Voith VL: Aggressive behavior in dogs and cats. Compend Contin Educ Pract Vet 1985; 7(11):949.
49. Borchelt PL, Voith VL: Dominance aggression in dogs. Compend Contin Educ Pract Vet 1986; 8(1):36.
50. Bowen J: Miscellaneous behaviour problems. In Horwitz DF, Mills DS, Heath S (eds): BSAVA Manual of Canine and Feline Behavioural Medicine. Quedgeley, Gloucester, England: British Small Animal Veterinary Association, 2002, p. 119.
51. Bradshaw JWS, Nott HMR: Social and communication behaviour of companion dogs. In Serpell J (ed): The Domestic Dog: Its Evolution, Behaviour and Interactions with People. Cambridge, England: Cambridge University Press, 1995, p. 115.
52. Bronson FH, Desjardins C: Steroid hormones and aggressive behavior in mammals. In Eleftheriou BE, Scott JP (eds): The Physiology of Aggression. New York: Plenum Press, 1971, p. 43.
53. Bruhwyler J, Chleide E: Comparative study of the behavioral, neurophysiological, and motor effects of psychotropic drugs in the dog. Biol Psychiatry 1990; 27:1264.
54. Cairns RE, Werboff J: Behavior development in the dog: An interspecific analysis. SCI 1967; 158(804):1070.
55. Campbell WE: Which dog breeds develop what behavioral problems. Mod Vet Pract 1972; 53:31.
56. Campbell WE: Social attraction: The ultimate tool for canine behavior control. Mod Vet Pract 1973; 54(5):73.
57. Campbell WE: When dog bites hand. Mod Vet Pract 1973; 54(5):78.
58. Campbell WE: The overprotective dog. Mod Vet Pract 1974; 55(9):738.
59. Campbell WE: The Santa syndrome. Mod Vet Pract 1974; 55(12):963.
60. Campbell WE: Correcting obnoxious behavior problems in dogs. Mod Vet Pract 1984; 65(12):933.
61. Campbell WE: Effects of training, feeding regimens, isolation and physical environment on canine behavior. Mod Vet Pract 1986; 67(3):239.
62. Campbell WE: Aggressive puppies. Mod Vet Pract 1987; 68(6):396.
63. Campbell WE: Leadership techniques for clients with dominant/aggressive puppies. Mod Vet Pract 1987; 68(7-8):445.
64. Canine geriatric behavior changes established. Vet Forum June 25, 1998:18.
65. Cases O, Seif I, Gumsby J, et al: Aggressive behavior and altered amounts of brain serotonin and norepinephrine in mice lacking MAOA. SCI 1995; 268:1763.
66. Chapman B, Voith V: Dog owners and their choice of a pet. American Veterinary Society of Animal Behavior meeting, Atlanta, July 20, 1986.
67. Chapman BL, Voith VL: Behavioral problems in old dogs: 26 cases (1984-1987). J Am Vet Med Assoc 1990; 196(6):944.
68. Chen C, Rainnie DG, Greene RW, et al: Abnormal fear response and aggressive behavior in mutant mice deficient for a-calcium-calmodulin kinase II. SCI 1994; 266:291.
69. Chun Y-T, Berkelhamer JE, Herold TE: Dog bites in children less than 4 years old. Pediatrics 1982; 69(1):119.

70. Clark GI, Boyer WN: The effects of dog obedience training and behavioural counseling upon the human-canine relationship. Appl Anim Behav Sci 1993; 37(2):147.

71. Clifford DH, Boatfield MP, Rubright J: Observations on fighting dogs. J Am Vet Med Assoc 1983; 183(6):654.

72. Connolly PB: Reproductive behaviour problems. In Horwitz DF, Mills DS, Heath S (eds): BSAVA Manual of Canine and Feline Behavioural Medicine. Quedgeley, Gloucester, England: British Small Animal Veterinary Association, 2002, p. 128.

73. Coppinger R, Feinstein M: 'Hark! Hark! The dogs do bark..' and bark and bark. Smithsonian 1991; 21(10):119.

74. Coppinger R, Zuccotti J: Kennel enrichment: Exercise and socialization of dogs. J Appl Anim Welfare Sci 1999; 2(4):281.

75. Correia C, Ruiz de la Torre R, Manteca X, et al: Accuracy of dog owners in the description and interpretation of canine body language during aggressive episodes. In Landsberg G, Mattiello S, Mills D (eds): Proceedings of the 6th International Veterinary Behaviour Meeting & European College of Veterinary Behavioural Medicine-Companion Animals European Society of Veterinary Clinical Ethology. Brescia, Italy: Fondazione Iniziative Zooprofilattiche e Zootecniche, 2007, p. 33.

76. Crowell-Davis SL: Identifying and correcting human-directed dominance aggression of dogs. Vet Med 1991; 86(10):990.

77. Crowell-Davis SL, Barry K, Ballam JM, et al: The effect of caloric restriction on the behavior of pen-housed dogs: Transition from unrestricted to restricted diet. Appl Anim Behav Sci 1995; 43(1):27.

78. Crowell-Davis SL, Barry K, Ballam JM, et al: The effect of caloric restriction on the behavior of pen-housed dogs: Transition from restricted to maintenance diets and long-term effects. Appl Anim Behav Sci 1995; 43(1):43.

79. Daniels TJ: The social organization of free-ranging urban dogs. I. Non-estrous social behavior. Appl Anim Ethol 1983; 10(4):341.

80. Daniels TJ, Bekoff M: Spatial and temporal resource use by feral and abandoned dogs. Ethol 1989; 81:300.

81. Dehasse J: The role of the family in behavioural therapy. In Horwitz DF, Mills DS, Heath S (eds): BSAVA Manual of Canine and Feline Behavioural Medicine. Quedgeley, Gloucester, England: British Small Animal Veterinary Association, 2002, p. 30.

82. DeNapoli JS, Dodman NH, Shuster L, et al: Effect of dietary protein content and tryptophan supplementation on dominance aggression, territorial aggression, and hyperactivity in dogs. J Am Vet Med Assoc 2000; 217(4):504.

83. DeNapoli JS, Dodman NH, Shuster L, et al: Correction: Effect of dietary protein content and tryptophan supplementation on dominance aggression, territorial aggression, and hyperactivity in dogs. J Am Vet Med Assoc 2000; 217(7):1012.

84. Dodds WJ: Apply systemic diagnostic plan to assess aggression: Behavior linked to thyroid disease. DVM 1992; 23(5):22.

85. Dodman NH, Donnelly R, Shuster L, et al: Use of fluoxetine to treat dominance aggression in dogs. J Am Vet Med Assoc 1996; 209(9):1585.

86. Dodman NH, Reisner I, Shuster L, et al: The effect of dietary protein content on aggression and hyperactivity in dogs. Appl Anim Behav Sci 1994; 39:185.

87. Dodman NH, Shuster L: Pharmacologic approaches to managing behavior problems in small animals. Vet Med 1994; 89(10):960.

88. Domínguez C, Ibáñez M, Bioñca EY, et al: Distribution of cases in a clinical ethology referral service in Spain. Proceed Third International Cong Vet Behav Med 2001:158.

89. Drobatz KJ, Smith G: Evaluation of risk factors for bite wounds inflicted on caregivers by dogs and cats in a veterinary teaching hospital. J Am Vet Med Assoc 2003; 223(3):312.

90. Dunbar I: Antiaggressive training for puppies. Pullman, WA, seminar, May 15, 1981.

91. Dunbar I: Personal communication, May 15, 1981.

92. Dunbar I: The control of anti-social behavior in dogs. Appl Anim Ethol 1982; 91(1):98.

93. Dunbar IF: The development of social hierarchies in domestic dogs. Appl Anim Ethol 1978; 4(3):290.

94. Edwards RA: Aggression in Golden Retrievers. Vet Rec 1991; 128(17):410.

95. Eichelman Jr BS, Thoa NB: The aggressive monoamines. Biol Psychiatry 1973; 6(2):143.

96. Elliot O, Scott JP: The development of emotional stress reactions to separation, in puppies. J Genet Psychol 1961; 99:3.

97. Fait L, Wilsson E: The effect of maternal deprivation between 6 and 10 weeks of age upon the behaviour of Alsatian puppies. Appl Anim Ethol 1979; 5(3):299.

98. Family life. Gaines Dog Research Progress. Summer 1975:8.

99. Fatjó J, Amat M, Manteca X: Animal behavior case of the month. J Am Vet Med Assoc 2003; 223(5):623.

100. Fatjó J, Amat M, Mariotti V, et al: Aggression in dogs: Analysis of 761 cases. In Mills D, Levine E, Landsberg G, et al (eds): Current Issues and Research in Veterinary Behavioral Medicine. West Lafayette, IN: Purdue University Press, 2005, p. 251.

101. Feddersen-Petersen D: Social behavior of wolves and dogs. Voorjaarsdagern, Amsterdam, Netherlands, April 22, 1994.

102. Flannigan G: Canine sibling rivalry: Characteristics, owner compliance and factors affecting prognosis for treatment outcome. Proc Am Coll Vet Behav Scientific Paper Session, July 2003.

103. Font EL: Spacing and social organization: Urban stray dogs revisited. Appl Anim Behav Sci 1987; 17(3-4):319.

104. Fox MW: Psychosocial and clinical applications of the critical period hypothesis in the dog. J Am Vet Med Assoc 1965; 146(10):1117.

105. Fox MW: Canine Behavior. Springfield, IL: Charles C Thomas, 1965.

106. Fox MW: Dog development rearing and training: Practical applications of research findings. Southwestern Vet 1966; 19:303.

107. Fox MW: Understanding Your Dog. New York: Coward, McCann & Geoghegan Inc, 1972.

108. Fox MW: The Dog: Its Domestication and Behavior. New York: Garland STPM Press, 1978.

109. Fox MW, Beck AM, Blackman E: Behavior and ecology of a small group of urban dogs (Canis familiaris). Appl Anim Ethol 1975; 1(2):119.

110. Fox MW, Spencer JW: Exploratory behavior in the dog: Experimental or age dependent? Dev Psychobiol 1969; 2(2):68.

111. Fox MW, Stelzner D: Approach/withdrawal variables in the development of social behavior in the dog. Anim Behav 1966; 14:362.

112. Fox MW, Stelzner D: The effects of early experience on the development of inter- and intra-species social relationships in the dog. Anim Behav 1967; 15:377.

113. Frank D: Animal behavior case of the month. J Am Vet Med Assoc 2005; 227(6):890.

114. Frank D: Diagnosis of separation anxiety. Am Vet Med Assoc Conv Proc 2006.

115. Frank H, Frank MG: On the effects of domestication on canine social development and behavior. Appl Anim Ethol 1982; 8(6):507.

116. Freedman DG, King JA, Elliot O: Critical period in the social development of dogs. SCI 1961; 133:1016.

117. Freedman DG, King JA, Elliot O: Critical period in the social development of dogs. In Scott JP (ed): Critical Periods. Stroudsburg, PA: Dowden, Hutchinson & Ross, Inc, 1978, p. 180.

118. Fuller JL: Cross-sectional and longitudinal studies of adjustive behavior in dogs. Ann N Y Acad Sci 1953; 56:214.

119. Fuller JL, Clark LD: Effects of rearing with specific stimuli upon postisolation behavior in dogs. J Comp Physiol Psychol 1966; 61(2):258.

120. Fuller JL, Clark LD: Genetic and treatment factors modifying the postisolation syndrome in dogs. J Comp Physiol Psychol 1966; 61(2):251.

121. Fuller JL, Clark LD: Genotype and behavioral vulnerability to isolation in dogs. J Comp Physiol Psychol 1968; 66(1):151.

122. Fuller JL, Fox MW: The behaviour of dogs. In Hafez ESE (ed): The Behaviour of Domestic Animals, 2nd ed. Baltimore: Williams and Wilkins, 1969, p. 438.

123. Gandelman R: Psychobiology of Behavioral Development. New York: Oxford University Press, 1992.

124. Gaultier E, Pageat P: Treatment of separation-related anxiety in dogs with a synthetic dog appeasing pheromone—Preliminary results. Am Vet Soc Anim Behav Annual Symp Anim Behav Res 2002; Meeting Proc:7.

125. Gentry C: When Dogs Run Wild: The Sociology of Feral Dogs and Wildlife. Jefferson, NC: McFarland & Co Inc, 1983.

126. Gilcrist J, Gotsch A, Annest JL, et al: Nonfatal dog bite-related injuries treated in hospital emergency departments—United States, 2001. MMWR Morb Mortal Wkly Rep 2003; 52(26):605.

127. Gittleman JL, Harvey PH: Carnivore home-range size, metabolic needs and ecology. Behav Ecol Sociobiol 1982; 10:57.

128. Guy NC, Luescher UA, Dohoo SE, et al: Canine household aggression? Results of a case-control survey. Am Vet Soc Anim Behav Proc 2000:8.

129. Guy NC Sanchez J, Luescher AU: Using multiple correspondence analysis to define groups of dogs (Canis familiaris) at risk for aggressive behaviour. In Mills D, Levine E, Landsberg G, et al (eds): Current Issues and Research in Veterinary Behavioral Medicine. West Lafayette, IN: Purdue University Press, 2005, p. 8.

130. Hanna TL, Selby LA: Characteristics of the human and pet population in animal-bite incidents recorded at two air force bases. Pub Health Rept 1981; 96:580.

131. Hare B, Brown M, Williamson C, et al: The domestication of social cognition in dogs. SCI 2002; 298(5598):1634.

132. Hart BL: Types of aggressive behavior. Canine Pract 1974; 1(1):6.

133. Hart BL: Aggressive behavior. Canine Pract 1976; 3(1):10.

134. Hart BL: More on aggressive behavior. Canine Pract 1976; 3(2):8.

135. Hart BL: Fighting between dogs in the owner's presence. Canine Pract 1977; 4(3):19.

136. Hart BL: Brain disorders and abnormal behavior. Canine Pract 1977; 4(4):10.

137. Hart BL: Three disturbing behavioral disorders in dogs: Idiopathic viciousness, hyperkinesis, and flank sucking. Canine Pract 1977; 4(6):10.

138. Hart BL: Sibling rivalry. Canine Pract 1979; 6(2):10.

139. Hart BL: Attention-getting behavior. Canine Pract 1979; 6(3):10.

140. Hart BL: Postparturient maternal responses and mother-young interactions. Canine Pract 1980; 7(1):10.

141. Hart BL: Progestin therapy for aggressive behavior in male dogs. J Am Vet Med Assoc 1981; 178(10):1070.

142. Hart BL, Hart LA: Selecting, raising and caring for dogs to avoid problem aggression. J Am Vet Med Assoc 1997; 210(8):1129.

143. Hepper PG: Sibling recognition in the domestic dog. Anim Behav 1986; 34(1):288.

144. Hopkins SG, Schubert TA, Hart BL: Castration of adult male dogs: Effects on roaming, aggression, urine marking, and mounting. J Am Vet Med Assoc 1976; 168(12):1108.

145. Horwitz D: Fights between household dogs. NAVC Clinician's Brief, December 2003:28.

146. Horwitz DF: Diagnosis and treatment of separation related disorders. Friskies PetCare Symposium: Small Animal Behavior Proceedings 1998:1.

147. Horwitz DF: Counseling pet owners on puppy socialization and establishing leadership. Vet Med 1999; 94(2):149.

148. Horwitz DF: Diagnosis and treatment of canine separation anxiety and the use of clomipramine hydrochloride (Clomicalm). J Am Anim Hosp Assoc 2000; 36(2):107.

149. Horwitz DF: Dealing with common behavior problems in senior dogs. Vet Med 2001; 96(11):869.

150. Horwitz DF: Separation-related problems in dogs. In Horwitz DF, Mills DS, Heath S (eds): BSAVA Manual of Canine and Feline Behavioural Medicine. Quedgeley, Gloucester, England: British Small Animal Veterinary Association, 2002, p. 154.

151. Horwitz DF: Puppy training and problem prevention. http://www.avma.org/conv/cv2002/cvnotes/CAn_Ped_PTP_HoD.asp, 7/3/2003.

152. Horwitz DF: Classical counter-conditioning as a treatment modality for dogs (Canis familiaris) showing aggression toward other dogs on walks. In Mills D, Levine E, Landsberg G, et al (eds): Current Issues and Research in Veterinary Behavioral Medicine. West Lafayette, IN: Purdue University Press, 2005, p. 207.

153. Houpt KA: Destructive behavior in dogs. Compend Contin Educ [Small Anim Pract] 1979; 1(3):191.

154. Houpt KA: Disruption of the human-companion animal bond: Aggressive behavior in dogs. In Katcher All, Beck AM (eds): New Perspectives on Our Lives with Companion Animals. Philadelphia: University of Pennsylvania Press, 1983, p. 197.

155. Houpt KA: Companion-animal behavior: A review of dog and cat behavior in the field, the laboratory and the clinic. Cornell Vet 1985; 75:248.

156. Houpt KA: Behavioral genetics of cats and dogs. http://www.avma.org/noah/members/convention/conv01/notes/04010101.asp, 6/11/2001.

157. Houpt KA, Beaver B: Behavioral problems of geriatric dogs and cats. Vet Clin North Am [Small Anim Pract] 1981; 11(4):643.

158. Houpt KA, Zicker S: Dietary effects on canine and feline behavior. Vet Clin North Am [Small Anim Pract] 2003; 33(2):405.

159. Hubrecht RC: Enrichment in puppyhood and its effects on later behavior of dogs. Lab Anim Sci 1995; 45(1):70.

160. Hunthausen W: Assessing the risk of injury of aggressive dogs. Proc AVSAB Annual Paper Presentations 2003:40.

161. Hunthausen WL: Preparation can ease introduction of new baby, pet into household; establishing routine essential. DVM 1990; 21(10):55.

162. Hunthausen WL: Rule out medical etiologies first in geriatric behavior problems. DVM 1991; 22(7):24.

163. Hunthausen WL: Identifying and treating behavior problems in geriatric dogs. Vet Med (Suppl) 1994; 89:688.

164. James WT: Social organization among dogs of different temperaments, terriers and beagles, reared together. J Comp Physiol Psychol 1951; 44:71.

165. James WT: Observations on the behavior of new-born puppies: II. Summary of movements involved in group orientation. J Comp Physiol Psychol 1952; 45:329.

166. Jewell PA: The concept of home range in mammals, Symp Zool Soc, London 1966; 18:85.

167. Joby R: The control of undesirable behaviour in male dogs using megestrol acetate. J Small Anim Pract 1984; 25:567.

168. Jones BA, Beck AM: Unreported dog bites and attitudes towards dogs. In Anderson RK, Hart BL, Hart LA: The Pet Connection: Its influence on Our Health and Quality of Life. Minneapolis: Center to Study Human-Animal Relationships and Environments, 1984.

169. Juarbe-Diaz SV: Personal communication, March 19, 2007.

170. King JN, Overall KL, Appleby D, et al: Results of a follow-up investigation to a clinical trial testing the efficacy of clomipramine in the treatment of separation anxiety in dogs. Appl Anim Behav Sci 2004; 89:233.

171. Kleiman DG, Eisenberg JF: Comparisons of canid and felid social systems from an evolutionary perspective. Anim Behav 1973; 21:637.

172. Knol BW: Behavioural problems in dogs. Problems, diagnoses therapeutic measures and results in 133 patients. Vet Q 1987; 9(3):226.

173. Knol BW: Influence of stress on the motivation for agonistic behaviour in the male dog: Role of the hypothalamus pituitary testis system. Thesis, Rijksuniversiteit te Utrecht Faculteit der Diergeneeskunde, 1989.

174. Kolata RJ, Kraut NH, Johnston DE: Patterns of trauma in urban dogs and cats: A study of 1000 cases. J Am Vet Med Assoc 1974; 164(5):499.

175. Lambert CA: Personal communication, August 23, 2006.

176. Landsberg G, Sherman Simpson B, Neilson J, et al: The effectiveness of fluoxetine chewable tablets in the treatment of canine separation anxiety. ACVB and AVSAB Scientific Paper and Poster Session 2007:25.

177. Landsberg G, Simpson B, Neilson J, et al: The effectiveness of fluoxetine chewable tablets in the treatment of canine separation anxiety. In Landsberg G, Mattiello S, Mills D (eds): Proceedings of the 6th International Veterinary Behaviour Meeting & European College of Veterinary Behavioural Medicine-Companion Animals European Society of Veterinary Clinical Ethology. Brescia, Italy: Fondazione Iniziative Zooprofilattiche e Zootecniche, 2007, p. 68.

178. Landsberg GM: Diagnosing dominance aggression. Can Vet J 1990; 31(1):45-6.

179. Landsberg GM: A veterinarian's guide to the correction of dominance aggression. Can Vet J 1990; 31(2):121.

180. Landsberg GM: The distribution of canine behavior cases at three behavior referral practices. Vet Med 1991; 86(10):1011.

181. Lauer EA, White WC, Lauer BA: Dog bites: A neglected problem in accident prevention. Am J Dis Child 1982; 136:202.

182. Lawson Jr RC: Change of environment causes problems. Mod Vet Pract 1985; 66(12):1011.

183. Lehner PN, McCluggage C, Mitchell DR, et al: Selected parameters of the Fort Collins, Colorado, dog population, 1970-1980. Appl Anim Ethol 1983; 10:19.

184. Lindell EM: Treatment of separation anxiety. Am Vet Med Assoc Conv Proc 2006.

185. Line S, Voith VL: Dominance aggression of dogs towards people: Behavior profile and response to treatment. Appl Anim Behav Sci 1986; 16:77.

186. Lohse CL, Selcer RR, Suter PF: Hepatoencephalopathy associated with situs inversus of abdominal organs and vascular anomalies in a dog. J Am Vet Med Assoc 1976; 168(8):681.

187. Lore RK, Eisenberg FB: Avoidance reactions of domestic dogs to unfamiliar male and female humans in a kennel setting. Appl Anim Behav Sci 1986; 15(3):261.

188. Lynch JJ: Psychophysiology and development of social attachment. J Nerv Ment Dis 1970; 151(4):231.

189. Man blamed for dog aggression. DVM 1980; 11(10):26.

190. Marcella KL: A note on canine aggression towards veterinarians. Appl Anim Ethol 1983; 10(1-2):155.

191. Marcus R, Stone RW: How much does pack disorder affect your clients' pets? Perhaps more than you think. Vet Forum August 1993:38.

192. Marder A, Engel J: Behavior problems after adoption. Am Vet Soc Anim Behav Annual Symp Anim Behav Res 2002; Meeting Proc: 6.

193. Marder AR: Animal behavior problems. American Veterinary Medical Association meeting, Las Vegas, July 24, 1985.

194. Marder AR: Aggression Rx: Make a specific diagnosis and use specific management methods. Pet Vet 1990; 2(3):43.

195. Marder AR: Treatment and management of aggression in shelter animals: Before and after adoption. http://www.avma.org/conv/cv2002/cvnotes/CAn_AnB_TMA_MaA.asp, 7/3/2002.

196. Markway D, Cornick-Seahorn J: Using $\alpha_2$-adrenergic agonists without aggression from the patient. Vet Forum December 2001:26.

197. Markwell PJ, Thorne CJ: Early behavioural development of dogs. J Small Anim Pract 1987; 28(11):984.

198. Mathews S: Paw grasping. Canine Pract 1983; 10(3):13.

199. McCrave EA: Diagnostic criterial of separation anxiety in the dog. Vet Clin North Am [Small Anim Pract] 1991; 21(2):247.

200. McIntire RW, Colley TA: Social reinforcement in the dog. Psychol Rep 1967; 20:843.

201. McKeown D, Luescher A: Canine competitive aggression-A clinical case of "sibling rivalry." Can Vet J 1988; 29(4):395.

202. Mertens PA: Canine aggression. In Horwitz DF, Mills DS, Heath S (eds): BSAVA Manual of Canine and Feline Behavioural Medicine. Quedgeley, Gloucester, England: British Small Animal Veterinary Association, 2002, p. 195.

203. Mertens PA: Aggression between household dogs. Am Vet Med Assoc Conv Proc, 2006.

204. Mertens PA, Lentz S, Fischer A, et al: Serotonin and 5-hydroxyindolacetic acid in cerebrospinal fluid, serum, and plasma in dominant-aggressive dogs and non-aggressive dogs. Am Vet Soc Anim Behav Proc 2000:11.

205. Millot JL, Filiatre JC: The behavioural sequences in the communication system between the child and his pet dog. Appl Anim Behav Sci 1986; 16:383.

206. Moffat K: Hints for handling the aggressive animal in every day appointments. Am Vet Med Assoc Conv Proc, 2006.

207. Morell V: Life at the top: Animals pay the high price of dominance. SCI 1996; 271(5247):292.

208. Moss SP, Wright JC: The effects of dog ownership on judgments of dog-bite likelihood. Amhrozoos 1987; 1(2):95.

209. Mugford RA: Aggressive behaviour in the English Cocker Spaniel. Vet Annual 1984; 24:310.

210. Muller G: Pseudo phobias in dogs. Proc Third International Cong Vet Behav Med 2001:114.

211. Murphee OD: Inheritance of human aversion and inactivity in two strains of the pointer dog. Biol Psychiatry 1973; 7-8:23.

212. Neilson J: Family feuds. Wild West Vet Conf Vet Syllabus 2002:585.

213. Neilson JC: Reconsidering the "dominant" dog. Wild West Vet Conf Vet Syllabus 2002:593.

214. Neilson JC, Eckstein RA, Hart BL: Effects of castration on problem behaviors in male dogs with reference to age and duration of behavior. J Am Vet Med Assoc 1997; 211(2):180.

215. Nelson RW: Diagnosis and treatment of canine hypothyroidism. Vet Quart 1996; 18(51):529.

216. Netto WJ, Planta DJU: Behavioural testing for aggression in the domestic dog. Appl Anim Behav Sci 1997; 52:243.

217. O'Farrell YO, Peachy E: Behavioural effects of ovariohysterectomy on bitches. J Small Anim Pract 1990; 31:595.

218. Overall K: Prevention of aggressive disorders. Canine Pract 1994; 19(1):19.

219. Overall K: Temperament testing and training: Do they prevent behavioral problems? Canine Pract 1994; 19(4):19.

220. Overall K: Teach clients to employ proper techniques to stop fighting dogs, avoid serious injury. DVM 1995; 26(7):15.

221. Overall K: Finding cause difficult in interdog aggression. DVM 1996; 27(3):145.

222. Overall K: Treatment of separation-related anxiety in dogs with clomipramine: Results from a multicenter, blinded, placebo-controlled clinical trial. Am Vet Soc Anim Behav Newsl 1997; 19(2):3.

223. Overall KL: Preventing behavior problems: Early prevention and recognition in puppies and kittens. Purina Specialty Review of Behavioral Problems in Small Animals 1992:18.

224. Overall KL: Canine aggression, part 1. Canine Pract 1993; 18(2):40.

225. Overall KL: Canine aggression. Canine Pract 1993; 18(3):29.

226. Overall KL: Canine aggression. Canine Pract 1993; 18(5):32.

227. Overall KL: Treating canine aggression. Canine Pract 1993; 18(6):24.

228. Overall KL: Early intervention by owner can help prevent inappropriate play aggression. DVM 1995; 26(9):45.

229. Overall KL: Dangerous dogs: Sometimes prognosis is poor. DVM 1996; 27(10):105.

230. Overall KL: Understanding and treating canine dominance aggression: An overview. Vet Med 1999; 94(11):976.

231. Overall KL: Using avoidance and passive behavior modification to treat canine dominance aggression. Vet Med 1999; 94(11):981.

232. Overall KL: Using active behavior modification to treat dominance aggression in dogs. Vet Med 1999; 94(12):1044.

233. Overall KL: Desensitizing dominantly aggressive dogs. Vet Med 1999; 94(12):1045.

234. Overall KL: The role of pharmacotherapy in treating dogs with dominance aggression. Vet Med 1999; 94(12):1049.

235. Overall KL: Biting an owner: Atypical behavior vs. dominance aggression. Vet Med 2001; 96(9):676.

236. Overall KL: Step 3: Dealing with dogs affected by separation anxiety. Vet Forum December 2001:40.

237. Overall KL: Medical differentials with potential behavioral manifestations. Vet Clin North Am [Small Anim Pract] 2003; 33(2):213.

238. Overall KL, Love M: Dog bites to humans—demography, epidemiology, injury, and risk. J Am Vet Med Assoc 2001; 218(12):1923.

239. Pageat P, Gaultier E: Current research in canine and feline pheromones. Vet Clin North Am [Small Anim Pract] 2003; 33(2):187.

240. Pal SK, Ghosh B, Roy S: Agonistic behaviour of free-ranging dogs *(Canis familiaris)* in relation to season, sex and age. Appl Anim Behav Sci 1998; 59(4):331.

241. Pal SK, Ghosh B, Roy S: Dispersal behaviour of free-ranging dogs *(Canis familiaris)* in relation to age, sex, season and dispersal distance. Appl Anim Behav Sci 1998; 61(2):123.

242. Panksepp J, Conner R, Forster PK, et al: Opioid effects on social behavior of kennel dogs. Appl Anim Ethol March 1983; 10:63.

243. Pawlowski AA, Scott JP: Hereditary differences in the development of dominance in litters of puppies. J Comp Physiol Psychol 1956; 49:353.

244. Penny NJ, Reid PJ: Canine aggression toward children: Are simulations valid tools? Proc Third International Cong Vet Behav Med 2001.

245. Peremans K, Audenaert K, Coopman F, et al: Estimates of regional cerebral blood flow and 5-HT2A receptor density in impulsive, aggressive dogs with $^{99m}$Tc-ECED and $^{123}$I-5-I-R91150. Eur J Nucl Med Mol Imaging 2003; 30(11):1538.

246. Perlson J: The Dog: An Historical Psychological and Personality Study. New York: Vantage Press, 1968.

247. Perry G, Seksel K, Beer L: Aggression: An analysis of the frequency of forms seen in an Australian behaviour practice and their interrelationships with other relevant factors. In Mills D, Levine E, Landsberg G, et al (eds): Current Issues and Research in Veterinary Behavioral Medicine. West Lafayette, IN: Purdue University Press, 2005, p. 280.

248. Pinson DM: Myocardial necrosis and sudden death after an episode of aggressive behavior in a dog. J Am Vet Med Assoc 1997; 211(11):1371.

249. Planta DJU: Testing dogs for aggressive biting behaviour: The MAG-test (sociable acceptable behaviour test) as an alternative for the aggression-test. Proc Third International Cong Vet Behav Med 2001:142.

250. Podberscek AL, Serpell JA: The English Cocker Spaniel: Preliminary findings on aggressive behaviour. Appl Anim Behav Sci 1996; 47(1-2):75.

251. Podberscek AL, Serpell JA: Environmental influences on the expression of aggressive behaviour in English Cocker Spaniels. Appl Anim Behav Sci 1997; 52(3-4):215.

252. Polsky R: Can aggression in dogs be elicited through the use of electronic pet containment systems? J Appl Anim Welfare Sci 2000; 3(4):345.

253. Polsky RH: How do you know if a dog's aggressive behavior can be changed? Vet Pract Staff 1993; 5(1):15.

254. Pongrácz P, Miklási Á, Kubinyi E, et al: Social learning in dogs: The effect of a human demonstrator on the performance of dogs in a detour task. Anim Behav 2001; 62(6):1109.

255. Pongrácz P, Miklási Á, Kubinyi E, et al: Interaction between individual experience and social learning in dogs. Anim Behav 2003; 65(3):595.

256. Pongrácz P, Miklósi Á, Timár-Geng K, et al: Verbal attention getting as a key factor in social learning between dog *(Canis familiaris)* and human. J Comp Psychology 2004; 118(4):375.

257. Practitioner's Exchange. J Am Vet Med Assoc 1997; 210(1):21.

258. Prato Previde E, Valsecchi P: Effect of abandonment on attachment behaviour of adult pet dogs. In Landsberg G, Mattiello S, Mills D (eds): Proceedings of the 6th International Veterinary Behaviour Meeting & European College of Veterinary Medicine-Companion Animals European Society of Veterinary Clinical Ethology. Brescia, Italy: Fondazione Iniziative Zooprofilattiche e Zootecniche, 2007, p. 31.

259. Professional Liability Insurance Trust: Dog bite costs for worker's comp. Personal communication, 2002.

260. Redding RW, Walker TL: Electroconvulsive therapy to control aggression in dogs. Mod Vet Pract 1976; 57(8):595.

261. Reinhard DW: Aggressive behavior associated with hypothyroidism. Canine Pract 1978; 5(6):69.

262. Reisner I: Use of lithium for treatment of canine dominance-related aggression: A case study. Appl Anim Behav Sci 1994; 39:190.

263. Reisner IR: Aggression in springer spaniels. American Veterinary Society of Animal Behavior meeting. Boston, August 2, 1992.

264. Reisner IR: Dominance-related aggression in English Springer Spaniels: A review of 53 cases. Appl Anim Behav Sci 1993; 37(1):83.

265. Reisner IR: Management of canine aggression. The Friskies Symposium on Behavior 1994:7.

266. Reisner IR: Canine aggression: Neurobiology, behavior and management. Friskies PetCare Symposium: Small Animal Behav Proc 1998:19.

267. Reisner IR: Differential diagnosis and management of human-directed aggression in dogs. Vet Clin North Am [Small Anim Pract] 2003; 33(2):303.

268. Reisner IR, Erb HN: Canine dominance-related aggression: Influences on course and outcome based on retrospective analysis. American Veterinary Medical Association meeting, Boston, August 2, 1992.

269. Reisner IR, Erb HN, Houpt KA: Risk factors for behavior-related euthanasia among dominant-aggressive dogs: 110 cases (1989-1992). J Am Vet Med Assoc 1994; 205(6):855.

270. Reisner IR, Houpt KA, Shofer FS: National survey of owner-directed aggression in English Springer Spaniels. J Am Vet Med Assoc 2005; 227(10):1594.

271. Reisner IR, Shofer FS, Nance ML: Aggression to children by the family pet: A retrospective study of 103 dogs referred to a university veterinary behavior clinic. ACVB and AVSAB Scientific Paper and Poster Session 2007:37.

272. Restraint of aggressive dogs. Mod Vet Pract 1978; 59(4):311.

273. Roll A, Unshelm J: Aggressive conflicts amongst dogs and factors affecting them. Appl Anim Behav Sci 1997; 52(3-4):229.

274. Rooney NJ, Bradshaw JWS: Social cognition in the domestic dog: Behaviour of spectators towards participants in interspecific games. Anim Behav 2006; 72(2):343.

275. Rooney NJ, Bradshaw JWS, Robinson IH: A comparison of dog-dog and dog-human play behaviour. Appl Anim Behav Sci 2000; 66(3):235.

276. Rooney NJ, Bradshaw JWS, Robinson IH: Do dogs respond to play signals given by humans? Anim Behav 2001; 61(4):715.

277. Ross S, Scott JP, Cherrier M, et al: Effects of restraint and isolation on yelping in puppies. Anim Behav 1960; 8:1.

278. Rubin HD, Beck AM: Ecological behavior of free-ranging urban pet dogs. Appl Anim Ethol 1982; 8(1-2):161.

279. Schalke E, Ott SA, von Gaertner AM, et al: Is there a difference? Comparison of Golden Retrievers and dogs affected by breed specific legislation regarding aggressive behaviour. In Landsberg G, Mattiello S, Mills D (eds): Proceedings of the 6th International Veterinary Behaviour Meeting & European College of Veterinary Behavioural Medicine-Companion Animals European Society of Veterinary Clinical Ethology. Brescia, Italy: Fondazione Iniziative Zooprofilattiche e Zootecniche, 2007, p. 62.

280. Schenkel R: Submission: Its features and functions in the wolf and dog. Am Zool 1967; 7:319.

281. Schoening B: Dangerous dogs in Germany—and how to define "normal aggression." Proc Third International Cong Vet Behav Med 2001:96.

282. Schwartz S: Separation anxiety syndrome in dogs and cats. J Am Vet Med Assoc 2003; 222(11):1526.

283. Scott JP: The effects of selection and domestication upon the behavior of the dog. J Natl Cancer Inst 1954; 15(3):739.

284. Scott JP: Critical periods in behavioral development. SCI 1962; 138(3544):948.

285. Scott JP: The evolution of social behavior in dogs and wolves. Am Zool 1967; 7:373.

286. Scott JP: Critical periods in behavioral development. In Scott JP (ed): Critical Periods. Stroudsburg, PA: Dowden, Hutchinson & Ross Inc, 1978, p. 70.

287. Scott JP: Critical periods for the development of social behavior in dogs. In Scott JP (ed): Critical Periods. Stroudsburg, PA: Dowden, Hutchinson & Ross Inc, 1978, p. 186.

288. Scott JP: The domestic dog: A case of multiple identities. In Roy MA (ed): Species Identity and Attachment: A Phylogenetic Evaluation. New York: Garland STPM Press, 1980.

289. Scott JP, Bronson F, Trattner A: Differential human handling and the development of agonistic behavior in Basenji and Shetland sheep dogs. Dev Psychobiol 1968; 1(2):133.

290. Scott JP, Fuller JL: Genetics and the Social Behavior of the Dog. Chicago: The University of Chicago Press, 1965.

291. Scott JP, Marston M-'V: The development of dominance in litters of puppies. Anat Rec 1948; 101:696.

292. Scott JP, Marston M-'V: Critical periods affecting the development of normal and maladjustive social behavior of puppies. In Scott JP (ed): Critical Periods. Stroudsburg, PA: Dowden, Hutchinson & Ross Inc, 1978, p. 162.

293. Scott JP, McCray C: Allelomimetic behavior in dogs: Negative effects of competition on social facilitation. J Comp Physiol Psychol 1967; 63(2):316.

294. Scott MD, Causey K: Ecology of feral dogs in Alabama. J Wildl Manage 1973; 37(3):253.

295. Seksel K, Coyle W, Chaseling S: Stresses associated with moving house with pets. Proc Third Internatl Cong Vet Behav Med 2001:47.

296. Serpell J, Jagoe JA: Early experience and the development of behaviour. In Serpell J (ed): The Domestic Dog: Its Evolution, Behaviour and Interactions with People. Cambridge, England: Cambridge University Press, 1995, p. 79.

297. Severance III CS: Innovar-Vet prompts unusual behavior. Mod Vet Pract 1976; 57(4):244.

298. Shepherd K: Development of behaviour, social behaviour and communication in dogs. In Horwitz DF, Mills DS, Heath S (eds): BSAVA Manual of Canine and Feline Behavioural Medicine. Quedgeley, Gloucester, England: British Small Animal Veterinary Association, 2002, p. 8.

299. Sherman CK, Reisner IR, Taliuferro LA, et al: Characteristics, treatment, and outcome of 99 cases of aggression between dogs. Appl Anim Behav Sci 1996; 47(1-2):91.

300. Sherman Simpson B, Landsberg G, Reisner I, et al: The effectiveness of fluoxetine chewable tablets with behavior management for the treatment of canine separation anxiety. ACVB and AVSAB Scientific Paper and Poster Session 2007:21.

301. Simpson BS: Canine separation anxiety. Comp Cont Educ 2000; 22(4):328.

302. Slabben JM, Rasa OAE: The effect of early separation from the mother on pups in bonding to humans and pup health. J South Afr Vet Assoc 1993; 64(1):4.

303. Stanford TL: Behavior of dogs entering a veterinary clinic. Appl Anim Ethol 1981; 7(3):271.

304. Stauffer VD: Aggressiveness following sedation. Mod Vet Pract 1977; 58(2):98.

305. Sueda K: Effect of owner compliance on the treatment of dominance-related aggression in dogs. Am Vet Soc Anim Behav Proc 2001:12.

306. Takeuchi Y, Houpt KA, Scarlett JM: Evaluation of treatments for separation anxiety in dogs. J Am Vet Med Assoc 2000; 217(3):342.

307. Taphorn C, Draper DO: Canine dominance aggression towards people. Iowa State Univ Vet 1991; 53(2):89.

308. Taylor A, Luescher UA: Animal behavior case of the month. J Am Vet Med Assoc 1996; 208(7):1026.

309. Thompson PG: The public health impact of dog attacks in a major Australian city. Med J Australia 1997; 167:129.

310. Topál J, Gácsi M, Miklási Á, et al: Attachment to humans: A comparative study on hand-reared wolves and differently socialized dog puppies. Anim Behav 2005; 70(6):1367.

311. Tuinier S, Verhoeven WMA, Van Praag HM: Serotonin and disruptive behavior: A critical evaluation of the clinical data. Hum Psychopharmacol 1996; 11:469.

312. Underman AE: Bite wounds inflicted by dogs and cats. Vet Clin North Am [Small Anim Pract] 1987; 17(1):195.

313. Van der Velden NA, DeWeerdt CJ, Brooymans-Schallenberg JHC, et al: An abnormal behavioural trait in Bernese Mountain Dogs (Berner Sennenhund). Tijdschr Diergeneesk 1976; 101(8):403.

314. Vas J, Topál J, Gácsi M, et al: A friend or an enemy? Dogs' reaction to an unfamiliar person showing behavioural cues of threat and friendliness at different times. Appl Anim Behav Sci 2005; 94:99.

315. Virga V, Houpt KA, Scarlett JM: Efficacy of amitriptyline as a pharmacological adjunct to behavioral modification in the management of aggressive behaviors in dogs. J Am Anim Hosp Assoc 2001; 37(4):325.

316. Vogel Jr HH, Scott JP, Marston M-'V: Social facilitation and allelomimetic behavior in dogs. l. Social facilitation in a non-competitive situation. Behaviour 1950; 2:121.

317. Voith VL: Fear-induced aggressive behavior. Canine Pract 1976; 3(5):14.

318. Voith VL: Aggressive behavior and dominance. Canine Pract 1977; 4(2):8.

319. Voith VL: Behavioural problems. In Chandler EA, Evans JM, Singleton WE, et al (eds): Canine Medicine and Therapeutics. Oxford, England: Blackwell Scientific, 1979, p. 395.

320. Voith VL: Intermale aggression in dogs. Mod Vet Pract 1980; 61(3):256.

321. Voith VL: Diagnosis and treatment of aggressive behavior problems in dogs. Proc Am Anim Hosp Assoc 1980:35.

322. Voith VL: Prognosis of treatment for aggressive behavior of dogs toward children. Mod Vet Pract 1980; 61(11):939.

323. Voith VL: An approach to ameliorating aggressive behavior of dogs toward children. Mod Vet Pract 1981; 62(1):67.

324. Voith VL: Profile of 100 animal behavior cases. Mod Vet Pract 1981; 62(6):483.

325. Voith VL: Diagnosing dominance aggression. Mod Vet Pract 1981; 62(9):717.

326. Voith VL: Treatment of dominance aggression of dogs toward people. Mod Vet Pract 1982; 63(2):149.

327. Voith VL: Procedures for introducing a baby to a dog. Mod Vet Pract 1984; 65(7):539.

328. Voith VL: Behavioral disorders. In Ettinger S (ed): Textbook of Veterinary Internal Medicine. Philadelphia: Saunders, 1989, p. 227.

329. Voith VL: Prevention and control of aggressive canine tendencies. Texas Veterinary Medical Association meeting, San Antonio, TX, February 1, 1992.

330. Voith VL: Use of crates in the treatment of separation anxiety in the dog. http://www.avma.org/conv/cv2002/cvnotes/CAn_AnB_UCT_VoV.asp, 7/3/2002.

331. Voith VL, Borchelt PL: Diagnosis and treatment of dominance aggression in dogs. Vet Clin North Am [Small Anim Pract] 1982; 12(4):655.

332. Voith VL, Borchelt PL: Separation anxiety in dogs. Compend Contin Educ 1985; 7(1):42.

333. Voith VL, Ganster D: Separation anxiety: Review of 42 cases. Appl Anim Behav Sci 1993; 37(1):84.

334. Voith VL, Karner P: Springer rage syndrome. Am Soc Vet Ethol meeting, July 19, 1982.

335. Voith VL, Marder AR: Canine behavioral disorders: Aggressive behavior problems. In Morgan RV (ed): Handbook of Small Animal Practice. New York: Churchill Livingstone, 1988, p. 1039.

336. Vollmer PJ: Conditioned avoidance response to the veterinary clinic in dogs: How it begins/How to prevent it. Vet Med Small Anim Clin 1977; 72(11):1719.

337. Vollmer PJ: Canine Socialization—Part 1. Vet Med Small Anim Clin 1980; 75(2):207.

338. Vollmer PJ: Canine Socialization—Part 2. Vet Med Small Anim Clin 1980; 75(3):411.

339. White MM, Neilson JC, Hart BL: Effects of clomipramine hydrochloride on dominance-related aggression in dogs. J Am Vet Med Assoc 1999; 215(9):1288.

340. Wilsson E: The social interaction between mother and offspring during weaning in German Shepherd dogs: Individual differences between mothers and their effects on offspring. Appl Anim Behav Sci 1984; 13(1-2):101.

341. Witnesses: Dog cared for abandoned baby. http://www.cnn.com/2005/WORLD/africa/05/09/dog.baby.ap/index.html, 5/9/2005.

342. Wolski TR: Preventing canine behavior problems. In Kirk RW (ed): Current Veterinary Therapy VIII: Small Animal Practice. Philadelphia: Saunders, 1983, p. 52.

343. Wright JC: The development of social structure during the primary socialization period in German Shepherds. Dev Psychobiol 1980; 13(1):17.

344. Wright JC: Canine aggression toward people: Bite scenarios and prevention. Vet Clin North Am [Small Anim Pract] 1991; 21(2):299.

345. Wright JC, Nesselrote MS: Classification of behavior problems in dogs: Distributions of age, breed, sex and reproductive status. Appl Anim Behav Sci 1987; 19 (1-2):169.

346. Young MS: Patterns of aggression in dogs. Vet Tech 1989; 10(2):110.

## Additional Readings

Adams GJ, Clark WT: The prevalence of behavioral problems in domestic dogs: A survey of 105 dog owners. Aust Vet Pract 1989; 19(3):135.

Arrowsmith CL, Bernader D, Waran N: Predicting dominance aggression. Is it possible and are there benefits? Am Vet Soc Anim Behav Proc 2001:18.

Althaus T: The development of a harmonic owner-dog relationship. J Small Anim Pract 1987; 28(11):1056.

Bauer EB, Smuts BB: Cooperation and competition during dyadic play in domestic dogs, *Canis familiaris.* Anim Behav 2007; 73(3):489.

Bebak J, Beck AM: The effect of cage size on play and aggression between dogs in purpose-bred Beagles. Lab Anim Sci 1993; 43(5):457.

Bekoff M, Diamond J, Mitton JB: Life history patterns and sociality in canids: Body size, reproduction, and behavior. Oecologia (Berl) 1981; 50:386.

Beata CA: Diagnosis and treatment of aggression in dogs and cats. http://www.ivis.org/advances/Behavior_Houpt/beata/chapter_frm.asp?LA=1, 9/17/2002.

Bleicher N: Physical and behavioral analysis of dog vocalizations. Am J Vet Res 1963; 24(100):415.

Borchelt PL: Separation-elicited behavior problems in dogs. In Katcher AH, Beck AM (eds): New Perspectives on Our Lives with Companion Animals. Philadelphia: University of Pennsylvania Press, 1983, p. 187.

Borchelt PL, Voith VL: Diagnosis and treatment of separation-related behavior problems in dogs. Vet Clin North Am [Small Anim Pract] 1982; 12(4):625.

Campbell WE: Cause of viciousness in dogs. Mod Vet Pract 1974; 55(2):78.

Campbell WE: Why do dogs bite? Mod Vet Pract 1974; 55(2):97.

Campbell WE: Dog-fighting dogs. Mod Vet Pract 1974; 55(10):813.

Campbell WE: Biologic clocks and canine neuroses. Mod Vet Pract 1974; 55(1):889.

Campbell WE: Understanding the shy dog. Mod Vet Pract 1975; 56(4):278.

Campbell WE: Chewing and aggression. Mod Vet Pract 1976; 57(6):474.

Campbell WE: Rote solutions. Mod Vet Pract 1976; 57(9):740.

Campbell WE: A biting case and fence jumping. Mod Vet Pract 1976; 57(10):854.

Campbell WE: Guard dog vs. family dog. Mod Vet Pract 1977; 58(7):626.

Campbell WE: The enigmatic biter. Mod Vet Pract 1985; 66(3):198.

Campbell WE: Preventing isolation-related destructive behavior in puppies. Mod Vet Pract 1987; 68(9-10):519.

Chapman B, Voith VL: Geriatric behavior problems not always related to age. DVM 1987; 18(3):32.

Clifford DH, Green KA, Scott JP: Do's and Don'ts Concerning Vicious Dogs. Chicago: AVMA Professional Liability Insurance Trust, 1993.

Clutton-Brock J, Jewell P: Origin and domestication of the dog. In Evans HE (ed): Miller's Anatomy of the Dog. Philadelphia: Saunders, 1993, p. 2l.

Connolly PB: Reproductive behaviour problems. In Horwitz DF, Mills DS, Heath S (eds): BSAVA Manual of Canine and Feline Behavioural Medicine. Quedgeley, Gloucester, England: British Small Animal Veterinary Association, 2002, p. 128.

Cooper JJ, Ashton C, Bishop S, et al: Clever hounds: Social cognition in the domestic dog *(Canis familiaris).* Appl Anim Behav Sci 2003; 81:229.

Cornwell JM: Dog bite prevention: Responsible pet ownership and animal safety. J Am Vet Med Assoc 1997; 210(8):1147.

Courreau J-F, Langlois B: Genetic parameters and environmental effects which characterize the defence ability of the Belgian shepherd dog. Appl Anim Behav Sci 2005; 91(3-4):233.

Davis KL, Gurski JC, Scott JP: Interaction of separation distress with fear in infant dogs. Dev Psychobiol 1977; 10(3):203.

Dehasse J: Pathological anticipatory defence behavior in dogs. Vet Q 1994; 16(51):515.

Denenberg S, Landsberg GM, Gaultier E: Evaluation of DAP's effect on reduction of anxiety in puppies *(Canis familiaris)* as well as its usefulness in improving learning and socialization. In Mills D, Levine E, Landsberg G, et al (eds): Current Issues and Research in Veterinary Behavioral Medicine. West Lafayette, IN: Purdue University Press, 2005, p. 225.

Denenberg S, Landsberg GM, Horwitz D, et al: A comparison of cases referred to behaviorists in three different countries. In Landsberg G, Mattiello S, Mills D (eds): Proceedings of the 6th International Veterinary Behaviour Meeting & European College of Veterinary Behavioural Medicine-Companion Animals European Society of Veterinary Clinical Ethology. Brescia, Italy: Fondazione Iniziative Zooprofilattiche e Zootecniche, 2007, p. 56.

Dodman NH, Miczek KA, Knowles K, et al: Phenobarbital-responsive episodic dyscontrol (rage) in dogs. J Am Vet Med Assoc 1992; 201(10):1580.

Draper DD: Improper puppy socialization and subsequent behavior. Iowa State Univ Vet 1976; 38(2):44.

Duxbury MM: Animal behavior case of the month. J Am Vet Med Assoc 2006; 229(1):44.

Duxbury MM: Animal behavior case of the month. J Am Vet Med Assoc 2006; 229(6):940.

Fallani G, Previde EP, Valsecchi P: Do disrupted early attachments affect the relationship between guide dogs and blind owners? Appl Anim Behav Sci 2006; 100:241.

Fatjó J, Martin S, Manteca X, et al: Animal behavior case of the month. J Am Vet Med Assoc 1999; 215(9):1254.

Feddersen-Petersen D: Social behavior of wolves and dogs. Vet Q 1994; 16(51):515.

Fox MW: Spontaneous displacement activities, compulsive behavior and abnormal social behaviour in the dog. Vet Rec 1964; 76(31):840.

Fox MW: Domestication and psychosocial development in the dog. Anim Hosp 1967; 3:87.

Fox MW: Comparative significance of agonistic behavior in canids. Am Zool 1970; 10:293.

Fox MW: Normal and abnormal behavioral development of the dog. In Kirk RW: Current Veterinary Therapy IV: Small Animal Practice. Philadelphia: Saunders, 1971, p. 506.

Fox MW: Overview and critique of stages and periods in canine development. Dev Psychobiol 1971; 4(1):37.

Fredericson E: Perceptual homeostasis and distress vocalization in puppies. J Personality 1952; 20:472.

Fuchs T, Gaillard C, Gebhardt-Henrich S, et al: External factors and reproducibility of the behaviour test in German shepherd dogs in Switzerland. Appl Anim Behav Sci 2005; 94:287.

Gaultier E: Separation-related behaviour problems: Diagnostic criteria identification using a cluster analysis. Proc Third Internatl Cong Vet Behav Med 1002:76.

Gaultier E, Bonnafous L, Vienet-Legué E, et al: Using multivariate analyses to emphasize behavioural patterns related or not to DAP treatment in newly adopted puppies. In Landsberg G, Mattiello S, Mills D (eds): Proceedings of the 6th International Veterinary Behaviour Meeting & European College of Veterinary Behavioural Medicine-Companion Animals European Society of Veterinary Clinical Ethology. Brescia, Italy: Fondazione Iniziative Zooprofilattiche e Zootecniche, 2007, p. 187.

Goddard ME, Beilharz RG: Genetics of traits which determine the suitability of dogs as guide-dog, for the blind. Appl Anim Ethol 1983; 9:299.

Goddard ME, Beilharz RG: A factor analysis of fearfulness in potential guide dogs. Appl Anim Behav Sci 1984; 12(3):253.

Goddard ME, Beilharz RG: Individual variation in agonistic behaviour in dogs. Anim Behav 1985; 33(4):1338.

Green JS, Woodruff RA: The use of three breeds of dog to protect rangeland sheep from predators. Appl Anim Ethol 1983; 11:141.

Hart BL: Problems with dogs from the animal shelters: The effects of early experience. Canine Pract 1974; 1(2):6.

Hart BL, Hart LA: Selecting the best companion animal: Breed and gender specific behavioral profiles. In Anderson RK, Hart BL, Hart LA (eds): The Pet Connection: Its Influence on Our Health and Quality of Life. Minneapolis: Center to Study Human-Animal Relationships and Environments, 1984, p. 180.

Haug LI, Beaver BV, Longnecker MT: Comparison of dogs' reactions to four different head collars. Appl Anim Behav Sci 2002; 79:53.

Horwitz DF: Behavior problems in senior dogs. http://www.avma.org/conv/cv2002/cvnotes/CAn_Ger_BPS_HoD.asp.

Hnatkiwsky JS: Tending two bitches injured during dog fighting. Vet Rec 1985; 117(8):190.

Hubrecht RC: A comparison of social and environmental enrichment methods for laboratory housed dogs. Appl Anim Behav Sci 1993; 37(4):345.

Hutson HR, Anglin D, Pineda GV, et al: Law enforcement K-9 dog bites: Injuries, complications, and trends. Ann Emerg Med 1997; 25(5):637.

Igel GJ, Calvin AD: The development of affectional responses in infant dogs. J Comp Physiol Psychol 1960; 53(3):302.

Jack DC: The veterinarian's role in canine aggression. Vet Pract News 2002; 14(5):22.

James WT, Gilbert TF: The effect of social facilitation on food intake of puppies fed separately and together for the first 90 days of life. Br J Anim Behav 1955; 3:131.

Jones-Baade RE: The influence of the owner on the development of aggressive behaviour in dogs. Proc Third Internatl Cong Vet Behav Med 2001:179.

King JD: Selective aggression. Vet Forum January 2002:52.

Lane JR, Bohon LM: Effect of telephone followup on client compliance in the treatment of canine aggression. In Mills D, Levine E, Landsberg G, et al (eds): Current Issues and Research in Veterinary Behavioral Medicine. West Lafayette, IN: Purdue University Press, 2005, p. 192.

Laven-Butler RD: Evaluating the effectiveness of systematic desensitization for the treatment of separation anxiety in the domestic dog. Australasian International Soc Appl Ethol meeting abstracts part 1, June 23, 1996.

Lindell EM: Diagnosis and treatment of destructive behavior in dogs. Vet Clin North Am [Small Anim Pract] 1997; 27(3):533.

Lindell EM: Aggression between dogs: Packing it in when dogs fight. http://www.avma.org/conv/cv2002/cvnotes/CAn_AnB_ABD_LiE.asp, 7/3/2002.

Lindstrom E: Territory inheritance and the evolution of group-living in carnivores. Anim Behav 1986; 34(6):1825.

McKiernan BC, Adams WM, Huse DC: Thoracic bite wounds and associated internal injury in 11 dogs and 1 cat. J Am Vet Med Assoc 1984; 184(8):959.

McMillan FD: Emotional pain management. Vet Med 2002; 97(11):822.

Meierhenry EF, Liu S-K: Atrioventricular bundle degeneration associated with sudden death in the dog. J Am Vet Med Assoc 1978; 172(12):1418.

Messent PR: Early behavioural development of the dog. Brit Vet J 1977; 133:191.

Miklósi, Topál J, Csányi V: Comparative social cognition: What can dogs teach us? Anim Behav 2004; 67(6):995.

Monks of New Skete: The Art of Raising a Puppy. Boston: Little, Brown and Co, 1991.

Moore RA: Educates owners. Mod Vet Pract 1985; 66(12):1010.

Neilson JC: Unruly and annoying behaviors in dogs and cats. http://www.avma.org/conv/cv2002/cvnotes/CAn_AnB_UAB_NeJ.asp, 7/3/2002.

New treatments uncovered for separation anxiety in older dogs. DVM 1996; 27(10):205.

Niebuhr BR, Levinson M, Nobbe DE, et al: Treatment of an incompletely socialized dog. Canine Pract 1977; 4(5):8.

Nobbe DE, Niebuhr BR, Levinson M, et al: Use of time-out as punishment for aggressive behavior. Canine Pract 1978; 5(2):12.

No call for poisons where dogs guard sheep: Anim Welfare Inst Information Rep 1980; 29(3):3.

Notari L, Antoni M, Gallicchio B, et al: Behavioural testing for dog *(Canis familiaris)* behaviour and owners' management I urban contexts: A preliminary study. In Mills D, Levine E, Landsberg G, et al (eds): Current Issues and Research in Veterinary Behavioral Medicine. West Lafayette, IN: Purdue University Press, 2005, p. 181.

O'Farrell V: Behaviour problems in the dog: Aggression towards people. Vet Annual 1990; 30:196.

Oswald M: Report on the potentially dangerous dog program: Multnomah County, Oregon. Anthrozoös 1991; IV(4):247.

Overall K: Anti-depressants can help in treatment of fearful aggression, elimination problem. DVM 1995; 26(1):95.

Overall K: Fearful aggression, anxiety case leads to intensive behavior modification protocol. DVM 1995; 26(5):65.

Overall KL: Diagnosing separation anxiety can be difficult for practicing veterinarians. DVM 1996; 27(4):145.

Overall KL: Anxiety-related disorder very correctable with proper diagnosis, treatment, follow-up. DVM 1996; 27(9):85.

Overall KL: Ten myths in dealing with an aggressive dog; Breeders need education, too. DVM Newsmagazine May 2001:22S.

Overall KL: Evaluation and management of behavioral conditions. http://www.ivis.org/special_books/braund/overall/chapter_frm.asp?LA=1, 9/17/2002.

Pageat P: The feeding behaviour in the dog: Functional relationships with dominance problems. Am Vet Soc Anim Behav Proc 2000:10.

Palestrini C, Michelazzi M, Cannas S, et al: Canine aggression: A survey in Northern Italy. In Mills D, Levine E, Landsberg G, et al (eds): Current Issues and Research in Veterinary Behavioral Medicine. West Lafayette, IN: Purdue University Press, 2005, p. 52.

Palestrini C, Previde EP, Custance DM, et al: Heart rate and behavioural responses of dogs *(Canis familiaris)* in the Ainsworth's Strange Situation Test: A pilot study. Proc Third Internatl Cong Vet Behav Med 2001:89.

Perry G, Seksel K, Beer L, et al: Separation anxiety: A summary of some of the characteristics of 61 cases seen at a Sydney, Australia behaviour practice. In Mills D, Levine E, Landsberg G, et al (eds): Current Issues and Research in Veterinary Behavioral Medicine. West Lafayette, IN: Purdue University Press, 2005, p. 203.

Pettijohn TF, Wong TW, Ebert PD, et al: Alleviations of separation distress in 3 breeds of young dogs. Dev Psychobiol 1977; 10(4):373.

Pfaffenberger CJ, Scott JP: The relationship between delayed socialization and trainability in guide dogs. J Genet Psychol 1959; 95:145.

Pimpolari L, Di Traglia M, Fantini C, et al: Influence of adoption on temperament in shelter dogs. In Landsberg G, Mattiello S, Mills D (eds): Proceedings of the 6th International Veterinary Behaviour Meeting & European College of Veterinary Behavioural Medicine-Companion Animals European Society of Veterinary Clinical Ethology. Brescia, Italy: Fondazione Iniziative Zooprofilattiche e Zootecniche, 2007, p. 45.

Plutchik R: Individual and breed differences in approach and withdrawal in dogs. Behaviour 1971; XL:302.

Polley DD: Shaping puppy personalities. Vet Forum February 1994:22.

Polsky RH: Factors influencing aggressive behavior in dogs. Calif Vet 1983; 37(10):12.

Polsky RH: Problem dogs or problem owners? Vet Pract Staff 1990; 2(5):7.

Polsky RH: Does thyroid dysfunction cause behavioral problems? Canine Pract 1993; 18(4):6.

Polsky RH: Recognizing dominance aggression in dogs. Vet Med 1996; 91(3):196, 200.

Polsky RH: Medical treatment of dominance aggression in dogs. Vet Med 1996; 91(5):416.

Provo Jr JW, Niebuhr BR, Nobbe DE: Aggressive behavior. Canine Pract 1980; 7(3):50.

Reimeis TJ, Lawler DF, Sutaria PM, et al: Effects of age, sex, and body size on serum concentrations of thyroid and adrenocortical hormones in dogs. Am J Vet Res 1990; 51(3):454.

Reisner I: An over view of aggression. In Horwitz DF, Mills DS, Heath S (eds): BSAVA Manual of Canine and Feline Behavioural Medicine. Quedgeley, Gloucester, England: British Small Animal Veterinary Association, 2002, 181.

Rieck D: Dog bite prevention from animal control's perspective. J Am Vet Med Assoc 1997; 210(8):1145.

Riegger MH, Guntzelman J: Prevention and amelioration of stress and consequences of interaction between children and dogs. J Am Vet Med Assoc 1990; 196(11):1781.

Sato A, Uetake K, Tanaka T: Relationship between rearing conditions and factors related to problem behaviours in pet dogs: A questionnaire survey in Japan. Proc Third Internatl Cong Vet Behav Med 2001:151.

Schalke E, Ott SA, von Gaertner AM, et al: Is breed specific legislation justified? Study of the results of the temperament test of Lower Saxony. In Landsberg G, Mattiello S, Mills D (eds): Proceedings of the 6th International Veterinary Behaviour Meeting & European College of Veterinary Behavioural Medicine-Companion Animals European Society of Veterinary Clinical Ethology. Brescia, Italy: Fondazione Iniziative Zooprofilattiche e Zootecniche, 2007, p. 47.

Schoening B, Bradshaw JWS: Applying ethological measures to quantify a dog's temperament: Are ethograms a valid instrument? In Landsberg G, Mattiello S, Mills D (eds): Proceedings of the 6th International Veterinary Behaviour Meeting & European College of Veterinary Behavioural Medicine-Companion Animals European Society of Veterinary Clinical Ethology. Brescia, Italy: Fondazione Iniziative Zooprofilattiche e Zootecniche, 2007, p. 41.

Scott JP: The social behavior of dogs and wolves: An illustration of sociobiological systematics. Ann N Y Acad Sci 1950; 51:1009.

Scott JP, Fuller JL: Research on genetics and social behavior. J Hered 1951; 72(4):191.

Scott JP, Marston M-'V: Social facilitation and allelomimetic behavior in dogs. II. The effects of unfamiliarity. Behaviour 1950; 2:135.

Scott JP, Marston M-'V: Critical periods affecting the development of normal and maladjustive social behavior of puppies. J Genet Psychol 1950; 77:25.

Seibert LM: Animal behavior case of the month. J Am Vet Med Assoc 2004; 224(11):1762.

Shull-Selcer EA, Stagg W: Advances in the understanding and treatment of noise phobias. Vet Clin North Am [Small Anim Pract] 1991; 21(2):353.

Smith MO, Turrel JM, Bailey CS, et al: Neurologic abnormalities as the predominant signs of neoplasia of the nasal cavity in dogs and cats: Seven cases (1973-1986). J Am Vet Med Assoc 1989; 195(2):242.

Tortora DF: Animal behavior therapy: The behavioral diagnosis and treatment of dominance-motivated aggression in canines: Part 1. Canine Pract 1980; 7(6):10.

Tortora DF: Animal behavior therapy: The behavioral diagnosis and treatment of dominance-motivated aggression in canines: Part 2. Canine Pract 1981; 8(1):13.

Tortora DF: Safety training: The elimination of avoidance-motivated aggression in dogs. J Exp Psychol Gen 1983; 112:176.

Tuber DS, Hothersall D, Peters MF: Treatment of fears and phobias in dogs. Vet Clin North Am [Small Anim Pract] 1982; 12(4):607.

Turner T: Tackling temperament in the Rottweiler. Vet Rec 1986; 118(8):198.

Uchida Y, Mizukoshi M, Ogata N: Canine aggression toward the owner in Japan. Proc Third International Cong Vet Behav Med, 2001.

Vanderlip SL, Vanderlip JE, Myles S: A socializing program for laboratory-raised canines. Lab Anim 1985; 14(1):33.

Venderlip SL, Vanderlip JE, Myles S: A socializing program for laboratory-raised canines; Part 2: The puppy socialization schedule. Lab Anim 1985; 14(2):27.

Voith VL: Destructive behavior in the owner's absence. Canine Pract 1975; 2(3):11.

Voith VL: Destructive behavior in the owner's absence. Canine Pract 1975; 2(4):8.

Voith VL: Fear-induced aggressive behavior. Canine Pract 1976; 3(6):14.

Voith VL: Treatment of fear reactions: Canine aggression. Mod Vet Pract 1979; 60(11):903.

Voith VL: Suggestions for introducing a dog to a new baby. Mod Vet Pract 1980; 61(10):866.

Voith VL: Separation anxiety in dogs. Kal Kan Forum 1984; 3(1):4.

Voith VL: Interdog aggression. Appl Anim Behav Sci 1995; 46(1-2):131.

Voith VL, Borchelt PL: The dog that cannot be left alone. Vet Tech 1985; 6(2):95.

Voith VL, Borchelt PL: The fearful dog. Vet Tech 1985; 6(9):435.

Voith VL, Riegger MH, Guntzelman J: Aggression in dogs. J Am Vet Med Assoc 1990; 197(7):807.

Vollmer PJ: Submissive urination. Vet Med Small Anim Clin 1977; 72(9):1435.

Vollmer PJ: Socially influenced aggression: The alpha syndrome. Vet Med Small Anim Clin 1978; 73(2):141.

Vollmer PJ: Avoidance responding in the show dog. Vet Med Small Anim Clin 1978; 73(7):568.

Vollmer PJ: Puppy-rearing—2: Establishing the leader-follower bond. Vet Med Small Anim Clin 1978; 73(8):994.

Vollmer PJ: Puppy-rearing—3: The leader-follower bond, part 2. Vet Med Small Anim Clin 1978; 73(9):1135.

Wells DL, Hepper PG: Prevalence of behaviour problems reported by owners of dogs purchased from an animal rescue shelter. Appl Anim Behav Sci 2000; 69(1):55.

West LW: Behavioral vices in dogs: Proper socialization of puppies. Mod Vet Pract 1985; 66(12):1010.

Young MS: Treatment of fear-induced aggression in dogs. Vet Clin North Am [Small Anim Pract] 1982; 12:645.

# Male Canine Sexual Behavior

Successful reproduction is critical for the survival of any species. In dogs, several aspects of sexual behavior also are important to allow the development of the various breeds. Although certain sexual behaviors are similar for all mammals, each species also has its own uniqueness. Additionally, individual differences can occur, even beginning before birth. To understand the abnormal cases, it is important to understand the normal sexual behavior in dogs.

## SEXUAL MATURATION

In males of most species, there is a surge of testosterone within a few days of birth that is responsible for masculinizing the brain, including those areas responsible for the male behaviors. This is called "the organizational effect of the hormone."[53] Without the testosterone influence at this time, the brain remains feminine regardless of which gonads are present. The exact time of this perinatal testosterone surge in male puppies is not well studied,[38] but it is known that at birth and for the first 20 days of life, testosterone levels in male puppies are approximately 2 mg/ml versus 0.1 mg/ml in the females.[44,48] Thereafter, levels gradually fall and do not rise again until puberty.[38,76] These levels do not explain the sexual differences, so it is assumed that the surge occurs prenatally.[45] Puppies experimentally castrated during the first few days postpartum and then injected with testosterone for 3 months developed almost the same as noncastrated puppies.[6] During the time of injections, these tiny puppies showed a preference for estrous females. This interest continued for at least 20 months. Early castrated puppies show no interest in estrous females unless they receive testosterone injections.

Behaviors such as mounting, pelvic clasps, and thrusts can appear in puppies as young as 3 to 6 weeks.[9,14,28,52] Instead of being sexual, however, these behaviors represent play. As with most adult behaviors that occur in puppies, these behaviors are abbreviated and out of context—a part of juvenile play. If puppies are deprived of opportunities to include these behaviors in play, their adult mating behaviors are adversely affected.[9,39]

Puberty in dogs comes at 6 to 18 months, occurring slightly later in males than in females.[9] In wolves puberty occurs at about 2 years.[27] In studies of Beagles, the first ejaculation occurred around 33 weeks of age.[76] Early ejaculates have large numbers of abnormal spermatozoa, but these numbers soon decrease.[76] All characteristics of the fluid part of the ejaculate are comparable with those of adults by 45 weeks of age.[76] Light deprivation may slow down maturation of the gonads,[55] as might other physical, environmental, and breed factors.[28]

The development of male behaviors at puberty is the expression of sexual dimorphism. As has already been mentioned, neonatal female puppies have low levels of testosterone, so it is not surprising that females occasionally show behaviors that are typically considered masculine. Part of the "female brain" remains in all males as well, so they can show varying amounts of behavior typically associated with females. Essentially all intact males show sexual mounting, thrusting, and raised-leg urination, but 40% of intact females also show mounting and thrusting, and 5% show raised-leg urination.[38,44] Other male traits tend to be dominance over owners, aggression to dogs, territorial defense, destructiveness, playfulness, general activity, and snapping at children.[45,46] It also has been shown that testosterone is necessary to produce interest in the vaginal secretions of estrus.[1] The distinction between maleness and femaleness is blurred, not absolute.[42] Removal of the gonads shifts the dimorphism somewhat toward the opposite sex. Dogs castrated at birth and injected with testosterone as adults will show more masculine behavior than either intact or neutered females but less than dogs castrated after sexual maturity.[8,38] The male sexually dimorphic behaviors in dogs include interest in estrous vaginal secretions, mounting, pelvic thrusting, ejaculation, urine marking, roaming, and intermale aggression.[36,42]

## PREMATING (COURTSHIP) BEHAVIOR

Male dogs are considered to be promiscuous breeders and receptive to an estrous bitch at any time of the year.[9,27] They may, however, occasionally show a preference for certain bitches, and they are more likely to reject individual females that are dominant or females of other breeds if their contact has been limited to one or two breeds.[9,39,77]

Premating (courtship) behavior begins when the male first picks up the scent of an estrous bitch. Apparently the odor can travel great distances, because dogs have been found at the home of an estrous female over 5 miles from the fenced yard where they usually stay. When in contact with estrous females, males display a lot of individual variation in behavior. Some show apparent indifference, and some give varied amounts of attention. Most follow the estrous female closely.[9,26,28,62] Free-ranging dogs tend to show the most elaborate courtship behaviors. A positive correlation has been found between the number of males attempting to mate and the length of time they show interest in the female.[30] In addition, when several males are around a female, they are more aggressive toward each other and tend toward hierarchy formation while she is in heat.[17] When the male and female remain close—a behavior called "running together"[27]—both dogs often show playful interactions including the play bow. He actively noses her ears and shows an increased amount of activity around her.

During the time the male is paying close attention to the female, he continues to be attracted to her reproductive odors (Fig. 5-1). There is a definite preference in male dogs for estrous females and for the urine and vaginal secretions from estrous females, as compared with the eliminative products from anestrous females or males.[7,19,21,30,62] He licks the perivulvar area (Fig. 5-2) and the bitch's urine spots with increased frequency, sampling odors through the vomeronasal organ. Flehmen, difficult to recognize because of the philtrum attaching the lips to the maxilla, may be shown as the dog samples the odors. The male also urine-marks frequently, usually on or near the female's urine spots.[21,56,62] Even then, his attention remains directed toward her.[9,28] One explanation for the male's urinary behaviors at this time is that his urine may help hide the identity or odor trail of the estrous female from other dogs.[22] If no estrous female is available, the male is 4 to 20 times more likely to investigate the face, anogenital area, and ears or body of an anestrous female than a male.[62]

Mounting the estrous bitch occurs directly from the rear 97% of the time by experienced males,

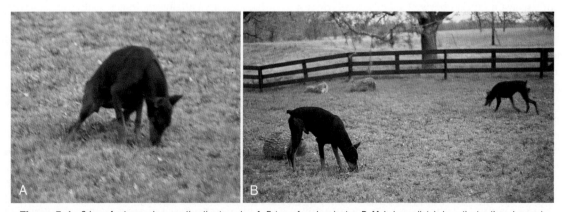

**Figure 5-1.** Odors of estrous urine are attractive to males. **A,** Estrous female urinates. **B,** Male immediately investigates the urine spot.

but the inexperienced ones and those raised in semi-isolation start at the rear only 39% of the time.[3] The rest of the time they start from the side, occasionally from the front, and work their way back.[9] How soon mounting will occur after the male finds the estrous female varies. It can be immediate or some time later based on individual and genetic differences in the style of sexual behavior.[39] The number of mounts made before mating begins can also vary. Only one mount may be made, or, for some dogs, several attempts.[39,57,78] Following a successful mount, the male pulls his forelimbs caudally in a behavior called clasping (Fig. 5-3). This action helps prevent the female from crouching or moving away by minimizing her ability to flex the coxofemoral joints.[9] Some males use an inhibited bite of the skin of the female's neck, the nape bite, as they mount.[28]

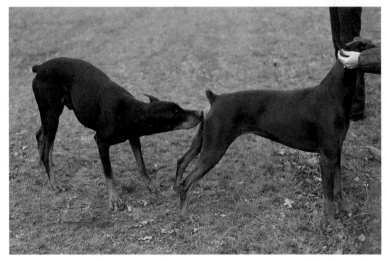

**Figure 5-2.** Male licking the perineum of an estrous female.

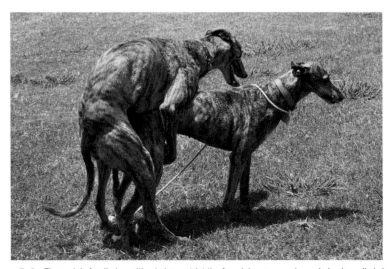

**Figure 5-3.** The male's forelimb position helps restrict the female's movements—a behavior called clasping.

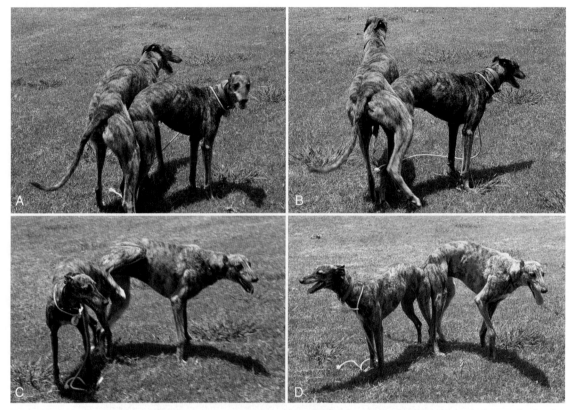

**Figure 5-4. A** to **D,** Once the tie occurs, the male dismounts, swings his leg over the female's back, and stands facing in the opposite direction.

## MATING BEHAVIOR

The mating phase of male reproductive behavior begins once the dog has successfully mounted the estrous female. Pelvic thrusts begin, and the glans penis enters the vulva by trial and error.[9,38,39] Intromission occurs successfully in 50% to 60% of mounts, unless the dog was raised under semi-isolated conditions. In that case, only 24% of mounts are associated with successful intromission.[3] This fact should be considered in cases of unsuccessful reproduction in pets that may have been raised away from other dogs.

Once intromission occurs, the rate of thrusting accelerates until the penis enters the vagina and the bulbus gland becomes fully erect.[9,28] At the same time, the constrictor vestibuli muscles of the female contract caudal to the bulbus glandis, and the two dogs are physically joined together in the unique canine event, the "copulatory tie" or "lock."[5,56,78] Only one of 15 males successfully achieves a tie during the first year of life, even after as many as 39 mounts.[30] After an intense 15 to 30 seconds of pelvic thrusts, the dog stops thrusting, and ejaculation begins.[78] The intense ejaculatory reaction stimulates the male component of the tie, and serum testosterone levels increase.[34] Stepping movements by the rear limbs occur and can be quite high during the 15 to 30 seconds of ejaculation.[39]

Within a minute or so after the pelvic thrusts stop, while the tie is maintained, the male dog will dismount to one side, swing a rear limb over the back of the female, and stand facing in the opposite direction from the female (Fig. 5-4). This action puts a twist in the penis, and the erection is maintained longer because of venous constriction.[9,31] The tie will last 10 to 30 minutes or more, during which time both dogs are relatively unresponsive to external activities and usually stand quietly.[9,26,28,39,57] Occasionally, a male dog may demonstrate a phantom tie, during which time the dogs stand motionless in a posture typical of a normal tie.[5]

Ejaculation occurs throughout most of the time the tie is maintained. The sperm-rich portion of ejaculate is usually produced during the first 2 minutes.[9,12] The first of three semen fractions in an ejaculate is a clear fluid. The sperm-rich second fraction usually comes during the 50- to 80-second point. The cloudy, white, third fraction comes during the remainder of the tie.[12]

Success at mating by any individual male depends on many factors, including the number of other males interested in the same female. In fact, a significant negative correlation exists between the number of males interested in a female and the copulatory success rate.[30] When one or two males are interested in a female, copulation occurs 75% to 80% of the time within 30 minutes. When three or more are interested, copulation occurs only 5% of the time, and 150 minutes may pass before it occurs.[30] Rejection rates of males by estrous females vary from 25% to 80%.[30] This rejection can be expressed in many ways, including aggression directed toward an approaching male or the female physically leaving an area.[30] When two equally dominant males try to mate, both fail.[30] Familiarity between the male and the estrous female is also important in mating success.[17]

## POSTMATING BEHAVIOR

Little physically based behavior occurs immediately after mating. As the venous blood drains from the bulbus glandis, that vascular structure eventually decreases in size until the two dogs are able to slip apart. The male usually licks his penis and prepuce briefly after separating.[9,28] Wild male canids may remain with a female through several copulations, perhaps the entire estrous period,[26] but human management of dog mating means dogs will show much more variation.

The refractory period is part of the postmating behavior. During this time, the male is not interested in estrous females. How long this disinterest lasts is highly variable and may have both a relatively

constant physiologic component and a psychologic one.[38] Psychologic factors include how often the male mated in the recent past and whether the estrous female is the same one just mated or represents a novel stimulus. At least over a short period, adult male dogs are usually capable of mating up to five times in 1 day.[9,38,52,73] If ejaculation occurs more than once or twice a day, however, the sperm count is cut in half by the fourth ejaculation despite libido remaining high.[12] Sperm output is also decreased if ejaculation occurs more than once every other day.[12]

## PARENTAL BEHAVIOR

Parental behavior in male domestic dogs is highly variable. Wild canids often remain close to the female and her young. They may even stand guard during times the mother leaves the immediate area.[66] The most common forms of infant care by wild canid males include grooming, playing, bringing escapees back, and resting with the young.[63] The male may also regurgitate food for the puppies.[66] Sometimes male domesticated dogs will show these behaviors, too. More commonly, however, the male dog is indifferent to the female and her young. Occasionally males will actually attack, and possibly kill, the puppies.[26]

## NEURAL AND HORMONAL REGULATION

Male behaviors are regulated by both neural and hormonal factors in the adult dog, with the former somewhat dependent on the latter. After masculinization of the brain from the perinatal testosterone surge, the full repertoire of mating behavior does not appear until puberty when testosterone is again present.

### Neurologic and Neuromuscular Regulation

Much information about the neurologic regulation of mating behavior has been learned from the cat, so the relevant canine behavior is often presumed rather than studied. The reader is referred to other references for this information.[11] In neurologic studies of canine copulatory behavior, researchers have found that lesions of the medial preoptic-anterior hypothalamus reduce mounting by juvenile male dogs and abolish copulatory behavior in adults.[37,49] Some of the more specific behaviors have other controls. For example, evidence suggests that the intense ejaculatory reaction and the copulatory tie are completely mediated at the spinal level.[32,36,38] Rhythmic contractions of the bulbocavernosus muscle help pump blood from the proximal corpus spongiosum distally, thus facilitating rapid engorgement of the bulbus glandis in the tie.[35] At the same time, the ischiourethral muscles contract tonically to facilitate erection by occluding venous return.[35] Both engorgement of the bulb and the copulatory tie are prevented if the ischiourethral muscle is severed or nerve function disrupted.[35]

Ejaculation appears to be inhibited by supraspinal structures and facilitated by neural disinhibition rather than neural excitation during sexual arousal.[32] Tactile stimulation of the body of the penis just proximal to the glans triggers ejaculation. Yet, without sexual excitement from the presence of an estrous bitch to suppress the normal tonic inhibition from the brain, ejaculation by tactile stimulation is difficult.[32,38] The postmating refractory period also has a neurologic component. It is at least partially associated with the refractoriness of spinal elements.[32] Overall, dogs are apparently more heavily dependent on cortical contributions to coital behavior than are rodents and other animals that have been studied more extensively.[4]

## Hormonal Regulation and Effects of Castration

The influence of hormones on adult male behaviors has been studied primarily after castration or after the use of exogenous progestins. In pet dogs, though, castration is still not common; only an estimated 12% are neutered.[67,79] Retention of a behavior after castration, and even after an adrenalectomy, is not caused by residual androgen, because testosterone is eliminated from the systemic circulation within 6 to 24 hours.[36,40,42,50,78] Castration results in a rapid decline in mounting behavior in one third of the dogs, a gradual decline in another one third, and no change in the behavior of the rest.[50]

Both experienced and inexperienced dogs may continue to mate for at least 8 months, and some even 2.5 years, after castration.[33,45,77] Although it takes longer for mounting to occur postcastration, it does not necessarily take longer for pelvic thrusts and other parts of the mating sequence.[33] Mating frequency drops to approximately half of precastration levels within 3 weeks.[36] Even if mounting occurs at precastration levels, the dog tends to become less successful with intromission, and experienced males take longer to mount.[33,36] Approximately 90% of dogs retain their ability to ejaculate 13 weeks postcastration.[36] Eighty percent will occasionally show the copulatory pattern at 15 weeks after surgery, and 60% show it 1 year later.[45]

Castration also affects other male sexually dimorphic behaviors in adult dogs. It is most effective in decreasing roaming behavior, which rapidly declines in 44% of dogs and gradually declines in another 50%.[40,42,50] Urine marking rapidly declines in 30% of dogs and gradually declines in 20% more.[40,50] Intermale aggression is also affected by castration in almost 63% of dogs; 38% show a rapid reduction in the behavior and 25% a more gradual decline.[40,50]

Progestins appear to cause reductions in the same behaviors, working at the level of the hypophyseal, hypothalamus, and peripheral target organs.[29] Little to no change occurs after castration in behaviors that are not sexually dimorphic, as would be expected for behaviors expressed equally by males and females.[42] Although aggression may be more common in males, it is possible that its onset is a function of male maturation and not of testosterone.[78]

Prepubertal castration continues to receive a lot of attention. Relative to the use of castration for existing behavior problems, it should be expected that the surgery would be most likely to affect male sexually dimorphic behaviors. As was previously noted, this is true—statistically significant improvement occurs in urine marking in the house, roaming, mounting, aggression toward family members, aggression toward other dogs in the household and to unfamiliar dogs, and aggression toward humans entering its territory.[47] The first three on the list are reduced by at least

**TABLE 5-1**  Comparison of behavior problems in male dogs neutered at 8 to 10 weeks versus 6 months or later

| | Aggression | | Overweight | | Intelligence (owner-defined) | | Medical problems | | Undesirable sexual behavior | |
|---|---|---|---|---|---|---|---|---|---|---|
| | % | CV | % | CV | % | CV | % | CV | % | CV |
| Male dogs neutered at 8+ weeks | 18 | — | 8 | — | 100 | — | 25 | — | 16 | — |
| Male dogs neutered at 6+ months | 54 | 3× | 21 | 2.6× | 64 | 0.6× | 50 | 2× | 78 | 4.9× |

Data from references 61, 74.
*%,* Likelihood of problem occurring; *CV,* comparative value of likelihood between age groups.

50% in 66% of the cases, and by 90% in 35% of cases.[47] Only 30% of the dogs showing some form of aggression had at least a 50% improvement,[47] as should be expected when all types of aggression are included, not just those associated with testosterone. Compared with puppies castrated at 6 months of age or later, those castrated at 8 weeks were much less likely to urinate when excited, be overly aggressive, achieve intromission, develop a copulatory tie, or have medical problems.[20,61,74] Male puppies castrated at 7 to 10 weeks are at least three times less likely to show behavior problems than dogs castrated at 6 months or later (Table 5-1). Some types of problems are more likely, such as psychogenic alopecia or noise phobias,[72] but other environmental factors may be involved instead. In addition, they are not predisposed to excessive weight gain,[15,61,70,71] although the relationship between weight gain and castration is still somewhat unclear.* The frequency and tendency to mount females is no different than seen in adult castrates.[45,60] If castration occurs between 7 weeks and 7 months, physeal closure is slowed, and the long-bone length becomes greater than in intact male dog controls.[70,71] The puppy castrates retain an infantile penis, prepuce, and os penis.[70,71]

Circulating testosterone levels are not hierarchy dependent in dogs.[58] This means that as a dog becomes more dominant within a group, his testosterone levels do not rise accordingly. What remains unclear, however, is if a dog's testosterone level affects his social status.[58]

Discussions have gone both ways as to whether early castration of a puppy helps or hurts its ability to perform various tasks later in life. Ongoing studies at Guide Dogs for the Blind have helped clarify this subject. In a study of 6396 dogs, of which 52.2% were male, the successful training and placing of guide dogs was 1.3 times better for those castrated at less than 6 months.[64,65]

## MALE SEXUAL BEHAVIOR PROBLEMS

Reluctance to mate is one of several problem behaviors for which owners of male dogs seek veterinary help. Dogs may refuse to show interest in an estrous bitch for many reasons. Improper socialization of the dog as a puppy by virtue of minimal to no contact with other dogs can result in a dog that does not recognize other dogs.[9,38] Poorly socialized dogs tend to play excessively and are very disoriented if they do mount a receptive female.[38] Inexperienced males often have difficulty around inexperienced or active females, and they may give up before achieving successful copulation.[9,78] A very submissive male is at a psychologic disadvantage with a very dominant or aggressive female. Conversely, the mere presence of a very dominant male may cause a submissive bitch to roll over or crouch down. Extreme variances in size may physically prevent successful coitus, such as if a Chihuahua and Great Dane attempt mating. Physical

*References 13, 15, 61, 70, 71, 74.

abnormalities of the reproductive tract can also make mating impossible or painful.[9]

Stress is minimized for male dogs when a specific breeding area is used consistently. It may also be helpful to restrain the female, so that she cannot leave or show aggression toward the male.

## Inappropriate Mounting

Dogs commonly mount dogs, other animals, objects, or people in a way that is considered unacceptable to the owner. For young, pubertal male dogs, excessive mounting is normal, as it is for pubertal males of many species.[9] One study found that 12.2% of all dogs show mounting behaviors. Of those, 73.3% were males, of which 56.1% were already castrated.[52] In older males that are physically confined, the mounting of inappropriate partners may be set off by the odors of estrus. Because the dog is unable to seek out the female in heat, it redirects the sexual behavior prompted by the estrous odors toward another target.

Another explanation of inappropriate mounting behavior is offered by the theory of dammed-up energy, which suggests that a normal behavior that is the least used will become the one that is the most easily triggered.[9] For the intact male dog that does not have an occasional opportunity to mate, sexual behaviors become the most easily expressed, even though the time, location, stimulus, or target are inappropriate. Inappropriate mounting is also simply an expression of the surplus energy that any energetic dog has, just as would be barking, pacing, or chewing.[10] It can also reflect a dominant social behavior or play.

True homosexual behavior is very rare in normal dogs.[2,9] Males mounting other males are more likely to be expressing play, investigation, curiosity, or grooming.[2] A male might direct mating behavior toward another male in the abnormal situations of (1) an extremely strong stimulus; (2) the complete, longstanding absence of a female; or (3) the feminization of another dog as a result of testicular tumors or external administration of drugs.[2] Males carrying the scent of an estrous female might also trigger mounting behavior by other males.[9] Male-male mounting occurs commonly as a dominant social behavior. Owners may mistake the mounting

for a sexual behavior because they fail to evaluate the context in which the behavior occurs[9] or the exact postures shown.

Though seldom recognized, rape by experienced, dominant, and physically powerful males can occur, and the victim is usually an inexperienced female.[30] In this case, the male will be persistent even if attacked and even if the female shows a submissive posture.[30]

Sometimes a dog shows sexual interest only in his dam, even if she has been neutered.[23,24] This condition has been described as resembling the Oedipus complex in humans.[23,24] It can occur if the two dogs have been separated for some time or if the male has become dominant in their social relations.

Mounting of individuals of other species occurs, too (Fig. 5-5).[24] This behavior is usually a result of poor socialization of the puppy toward its own species,[24] or it can be shown by a male dog approaching puberty. It is frequently preceded by play-like courtship behaviors.[14] Any species can serve as a potential target, including pigs,[69] cats, and people. Of behavior cases where mounting was complained of as a problem, slightly over half involved dogs mounting people,[51] and the target is usually a leg or foot.

A number of treatments have been tried for inappropriate mounting behavior, but results are inconsistent.[39] Punishment for a behavior considered

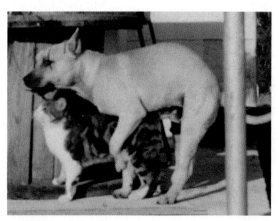

**Figure 5-5.** A 5-month-old male puppy directs mounting behavior and erection toward a cat.

normal by the dog usually does not work. Castration does not always eliminate mounting, as was already mentioned, but it is a logical first step. Progestin therapy can help in some cases, even when castration did not control the problem, but long-term use of these drugs is not desirable. Many dogs that mount individuals of other species can be prevented from doing so by decreasing the excitement that tends to trigger the behavior, such as excessive petting or physical interaction with the dog.[14] Moving away from the dog so that it slides off may stop the problem. For the persistent individual, extra exercise gets rid of extra energy and tends to reduce the frequency of the mounting behavior. Another technique that can be tried is to ask for a conflicting behavior like "sit" or "down." The inappropriate behavior can no longer be performed when the dog obeys the command, and the owner can reward the acceptable behavior.

## Masturbation

Masturbation is closely associated with unacceptable mounting behavior and may occur in similar situations. The behavior usually includes mounting and pelvic thrusts with stimulation of the prepuce and penis on an object. Full erection and expulsion of prostatic fluid may also occur.[9] Mounting can be directed toward individuals or inanimate objects, such as a wadded-up throw rug or a fuzzy slipper (Fig. 5-6).[9] Masturbation is more likely to occur in excitable or active intact males that are isolated

from their own species.[25] Like inappropriate mounting, then, masturbation could be explained by the theory of dammed-up energy. Also, masturbation may be more likely to occur if the dog is sensitized by estrous odors from a nearby bitch, or it can be self induced with genital grooming.[25,68] The typical case history for a masturbating dog reveals a dog that becomes overly excited in the presence of visitors and, after the initial excitement, attempts to mount the owner's leg or a nearby object such as a throw rug.

Controlling masturbation can be difficult and may require several approaches. This behavior may have anxiety reduction as its own internal reward, so punishment is neither appropriate nor likely to be successful. Castration helps in some cases, but not all. Progestins help a few more of the affected dogs but are not a long-term solution. Discarding the inanimate object that is mounted may be possible, although some dogs simply find another target. Lots of regular exercise minimizes energy reserves for inappropriate behaviors, as will a diet of 18% to 22% protein instead of one with a higher protein level. If specific events are likely to trigger the behavior, it may be possible to use heavy exercise immediately before the triggering event or to isolate the dog away from the triggering event by confining it to a crate, another room, or a fenced yard. Diversion and giving a command for a conflicting behavior are other techniques that can be tried.

## Penile Problems

Occasionally a dog will protrude the penis, have an erection, but be unable to retract the penis back into the prepuce. This occurs most frequently in Maltese.[53] At the other end of the spectrum is the dog that cannot protrude the penis from the prepuce. The resulting pain during an erection can result in aggression.[53] A quiet environment and penile lubrication may help the penis retract into the prepuce, but in both cases, surgery is often necessary to enlarge the preputial orifice.

## Crotch Sniffing

Male dogs from most large breeds tend to push their noses into the perineal area of women upon first meeting them. Although it is quite objectionable

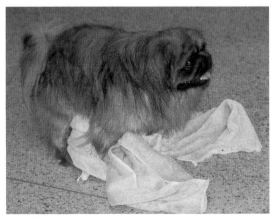

**Figure 5-6.** A Pekingese masturbating on a wadded-up towel.

to humans, the behavior is based on normal dog behavior. Normal greeting behaviors between dogs include anogenital and inguinal investigative behaviors, because these are areas of concentrated scents. The odors of vaginal discharge would make a woman's underwear of interest to olfactory-oriented dogs. Crotch-sniffing behavior is difficult to stop, so prevention is most appropriate. Restraint until the dog is used to the visitor minimizes the expression of this behavior. Currently no published studies exist on the effectiveness of castration in eliminating this behavior.

## Deficient Male Behavior

There are times when a dog may show no interest in breeding. Although the usual cause is that the female is not in estrus, other things can present the same way. Fear of the environment or of a high-ranking female, the lack of experience, the lack of play mounting as a puppy, or poor communication skills are other reasons.[53] A shy but experienced bitch and familiarization with the surroundings can help in these cases.

## Cryptorchidism

The retention of one or both testicles within the body cavity occurs occasionally in dogs. No studies have been published on behavioral implications of this condition in dogs, but it is likely that such implications are similar to those known in other species. In horses, for example, the higher temperature of the internal testicles results in increased production of testosterone at the expense of sperm maturation. A corresponding increased intensity of male sexual behaviors, activity levels, and aggressiveness is associated with this higher level of testosterone.[16]

## Drugs' Effect on Male Sexual Behavior Problems

A number of drugs are known to have a negative effect on male reproduction.[18] Although the list in Table 5-2 is probably not complete, it should serve to point out that the possibility of this side effect should be considered when prescribing drug therapy for a dog standing at stud.

Progestins have been used for several years to treat excessive male sexual behavior.[75] The current

| TABLE 5-2 | A partial list of drugs that negatively affect male behaviors |
|---|---|
| **Drug** | **Effect** |
| Amphotericin B | Inhibits spermatogenesis |
| Anabolic steroids | Metabolize to testosterone; therefore, castrates may act intact |
| Antineoplastics | Results in aplasia of germinal epithelium |
| Ketoconazole | Lowers serum testosterone |
| Nitrofurans | Inhibits spermatogenesis |
| Progestins | Lowers serum testosterone |
| Vasopressors | Results in testicular ischemia |

concern about the long-term use of progestins is in regard to their many side effects. Thus, these drugs are best used for short-term intervention to break a pattern or until environmental changes also can be accomplished. Progestins suppress male sexually dimorphic behaviors that would be affected by castration.[41,43,54,59] Sometimes they also can result in changes after castration.[78] The antianxiety calming effect of progestins can be particularly helpful if the male sexual behavior is stress induced.[41] When progestins are used to reduce mounting, roaming, or urine marking in the house, 72% to 74% of dogs improve after the onset of treatment.[54] After 3 months of progestin treatment, the success rate is approximately 50% for reducing mounting and roaming and 33% for reducing urine marking.[54]

## References

1. Anisko JJ: Hormonal substrate of estrous odor preference in Beagles. Physiol Behav 1977; 18(1):13.
2. Barton A: Sexual inversion and homosexuality in dogs and cats. Vet Med 1959; 54:155.
3. Beach FA: Coital behavior in dogs. III. Effects of early isolation on mating in males. Behavior 1968; 30(2):218.
4. Beach FA: Locks and beagles. Am Psychol 1969; 24(11):971.
5. Beach FA: Coital behavior in dogs. IX. Sequelae to "coitus interruptus" in males and females. Physiol Behav 1970; 5(3):263.
6. Beach FA, Buehler MG, Dunbar IF: Development of attraction to estrous females in male dogs. Physiol Behav 1983; 31(3):293.
7. Beach FA, Gilmore RW: Response of male dogs to urine from females in heat. J Mammal 1949; 30:391.

8. Beach FA, Kuehn RE, Sprague RH, et al: Coital behavior in dogs. XI. Effects of androgenic stimulation during development on masculine mating responses in females. Horm Behav 1978; 3(2):143.

9. Beaver BV: Mating behavior in the dog. Vet Clin North Am 1977; 7(4):723.

10. Beaver BV: Therapy of behavior problems. In Kirk RW (ed): Current Veterinary Therapy VIII: Small Animal Practice. Philadelphia: Saunders, 1983, p. 58.

11. Beaver BV: Feline Behavior: A Guide for Veterinarians. Philadelphia: Saunders, 2002.

12. Boucher JH, Foote RH, Kirke RW: The evaluation of semen quality in the dog and the effects of frequency of ejaculation upon semen quality, libido, and depletion of sperm reserves. Cornell Vet 1958; 48(1):67.

13. BSAVA Congress Report: Sequelae to bitch sterilisation: Regional survey. Vet Rec 1975; 96:371.

14. Campbell WE: Mounting and other sex-related problems. Mod Vet Pract 1975; 56(6):420.

15. Crenshaw WE, Carter CN: Should dogs in animal shelters be neutered early? Vet Med 1980; 90(8):756.

16. Cryptorchidism in dogs. Mod Vet Pract 1976; 57(2):137.

17. Daniels TJ: The social organization of free-ranging urban dogs. II. Estrous groups and the mating system. Appl Anim Ethol 1983; 10:365.

18. Davis LE: Adverse effects of drugs on reproduction in dogs and cats. Mod Vet Pract 1983; 64(12):969.

19. Doty RL, Dunbar I: Attraction of Beagles to conspecific urine, vaginal, and anal sac secretion. Physiol Behav 1974; 12:825.

20. Dunbar IF: Behaviour of castrated animals. Vet Rec 1975; 96:92.

21. Dunbar IF: Olfactory preferences in dogs: The response of male and female Beagles to conspecific odors. Behav Biol 1977; 20:471.

22. Dunbar IF, Buehler MG: A masking effect of urine from male dogs. Appl Anim Ethol 1980; 6:297.

23. Fox MW: A sociosexual behavioral abnormality in the dog resembling Oedipus complex in man. J Am Vet Med Assoc 1964; 144(8):868.

24. Fox MW: Spontaneous displacement activities, compulsive behaviour and abnormal social behaviour in the dog. Vet Rec 1964; 76(31):840.

25. Fox MW: Control of masturbation in dogs. Mod Vet Pract 1967; 48(9):68.

26. Fox MW: Understanding Your Dog. New York: Coward, McCann & Geoghegan, Inc, 1972.

27. Fox MW: The Dog: Its Domestication and Behavior. New York: Garland STPM Press, 1978.

28. Fuller JL, Fox MW: The behavior of dogs. In Hafez ESE (ed): The Behaviour of Domestic Animals, 2nd ed. Baltimore: Williams & Wilkins, 1969, p. 438.

29. Gerber HA, Jöchle W, Sulman FG: Control of reproduction and of undesirable social and sexual behaviour in dogs and cats. J Small Anim Pract 1973; 14:151.

30. Ghosh B, Choudhuri DK, Pal B: Some aspects of sexual behaviour of stray dogs, *Canis familiaris*. Appl Anim Behav Sci 1984; 13(1-2):113.

31. Grandage J: The erect dog penis: A paradox of flexible rigidity. Vet Rec 1972; 91(6):141.

32. Hart BL: Sexual reflexes and mating behavior in the male dog. J Comp Physiol Psychol 1967; 64(3):388.

33. Hart BL: Role of prior experience in the effects of castration on sexual behavior of male dogs. J Comp Physiol Psychol 1968; 66(3):719.

34. Hart BL: Alteration of quantitative aspects of sexual reflexes in spinal male dogs by testosterone. J Comp Physiol Psychol 1968; 66(3):726.

35. Hart BL: The action of extrinsic penile muscles during copulation in the male dog. Anat Rec 1972; 173(1):1.

36. Hart BL: Gonadal androgen and sociosexual behavior of male mammals: A comparative analysis. Psychol Bull 1974; 81:383.

37. Hart BL: Medial preoptic-anterior hypothalamic area and sociosexual behavior of male dogs: A comparative neuropsychological analysis. J Comp Physiol Psychol 1974; 86(2):328.

38. Hart BL: Normal behavior and behavioral problems associated with sexual function, urination, and defecation. Vet Clin North Am 1974; 4(3):589.

39. Hart BL: Normal sexual behavior and behavioral problems in the male dog. Canine Pract 1975; 2(2):11.

40. Hart BL: Behavioral effects of castration. Canine Pract 1976; 3(3):10.

41. Hart BL: Indications for progestin therapy for problem behavior in dogs. Canine Pract 1979; 6(5):10.

42. Hart BL: Problems with objectionable sociosexual behavior of dogs and cats: Therapeutic use of castration and progestins. Compend Contin Educ Pract 1979; 1:461.

43. Hart BL: Progestin therapy for aggressive behavior in male dogs. J Am Vet Med Assoc 1981; 178(10):1070.

44. Hart BL: Advising clients on selecting and socializing dogs: Effects of gonadectomy. American Veterinary Medical Association meeting, Minneapolis, July 17, 1993.

45. Hart BL, Eckstein RA: The role of gonadal hormones in the occurrence of objectionable behaviours in dogs and cats. Appl Anim Behav Sci 1997; 52(3-4):331.

46. Hart BL, Hart LA: Selecting pet dogs on the basis of cluster analysis of breed behavior profiles and gender. J Am Vet Med Assoc 1985; 186(11):1181.

47. Hart BL, Hart LA: Selecting, raising and caring for dogs to avoid problem aggression. J Am Vet Med Assoc 1997; 210(8):1129.

48. Hart BL, Ladewig J: Serum testosterone of neonatal male and female dogs. Biol Reprod 1979; 21:289.

49. Hart BL, Ladewig J: Accelerated and enhanced testosterone secretion in juvenile male dogs following medial preoptic-anterior hypothalamic lesions. Neuroendocrinology 1980; 30:20.

50. Hopkins SG, Schubert TA, Hart BL: Castration of adult male dogs: Effects on roaming, aggression, urine marking, and mounting. J Am Vet Med Assoc 1976; 168(12):1108.

51. Houpt KA: Problems in maternal and sexual behaviors. American Veterinary Medical Association meeting, Minneapolis, July 18, 1993.

52. Houpt KA: Sexual behavior problems in dogs and cats. Vet Clin North Am [Small Anim Pract] 1997; 27(3):601.

53. Houpt KA: Sexual and maternal behavior problems: More common than you think. Am Vet Med Assoc Convention Proceedings, July 2006.

54. Joby R: The control of undesirable behaviour in male dogs using megestrol acetate. J Small Anim Pract 1984; 25:567.

55. Kirk GR, Kirby R, Cox VS, et al: The effects of light deprivation on the development of the gonads in the dog. J Am Anim Hosp Assoc 1976; 12(4):528.

56. Kleiman D: Reproduction in the canidae. Int Zoo Yearbook 1968; 8:2.

57. Kleiman DG, Eisenberg JF: Comparisons of canid and felid social systems from an evolutionary perspective. Anim Behav 1973; 21:637.

58. Knol BW: Influence of stress on the motivation for agonistic behaviour in the male dog: Role of the hypothalamus pituitary testis system. Thesis: Rijksuniversiteit te Utrecht, Faculeit der Diergennskunde, 1989.

59. Knol BW, Egberink-Alink ST: Treatment of problem behaviour in dogs and cats by castration and progestagen administration: A review. Vet Q 1989; 11(2):102.

60. LeBoeuf BJ: Copulatory and aggressive behavior in prepubertally castrated dogs. Horm Behav 1970; 1(2):127.

61. Leiberman LL: A case for neutering pups and kittens at two months of age. J Am Vet Med Assoc 1987; 191(5):518.

62. Macdonald DW: The carnivores: Order Carnivora. In Brown RE, Macdonald DW (eds): Social Odours in Mammals, vol 2. Oxford, England: Clarendon Press, 1985, p. 619.

63. Malcolm JR: Paternal care in canids. Am Zool 1985; 25:853.

64. Olson PN, Pouliot M: Guide dog schools: A model for interdisciplinary studies on canine behavior. Proc Third International Congress Vet Behav Med 2001:69.

65. Olson PN, Pouliot M: New concepts in addressing canine behavior: Guide dog schools as a model. http://www.avma.org/conv/cv2002/CAn_AnB_NCA_OlP.asp, 7/3/2007.

66. Pal SK: Parental care in free-ranging dogs, *Canis familiaris*. Appl Anim Behav Sci 2005; 90:31.

67. Pet sterilization. Bull Inst Study Anim Probl 1979; 1(3):4.

68. Pritchett HD: Abnormal sex behavior in a dog. Canad J Comp Med 1939; 111(10):289.

69. Pritchett HD: Abnormal sex behaviour in a dairy bull, a dog, a goat and a sow. North Am Vet 1944; 25:359.

70. Salmeri KR, Bloomberg MS, Scruggs SL: Prepubertal gonadectomy in the dog: Effects on skeletal growth and physical development. Proc World Small Anim Vet Assoc/British Small Anim Vet Assoc 1989, p. 229. In Alpo Vet Clinic Briefs 1990; 8(2):2.

71. Salmeri KR, Bloomberg MS, Scruggs SL, et al: Gonadectomy in immature dogs: Effects on skeletal, physical, and behavioral. J Am Vet Med Assoc 1991; 198(7):1193.

72. Scarlett JM: The best time to neuter dogs: Long-term risks and benefits of early neutering. http://www.avma.org/conv/cv2002/cvnotes/CAn_PSN_TND_SpV.asp, 7/3/2002.

73. Smithcors JF: Sexual capacity of males. Mod Vet Pract 1977; 58(7):579.

74. Spaying/neutering dogs at 8 weeks of age. DVM Manage Consult Rep 1988; 19(5):1.

75. Stabenfeldt GH: Physiologic, pathologic and therapeutic roles of progestins in domestic animals. J Am Vet Med Assoc 1974; 164(3):311.

76. Taha MA, Noakes DE, Allen WE: Some aspects of reproductive function in the male beagle at puberty. J Small Anim Pract 1981; 22(10):663.

77. Voith VL: Effects of castration on mating behavior. Mod Vet Pract 1979; 60(12):1040.

78. Voith VL: Behavioural problems. In Chandler EA, Evans JM, Singleton WB, et al (eds): Canine Medicine and Therapeutics. Oxford, England: Blackwell Scientific, 1979, p. 395.

79. Wilbur RH: Pets, pet ownership and animal control: Social and psychological attitudes, 1975. Proc Natl Conf Dog Cat Control, Denver, February 3-5, 1976, p. 21.

## Additional Readings

Alexander SA, Shane SM: Characteristics of animals adopted from an animal control center whose owners complied with a spaying/neutering program. J Am Vet Med Assoc 1994; 205(3):472.

Antelyes J: Masturbation in household pets. Mod Vet Pract 1971; 52:53.

Bardens JW: Combined estrogen-androgen steroid therapy in canine practice. North Am Vet 1957; 38:93.

Beach FA, Buehler MG, Dunbar IF: Competitive behavior in male, female, and pseudohermaphroditic female dogs. J Comp Physiol Psychol 1982; 96(6):855.

Beach FA, Kuehn RE: Coital behavior in dogs. X. Effects of androgenic stimulation during development of feminine mating responses in females and males. Horm Behav 1970; 1:347.

Blackshaw JK: Abnormal behaviour in dogs. Aust Vet J 1988; 65(12):393.

Dunbar IF, Buehler MG, Beach FA: Developmental and activational effects of sex hormones on the attractiveness of dog urine. Physiol Behav 1980; 24(2):201.

Gerber HA, Sulman FG: The effect of methyloestrenolone on oestrus, pseudo-pregnancy, vagrancy, satyriasis, and squirting in dogs and cats. Vet Rec 1964; 76(39):1089.

Hart BL: Effects of neutering and spaying on the behavior of dogs and cats: Questions and answers about practical concerns. J Am Vet Med Assoc 1991; 198(7):1204.

Immegart HM, Threlfall WR: Evaluation of intratesticular injection of glycerol for nonsurgical sterilization of dogs. Am J Vet Res 2000; 61(5):544.

Lieberman LL: Advantages of early spaying and neutering. J Am Vet Med Assoc 1982; 181(5):420.

Vollmer PJ: Canine socialization. Part 2. Vet Med Small Anim Clin 1980; 75(3):411.

# Female Canine Sexual Behavior

Reproductive behaviors of a female dog are not generally understood by the public. A survey of owners relinquishing their dog to an animal shelter revealed that 43% of them did not realize a dog would have two estrous cycles per year.[136] In addition, 61% either believed or were not sure if a bitch was better off having at least one litter before she had an ovariohysterectomy.[136] Because 59.7% of the dogs relinquished were acquired at no cost,[136] and because they are less likely to have been neutered,[110] it suggests many dog owners do not want to invest in their dog. It is important for veterinarians to educate new dog owners about good care, especially relative to reproduction.

## PRENATAL INFLUENCES

Differences between male and female dogs become most obvious after puberty, but subtle differences can be detected even in the very young. As mentioned in the last chapter, the brain must be exposed to a testosterone surge around the time of birth for male characteristics to develop. Without that exposure, the brain develops as a female.[78,80] If female puppies are given testosterone before or just after birth and tested as adults against normal males and females, the results suggest a definite shift toward maleness.[12,15,16] Conversely, male puppies deprived of the perinatal testosterone show a definite shift toward femaleness.[78] This early influence on the infant brain determines what adult sexual behavior will emerge when the gonadal hormones are activated at puberty.

Hormones can influence developing fetuses in another way. It has been shown in several species that typically give birth to multiple offspring in each pregnancy that female fetuses positioned near a male fetus,[47,114] and being "upstream" in the uterine blood flow, have increased chances of

contacting androgens from male fetuses.[96,133,161,162] This can help explain the gradual progression between male and female in behavior, as well as appearance, in sexual dimorphism. Obviously surgical neutering affects this too.

Other than reproductive behaviors, three traits have been described as sexually dimorphic for the female dog—ease of training, tendency to seek more attention, and the ease of housebreaking.[87]

## SEXUAL MATURATION

Sexual maturation can actually take place over a wide age range—from 1.5 to 24 months.[20,68,143] The most common age for puberty is 6 to 9 months.[22,65] In one study, however, the average age of first estrus was 42.4 days (± 15.7).[143] Considerable breed variation exists in regard to puberty, but it usually occurs in dogs considerably earlier than it does in the wolf, for which the first estrus is around 22 months of age.[32] The age of onset of first estrus in dogs is 7.8% heritable.[143] Occasionally the first proestrus signs may end abruptly without leading to a standing estrus. This cessation of signs is usually followed in 2 to 3 months by the first complete proestrus-estrus-metestrus series.[20,70] The earlier partial sequence probably indicates follicular activity without ovulation accompanied by corresponding hormonal insufficiencies.[167]

Various features of the first complete estrous period differ from those of the second and subsequent ones. Not only are serum hormone concentrations lower during the first cycle, but the durations of proestrus and estrus are shorter.[39] In breeding colonies, it has been determined that the optimal breeding age for a dog is 2 to 3.5 years.[100] At this age a bitch can wean the most puppies/litter (average of 4.28 puppies) with the lowest puppy mortality (8.5%).[100] For bitches 7 years of age, weaned litter size is 1.22 puppies, and mortality approaches 40%. For those 9 years of age, 0.6 puppies/litter are weaned, and mortality is almost 80%.[100]

## REPRODUCTIVE CYCLES

The idea of a reproductive cycle occurring every 6 months is a misconception. In fact, there are more exceptions to the "normal" cycle than a general statement will allow. The estrous cycle of the bitch is unique among domestic animals because every phase is prolonged.[98] The bitch has between one and three estrous periods each year.[20,51,159] Although an average estrous cycle is said to last 6 months, the actual duration can vary between 4 and 12 months.[22] No evidence of a seasonal nature to the estrous cycle in dogs exists overall,[99,143,146,152] but certain breeds might have a slight tendency to be in estrus in early fall[69] or late winter–early spring.[44,99,152,158] In contrast, wolves and most other wild canids are seasonal breeders, with a single estrous period in early spring.[20,32,102] Evidence also suggests that some estrous synchronization occurs in bitches housed together.[65]

The duration of proestrus, estrus, and vaginal bleeding is the same across various breeds, ages, and mated versus unmated bitches.[26] Proestrus can last 1 to 27 days but typically lasts 5 to 10 days.[20,26] External signs include vulvular swelling and a bloody discharge, plus an unwillingness to stand for mounting. Estrus has a mean duration of 9 to 13 days, with a range of 4 to 24 days.[20,26,45,89,126] Vaginal bleeding continues from proestrus until day 9 of estrus, although in an occasional dog it might continue into metestrus.[26] It is felt that the combined duration of a normal proestrus and estrus should not exceed 21 days.[153]

Metestrus lasts 80 to 140 days and initially may include a dark vaginal discharge.[20,99] Although the entire estrous cycle ranges from 4 to 12 months, it averages 218 days in laboratory Beagles.[43,143] The length of the cycle was only 43% repeatable in bitches, but heritability of when estrus recurred was relatively high, at 38%.[143] Significant differences exist in the length of the entire estrous cycle across various breeds; however, these differences are unrelated to the average size or weight of breed

members.[44] In one study of seven breeds, German Shepherds had the shortest interestrous interval— $149 \pm 28.5$ days.[146] Another study indicated metestrus varies by breed, but not by size.[99]

### Vaginal Smears

Much has been written about being able to follow an estrous cycle noninvasively by using vaginal smears.* Changes in the vaginal epithelium, and thus in the vaginal smears, are caused by hormonal changes associated with ovarian and pituitary activity. The behaviors associated with the estrous cycle also are related to the hormonal changes, but more variation occurs in behavioral sequences than in vaginal cytology. Thus, vaginal smears are a more accurate method of determining hormonal activity than are behavioral measurements, body temperature changes,[43] or body weight fluctuations.[27]

## MATING BEHAVIORS

### Proestrous Behaviors

Proestrus is characterized by rapid follicular development and an increase in estrogen. These changes result in swelling of the vulva, congestion of the reproductive tract, and a bloody vaginal discharge.[126,165] The behavior of the bitch becomes increasingly restless as she falls under estrogen's influence, and behaviors gradually approach those of standing estrus.[46] The female will begin to play bow and show submissive behavior toward the male.[93] As ovulation approaches, the female will show an increased frequency of urination, more licking of the vulva, and a greater attraction to males, and she will spend more time with nearby males.[20,66] More time is spent investigating male dogs and their urine as compared with time spent investigating female dogs and female dog urine.[57] When first approached, the female will usually stand quietly while the male smells her but crouch down if he attempts to mount.[22] When in proestrus, a bitch may even show aggression toward the male.[22,153]

---

*References 25, 28, 42, 55, 66, 89, 90, 138, 139.

## Estrous Behaviors

The behaviors of estrus include all aspects of courtship, mating, and postmating rituals. Initial mate selection can be more than a random act of mating with whichever male happens to be nearby. During their first estrus, females tend not to show active courtship solicitation, although they may identify preferred mates.[74] Variations in behavior are more likely to occur during the first estrus period than in subsequent ones.[167] These behavioral variations are probably related to hormonal insufficiencies or irregularities.[51,167] Only 10% of females will actively avoid or attack specific males during the first estrus.[74] Most older females show some amount of preference for certain males.* The preferences and aversions shown by individual estrous bitches may be different than the social affinity between the same dogs when the female is anestrus.[10] Preferences tend to persist from one estrus to the next.[10] If housed away from males, an estrous female seldom rejects a male.[44] Favored males often were raised around or lived with the female.[10,53] During the first heat, the female does not let a littermate sniff, lick, or mount her unless he persists more than 30 minutes.[74] By the second estrus, she may reject half the males that were accepted during the first heat, but there are usually twice as many males around.[74] She will not allow unfamiliar males to mate with her.[53]

The relative dominance between the dogs can influence whether a successful mating will occur. A dominant female may not let a subordinate male mount.[64] Conversely, a dominant male may be shown extremely submissive postures by a subordinate female, or he may inhibit a submissive male from mating merely by being present.[64]

Premating behaviors include seeking out males and increased vocalization, restlessness, and exploration. By the time of estrus, the bitch is usually being followed by two to eight males.[74] The rate of scent marking by the bitch in the presence of a male, which may include a leg-lift urination posture,[80] will at least double.[74] Overmarking by the male also increases.[109] The time spent searching for food

decreases, interest in male urine and anal sac odors increases, and 70% to 80% of her time is spent with potential partners.[56,74] If only one or two males are present, a bitch may show soliciting behavior. This behavior includes physical contact with the male, and if there is no response, the bitch will present the perineum with the tail up to the male's nose. That behavior is often sufficient to induce the male courtship behaviors. If the male shows interest, the female may run a short distance away. If the male shows minimal interest, the bitch may continue the teasing behavior by sniffing and licking the male's anogenital area and by investigating his face, inguinal area, and penis. She may mount the male, and although this generally is a strong soliciting behavior, it may take between 2 and 29 mounts before the male responds by mounting or leaving.[74]

By definition, estrus is the time when the bitch will stand for the male, although this behavior is strongly influenced by the hormonal state and environmental factors. The female also shows more interest in odors associated with male dogs when she is in estrus.[57] The word *estrus* is said to come from *oistros,* which means "mad desire."[66] Preferences may be displayed for certain familiar males, and rejection of others can also occur.[9,10,17,53] Over half of males are unsuccessful.[51] While the male mounts, the bitch stands quietly with her tail flagged to one side.[79] Once the tie occurs and the male dismounts, the bitch may remain standing quietly, pull against the tie, or forcefully throw the male off balance.[20] This twisting and turning usually lasts 5 to 30 seconds, and the female may actually roll over once or twice.[78] Studies suggest the twisting and turning reaction is a spinal reflex evoked by clitoral stimulation.[78] Excessive salivation may also be seen, in which saliva comes out of the corners of her mouth (Fig. 6-1).[20] Unlike males, most females will tie at least once during their first year.[74] Should the mount not result in a long tie, the estrous female will become very active and sexually aggressive toward the male.[11,70] She will bump him, investigate his inguinal and perineal areas, mount him, and present her perineum to him. She may mate once or twice daily for 2 to 5 days.[103]

Female dogs will mount other females more often when the mounted animal is in estrus, but the

*References 9, 10, 17, 32, 64, 74, 78, 103, 159.

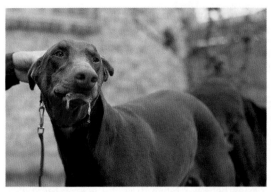

**Figure 6-1.** Estrous bitch showing the excessive salivation associated with mating.

frequency is not related to the hormonal state of the one doing the mounting.[19,46] When a female mounts a male, the female usually is in estrus.[19]

## Odor

Odors are significant communication signals for canids. Sexually experienced males spend more time investigating estrous urine and vaginal secretions than diestrous urine, male urine, vaginal secretions, or anal sac odors.[13,56] Volatile compounds in urine from an estrous bitch are different from those in an anestrous one. The active principle has been identified as methyl-*p*-hydroxybenzoate.[1,75,76,109] Other major constituents are methyl propylsulfide, methyl butylsulfide, and acetone.[137] Both of the sulfides are somewhat higher during proestrus and estrus than during metestrus or anestrus.[137]

## Metestrous Behaviors

During metestrus, the bitch again is unreceptive to the male. Because this is the time the corpus lutea are maintained, maximal plasma progesterone levels occur. A gradual decline in progesterone then follows over the 50- to 60-day period.[45] Estrous females may be attractive to metestrous females, resulting in mounting by the metestrous individuals.[45]

## Other Species

Many canids are close genetically, which allows for opportunities of crossbreeding. Crossbreeding can occur by artificial breeding or if the dog and wild species member are tolerant of each other's species, usually through socialization. Dog crossbreeding with wolves, coyotes, and jackals will produce fertile offspring, but dog crossbreeding with foxes will not.[71]

In canids of all species, including the domestic dog, large females produce young that are larger than those of small females.[23] Relative to the mother's own body weight, though, large females allocate fewer resources to bringing a large pup to term.[23]

## PREGNANCY

At birth a female puppy has approximately 700,000 ova.[126] This number decreases to 250,000 at puberty, 33,000 at 5 years of age, and 500 at 10 years.[126] These figures reflect the decreasing fertility rates and litter sizes that occur with age, too. It has been shown that successful pregnancy is related to many things. Ovulation usually occurs 1 to 2 days after the bitch will stand for breeding.[88] By the end of estrus, histologic evaluations indicate that 93.5% of ovarian follicles have ruptured.[164] Breeding success for the species as a whole occurs because each bitch has two or three estrous cycles a year and a generally good conception rate. The probability of pregnancy is helped both by the release of most eggs and by a typical intrauterine life span for sperm of 48 ± 12 hours and a maximum possible of 6 days.[48,138] It can be argued that the normal reproductive state of a female dog is being pregnant or caring for puppies.

Once ovulation occurs, the corpus luteum reaches maximum size in 4 to 8 days, approximately 7 days before fetal implantation, and remains visible on the ovarian surface for 16 weeks.[22,88,165] The high progesterone levels from the corpus luteum maintain pregnancy for 51 to 80 days, with the average length of time being 62 to 65 days.[48,117,124,151] Normally, there is a sharp fall in progesterone 36 to 48 hours postpartum, suggesting a role for decreasing progesterone levels in parturition.[49] Onset of parturition is partially affected by litter size, as well as by length of pregnancy and hormonal state.[48,117] Because the corpus luteum remains regardless of whether pregnancy occurs, false pregnancies might be considered normal. Because they are considered abnormal to most dog owners, however, they will be discussed under the "Female Sexual Behavior Problems" section of this chapter.

As the end of a normal pregnancy approaches, the bitch begins to show external signs, including behavior changes. She will seek a quiet area with some type of appropriate nesting material. An instinctive tendency to dig is present, inherited from canine ancestors that dig their own nest sites.[117] As the female's restlessness increases, she will frequently rearrange bedding material, especially in the days immediately before parturition. The bitch's appetite will decrease during this time as well.[30]

In the 12 to 24 hours before the actual onset of labor, there is a dramatic increase in restlessness.[30] The bitch will shred nesting material by digging and tearing it. She will get up and lie down, ask to go in and out (in the case of a house dog), and posture as if for urination. She will show an increased friendliness toward favored individuals but an increased aggression toward strangers, which is probably a remnant behavior of protecting the nest site.[30] Dogs that are extremely attached to their owners may become distressed if the person leaves the area of the nest site.[117] For these dogs, the stress of separation may be so great as to cause them to leave a chosen site and whelp near the owner instead.

## Parturition

### The Contraction Phase

Parturition is divided into four phases and is similar to that of other multiparous mammals. As the birth of each puppy becomes imminent, the bitch will show a specific series of behaviors that last 1 to 10 minutes. These are the external signs of the first phase—the *contraction phase.*[22] Activity decreases, with the bitch spending more time sitting or lying on her side, perhaps with her back pressed against something firm.[30,117] She may also seek out a nest site, although this may have been done already in the preceding few days. Respirations increase to 100 to 175 breaths per minute for periods lasting from a few seconds to longer than a minute.[30] These increased respiratory rates alternate with normal rates of 16 to 20 breaths per minute and an intermediate rate of 40 to 60 breaths per minute,[30] and are probably related to times of active uterine

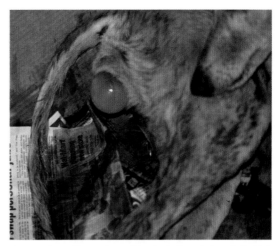

**Figure 6-2.** The expulsion of the chorioallantois through the birth canal causes an external bulging of the vulva.

contractions. At least in some animals, these contractions help position the fetus for delivery. The cervix dilates during this phase for the first puppy. The contraction phase may be very brief or as long as 36 hours in a nervous bitch[67] but typically lasts 6 to 12 hours.[91]

### The Emergence Phase

In the *emergence phase,* the bitch may shiver, have occasional twitching of the rear limbs, and with a few strong uterine contractions, push the puppy into the birth canal. Externally, a bulge appears just above the vulva as the fetus nears its exit (Fig. 6-2). The chorioallantois will begin to protrude from the vulva and often breaks to release its watery contents.[22] The emergence phase usually lasts a few seconds, but if it is prolonged, the bitch may start removing the fetal membranes before the puppy is completely out.[30]

### Delivery

Uterine contractions and forceful straining of abdominal muscles result in expulsion of the puppy (Fig. 6-3). This is the *delivery,* or third, *phase* of parturition. The mother's attention is immediately given to licking up fetal fluids on the puppy, herself, and the nest material.[83] In so doing, she cleans up the puppy, removes remaining amnionic membranes, and stimulates the first respirations in the

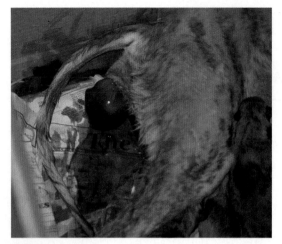

**Figure 6-3.** The delivery phase of parturition is associated with the expulsion of a puppy.

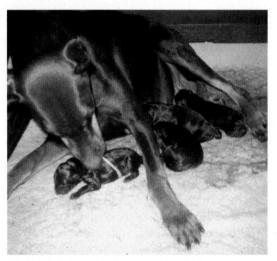

**Figure 6-4.** The bitch chews through the umbilical cord of her newborn puppy.

newborn. The bitch will chew through the umbilical cord and eat the fetal membranes (Fig. 6-4). Some authors combine the emergence and delivery phases into one—that of expelling the fetus.[67,83,117]

### The Placental Phase
Eventually the alternating periods of rest and puppy-oriented attention give way to the *placental*, or fourth, *phase*. Uterine contractions resume and result in the expulsion of the placenta. Bitches normally eat the placenta after its delivery. Even

though this behavior is not necessary in dogs, eating of fetal membranes probably serves specific purposes in wild canids. First, it provides a source of protein to the mother—necessary because she uses up a considerable amount of energy in parturition,[30] and she will not be able to hunt for several days. Second, it removes the tissue from the nest site so it does not become an attractant for potential predators. Removal of the membranes also helps with sanitation to minimize the risk of infection.[30] Perhaps it helps eliminate some thirst for the new mother, too.[30] What actually triggers the behavior in canids remains unknown, but perhaps it is an odor.[30]

In multiparous animals like dogs, multiple births can mean that a second, or even third puppy could be delivered before the first one's placenta is expelled, and this is more likely to occur if the puppies have been carried in opposite uterine horns.[67] When a puppy is expelled from one uterine horn, the next puppy will come from the opposite horn 78.2% of the time.[156] And then, one, two, or even three placentas may come at one time. Thus, the phases of parturition associated with the delivery of more than one puppy may overlap in their sequencing. Once a puppy has been born, the bitch's attention may be directed toward removal of fetal fluids from the nest site, even to the point of ignoring the new arrivals.

In uncomplicated births, the time for delivery of four to five puppies averages 3.0 to 3.5 hours, with irregular delivery intervals of 10 to 60 minutes between births. Giving birth to 11 puppies can take 2 to 15 hours, with an average of about 9 hours.[117] Review of registration records indicates the average litter size is 4.73 puppies, with a sex ratio of 1.024 male puppies to 1.0 female.[130] Small dogs like Papillons, Norwich Terriers, English Toy Spaniels, Brussels Griffins, and Pomeranians have the smallest litters.[152] And, as might be expected, the bigger dogs have the largest average litter size, including English Foxhounds, Irish Setters, Irish Water Spaniels, and Golden Retrievers.[152] They also have a greater percentage of male puppies.[152] Free-ranging dogs are influenced by a broader range of genetic influences. Their average litter size is 5.83 puppies with 1.69 male puppies to 1.0 females.[124]

During parturition, the bitch is insensitive to the distress calls of the neonates[30] but she is sensitive to other disturbances. It is not until after all the puppies are born that the bitch begins responding to the puppy cries.[22,30,67,70,117] If a single disturbance occurs during a time with no to minimal uterine contractions, either contractions do not begin, or else a fetus is not expelled at the next expected interval.[30] If the disturbance occurs during labor, the puppy may not be expelled, and one or more ineffective bouts of uterine contractions will follow.[30] Long disturbances are disruptive to the birthing process. In addition to stopping labor, the bitch often shows aggression, agitation, and apprehension.[30] Disturbance also increases the likelihood that she may injure one or more of her newborn puppies. Parturition resumes in 15 to 60 minutes after a disturbance unless there are repeated disturbances. Such disturbances can result in delays as long as 6 hours, even with a puppy already in the birth canal.[30] Strong but ineffective uterine contractions may be accompanied by vigorous grooming of puppies, as if the behavior were being directed at a phantom newborn.[30]

Bitches will usually treat puppies that are born dead the same as those born alive until their bodies cool.[30] Then the bitch may push away the lifeless body, eat it, or bury it.[30,117]

Puppies are influenced by the dam in more ways than genetics. At birth, puppies from large litters will weigh less than those from small litters, but during the next several weeks things will change. Those born to a bitch during her first 1.5 years will weigh 25% more at weaning than those born during the following 4.5 years.[169] Puppy weight does affect behavior and ability to thrive. Large female puppies are more active and explore more. They will score higher on defense drive and hardiness as adults, too.[169]

## MATERNAL BEHAVIOR

### Maternal-Young Interactions

During the first 12 hours after the completion of parturition, the new mother rarely leaves the puppies and she is extremely protective of them, especially toward strangers.[30] This extreme reaction may be a way to release her inhibition—that is, the prey-like appearance of the puppies and her hormonal state would normally trigger aggression, but this aggressive instinct is inhibited. She may let familiar people handle her puppies, but even then the bitch remains nervous until the puppies are replaced.[100] Removed puppies are licked more than those left alone.[129]

During the first week, the bitch hardly leaves the puppies. By 2 weeks postpartum, she will remain outside the nest box for 2 to 3 hours at a time.[70] When in the box, the new mother grooms the puppies frequently and nurses them often. Puppies will spend a maximum of 27.54 minutes per nursing bout during the first week.[124] She will also rest with the puppies, a behavior that helps her offspring maintain body temperature when they are incapable of doing so on their own.

During the first few weeks, the bitch is relatively insistent that the puppies remain where they were whelped. She will take the puppy away from someone who picks it up, or she will retrieve the entire litter from a new location if they have been moved.[30,70] She may not retrieve an individual puppy that has wandered off on its own even if it uses distress cries. For most puppies, that is not a problem because the owners are more than willing to retrieve a wanderer.

Some newborns do not thrive. A bitch may reject such a puppy because of its low body temperature, lack of movement, or some other reason that is not clear to us.[60] This rejection may be expressed by ignoring the puppy, shoving it out of the nest box, killing it, or burying it away from the nest box (Fig. 6-5). Such behavior can be very upsetting to owners, but in nature it would minimize the attraction of predators to the other youngsters and avoid wasting precious energy resources of the mother on a neonate that would probably not have a good chance for long-term survival.

As the puppies grow older, the dam spends less time with them. In part, this gradual change of behavior may be caused by hormonal alterations, but it also has to do with physical changes in the puppies. Exchanging some of a bitch's puppies with very young puppies from another litter causes a dramatic change in her behavior. All indices of

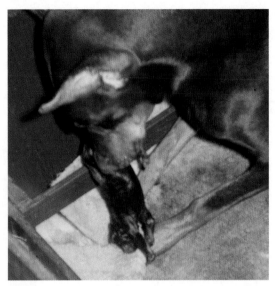

**Figure 6-5.** A bitch attempts to bury a newborn puppy under the carpet of the whelping box.

maternal behavior increase, from puppy grooming to nursing bouts.[104,105]

Mother-young interactions change over time. Initially, the appearance of the young may prompt the appearance of submission by the mother.[168] Lactating bitches also show a smaller adrenocortical response to stress than do nonlactating dogs. This lessened response to stress is another reason they tend to remain calm and provide for their young in circumstances that would produce stress behavior otherwise.[99] Then, when the puppies are approximately 4 weeks of age, there is a change in this relationship. The mother is gone more and becomes increasingly less likely to respond to the puppies' attempts to nurse, often standing to prevent it (see Chapter 7, Fig. 7-2). She also becomes more aggressive toward the puppies, using an inhibited bite to emphasize to them her reduced interest in their nursing attempts.[168] Her actions are usually followed by a submissive response from the puppies, to which she responds by licking them (Fig. 6-6).[168] The puppies may continue to nurse until 10 to 11 weeks of age when time spent nursing reaches a minimum of 2.22 minutes per session.[124] By 10 weeks, all puppies move away from the

dam's inhibited aggressive actions,[31] as would be expected with the development of parent-offspring conflicts.[155] There is a natural conflict that occurs over the length and amount of parental investment. Longer and more intense care for the puppies gives them a better chance for survival, but it also means a longer time of limited resources for the bitch. Early weaned puppies are more likely to develop behavior problems, particularly those associated with fear or anxiety.[112,128] The benefits of remaining with the mother after weaning also have been demonstrated experimentally. Puppies that stayed with their dam from the sixth to tenth weeks showed better development of motor abilities and agility, were less distressed by isolation, and were less likely to approach people.[59]

## Infant Adoption

Fostering puppies is usually not a problem for a bitch with a litter, even if the young are a few weeks older than her own litter.[84] Because all wolves in a pack share in cub care and are all genetically part of the same family, there is no advantage to a female wolf recognizing only her own cubs.[84] This wolf behavior has probably been retained to some extent in modern dogs and makes fostering unrelated puppies much easier.

## Care by Others

Wild canids often share duties for care of the young. Related females may stand guard over and play with the youngsters while the mother goes hunting. Because of false pregnancies, these females may even produce milk and share nursing duties. This sharing is less common in the dog, but the reason may be more a function of how dogs are kept (a lack of opportunity) rather than a lack of the behavior.

Male dogs can respond in a broad range of ways to the presence of puppies, so it is best to use caution about keeping a male near a litter. The initial reaction is usually one of curiosity. After the initial investigating, the behavior can go to one extreme or another. Some males will patiently lie among the puppies, regurgitate food, and/or guard puppies, even those that are not their own. At the other extreme is the male that kills any puppy. Most male behavior falls somewhere in between.

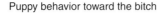

Puppy behavior toward the bitch

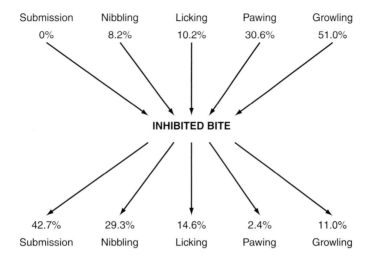

| Submission | Nibbling | Licking | Pawing | Growling |
|---|---|---|---|---|
| 0% | 8.2% | 10.2% | 30.6% | 51.0% |

**INHIBITED BITE**

| 42.7% | 29.3% | 14.6% | 2.4% | 11.0% |
|---|---|---|---|---|
| Submission | Nibbling | Licking | Pawing | Growling |

Puppy response from the bitch's behavior

**Figure 6-6.** Puppy behaviors and their relationship to inhibited bites by the female. (From reference 168.)

## NEUROLOGIC AND HORMONAL CONTROLS

Both neurologic and hormonal factors control female sexual behavior in most animal species. Unfortunately, the neurologic control of female behavior is not well studied in the dog. The cat has been one of the main research models used, so the reader is referred to other sources for a better understanding of the role of the central nervous system in female sexual behavior.[21]

## Hormones

### Estrogen

In intact female dogs, serum levels of estrogen and its related compounds, like estradiol-17β, begin increasing at the onset of proestrus and peak near or on the first day of estrus.[*] They then fall rapidly to 30 to 80 pg/ml by the start of estrus.[4,58] The drop continues throughout estrus, reaching the lowest point after 10 to 14 days.[58,113] After that, levels begin to rise again.[113] The duration of estrus is not

related to the length of time estrogen levels were raised but rather to the peak amounts of estrogen.[77] The amount of estrogen in the peripheral blood during anestrus is insignificant.[77]

Paralleling the estrogen rise in proestrus are the uterine changes that help with sperm transport and maintenance.[5] These include the development of crypts and the differentiation of glandular epithelial cells into mucus-secreting ones.[5] Estrogen levels in the urine are much lower than in the plasma, but a significant correlation exists between the two.[7,8]

### Progesterone

Progesterone levels begin increasing during proestrus about 2 days before the onset of estrus, and they peak between 15 and 25 days after the start of estrus.[77,113] Some studies indicate that regardless of whether a bitch is pregnant, progesterone levels gradually fall to a low around day 65 to 80.[4,80,113,151] Other studies suggest considerable progesterone variations.[5,58,166] Uterine changes during the time of maximum progesterone levels include the hypertrophy and hyperplasia of the glandular epithelium.[5] These changes would support fetal implantation. Progesterone levels remain low throughout anestrus.[113]

*References 4, 8, 58, 77, 80, 116, 166.

## Luteinizing Hormone

Plasma luteinizing hormone (LH) levels are the best measurable indication of ovulation.[127] A sharp, tenfold increase in LH values occurs at or just before the onset of estrus, with ovulation regularly following in 2 days—the second or third day of estrus.* This LH peak is 8 days before the onset of diestrus.[90]

## Testosterone

Serum testosterone levels rise during proestrus and peak about the same time as LH.[120] Near the start of estrus, testosterone levels are four times higher than resting levels.[120]

## External Hormones

Supplementation by external hormones has been tried in a variety of forms, doses, protocols, and combinations in efforts to bring on estrus, prevent it, or prevent pregnancies. Overall, the success rates are low. Reported results are inconsistent, and most of the drugs used have significant side effects.

Approaches to controlling the onset of estrus include the use of synthetic progestins,† testosterone, mibolerone,[106,141,144,147] and norspiroxenone.[115] The chemical induction of estrus with or without the attraction of a male or successful mating usually depends on a natural hormone, such as pregnant mare serum gonadotropin,[37,145,154,170,171] human chorionic gonadotropin,[37,145,154,170] hypothalamic gonadotropin-releasing hormone,[38] follicle-stimulating hormone,[140] estradiol,[14,40,50] or estrogen.[18] Those investigating the termination of pregnancy or prevention of fetal implantation have also tried several products, but their research focuses mainly on estrogens and prostaglandins. For the most current recommendations regarding chemical manipulation of estrus or pregnancy, the reader should consult a recent theriogenology book.

Many protocols have been tried, and new research continues to address the pet overpopulation problem. It is estimated that 31% to 57% of the owned female dogs in the United States have had an ovariohysterectomy.[110,125,163] There is a higher likelihood that a licensed dog will be sterilized (40.3% versus 26.0%) and a reduced chance if the dog is rural (20.8%) or turned into an animal shelter (17.7%).[110] Factors like estral bleeding and male dogs hanging around are strong incentives for the surgery. Reasons for not neutering female dogs include interest in breeding (44%), expense of the surgery (26%), and concern about weight gain or personality changes (26%).[125] Unfortunately, it takes a surgical sterilization rate of approximately 85% to have any effect on free-roaming dog populations.[118,130] The overpopulation problem is unlikely to be solved with the addition or sole use of nonsurgical techniques. Without addressing the primary cause of pet overpopulation—apparent public apathy or lack of awareness[2,136]—no major changes can be made.

## Surgical Removal of Hormone Sources

Prepubertal neutering has become a subject of much interest. Behavioral studies on puppies neutered at a very young age suggest that for a family pet, there are minimal to no physical or behavioral differences in these puppies as compared with those surgically altered at or after the onset of puberty.* By 2 years after ovariohysterectomy, pet dogs neutered at age 7 to 10 weeks are considered by owners to be smarter than dogs neutered at 6 months or later. This correlates with the finding in guide dogs that dogs neutered before 6 months of age are 1.3 times more likely to be successfully trained.[122,123] Undesirable behavioral side effects are reported in one study to be lower in those spayed early (Table 6-1). Another long-term study did not show behavioral differences between the two groups.[97] In the early-neuter group, 32% developed behavior problems, whereas in the older group, 38% did so. In both groups aggression was the most common concern. A third study showed that early neutering decreased separation anxiety and the tendency to escape from home but increased the risk of noise phobia and urination if frightened.[149] Only dogs

---

*References 88, 113, 126, 127, 142, 164.
†References 29, 34, 36, 72, 73, 107, 131, 132, 145, 151, 157.

*References 52, 108, 134, 135, 148, 150

| TABLE 6-1 | Comparison of behavior problems in female dogs neutered at 8 to 10 weeks compared with 6 months or later | | | | | | | | | |
|---|---|---|---|---|---|---|---|---|---|---|
| | Aggression | | Overweight | | Intelligence (owner-defined) | | Medical problems | | Excited urination | |
| | % | CV | % | CV | % | CV | % | CV | % | CV |
| Female dogs neutered at 8 weeks | 16 | — | 5 | — | 95 | — | 16 | — | 10 | — |
| Female dogs neutered at 6+ months | 32 | 2× | 50 | 10× | 68 | 0.7× | 55 | 3.4× | 59 | 5.9× |

Data from references 108, 150.
%, Likelihood of problem occurring; *CV,* comparative value of likelihood between age groups.

that were already showing some aggression and had an ovariohysterectomy before 12 months of age showed an increase in dominance aggression as they got older.[86,94] Female dogs that undergo prepubertal neutering are not predisposed to excessive weight gains.[52,108,134,135] Weight changes are, however, associated with stages of the estrous cycle.[27] Physical maturation is delayed by early neutering, and the vulvas tend to remain more immature.[134,135]

When the female dogs neutered at or after puberty were compared to intact controls, several differences were noted. One difference was a significantly greater tendency for dominance aggression to be shown toward family members by the neutered females.[119] What is not clear about the study is whether the surgery was performed in more of these dogs because aggression had already been identified as a problem, or whether there is a direct cause-effect relation. Ovariohysterectomized bitches also showed significantly more excitement in the car and a less discriminate appetite than did the intact ones, even immediately postsurgery.[95,119] This latter point may be relevant to the overweight/obesity rate of 38% to 50% reported in spayed females.[35,108]

## FEMALE SEXUAL BEHAVIOR PROBLEMS

### Pseudocyesis

Pseudocyesis (false pregnancy, phantom pregnancy, pseudopregnancy) involves hormonal changes consistent with pregnancy that result in psychological or behavioral changes. Because the corpus lutea secrete progesterone for approximately 60 days postovulation in a bitch, the hormonal state during this time is the same for pregnant and nonpregnant females.[80,101,121,126,160] No apparent luteolytic agent is produced to terminate the corpus lutea in the absence of fertilization.[98] Pseudocyesis might therefore be considered normal for the nonpregnant dog.[80,93,126] It has been hypothesized that this condition is an adaptive response to allow nonbreeding females to help raise offspring of the breeding female.[54] Associated physical and behavioral changes are very broad in scope, ranging from none all the way to the equivalent of pregnancy. Included can be nervousness, guarding an area, making a nest (66.1% of nonpregnant females), abdominal distention, mammary gland development with or without lactation (78.6%), external signs of labor, self-nursing, and guarding or carrying a stuffed toy or other object (53.6%).[33,54,80,160] Following a true pregnancy, behavior will return to normal in 4 to 8 weeks when nursing stops. Because the behaviors of pseudocyesis are typical of normal behaviors that start about the time progesterone levels decrease, it is reasonable to expect that up to 8 weeks may be needed for the changes of pseudocyesis to gradually stop. Almost 80% of nonpregnant intact bitches will show some of these signs postestrus.[54,111] Up to 67% of affected females will show recurrent pseudocyesis with subsequent estrous cycles.[54]

Many owners want the unusual behaviors to stop, but until the dog's bodily response to the hormone changes runs its course, the best treatment is no treatment. Progestins will stop the behaviors of pseudocyesis by putting the dog back into "pregnancy." The down side to this treatment is that each time it ends, the signs of pseudocyesis return in 10% to 15% of these dogs.[3] An ovariohysterectomy within 3 months after estrus can also result in a sharp drop in progesterone and signs of pseudocyesis, including lactation, by 4 days post-surgery.[101] A hysterectomy alone can prolong luteal activity, because there is no longer a uterine feedback mechanism.[151] It is suggested that this surgery be postponed at least 3 months past estrus,[3] or until signs of pseudocyesis end, whichever is longest. Dogs that show external signs of pseudocyesis develop pyometra less often than those that do not.[60]

## Abnormal Maternal Behavior

The amniotic fluid is important to the female for helping her learn which are her puppies. A puppy that has been dried off by people is more likely to be rejected.[94,129] It may be necessary to wet the newborn, being careful that it stay warm, and present it to the dam to try to have her accept it.

In the worst case scenario, some bitches will kill their puppies—a trait seen more in Jack Russell Terriers.[94] Because this is a breed that hunts small prey, it has been hypothesized that these bitches fail to recognize puppies as dogs and treat them as rats instead.[94]

Cannibalism of a new puppy by its mother is probably the most upsetting behavior an owner can witness. As has already been mentioned, a bitch will occasionally eat a rejected puppy even when the reason for its rejection is not obvious. A bitch might at times be overzealous in cleaning up a newborn puppy and chew into its abdominal cavity while shortening the umbilical cord.[51,62,91] Care must be taken to be sure she is not going to eat the whole puppy or more than one puppy. Cannibalism requires permanent separation of the puppies from this mother.

A bitch may also ignore her puppies. This is most common if the puppies are born before 57 days of gestation.[51,62] It is probably more likely in first-litter bitches,[91] when the bitch is very owner-dependent, if a cesarean section is done, and when there are frequent environmental disturbances.

Puppies can be hurt if the mother is not careful when she moves or retrieves them. The distressed bitch may constantly carry her puppies from one place to another. Such behavior is stressful to them and could result in their being hurt or chilled. Possible injury may also occur to puppies when they are 3 to 4 weeks of age. This is a time when maternal-young relationships begin to change and solid food is first introduced.[61]

## Abnormal Sex Partners

True homosexual behavior is rare in adult dogs.[6,20] Frequently, owners have made the assumption that homosexual behavior was happening when the dog was actually showing investigative, play, dominance, or grooming behavior.[6] Careful observation or history-taking is necessary to put the specific behavioral series in perspective of the environmental situation. For example, mounting can be sexual, play, or dominance related. Although all three types of mounting behaviors may look similar, past and present happenings can help the observer determine the context, and therefore the type, of behavior. Mounting and pelvic thrusts are shown by up to 40% of intact female dogs.[85] In one study of 356 problem-behavior cases, 46% involved a dog mounting a dog, person, or other object.[92] Forty cases of the 356 involved females, including 10 neutered females.[92] Most incidences of mounting done by intact females occur during estrus.[92]

Two possible explanations have been given for female dogs showing masculine behavior. The first explanation is that because sexual dimorphism is a relative thing, environmental and social factors that occasionally arouse male behavior in castrated males may do so in females if intense enough.[82] A second explanation is based on the "womb-mate" effect.[82] In this case, it is speculated that a female fetus positioned between two male fetuses in the uterus may get enough androgen to cause some behavioral masculinization.[82]

Mounting of people by female dogs is less common than by males, but it is just as objectionable to owners. If certain types of activities are likely to stimulate mounting, the easiest treatment may be to keep the dog away from those activities. If avoiding certain situations is impossible or undesirable, the owner may be able to use high-activity games to get rid of the dog's extra energy in more acceptable ways.

## Masturbation

Masturbation is occasionally shown by both intact and neutered female dogs, and it can take several forms. The dog may mount an object and show pelvic thrusting while rubbing the perineum against the object.[63] She may also rub her vulva on the floor or ground while swinging back and forth by bracing her front limbs.[20] A third form of masturbation occurs when the dog licks her external genitalia excessively.[63] Excitement often precipitates the activities of masturbation. The behavior probably provides an internal reward for the dog, because if its development is not inhibited early, masturbation becomes very difficult to eliminate later.[63]

Several tactics can be tried to stop masturbation. Increased exercise, especially immediately before a predictable excitatory stimulus, reduces the excitement and the amount of energy available. Putting the dog in another room as an excitatory event occurs may defuse the stimulus, and if it does not, the behavior is at least unobserved by the owner or house guests. Because mounting and pelvic thrusts are a male sexually dimorphic behavior prompted in the female by certain stimuli, short-term use of a progestin may be helpful to stop the behavior early. More important, however, is the need for environmental changes, including the provision of more exercise.[24,81]

## Other Problems

Unusual behaviors can be related to medical problems, too. For example, urinary tract, anal sac, and vaginal infections can result in odors that attract male dogs. Tumors, like granulosa cell tumors, might result in a bloody discharge similar to that of estrus.[41] Estrous behavior is occasionally observed in pregnant bitches and in the ovariohysterectomized animal.[93] Hormone levels should be measured to help determine what is going on. Pregnancy can be confused with pyometra, especially in bitches that do not show obvious signs of estrus. Instead, "anestrus" may be the unusual case of a silent estrus, a bitch that has previously been surgically neutered, or reflect a medical condition. As with other types of behavior problems, abnormal sexual behavior can have a medical basis, so differential diagnoses must consider hormonal, medical, and behavioral etiologies.

## References

1. Albone ES: Mammalian Semiochemistry: The Investigation of Chemical Signals Between Mammals. New York: John Wiley & Sons Inc, 1984.
2. Alexander SA, Shane SM: Characteristics of animals adopted from an animal control center whose owners complied with a spaying/neutering program. J Am Vet Med Assoc 1994; 205(3):472.
3. Allen WE: Pseudopregnancy in the bitch: The current view on aetiology and treatment. J Small Anim Pract 1986; 27:419.
4. Austad R, Lunde A, Sjaastad ØV: Peripheral plasma levels of oestradiol-17β and progesterone in the bitch during the oestrous cycle, in normal pregnancy and after dexamethasone treatment. J Reprod Fertil 1976; 46(1):129.
5. Barrau MD, Abel Jr JH, Verhage HG, et al: Development of the endometrium during the estrous cycle in the bitch. Am J Anat 1975; 142(1):47.
6. Barton A: Sexual inversion and homosexuality in dogs and cats. Vet Med 1959; 54:155.
7. Batchelor A, Bell ET, Christie DW: Urinary oestrogen levels in the Beagle bitch. J Endocrinol 1971; 51(2):xxvi.
8. Batchelor A, Bell ET, Christie DW: Urinary oestrogen excretion in the beagle bitch. Br Vet J 1972; 128(11):560.
9. Beach FA: Locks and beagles. Am Psychol 1969; 24(11):971.
10. Beach FA: Coital behavior in dogs. VIII. Social affinity, dominance and sexual preference in the bitch. Behaviour 1970; 36:131.
11. Beach FA: Coital behavior in dogs. IX. Sequelae to "coitus interruptus" in males and females. Physiol Behav 1970; 5(3):263.
12. Beach FA, Buehler MG, Dunbar IF: Competitive behavior in male, female, and pseudohermaphroditic female dogs. J Comp Physiol Psychol 1982; 96(6):855.
13. Beach FA, Gilmore RW: Response of male dogs to urine from females in heat. J Mammal 1949; 30:391.
14. Beach FA, Johnson AI, Anisko JJ, et al: Hormonal control of sexual attraction in pseudo hermaphroditic female dogs. J Comp Physiol Psychol 1977; 91:711.
15. Beach FA, Kuehn RE: Coital behavior in dogs. X. Effects of androgenic stimulation during development of feminine mating responses in females and males. Horm Behav 1970; 1:347.
16. Beach FA, Kuehn RE, Sprague RH, et al: Coital behavior in dogs. XI. Effects of androgenic stimulation during development on masculine mating responses in females. Horm Behav 1972; 3(2):143.
17. Beach FA, LeBoeuf BJ: Coital behaviour in dogs. I. Preferential mating in the bitch. Anim Behav 1967; 15:546.
18. Beach FA, Merari M: Coital behavior in dogs. V. Effects of estrogen and progesterone on mating and other forms of social behavior in the bitch. J Comp Physiol Psychol 1970; 70(1):1.
19. Beach FA, Rogers CM, LeBouf BJ: Coital behavior in dogs: Effects of estrogen on mounting by females. J Comp Physiol Psychol 1968; 66(2):296.

20. Beaver BV: Mating behavior in the dog. Vet Clin North Am 1977; 7(4):723.

21. Beaver BV: Feline Behavior: A Guide for Veterinarians, 2nd ed. Philadelphia: Saunders, 2003.

22. Beaver BV: The Veterinarian's Encyclopedia of Animal Behavior. Ames: Iowa State University Press, 1994.

23. Bekoff M, Diamond J, Milton JB: Life history patterns and sociality in canids: Body size, reproduction, and behavior. Oecologia (Bed) 1981; 50:386.

24. Belaiche AD, Hart BL: Behavior problems. Canine Pract 1977; 4(5):6.

25. Bell ET, Bailey JB, Christie DW: Studies on vaginal cytology during the canine oestrus cycle. Res Vet Sci 1973; 14(2):173.

26. Bell ET, Christie DW: Duration of proestrus, oestrus, and vulval bleeding in the beagle bitch. Br Vet J 1971; 127(8):xxv.

27. Bell ET, Christie DW: Bodyweight changes during the canine oestrous cycle. Br Vet J 1971; 127(10):460.

28. Bell ET, Christie DW: The evaluation of cellular indices in canine vaginal cytology. Br Vet J 1971; 127(12):xiii.

29. Bigbee HG, Hennessey PW: Megestrol acetate for postponing estrus in first-heat bitches. Vet Med Small Anim Clin 1977; 72(11):1727.

30. Bleicher N: Behavior of the bitch during parturition. J Am Vet Med Assoc 1962; 140:1076.

31. Bleicher N: Physical and behavior analysis of dog vocalization. Am J Vet Res 1963; 24(100):415.

32. Borchelt P, Voith VL: Dominance aggression in dogs. Compend Contin Educ Pract Vet 1986; 8(1):36.

33. Brown JM: Efficacy and dosage titration study of mibolerone for treatment of pseudopregnancy in the bitch. J Am Vet Med Assoc 1984; 184(12):1467.

34. Bryan HS: Parenteral use of medroxyprogesterone acetate as an antifertility agent in the bitch. Am J Vet Res 1973; 34(5):659.

35. BSAVA Congress Report: Sequelae to bitch sterilisation: Regional survey. Vet Rec 1975; 96:371.

36. Burke TJ, Reynolds Jr HA: Megestrol acetate for estrus postponement in the bitch. J Am Vet Med Assoc 1975; 167(4):285.

37. Chaffaux S, Locci D, Poruois M, et al: Induction of ovarian activity in anoestrous beagle bitches. Br Vet J 1984; 140(2):191.

38. Chakraborty PK, Fletcher WS: Responsiveness of anestrous Labrador bitches to GnRH. Proc Soc Exper Biol Med 1977; 154(1):125.

39. Chakraborty PK, Panko WB, Fletcher WS: Serum hormone concentrations and their relationships to sexual behavior at the first and second estrous cycles of the Labrador bitch. Biol Reprod 1980; 22(2):227.

40. Chakraborty PK, Wildt DE, Seager SWJ: Induction of estrus and ovulation in the cat and dog. Vet Clin North Am [Small Anim Pract] 1982; 12(1):85.

41. Cheng N: Aberrant behavior in a bitch with a granulosa-theca cell tumour. Aust Vet J 1992; 70(2):71.

42. Christie DW, Bailey JB, Bell ET: Classification of cell types in vaginal smears during the canine oestrous cycle. Br Vet J 1972; 128(6):301.

43. Christie DW, Bell ET: Changes in rectal temperature during the normal oestrous cycle in the Beagle bitch. Br Vet J 1970; 127:93.

44. Christie DW, Bell ET: Some observations on the seasonal incidence and frequency of oestrus in breeding bitches in Britain. J Small Anim Pract 1971; 12(3):159.

45. Christie DW, Bell ET: Endocrinology of the oestrous cycle in the bitch. J Small Anim Pract 1971; 12(7):383.

46. Christie DW, Bell ET: Studies on canine reproductive behavior during the normal oestrous cycle. Anim Behav 1972; 20(4):621.

47. Clemens LG, Gladue BA, Coniglio LP: Prenatal endogenous androgenic influences on masculine sexual behavior and genital morphology in male and female rats. Horm Behav 1978; 10:40.

48. Concannon P, Whaley S, Lein D, et al: Canine gestation length: Variation related to time of mating and fertile life of sperm. Am J Vet Res 1983; 44(10):1819.

49. Concannon PW, Powers ME, Holder W, et al: Pregnancy and parturition in the bitch. Biol Reprod 1977; 16(4):517.

50. Concannon PW, Weigand N, Wilson S, et al: Sexual behavior in ovariectomized bitches in response to estrogen and progesterone treatments. Biol Reprod 1979; 20(4):799.

51. Connolly PB: Reproductive behaviour problems. In Horwitz DF, Mills DS, Heath S (eds): BSAVA Manual of Canine and Feline Behavioural Medicine, Quedgeley, Gloucester, England: British Small Animal Veterinary Association, 2002, p. 128.

52. Crenshaw WE, Carter CN: Should dogs in animal shelters be neutered early? Vet Med 1980; 90(8):756.

53. Daniels TJ: The social organization of free-ranging urban dogs. II. Estrous groups and the mating system. Appl Anim Ethol 1983; 10:365.

54. Darder P, López J, Fatjó JF, et al: Pseudopregnancy in the bitch: An epidemiological study. In Mills D, Levine E, Landsberg G, et al (eds): Current Issues and Research in Veterinary Behavioral Medicine. West Lafayette, IN: Purdue University Press, 2005, p. 243.

55. Dore MA: The role of the vaginal smear in the detection of metoestrus and anoestrus in the bitch. J Small Anim Pract 1978; 19(10):561.

56. Doty RL, Dunbar I: Attraction of beagles to conspecific urine, vaginal, and anal sac secretion. Physiol Behav 1974; 12:825.

57. Dunbar IF: Olfactory preferences in dogs: The response of male and female beagles to conspecific odors. Behav Biol 1977; 20:471.

58. Edqvist L-E, Johansson EDB, Kasström H, et al: Blood plasma levels of progesterone and oestradiol in the dog during the oestrous cycle and pregnancy. Acta Endocrinol 1975; 78(3):554.

59. Fält L, Wilsson E: The effect of maternal deprivation between 6 and 10 weeks of age upon the behaviour of Alsatian puppies. Appl Anim Behav Ethol 1979; 5(3):299.

60. Fidler IJ, Brodey RS, Howson AE, et al: Relationship of estrous irregularity, pseudopregnancy, and pregnancy to canine pyometra. J Am Vet Med Assoc 1966; 148(8):1043.

61. Fox MW: Maternal aggression in the dog. Vet Rec 1964; 76(27):754.

62. Fox MW: Spontaneous displacement activities, compulsive behaviour and abnormal social behaviour in the dog. Vet Rec 1964; 26(31):840.

63. Fox MW: Control of masturbation in dogs. Mod Vet Pract 1967; 48(9):68.

64. Fox MW: Understanding Your Dog. New York: Coward, McCann & Geoghegan Inc, 1972.

65. Fox MW: The Dog: Its Domestication and Behavior. New York: Garland STPM Press, 1978.

66. Frankland AL: Vaginal cytology and reproductive behaviour in the bitch. Br Vet J 1972; 128(9):478.

67. Freak MJ: I. Abnormal conditions associated with pregnancy and parturition in the bitch. Vet Rec 1962; 74(48):1323.

68. Freshman J: Canine and feline reproduction. Texas Veterinary Medical Association meeting, Fort Worth, TX, January 31, 1997.

69. Fuller JL: Photoperiodic control of estrus in the Basenji. J Heredity 1956; 47:179.

70. Fuller JL, Fox MW: The behaviour of dogs. In Hafez ESE (ed): The Behaviour of Domestic Animals, 2nd ed. Baltimore: Williams & Wilkins, 1969, p. 438.

71. Gentry C: When Dogs Run Wild: The Sociology of Feral Dogs and Wildlife. Jefferson, NC: McFarland & Co Inc, 1983.

72. Gerber HA, Jöchle W, Sulman FG: Control of reproduction and of undesirable social and sexual behaviour in dogs and cats. J Small Anim Pract 1973; 14:151.

73. Gerber HA, Sulman FG: The effect of methyloestrenolone on oestrus, pseudo-pregnancy, vagrancy, satyriasis and squirting in dogs and cats. Vet Rec 1964; 76(39):1089.

74. Ghosh B, Choudhuri DK, Pal B: Some aspects of the sexual behaviour of stray dogs *Canis familiaris*. Appl Anim Behav Sci 1984; 13(1-2):113.

75. Goodwin M, Gooding KM, Regnier F: Sex pheromone in the dog. SCI 1979; 203(4380):559.

76. Gorman ML, Trowbridge BJ: The role of odor in the social lives of carnivores. In Gittleman JL (ed): Carnivore Behavior, Ecology and Evolution. Ithaca, NY: Comstock Publishing Associates, 1989, p. 57.

77. Hadley JC: Total unconjugated oestrogen and progesterone concentrations in peripheral blood during the oestrous cycle of the dog. J Reprod Fertil 1975; 44(3):445.

78. Hart BL: Normal behavior and behavioral problems associated with sexual function, urination, and defecation. Vet Clin North Am 1974; 4(3):589.

79. Hart BL: Normal sexual behavior and behavioral problems in the male dog. Canine Pract 1975; 2(2):11.

80. Hart BL: Gonadal hormones and behavior of the female dog. Canine Pract 1975; 5(2):8.

81. Hart BL: Deviant sexual behavior of the spayed bitch. Mod Vet Pract 1976; 57:663.

82. Hart BL: Problems with objectionable sociosexual behavior of dogs and cats: Therapeutic use of castration and progestins. Compend Contin Educ 1979; 1:461.

83. Hart BL: Maternal behavior in the twentieth century. Canine Pract 1979; 6(6):18.

84. Hart BL: Postparturient maternal responses and mother-young interactions. Canine Pract 1980; 7(1):10.

85. Hart BL: Advising clients on selecting and socializing dogs: Effects of gonadectomy. American Veterinary Medical Association meeting, Minneapolis, July 17, 1993.

86. Hart BL, Eckstein RA: The role of gonadal hormones in the occurrence of objectionable behaviours in dogs and cats. Appl Anim Behav Sci 1997; 52(3-4):331.

87. Hart BL, Hart LA: Selecting pet dogs on the basis of cluster analysis of breed behavior profiles and gender. J Am Vet Med Assoc 1985; 186(11):1181.

88. Holst PA, Phemister RD: The prenatal development of the dog: Preimplantation events. Biol Reprod 1971; 5(2):194.

89. Holst PA, Phemister RD: Onset of diestrus in the Beagle bitch: Definition and significance. Am J Vet Res 1974; 35(3):401.

90. Holst PA, Phemister RD: Temporal sequence of events in the estrous cycle of the bitch. Am J Vet Res 1975; 36(5):705.

91. Hoskins JD: DVMs can help clients understand behaviors during, after delivery. DVM June 2001:2S.

92. Houpt KA: Problems in maternal and sexual behaviors. American Veterinary Medical Association meeting, Minneapolis, July 18, 1993.

93. Houpt KA: Sexual behavior problems in dogs and cats. Vet Clin North Am [Small Anim Pract] 1997; 27(3):601.

94. Houpt KA: Sexual and maternal behavior problems: More common than you think. Am Vet Med Assoc Conv Proc, 2006.

95. Houpt KA, Coren B, Hintz HF, et al: Effect of sex and reproductive status on sucrose preference, food intake, and body weight of dogs. J Am Vet Med Assoc 1979; 174(10):1083.

96. Houtsmaller EJ, Slob AK: Masculinization and defeminization of female rats by males located caudally in the uterus. Physiol Behav 1990; 48(4):555.

97. Howe LM, Slater MR, Boothe HW, et al: Long-term outcome of gonadectomy performed at an early age or traditional age in dogs. J Am Vet Med Assoc 2001; 218(2):217.

98. Jöchle W: Pet population control: Chemical methods. Canine Pract 1974; 1-2:8.

99. Jöchle W, Andersen AC: The estrous cycle in the dog: A review. Theriogenology 1977; 7(3):113.

100. Johnson CA, Grace JA: Care of newborn puppies and kittens. Forum 1987; 6(1):9.

101. Johnston SD: Signs of pseudocyesis following ovariohysterectomy. Mod Vet Pract 1978; 59(7):490.

102. Kleiman D: Reproduction in the canidae. Int Zoo Yearbook 1968; 8:3.

103. Kleiman DG, Eisenberg JF: Comparisons of canid and felid social systems from an evolutionary perspective. Anim Behav 1973; 21:637.

104. Korda P, Brewinska J: The effect of stimuli emitted by sucklings on tactile contact of the bitches with sucklings and on number of licking acts. Acta Neurobiol Exp 1977; 37:99.

105. Korda P, Brewinska J: The effect of stimuli emitted by sucklings on the course of their feeding by bitches. Acta Neurobiol Exp 1977; 37:117.

106. Krzeminski LF, Sokolowski JH, Dunn GH, et al: Serum concentrations of mibolerone in Beagle bitches as influenced by time, dosage form, and geographic location. Am J Vet Res 1978; 39(4):567.

107. Lake SG: Controlling oestrus in the dog. Vet Rec 1977; 101(26-27):530.

108. Lieberman LL: A case for neutering pups and kittens at two months of age. J Am Vet Med Assoc 1987; 191(5):518.

109. Macdonald DW: The carnivores: Order Carnivora. In Brown RE, Macdonald DW (eds): Social Odours in Mammals, vol 2, Oxford, England: Clarendon Press, 1985, p. 619.

110. Mahlow JC: Estimation of the proportions of dogs and cats that are surgically sterilized. J Am Vet Med Assoc 1999; 215(5):640.

111. Mann CJ: Some clinical aspects of problems associated with oestrus and with its control in the bitch. J Small Anim Pract 1971; 12(7):391.

112. Marder A, Engel J: Behavior problems after adoption. AVSAB Ann Symp Anim Behav Res 2002 Meeting Proc:6.

113. Masken JF: Circulating hormone levels in the cycling beagle. Gaines Dog Research Progress 1973; Winter:7.

114. Meisel RL, Ward IL: Fetal female rats are masculinized by male littermates located caudally in the uterus. SCI 1981; 213:239.

115. Mellin TN, Orczyk GP, Hichens M, et al: Chemical inhibition of estrus in the Beagle. Theriogenology 1976; 5(4):165.

116. Mellin TN, Orczyk GP, Hichens M, et al: Serum profiles of luteinizing hormone, progesterone and total estrogens during the canine estrous cycle. Theriogenology 1976; 5(4):175.

117. Naaktgeboren C: Some aspects of parturition in wild and domestic Canidae. Int Zoo Yearbook 1968; 8:8.

118. Nasar R, Mosier JE, Williams LW: Study of the feline and canine populations in the greater Las Vegas area. Am J Vet Res 1984; 45:282.

119. O'Farrell V, Peachey E: Behavioural effects of ovariohysterectomy on bitches. J Small Anim Pract 1990; 31:595.

120. Olson PN, Bowen RA, Behrendt MD, et al: Concentrations of testosterone in canine serum during late anestrus, proestrus, estrus, and early diestrus. Am J Vet Res 1984; 45(1):145.

121. Olson PN, Bowen RA, Behrendt MD, et al: Concentrations of progesterone and luteinizing hormone in the serum of diestrous bitches before and after hysterectomy. Am J Vet Res 1984; 45(1):149.

122. Olson PN, Pouliot M: Guide dogs schools: A model for interdisciplinary studies on canine behaviour. Proc Third International Cong Vet Behav Med 2001:69.

123. Olson PN, Pouliot M: New concepts in addressing canine behavior: Guide dog schools as a model. http://www.avma.org/conv/cv2002/cvnotes/CAn_AnB_NCA_OlP.asp, 7/3/2002.

124. Pal SK: Parental care in free-ranging dogs, *Canis familiaris*. Appl Anim Behav Sci 2005; 90:31.

125. Pet sterilization. Bull Inst Study Anim Probl 1979; 1(3):4.

126. Phemister RD: Nonneurogenic reproductive failure in the bitch. Vet Clin North Am 1974; 4(3):573.

127. Phemister RD, Holst PA, Spano JS, et al: Time of ovulation in the Beagle bitch. Biol Reprod 1973; 8(1):74.

128. Pierantoni L, Verga M: Behavioural consequences of premature maternal separation and of a lack of stimulation during the socialization period in dogs. In Landsberg G, Mattiello S, Mills D (eds): Proceedings of the 6th International Veterinary Behaviour Meeting & European College of Veterinary Behavioural Medicine-Companion Animals European Society of Veterinary Clinical Ethology. Brescia, Italy: Fondazione Iniziative Zooprofilattiche e Zootecniche, 2007, p. 102.

129. Piñol MJ, Cornelles S, Fatjó J, et al: Effects of early separation and handling of puppies on maternal licking in the bitch. In Mills D, Levine E, Landsberg G, et al (eds): Current Issues and Research in Veterinary Behavioral Medicine. West Lafayette, IN: Purdue University Press, 2005, p. 295.

130. Polydorou K: Stray-dog control on Cyprus: Primitive and humane methods. Int J Study Anim Prob 1983; 4:146.

131. Prole JHB: The control of oestrus in racing Greyhound bitches using norethisterone acetate. J Small Anim Pract 1974; 15(4):213.

132. Prole JHB: The effect of the use of norethisterone acetate to control oestrus in Greyhound bitches on subsequent racing performance and fertility. J Small Anim Pract 1974; 15(4):221.

133. Richmond G, Sachs BD: Further evidence for masculinization of female rats by males located caudally in utero. Horm Behav 1984; 18:484.

134. Salmeri KR, Bloomberg MS, Scruggs SL: Prepubertal gonadectomy in the dog: Effects on skeletal growth and physical development. Proc World Small Anim Vet Assoc Br Small Anim Vet Assoc, as reported in Alpo Veterinary Clinic Briefs 1990; 8(2):2.

135. Salmeri KR, Bloomberg MS, Scruggs SL, et al: Gonadectomy in immature dogs: Effects on skeletal, physical, and behavioral development. J Am Vet Med Assoc 1991; 198(7):1193.

136. Scarlett JM, Salman MD, New Jr JG, et al: Reasons for relinquishment of companion animals in U.S. animal shelters: Selected health and personal issues. J Appl Anim Welfare Sci 1999; 2(1):41.

137. Schultz TH, Kruse SM, Flath RA: Some volatile constituents of female dog urine. J Chem Ecol 1985; 11(2):169.

138. Schulte AP: Canine vaginal cytology. I. Technique and cytological morphology. J Small Anim Pract 1967; 8(6):301.

139. Schulte AP: Canine vaginal cytology. II. Cyclic changes. J Small Anim Pract 1967; 8(6):307.

140. Shille VM, Thatcher MJ, Simmons KJ: Efforts to induce estrus in the bitch, using pituitary gonadotropins. J Am Vet Med Assoc 1984; 184(12):1469.

141. Simmons JG, Hammer CE: Inhibition of estrus in the dog with testosterone implants. Am J Vet Res 1973; 34(11):1409.

142. Smith MS, McDonald LE: Serum levels of luteinizing hormone and progesterone during the estrous cycle, pseudopregnancy, and pregnancy in the dog. Endocrinology 1974; 94:404.

143. Smith WC, Reese Jr WC: Characteristics of a Beagle colony. I. Estrous cycle. Lab Anim Care 1968; 18(6):602.

144. Sokolowski JH: Evaluation of estrous activity in bitches treated with mibolerone and exposed to adult male dogs. J Am Vet Med Assoc 1978; 173(8):983.

145. Sokolowksi JH, Medernach RW, Helper LC: Exogenous hormone therapy to control the estrous cycle of the bitch. J Am Vet Med Assoc 1968; 153(4):425.

146. Sokolowski JH, Stover DG, VanRavenswaay F: Seasonal incidence of estrus and interestrous interval for bitches of seven breeds. J Am Vet Med Assoc 1977; 171(3):271.

147. Sokolowski JH, Zimbelman RG: Evaluation of selected compounds for estrus control in the bitch. Am J Vet Res 1976; 37(8):939.

148. Spain CV: The best time to neuter dogs: Long-term risks and benefits of early neutering. http://www.avma.org/conv/cv2002/cvnotes/CAn_PSN_TND_SpV.asp, 7/3/2002.

149. Spain CV, Scarlett JM, Houpt KA: Long-term risks and benefits of early-age gonadectomy in dogs. J Am Vet Med Assoc 2004; 224(3):380.

150. Spaying/neutering dogs at 8 weeks of age. DVM Manage Consult Rep 1988; 19(5):1.
151. Stabenfeldt GH: Physiologic, pathologic and therapeutic roles of progestins in domestic animals. J Am Vet Med Assoc 1974; 164(3):311.
152. Tedor JB, Reif JS: Natal patterns among registered dogs in the United States. J Am Vet Med Assoc 1978; 172(10):1179.
153. Threlfall WR: Estrous cycle (normal and abnormal): What is clinically normal? http://www.avma.org/conv/cv2002/cvnotes/CAn_The_ECN_ThW.asp, 7/3/2002.
154. Thun R, Watson P, Jackson GL: Induction of estrus and ovulation in the bitch, using exogenous gonadotropins. Am J Vet Res 1977; 38(4):483.
155. Trivers RL: Parent-offspring conflict. Am Zool 1974; 14:249.
156. Van der Weyden GC, Taverne MAM, Okkens AC, et al: Intra-uterine position of canine fetuses and their sequence of expulsion at birth. J Am Vet Med Assoc 1982; 180(8):901.
157. Van Os JL, Oldenkamp EP: Oestrus control in bitches with proligestone, a new progestational steroid. J Small Anim Pract 1978; 19(9):521.
158. Vig MM, Blackledge GT: Automobile accidents correlate with estrus in dogs. J Am Vet Med Assoc 1982; 181(4):372.
159. Voith VL: Behavioural problems. In Chandler EA, Evans JM, Singleton WB, et al (eds): Canine Medicine and Therapeutics. Oxford, England: Blackwell Scientific, 1979, p. 395.
160. Voith VL: Functional significance of pseudocyesis. Mod Vet Pract 1980; 61:75.
161. Vom Saal FS: Variation in phenotyped due to random intrauterine positioning of male and female fetuses in rodents. J Reprod Fert 1981; 62:633.
162. Vom Saal FS, Bronson FH: In utero proximity of female house mouse fetuses to males: Effect on reproductive performance during later life. Biol Reprod 1978; 19:842.
163. Wilbur RH: Pets, pet ownership and animal control: Social and psychological attitudes. Proc Natl Conf Dog Cat Control, Denver, February 3-5, 1976, p. 21.
164. Wildt DE, Chakraborty PK, Panko WB, et al: Relationship of reproductive behavior, serum luteinizing hormone and time of ovulation in the bitch. Biol Reprod 1978; 18(4):561.
165. Wildt DE, Levinson CJ, Seager SWJ: Laparoscopic exposure and sequential observation of the ovary of the cycling bitch. Anat Rec 1977; 189(3):443.
166. Wildt DE, Panko WB, Chakraborty PK, et al: Relationship of serum estrone, estradiol-17β and progesterone to LH, sexual behavior and time of ovulation in the bitch. Biol Reprod 1979; 20(3):648.
167. Wildt DE, Seager SWJ, Chakraborty PK: Behavioral, ovarian and endocrine relationships in the pubertal bitch. J Anim Sci 1981; 53(1):182.
168. Wilsson E: The social interaction between mother and offspring during weaning in German shepherd dogs: Individual differences between mothers and their effects on offspring. Appl Anim Behav Sci 1984; 13(1-2):101.
169. Wilsson E, Sundgren P-E: Effects of weight, litter size and parity of mother on the behaviour of the puppy and the adult dog. Appl Anim Behav Sci 1998; 56(2-4):245.
170. Wright PJ: The induction of oestrus and ovulation in the bitch using pregnant mare serum gonadotrophin and human chorionic gonadotrophin. Aust Vet J 1980; 56(3):137.
171. Wright PJ: The induction of oestrus in the bitch using daily injections of pregnant mare serum gonadotrophin. Aust Vet J 1982; 59(4):123.

## Additional Readings

Brodey RS, Fidler IJ, Howson AE: The relationship of estrous irregularity, pseudopregnancy, and pregnancy to the development of canine mammary neoplasms. J Am Vet Med Assoc 1966; 149(8):1047.

Burke TJ: Pharmacologic control of estrus in the bitch and queen. Vet Clin North Am [Small Anim Pract] 1982; 12(1):79.

Campbell WE: Social aspects of whelping and litter care. Mod Vet Pract 1974; 55(5):404.

Campbell WE: Pot pourri. Mod Vet Pract 1977; 58(2):167.

Catton DG: Chemotherapeutic oestrus control in the bitch and latest advances. J S Afr Vet Assoc 1980; 51(4):213.

Christie DW, Bell ET: Changes in the dimensions of the uterus of the Beagle bitch during the oestrous cycle. J Small Anim Pract 1972; 13(2):97.

Davis LE: Adverse effects of drugs on reproduction in dogs and cats. Mod Vet Pract 1983; 64(12):969.

Donovan CA: Canine anal glands and chemical signals (pheromones). J Am Vet Med Assoc 1969; 155(12):1995.

Evans JM, Uvarov O, Valliance DK: Hormonal control of the oestrus cycle in the bitch. Vet Rec 1969; 85(8):233.

Gobello C, Castex G, Corrada Y: Use of cabergoline to treat primary and secondary anestrus in dogs. J Am Vet Med Assoc 2002; 220(11):1653.

Hansen BD, Hardie EM, Carroll GS: Physiological measurements after ovariohysterectomy in dogs: What's normal? Appl Anim Behav Sci 1997; 51(1-2):101.

Hardie EM, Hansen BD, Carroll GS: Behavior after ovariohysterectomy in dogs: What's normal? Appl Anim Behav Sci 1997; 51(1-2):111.

Igel GJ, Calvin AD: The development of affectional responses in infant dogs. J Comp Physiol Psychol 1960; 53(3):302.

Joshua JO, Taylor DR: Unusual behaviour in the bitch. Vet Rec 1972; 90(6):163.

Kirk GR, Kirby R, Cox VS, et al: The effects of light deprivation on the development of the gonads in the dog. J Am Anim Hosp Assoc 1976; 12(4):528.

Kirkwood JK: The influence of size on the biology of the dog. J Small Anim Pract 1985; 26:97.

Lieberman LL: Advantages of early spaying and neutering. J Am Vet Med Assoc 1982; 181(5):420.

Malm K, Jensen P: Regurgitation as a weaning strategy—A selective review on an old subject in a new light. Appl Anim Behav Sci 1993; 36(1):47.

Olson PN, Johnston SD: New developments in small animal population control. J Am Vet Med Assoc 1993; 202(6):904.

Pearson RE: Unusual maternal behaviour in the bitch. Vet Rec 1972; 90(2):50.

Robinson R: Relationship between litter size and weight of dam in the dog. Vet Rec 1973; 92(9):221.

Sokolowski JH: False pregnancy. Vet Clin North Am [Small Anim Pract] 1982; 12(1):93.

Spain CV, Scarlett JM, Cully SM: When to neuter dogs and cats: A survey of New York state veterinarians' practices and beliefs. J Am Anim Hosp Assoc 2002; 38(5):482.

Spanel-Borowski K, Thor-Wiedemann S, Pilgrim C: Cell proliferation in the dog (Beagle) ovary during proestrus and early estrus. Acta Anat (Basel) 1984; 118(3):153.

Stopforth A: Unusual maternal behaviour in the bitch. Vet Rec 1972; 90(4):109.

Verhage HG, Abel Jr JH, Tietz Jr WJ, et al: Development and maintenance of the oviductal epithelium during the estrous cycle in the bitch. Biol Reprod 1973; 9(5):460.

Vomachka AJ, Lisk RD: Androgen and estradiol levels in plasma and amniotic fluid of last gestational male and female hamsters: Uterine position effects. Horm Behav 1986; 20:181.

# CHAPTER 7

# Canine Ingestive Behavior

A lot is known about ingestive behaviors of dogs, but much of this information remains hidden within the confines of the major dog food manufacturers. Independent research is providing some interesting observations that are useful in understanding all dogs.

## SUCKLING BEHAVIOR

Nursing by neonates is the start of a dog's eating behavior. During most of parturition, the bitch shows little interest in nursing any of her puppies. Once they all have been born, though, she quietly presents her mammary surface to them. Newborn puppies have little strength and coordination, so their first attempts to nurse are clumsy and awkward. Because of the rooting reflex, puppies burrow into any warm, soft surface they encounter. This warm, soft surface is usually the littermates or the dam, so this reflex helps ensure that the puppies will find food and warmth. As their heads bob up and down during nursing bouts, they also swing back and forth. The rear limbs move, too, as the puppies try to remain in an upright position. After touching a nipple, the neonate will make several attempts to grasp it and then make several attempts to nurse before being able to achieve proper suction.[20,61] Some puppies seem more proficient than others, and most will perfect the technique as they get older.

While the puppy nurses, it makes a rhythmic, kneading movement of its forelimbs against the bitch's mammary region. This kneading motion may serve one or more purposes. Newborn puppies have a blocky appearance to their face, and the nose does not elongate until the puppy is a few weeks old. Considering the fact that the kneading occurs during sucking and is most consistent in very young puppies, one might speculate that it helps push the mother's abdomen away from the youngster's nose.[55] A second function might be to help stimulate milk flow via massage of the mammary gland,[20] although, in theory at least, massage should come later, as larger puppies require more milk. Also, massage should occur in a suckle-knead-suckle-knead cycle. By 17 days of age, forelimb thrusting is no longer seen in the puppies, and by 21 days, their sucking is no longer rhythmic but has become noisy and irregular instead.[55]

The lip sucking reflex (Fig. 7-1) helps ensure that newborns will try to nurse on soft projections. It is independent of hunger or food intake.[89] If, however, the puppy's stomach is filled via stomach tube just before being allowed to suckle, the full puppy will spend significantly less time sucking than a puppy that was not full to begin with.[137] Sucking can also be non-nutritional, as food-satiated puppies commonly fall asleep while showing sucking behaviors. They also will show sucking behavior again if someone disturbs their sleep. This type of non-nutritional sucking has been called a "comfort behavior."

During the first 3 weeks, the mother initiates all nursing sessions. She makes the approach, presents the mammary area, and arouses the puppies by licking them. [53] The puppies do not have preferred nipple positions.[61,73]

Each day a puppy ages brings changes in needs and physiology. Many bacteria are already present in the stomach on the first day.[142] In puppies younger than 8 days of age, the stomach usually contains 1 to 5 ml of milk and is very alkaline.[131] This condition of the stomach may indicate a need for frequent sucking bouts. The average daily intake is 175 g per day (150 to 175 ml).[123] After the eighth day, the puppy's stomach will hold 10 to 20 ml,[142] and milk intake reaches a peak at 26 days.[123] At this time, milk can provide 1.5 kcal/g gross energy, and the average bitch can produce 1050 g per day of milk (approximately 1 L).[123]

## TRANSITIONAL INGESTIVE BEHAVIOR

By 4 weeks after birth, puppies start developing the eating behaviors that they will use as adults, yet they continue nursing, too. This is the age at which the young should be introduced to semisolid food. It is also a time when the bitch becomes less cooperative in nursing bouts, so the puppies are more apt to solicit the mother to nurse. She usually cooperates with the solicitations by lying down. After day 30, the young initiate all nursing bouts.[73] The bitch is

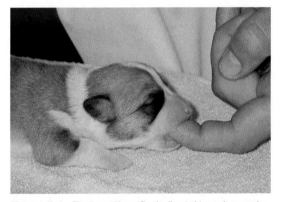

**Figure 7-1.** The lip sucking reflex is directed toward any projection, including fingers.

apt to restrict the length of these periods, be gone longer, and even show aggression to the puppies if they attempt to nurse more often than she wishes them to.[21,61,110] Their solicitation attempts become increasingly unsuccessful during this period, with the mother remaining standing for the ever shorter nursing bouts (Fig. 7-2). She might even lie down and hide her nipples against the floor.[73]

In wolves, this is also a time of increased nursing demands by the cubs. To meet this need and help ensure survival of the cubs, the nonpregnant females go through pseudocyesis about the same time that the dominant female is pregnant. Nursing can then stimulate lactation in females that are not the cub's mother.[72]

For most puppies, their first solid food is some variety of commercial dog food, either canned or moistened to make it compatible to deciduous teeth and soft gums. Deciduous teeth are in place by 3 weeks and are not replaced until 16 to 26 weeks.[107] Care is necessary during this transitional period because sometimes a bitch will aggressively compete with her puppies for available food.[61] If she is well fed, this competition for food is unlikely to occur. Variance in flavors in puppy diets is not particularly important to long-term diet preferences in adult dogs,[52] but it does help prevent some

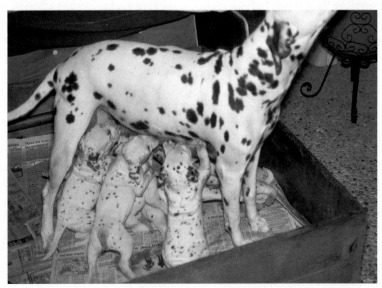

**Figure 7-2.** The bitch stands so that nursing is more difficult for the puppies.

individuals from becoming picky eaters. Considerable individual variation exists in the amount of milk and solid-food intake by puppies during the transitional period. A significant correlation exists, however, between solid-food intake and the weight of the puppy.[108]

In wolves, semisolid food is introduced to the cubs at 3 to 4 weeks, when the mother and other pack members are stimulated to regurgitate by face licking from the cubs. This behavior allows the adults to carry large amounts of food for the cubs without it being stolen, and it means the young are not exposed to the dangers of traveling with the adults as they hunt large herbivores.[96,107] Eating regurgitated food also facilitates the transition from suckling to eating solid food.[106] The same type of regurgitation behavior occurs in some dogs.[15,106] Almost two thirds of pet dog breeds have displayed regurgitation for puppies on occasion.[106] Almost all free-ranging bitches will regurgitate for their puppies and males will occasionally do so too.[128] The age of the puppies when the behavior starts varies but usually occurs at 3 to 6 weeks (Fig. 7-3). Although 78% of the time it is the mother that regurgitates food for the puppies, other dogs may be involved.[96,106,107] The sire is involved 3% of the time, and other nearby dogs the remainder of the time.[106] It takes more effort by the puppies to get other dogs besides the mother to regurgitate.[106] The puppies initiate the regurgitation 15% of the time, the adult dog initiates it 29%, and both are equally involved 56% of the time.[106]

Many owners fail to realize that the regurgitation of stomach contents by an adult dog in the presence of appropriately aged puppies is normal and, furthermore, may not be limited to the mother of the puppies. Therefore, in the history-taking for any dog presented for vomiting or regurgitation, it is important to discover if the dog is around young puppies.

While the litter remains together, competition for food increases food intake by each puppy until dominance relations have been established.[55,61] Puppies will normally eat 14% to 50% more when fed as a group than when fed individually.[61,91] If a single puppy is fed until it is "full," it will eat 30% to 200% more if its hungry littermates are then allowed to eat.[61,91] After dominance is established, social facilitation becomes important.[90] When social relations develop between group members that are fed together, the dogs will eat more in the group than if fed alone,[71,78,90,91] but dominant puppies, simply with their presence, may inhibit some of their littermates from eating as much.

Even though weaning is complete at 7 to 10 weeks in dogs and wolves,[107,110] young wolves are

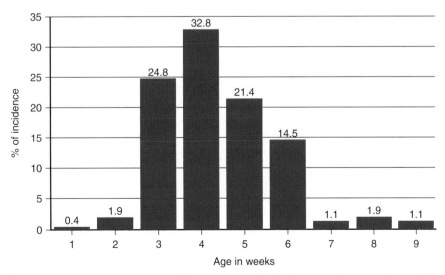

**Figure 7-3.** Age of puppies when regurgitation from food solicitation first occurs. (Data from reference 106.)

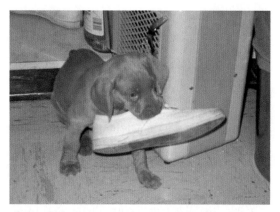

**Figure 7-4.** Oral exploration is a normal part of puppy learning.

not capable of hunting large prey until they are at least 4 months of age.[107] To learn the necessary skills and develop appropriate strength, wolf cubs usually do not become independent until 4 to 6 months.[107]

## Non-Nutritional Chewing

Puppies show oral behaviors that are not associated directly with eating. Mouthing behaviors are a normal canine form of exploration and investigation that begin at the onset of socialization—around 3 weeks.[55,78] By chewing, licking, carrying, tugging, and even swallowing small objects, a puppy can gain sensory information about its environment (Fig. 7-4). The actual relationship of chewing on objects to teething remains unclear.[78] Certain breeds seem to show these behaviors more. Those with mouth-oriented adult traits, like Labrador Retrievers and German Shepherds, are more likely to show a lot of oral activity as puppies. Thus, control measures must be taken so that the mouthing behavior does not become a problem. The use of a crate for young puppies controls their access to objects so their oral activity can be directed to two or three likable chew-toys. Chew-toys can be made more attractive by smearing them with food or by tucking food in the crevices. Praise should be used when the puppy plays with the toy, and a "No" and replacement with an acceptable toy should be used for incidences of inappropriate chewing.[86]

Coprophagy is also a normal behavior in puppies for a short period.[55] Eating the feces from another dog may help a puppy establish normal flora in the intestinal tract, and diet can affect intestinal flora.[2] Coprophagy in puppies may simply represent an exploratory behavior. In either case, the owner should not punish the behavior. Instead, the puppy's attention could be diverted to another activity or access prevented to the feces of other dogs.

## ADULT INGESTIVE BEHAVIOR

Once dominance has been established, juvenile eating behaviors are gradually replaced by adult ones. Most wild canids survive with a feast-or-famine type of food intake, because the successful hunting of large game is sporadic.[14,27,61,75,124] The tendency with this pattern is to overeat when food is plentiful to get past the times when it is scarce. Dogs tend to retain the feast-or-famine characteristics and will eat more calories than necessary if food is available. When free-choice dry food is available, dogs tend toward eating several meals per day within just a few days.[25,133] Individually housed dogs eat whenever fresh food is offered and usually will eat three to six meals per day.[78,133] If the dogs are kept in groups instead of singly, however, their tendency is to eat nine to twelve meals per day.[78,82] In general, dogs tend to eat more than they need for maintenance,[61,92] and it has even been hypothesized that a second set point for body weight may develop when highly palatable food is routinely offered.[78] Approximately 70% of dogs will eat a great deal more than they are used to eating if the food is available.[25]

Pet-feeding patterns of dog owners have been studied.[33,48,130,141] Only 26% of dog owners feed their pet once a day; others feed their pets more often. Even the dogs that are fed just once a day get treats in addition to their meal. Figure 7-5 shows what types of food—dry and canned dog food, treats, table food, and so forth—are provided.

There are apparently a number of controls for food intake by dogs. For a short time, distention resulting from the bulk of the food is the major factor for limiting intake.[55,78,94,139] Caloric content,[55,93] body temperature,[49,78] ambient temperature,[47,78,133] stress,[57] oropharyngeal sensory input,[94,97] timing of the food availability,[133] olfaction,[78] taste and texture,[75,78] and intestinal chemoreceptors[78] also can

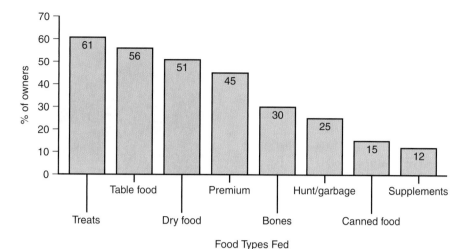

**Figure 7-5.** Feeding characteristics of dogs. (Data from reference 141.)

be restrictive. Food intake will decrease 4% for every 10° F (2° C) rise in environmental temperature.[47] The influences of smell on the perception of taste appear to involve a cognitive mechanism.[74] Taste appears to influence the perception of smell as well, probably by way of oropharynx to nasopharynx.[74] The tendency to adjust daily intake from bulk to caloric needs is modified only slowly.[93]

## Food Preferences

Several studies have been reported on the relative preferences of various foods by dogs. It is important to remember that these preferences are relative, although individual food preferences do exist. A palatable food is one that has some probability of being eaten under some specific conditions.[66] Preference has to do with the likelihood that one of two available foods will be eaten under very specific conditions.[66] Many types of meals are palatable under certain conditions and not others, and foods that are sometimes regarded as unpalatable can even be highly desirable when the dog is hungry.[97] This fact is particularly relevant in regard to dogs that must forage for all or part of their food. Even within the components of garbage, a preference ranking can be determined.[16]

Comparison of food preferences indicates that dogs prefer meat to a food that is high-protein and fatty but nonmeat (Fig. 7-6).[78,83] The descending

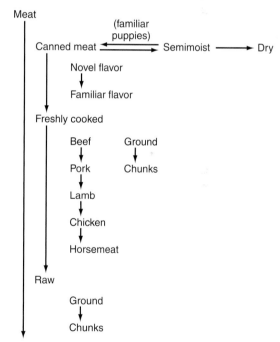

**Figure 7-6.** General taste preferences of dogs. (Data from references 78, 83.)

preference order for meat is beef, pork, lamb, chicken, and horsemeat.[78,83,103,149] Canned food is usually preferred to semimoist food, and that to dry kibble.[78,95,143,149] Canned meat is preferred to the same meat freshly cooked, and the freshly cooked meat is preferred to raw.[78,83,103,149] Ground meat is preferred to meat chunks by dogs, and warm rates better than cold.[83]

A novel canned flavor is preferred initially 90% of the time to a long-term familiar food.[52,78,95,159] This is true too in puppies fed a specific food from weaning until 6 months and then offered a novel one.[84] If given choices early, palatability and the maternal affect of a dam's diet flavoring her milk may negate the draw of a novel food.[78] If a puppy is familiar with semimoist food, it will prefer it to canned foods.[78]

Dogs prefer sweet to bland tastes,[83,149] so sweet tastes also can be rated by preferences. The predominant taste bud units of the facial nerve of a dog are the type A ones that respond to amino acids.[27] Many of these amino acids are described as "sweetish" by people.[27] Glucose ranks as the most liked, followed by fructose, sucrose, and table sugar.[34,58] Even though sucrose is liked by dogs,[65,80,95] fructose ranks higher than sucrose, the opposite of humans and pigs.[78] Saccharin and maltose are not liked.[65,78] Dogs tend to overeat sweet foods.[158] As natural foods do not contain a lot of sweets, nature has developed no method to limit intake of sweet foods.

When the sense of smell is lost through disease, trauma, or experimental manipulation, palatability and preferences are also affected. The preference for meat or sucrose over a bland cereal remains, but preferences in between are eliminated.[78,83]

Although food preferences rarely pose a problem for dogs, a puppy's early experience with solid food can influence its choices later. If fed limited diets before 6 months of age, a puppy may continue to choose to eat that particular diet as an adult.[71,149] Even later a dog can acquire a preference for a certain food if it is exposed to the odor of that food on the breath of another dog that ate that same food.[105] Antidotal reactions to certain are dogs that become very distressed when lamb is cooked.[60] Some of these dogs will eat lamb but others will not.

## Plant (Grass) Eating

Most owners have observed their dogs eating grass or other plants (Fig. 7-7). Grass eating represents a normal behavior that if carried to excess can be considered a problem. Grass is eaten more often

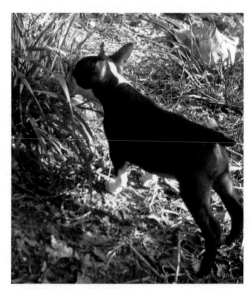

**Figure 7-7.** Grass eating by a dog is a normal behavior.

that other types of plants, and there is no correlation with the frequency of eating plants to sex, breed, diet, internal parasite load, or other behavioral problems.[145] Instead, the behavior is related to that seen in wolves. Wolves eat large ungulates, with the viscera being a favorite portion of the prey. In eating the abdominal contents, a wolf normally takes in some partially digested vegetable matter. Carnivores lack the ability to break the beta-bonds of cellulose to glucose, which is then converted to volatile fatty acids for absorption, so they depend on a partially digested form instead.[9,14] Yet, most dogs will routinely eat small amounts of grass without adverse effects. Problems arise only if the dog has not had access to vegetable matter for a while, as can occur over winter.[9,14] They then tend to eat large amounts of grass when they have access to it again. Since they cannot digest this material, it remains as a gastrointestinal irritant until the dog either vomits it up or passes it in the feces.

Apparently some dogs learn to associate plant eating with vomiting and seek out plants at times when they are not feeling well.[9,14] The incidence of plant-associated vomiting can be minimized by supplementing the dog's diet with small amounts of fresh grass or with cooked vegetables (cooking starts the breakdown of cellulose).[9,14] Because some plants are poisonous to dogs, it is best to prevent access to any poisonous or favorite household plants.[119]

## Hunting (Predatory) Behavior

Ancestral feeding patterns still play a role in the dog's ingestive behavior. The order Carnivora literally means "eaters of flesh."[149] Canids have developed sophisticated pack-hunting techniques.[96] As the size of the prey hunted by wolf ancestors for their primary food source increased, hunting techniques changed. Pack sizes now typically range from 2 to 12 members, although they can be larger.[114] Group hunting allows a pack to locate, chase, kill, and eat large animals more efficiently.[114] In theory an individual would have more food available per meal than does a pack member; however, the advantages of group hunting increase the likelihood the hunt will be successful. Also, scavengers are more successful against the individual hunter, so total take is less.[157]

For *Canis lupus,* the gray wolf, certain prehunt behaviors are typical. As the pack members get together, there is much tail wagging and activity to motivate the leaders to hunt.[114] Once prey is located, the hunting behavior sequence begins. At first, the wolves will stalk the prey animal to get as close to it as possible. Then comes the encounter. As the wolves and prey confront each other, large prey tend to stand their ground, whereas smaller ones tend to bolt.[114] The hunters will rush toward the retreating animal. A chase can get up to a speed of 35 to 40 miles per hour and usually does not go for more than 2 miles.[114] Success at catching prey from this chase varies from 25% to 63%.[114]

When the wolves catch smaller prey, they typically throw it down and tear anywhere at its flesh.[114] Larger prey are usually attacked from behind in the rump, flank, or rear limbs by several wolves, as one wolf holds the nose of the prey.[114] During feeding of the downed animal, pack members tend to stand side by side around the carcass and usually start on the rump and abdomen, tearing in every direction.[114] Food is eaten quickly. If space is limited, higher ranking members eat first, juveniles eat last.[27] A correlation exists between the size of the prey and either the size of the predator or the

number of cooperative predators of the same species.[55] All canids have a tendency to bury extra food after they are satiated.[129]

By 4 weeks of age, some wolf cubs will begin showing predatory behavior toward rats.[55] Within a few days of starting this behavior, they will crush the rat immediately and weakly shake it.[55] Shaking behaviors will eventually be used to stun smaller prey while strengthening the predator's grip on its prey.[129] Cubs rarely play with their prey in the presence of another wolf.[55] They also prefer prey that move and make noise.[55]

The point of discussing hunting behavior in the wolf is that much of the same behavior is shown by dogs, including orientation toward the prey and attack sites. When dogs attack larger animals, the wounds are often in the perineum and area of the tailhead.[3] Slightly smaller victims of dog attacks, like calves, sheep, or ponies, have a predominance of wounds to the rear limbs, head, or neck. The opportunity to successfully stalk is not common for dogs, because truly feral populations are not common, and most dogs do not have access to prey.

Dogs will chase moving objects because prey-chasing behavior is initiated by the sight of something moving rapidly away. The intensity of the urge to pursue increases with the length of the pursuit.[129] This is why the dog may chase the family cat when it is in its yard but ignore the cat in the house. Prey-shaking behavior likewise increases with the length of the pursuit. If no chase is initiated, or if the chase is short, prey shaking is likely to be minimal or absent. For example, a rabbit placed immediately in front of a dog is probably much safer than one given a 20-foot head start.

Unlike wolves, the presence of another dog increases the incidence of play directed toward prey. This play behavior includes a lot of prey shaking and throwing of the prey in the air, as well as pawing and nosing.[56] Puppies younger than 10 weeks of age typically show attempts to pin down the prey with their front limbs—the forelimb stab—with and without a vertical leap.[58] They also show all the various aspects of adult predatory behaviors in fragmented sequences associated with other play behaviors.[58] Another feature of the puppy form of play is the inhibited bite.[58] Movements and sounds reinforce the various behaviors, and immobility is responded to by nosing and pawing. When the prey tries to escape, its movements are followed by the chase or blockage of escape.[56] Even a dead rat will be played with by laying it between the forepaws, nosing, nipping, and tossing it in the air.[56] Dominance is not asserted over possession of prey in dogs, which is different than in other canids.[56]

During a biting attack on prey, all canids will flatten their ears and partially close their eyes.[56] When they are striking with a forepaw, their head and neck are raised and arched and the ears pricked upward.[56] As with other consummatory behaviors, such as mating and eliminating, the undisturbed canid shows a "consummatory facial expression" with ears partially flattened and eyes partially or fully closed, a pleasure face (see Chapter 3, Fig. 3-5).[56]

Selective breeding has produced many variations in play behavior. It has been suggested that dogs are the neotenic descendants of some canid ancestor, which means that behaviors like herding or guarding represent the retardation of development that led to the retention of certain ancestral juvenile or embryonic characteristics.[38] According to this theory, the livestock-guarding dogs would represent the most juvenile forms because of their physical features of floppy ears and domed skulls.[38] The herding dogs have a somewhat less juvenile form, with more adult-shaped skulls and half-erect ears.[38] When dogs of various breeds are field tested with goats, most react by barking, stalking, chasing, and attacking.[63] Basenjis regularly attack as a pack.[63] Other dogs show attack inhibition, which apparently is genetically programmed to take effect at a certain stage of predation. Both sight and smell hounds excel in the tracking or trailing aspect of predation but are less likely to go beyond this point in the behavior sequence. Sheep and cattle dogs have been observed to stop at herding or driving, whereas dogs like Boarhounds and Terriers continue on to the attack/kill stage. Retrievers have the tendency to provision cubs or mates.[38,58] Another variation of selective breeding is the dog that guards one species (such as sheep) but will attack other species (like coyotes) as potential predators.[38] Stalking and pointing tend to be traits of setters and pointers. Diet has been shown to affect the performance too,

with some commercial products resulting in more birds while bird hunting.[44]

Large herbivores are not the only prey for canids. Dogs will go after rabbits, cats, birds, and occasionally even fish.[148] Other small species unique to certain locations also might be consumed, such as poultry, iguanas, or tortoises.[7,62] It is suggested that because more than one type of wolf gives rise to dogs, their adaptability to different types of food may be a result of that background.[149] No correlation has been found between hunting efficiency and the social rank, size, or sex of the hunter.[24] Studies of stomach contents and feces analysis from a feral dog population of free-ranging dogs revealed a variety of foodstuffs, indicating the dogs had been acting as both predators and scavengers. Foods of animal origin included rabbits, mice, songbirds, carrion, and insects.[62,138] Other items that dogs can consume include foods of plant origin like grass, leaves, and fruits (especially persimmons).[62,138] Maggots, a find in 40% of the samples, indicate that dogs commonly eat decaying tissues.[62] With more than 1 million wild animals becoming road kill each year in the United States,[62] free-ranging and feral dogs are likely to drag off this readily available food source without detection. Trash also has become a major source of food for dogs.[62,125,138] Not only is the uncontrolled dog a nuisance because it breaks open garbage bags, but garbage can be a major food source for some dog populations.[62,125,136]

## WATER CONSUMPTION

Drinking has two components—the behavior and the underlying process that results in water consumption. A dog laps water with its tongue. The tongue is curled backward and serves as a ladle to lift the water into the mouth (Fig. 7-8). Because the curl is almost flat across instead of cup-shaped, much of the water spills out from the sides before the dog can get it into the mouth. Depending on the rate of lapping, size of the tongue, size of the water dish, and distance between the mouth and the water, a dog can dribble water over a large area or keep almost all of it in the water bowl.

The amount a dog drinks each day depends on a number of factors, but the most significant is size.

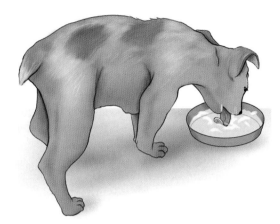

**Figure 7-8.** The dog's tongue curls backward while it drinks, but the flat curl allows water to run off the corners.

The average dog takes in approximately 1100 ml of water per day.[61] Of this amount, approximately half comes from eating food and the other half from drinking.[61] On average, a dog drinks nine times per day, averaging 60 ml per time.[61] As ambient temperature increases, so does water consumption.[133] The regulation of water consumption depends on several things. For a short period, the amount of water passing through the mouth and pharynx can bring a temporary end to drinking.[17] A second factor that helps inhibit drinking is distention of the stomach.[150] Subsequent permanent satiation follows intestinal absorption[150] that exactly replenishes the body's water deficit,[132,134] rebalances plasma sodium levels,[76,131,163] and helps restore extracellular electrolyte levels.[36] Cholecystokinin, which is released when high-protein or fatty foods are eaten, stimulates gallbladder contraction, increases pancreatic enzyme secretion, and acts as a satiety agent.[82]

## NEURAL AND HORMONAL REGULATION

Several related neurohormonal responses are associated with eating. Gastin, adrenocorticotropic hormone, prolactin, growth hormone, oxytocin, and insulin are released with digestion.[151,152,153] The output of somatostatin, an inhibitory peptide, is reduced.[151] Pregnancy and lactation are associated with changes in the gastrointestinal hormones that may increase digestive and anabolic capacity.[102] During pregnancy, the levels of gastrin, somatostatin, and cholecystokinin increase.[102] Somatostatin levels remain elevated during the first week or so of lactation; gastrin and cholecystokinin increase in response to suckling.[102,151] Insulin and prolactin levels also rise in response to suckling by young.[151,152] Oxytocin levels rise in response to suckling by young, eating by the bitch, and the presence of food in the gastrointestinal tract.[151,153]

Within the brain, several areas of the hypothalamus affect eating behaviors. The "satiety center" in the ventromedial hypothalamus helps stop the desire for food and is responsible for adipose regulation.[99] Experimental stimulation of the ventromedial hypothalamus causes anorexia, and destruction of this area causes hyperphagia. The lateral hypothalamus, or "feeding or hunger center," is associated with glucose availability.[82] Stimulation of this area causes great increases in food intake, even in the satiated. On the other hand, destruction of the lateral hypothalamus results in aphagia. Much of the research relating to the central regulation of eating behaviors has been done in the cat, and the reader is directed to other references for more detailed information.[12] The pontine parabrachial nucleus is important for the acquisition of taste aversion.[18]

Other inputs influence eating behaviors directly or indirectly: environmental temperatures, osmotic pressures in the small intestines, social facilitation, and the taste and smell of food, to name a few.[82] Flavor validation is primarily based on olfaction, as can be shown when a trained dog loses as much as 75% of its ability to select a specific meat when made anosmic.[81]

Psychodietetics is the study of behavior and diet.[5] Understanding the relationship between the two can be difficult and constantly undergoes modification as researchers gather new information. Of most interest at the current time is the dietary influence of the amino acids on the neurotransmitters. Tryptophan becomes 5-hydroxytryptophan, which becomes serotonin. Tyrosine is changed to dihydroxyphenylalanine and then to dopamine, which can change to noradrenaline, and that to adrenaline.

The third pathway is histidine, which becomes histamine. The last pathway is lecithin, to choline, to acetylcholine, and back to choline. From the amino acids of tryptophan, tyrosine, lecithin, and histidine come six neurotransmitters—serotonin, dopamine, noradrenaline, adrenaline, acetylcholine, and histamine (see Chapter 2, Box 2-1).[5]

# INGESTIVE BEHAVIOR PROBLEMS

The actual incidence of behavior problems that involve the use of the mouth is unknown. If obesity is included, the incidence is probably greater than 50% of all dogs. If obesity is excluded, the various eating problems combine to approximately 1.4% to 4% of all dogs[1,6,13,19] and up to 5.3% to 38% when destructive chewing is included.[1,13,35,88] In dogs older than 9 years of age, destructive behaviors are almost exclusively associated with separation anxiety.[35]

## Polyphagia

Excessive eating and compulsive eating (polyphagia) can be related to a number of behavioral or medical conditions. This behavior is common in old dogs when a new dog is introduced into a home.[78] Diabetes mellitus is also associated with polyphagia, because the eating-related hypothalamic centers are apparently nonresponsive to blood glucose levels and react as if they needed higher levels.[79]

## Obesity

By far, the largest oral-related behavior problem in dogs today is obesity, defined as an excessive accumulation of body fat sufficient to impair body functions.[50] The incidence of obesity has been estimated at 20% to 44% of pet dogs.* Several factors tend to be associated with obesity. Females are more likely than males to be obese,[69,100,112,122] and ovariohysterectomized females more so than intact ones.[4,80,82,100] Middle-aged dogs are approximately twice as likely to be obese than are younger dogs.[100,112,122] Dogs that get treats, table scraps, or home-cooked meals also have a higher incidence of obesity.[100,112,122]

The owners' perceptions also affect the dog. Almost one third of the owners of obese dogs consider their dog's weight to be normal.[112,122] Almost half of obese owners and a quarter of nonobese owners have dogs that are obese.[100,112,122] Owners older than 40 years of age are almost twice as likely to have an obese pet as younger owners.[100,112,122] Obesity in dogs varies by breed, so it may be partially controlled by a genetic predisposition.[82,100,112,122] Breeds specifically noted for being overweight include American Cocker Spaniels,[100,122] Labrador Retrievers,[100,122] Collies,[100,122] Cairn Terriers,[100,122] West Highland White Terriers,[77,122] Scottish Terriers,[77,122] and Beagles.[78]

Because dogs evolved from the wolf, they retain many of the behaviors associated with their ancestor, including a feast-or-famine eating pattern. If food is available, most dogs will continue eating until they can hold no more.[71,121] Each time food is presented, a dog may eat as if it does not know when its next meal will come, even though it is fed at the same time every day. Obesity also comes about because of a combination of factors, such as genetic predisposition, the availability of highly palatable and calorically dense foods, and the tendency of many owners to give high-calorie treats to their dog.[71,77] Modern dogs also get less exercise than their wild relatives. Without having to make long trips to hunt prey, they expend fewer calories, so fewer are needed for maintenance. Some animal models of obesity suggest there can also be a defective gene expression, an example being adipocyte secretion of adipsin into the blood.[135]

Prevention of or treatment for obesity is usually dependent on the owner. The hardest task is to convince the owner and everyone else in the household that the dog has a problem.[69,100] Owners like to reward their dogs, even if it is for something as simple as just being a dog or for begging.[69,77] Instead of food, rewards can be verbal praise, petting, or playing with toys.[121] Owners should limit the times and locations where the dog is fed, and all food should be placed in the dog's dish instead of fed by hand or offered on dishes used by humans.[121] This helps remind owners not to overfeed, and it decreases the dog's tendency to beg at the table. Of course, the traditional recommendations of reducing daily

---

*References 4, 69, 77, 78, 82, 84, 100, 112, 122.

caloric intake and increasing the amount of exercise the dog gets are the major parts of weight management.[23,50,69,100] Pharmacologic suppression of appetite has not been useful for treating canine obesity,[23,77,78,100] but the newer weight control product can be useful for the truly obese dog.

## Pica

Pica is an abnormal craving to eat nonfood items, unusual foods, or non-nutritive items.[14,26,77,126] The list of items that dogs have eaten is extensive. It includes toys, jewelry, dirt, house plants, electric cords, marbles, antifreeze, clothing, pencils, coins, rocks, linoleum, blankets, chairs, underwear, balls, and many other things. In some cases, as when a dog eats a knife, the object may be coated with juices of meats or other real food attractants, so the item is eaten accidentally. It is important to differentiate these cases from cases of true pica. It is also important to differentiate pica from destructive chewing, where objects are torn apart and not eaten.

The causes of pica are numerous. Brain lesions involving the hypothalamus and extreme nutritional deficiencies have been associated with pica.[14] With the intense fixation some dogs have toward a specific target, obsessive-compulsive disorders may be manifested with this behavior. Preference for antifreeze over water has been given as a reason dogs are so likely to drink it; however, experimental data do not support this hypothesis.[111] Attention seeking, play solicitation, and response to stress also have been suggested as other causes of pica.[26,144] Humans have certainly been known to eat more often when stressed. If a dog has been mouth-oriented since it was a puppy and normal dog food is not available, it is reasonable that stress could be expressed orally toward nonfood items. Although some of these dogs might simply engage in destructive chewing, others ingest the materials.

Treatment for pica may be easy or complicated, depending on severity and duration. Keeping the dog away from preferred materials is the only sure way to prevent pica from occurring again. This can mean picking up a favorite target, confining the dog away from the object, or even muzzling the dog, as with the cage or basket muzzles, when appropriate. Once pica starts, early intervention allows the owner to interrupt the behavior and either provide an acceptable substitute or direct the dog to a more appropriate behavior.[126] Taste aversion and controlled access can be particularly useful at this time. If there have been recent changes in the home that indicate stress is part of the cause, antianxiety medications may be helpful while efforts are made to tighten up the dog's overall schedule, including providing more exercise. As the behavior becomes chronic, it becomes more programmed to occur and much harder to extinguish. Prevent access to material the dog likes to eat, perhaps with the addition of a tricyclic antidepressant or selective serotonin reuptake inhibitor, if an obsessive compulsive problem is suspected.

## Upsetting Garbage

Garbage can raids are commonly made by dogs. Over 50% of the garbage bags are broken into within 24 hours of being set out for pickup, and most of the animals that break into them are owned dogs.[77,162] Scavenging through human trash is an important food-gathering activity of feral dogs as well.[59] The attractant seems to be food. Items commonly found in human garbage have been tested in paired trials to determine what the favorite components are. It is no surprise that meats were preferred to nonmeat items or that fresh odors rated higher than those aged 72 hours.[16] Fried liver with onions and baked chicken topped the fresh and aged list of favorites.[16] Raw liver was the highest ranking uncooked meat, but it only ranks twelfth of 26 items.[16]

A great deal of time and effort has gone into finding a repellent for dogs in an effort to keep them from scattering garbage or to keep them out of that which has already been scattered. Other uses could repel dogs from a specific livestock pen, the yard, or a flower bed. No commercial product offers long-term success as yet. Scent gland secretions from rattlesnakes or other reptiles have not been successful.[160,161] Capsaicin, the irritant in red chili pepper, will repel coyotes for a while.[147] Other chemicals that have shown some repellent activity include β-chloroacetyl chloride[98]; cinnamaldehyde[98]; 1 carvone (0.1), 1-naphthalene thiol (0.05) [98]; methyl nonyl ketone[162]; and methyl nonyl ketone combined with cinnamic aldehyde.[162] The bottom line of many of the studies is that results of repellent in the laboratory can be very different than those in the field, so promising products need to be tested in both situations.[162] Spray repellents have been reported to actually attract dogs to garbage, perhaps because the dogs use it as an olfactory clue to the availability of garbage.[77]

## Effects of Dietary Reduction

When caloric restrictions are imposed to treat obesity, behaviors may be negatively affected. Small dogs put on very severe diets show an initial increase in general activity immediately prior to feeding.[41,42] A decrease in activity follows as the restriction continues.[41,42] Overall, severe caloric restrictions—that is, those approaching half of what is needed for maintenance—may actually be counterproductive because of the reduced activity levels that accompany them.[41,42] These responses can be minimized, which also makes an owner more likely to comply with the protocol, if the reductions in amounts occur very gradually over a several-week period. Fights among dogs on calorie-restricted diets drop from 0.12 to 0.0 incidents per hour.[43]

Quality of the diet also affects behavior.[39] As the quality increases, food guarding increases. In hyperactive, livestock-guarding dogs, it may be necessary to reduce the digestibility of the food eaten to prevent the development of predatory motor patterns, an undesirable trait.[39]

## Anorexia

Anorexia is the loss of the desire to eat, so it is necessary to differentiate between a dog that wants to eat but cannot and a dog that has no interest in food at all. In the former case, consideration should be given to the possibility of pain. This pain could be from cranial fractures, bad teeth, cervical vertebral instability, or from other sources that punish the dog with each attempt it makes to eat. Eventually the dog quits eating even though salivation and some interest remain. When a dog has no interest in the food at all, several possible causes should be investigated.[77] Anorexia is usually associated with illness—wherein appetite is suppressed by fever, nausea, or cachexia—or with psychogenic influences (anorexia nervosa) such as separation anxiety.

A few dogs refuse to eat because they are holding out for a better-tasting morsel.[78]

Some dogs show partial anorexia. If the owner puts food down and then leaves the house, the dog may not touch the food until the owner's return. Then it immediately runs to the food bowl to eat. A second type of partial anorexia is seen in dogs that are light eaters. This behavior is a normal variation and should be accepted rather than treated. A reduction in food intake is commonly associated with estrus and pseudocyesis.[26,127] A third type of dog may not like a particular dog food and is willing to wait for something better. In this case, the dog may actually be rewarded for its anorexic behavior when the owner starts offering treats and special foods to induce it to eat.[26,78]

When intervention for anorexia should start is not a very exact science. It is rare that a healthy dog will starve to death rather than eat, but outwaiting the dog can be difficult for some owners. When boarded, some dogs refuse to eat anything until the owner returns or until they form a relationship with one of the employees. This behavior is very distressing to owners, who always notice the weight loss upon their return. Future problems in these cases may be prevented by gradually having the dog become accustomed to a boarding facility and its staff for small periods of time over several weeks. Other options might be to have a house/pet sitter, leave the dog with friends or family, or take it along instead of boarding it. In most situations where stress seems to cause the anorexia, careful handling or antianxiety drugs can be helpful in the short term. Diazepam has been reported as the drug of choice,[77,78] but other anxiolytic drugs can be used, such as mirtazapine[117] and ciproheptadine.

## Polydipsia and Adipsia

Polydipsia is fairly common in dogs. It can be secondary to a medical problem, such as diabetes mellitus or chronic renal failure. It can also be secondary to a behavior problem, such as separation anxiety, fear-associated drooling, or excessive panting. Polydipsia also can be a primary behavior problem, as in a displacement activity or psychogenic polydipsia.[77,113] Adipsia is rare. Dogs may not want to drink water that tastes bad or is contaminated, but they will usually drink right away if given clean water. High serum sodium levels can impair thirst perception as an osmoreceptor function.[40]

## Coprophagy

A very common complaint made by dog owners is that their pet is eating feces, coprophagy. The feces can be from canine or other sources.[14,71,77,78] Most often coprophagy refers to the dog eating its own feces or that from another dog. The eating of dog feces may be under the control of different neurochemicals than is the eating of feces from another species.[126] In reality, coprophagy is uncommon, occurring in less than 10% of dogs,[43] but it is usually very upsetting to owners. Eating feces is a normal behavior in a bitch that licks the urine and feces away from her young puppies. The behavior may also be a normal method for a puppy to explore its environment or establish intestinal micro flora.[15,71,118,126]

Medically related causes must be considered, such as a poor diet,[126] pancreatic enzyme deficiency,[126] intestinal parasites,[22] malabsorption,[22] vitamin deficiencies,[140] or hydrocephalus. Ruling out medical causes is important. In addition to the complete blood count, blood chemistry panel, urinalysis, and thyroid profile, recommended tests include amylase, lipase, canine trypsin-like immunoreactivity (cPLI), cobalamin, folate, fecal fat, fecal trypsin, fecal muscle fiber, trace minerals, fecal float, and fecal stain.[119,140] Coprophagy in adult dogs seems to be more common in those that do not get much exercise, are kept in a barren environment, or are small.[15,119]

Once coprophagy has been diagnosed and medical causes systematically ruled out, treatment of the behavior problem can be directed in several ways. The yard needs to be kept clean of fecal piles to minimize the attraction, especially to young dogs.[126] If the problem is relatively new, coprophagy may be stopped simply by changing the character of the feces. This can be done by changing the diet of the dog whose feces is eaten. Owners also can change the taste of the feces with additives like monosodium glutamate (meat tenderizers, For-Bid),[118] pineapple, trypsin supplements, or crushed breath mints.[146]

A second method of stopping coprophagy is to make the feces undesirable after it has been voided by means of taste-aversion techniques as described in Chapter 2. It is hard to imagine that feces could be made less desirable than it already is, but faithful treatment of each feces pile after the initial lesson in aversion with hot sauce, pepper, kerosene, steak sauce, monosodium glutamate, or other bad taste may deter those dogs in which the problem is not yet deeply ingrained.[23,71,78,126] Apomorphine or other emetics in the feces may successfully induce vomiting, and the vomiting may inhibit further coprophagy in some dogs.[71,78,126] Also during this time of topically treating the feces, if the dog gets access to untreated feces it is an important intermittent reinforcement of the wrong behavior.

Coprophagy also can be addressed by preventing access to feces—the only method that will consistently work. Dogs should be walked on leash when taken out to eliminate so the owner controls the situation.[77,78,126,146] While the dog is under leash control, the owner can topically treat fresh feces with the pepper sauce or other product,[77] or the dog can be given a food reward immediately after defecating and thereby counterconditioned to expect the food rather than go after the feces.[67] Muzzling the dog with a rigid type of muzzle is another way to prevent it from getting to the feces.[126]

Cat feces is something many dogs seek out. It is high in protein and so can have dietary appeal.[15] Cat litterboxes should be put up high, covered, or put it in a room where the dog is not allowed. If this type of management makes litterbox accessibility too difficult for the cat, it may be necessary to ignore the dog's coprophagy. The behavior is aesthetically unpleasant to the owners, but to the dog, it is rewarding and usually not harmful.

Dogs will eat ungulate feces, particularly from horses (Fig. 7-9). This feces may offer special types of nutrition, like enrichment from large intestinal fermentation,[77,78] partially digested vegetable matter, as was discussed under "Plant (Grass) Eating,"[15] or B vitamins.[126] This type of coprophagy can be difficult to control unless the dog is prevented from being around the feces. As would be expected with a highly desirable food, most dogs will sneak opportunities to get horse feces if the owner reprimands too much.

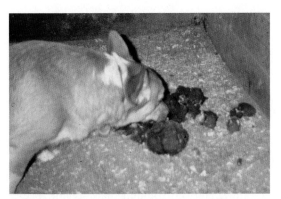

**Figure 7-9.** Dogs commonly eat horse feces.

## Destructive Chewing

Dogs engage in destructive chewing for a number of reasons, making it a very common problem.[87] Puppies from mouth-oriented breeds are presented as behavior problems because of chewing furniture, window sills, shoes, socks, kitchen cabinets, or barrier gates. This behavior is a natural outlet for play and exploration that needs to be channeled elsewhere very early.[8,101] These same puppies, usually from large breeds, have a lot of energy that needs to be expended. If that energy does not get used physically, it is likely to be used orally. Emphasis for mouth activities can also be increased by owners who encourage mouth-oriented activities, like tug-of-war games and chew objects of toys, old socks, or shoes.[8,87] It is also a common problem in dogs older than 4 months of age that are adopted from an animal shelter.[109]

Mouthing behaviors in puppies have not been specifically linked to teething, and in fact, tend to continue long after all the permanent teeth are in place. Because these mouth-oriented behaviors are normal for puppies, the puppy should not be punished. They should be supervised, so if caught in the act of chewing, the puppy's attention can be diverted[8,119] or an acceptable substitution made as with a rawhide chew. In anticipation of a problem, it is easier to confine the puppy where it cannot get into trouble. It is common for puppy chewing to continue for 1½ years, so proper crate training is useful to save property as well as to housebreak young dogs. Puppies can also be tethered to the owner to be sure they do not get into trouble when out of the crate. Specific items that may be particularly dangerous to the puppy, like electrical cords, can be treated with a bad-tasting substance and avoidance taught by taste aversion. The treated object is then put in the puppy's mouth and the puppy rewarded as soon as the object is spit out.[156] Alternatively, home improvement stores sell protective covers for electrical cords.[119] A mouthy puppy can try an owner's patience severely, but hard work to channel the chewing to a few specific toys is time well spent in the long run.

Destructive chewing can also start in young adults with no previous chewing problem. History taking should seek out precipitating events and when they occurred.[154] Stressful events, like the arrival of a new baby, a change of schedule creating separation anxiety, the erection of a barrier, the use of inappropriate punishment, a delay in feeding times, or a lack of environmental stimulation can result in destructive chewing. It is important to distinguish destructive chewing caused by separation anxiety or thunderstorm phobias from other types. It may be necessary to videotape the dog's behavior when the owner leaves to do this.

When the problem of destructive chewing is not associated with separation anxiety or phobias, several approaches to treatment are possible, but the best is to remove the source of the problem, if possible. Many approaches discussed elsewhere for other behavior problems can be applied. Stress created by the presence of new babies and separation anxiety are social behavior problems. Chewing through a fence is an escape behavior, just as is digging under or climbing over the fence.

Some general recommendations are helpful. First, be sure that the owner is not accidently rewarding the behavior with attention. For some dogs, negative attention may be better than none at all. A specific schedule or routine should be established to allow for day-to-day continuity. Routine helps minimize the stressful impact on the dog of changes in the owner's life. The dog's routine not only involves feeding schedules and elimination times but also specific times of interaction with owners, during which the dog is rewarded for correct obedience or performance tricks.[154] Another important part of the dog's routine is exercise. This period of exercise should be long enough to use up excess energy,[154] so there will be less energy to direct toward destructive chewing.

The dog should gradually get used to a crate or muzzle, or both, so that the dog views them as normal additions to its environment. Without a gradual introduction, the dog may panic and frantically claw at confinement. Chewing on one or two acceptable toys should be encouraged while the owner is home. When the owner is gone, the dog should be crated and a rawhide chew given as a reward for going in the crate.

Chewing on unacceptable things can be discouraged by taste aversion. When owners catch the dog in the act of destructive chewing, they can chase the dog with a hissing spray, as from a spray deodorant. They should not corner the dog. After that experience, the odor can be used to coat the wrongfully chewed item as a form of smell aversion.[31] Another approach is to substitute an acceptable chew-toy each time the dog starts chewing the wrong item.[29] This approach obviously requires careful monitoring of the dog, but it is a good technique with young puppies. It teaches what objects are acceptable to chew and which ones are not. Another technique involves controlling access to the unacceptable things that the dog likes to chew and using remote punishment. Here, the dog views the punishment as coming from the item and does not make a connection to the owner. Each time it begins to chew the specific item, the punishment occurs. Punishment can be provided by taste or odor aversion, coating the object with sticky tape, or placing the object where, to reach it, the dog must break a light beam that remotely turns on an electric switch that activates an electric hair dryer or blower. An unlimited number of situations can be set up to consistently punish in a specific circumstance. Owners also need to remember to reward desirable behaviors with random rewards. Punishment alone, especially for a normal behavior that the owner does not like, is very stressful to the dog.

Medical problems should also be considered as differential diagnoses for destructive chewing. Hepatoencephalopathies, gastritis/esophagitis, or mouth pain are some to consider.[87,104] These need to be ruled out before a treatment plan is determined.

## Unacceptable Prey Chasing

The instinct for predation is strong in dogs, and breed tendencies toward this behavior have also developed.[8] Because the chase itself has a certain amount of self-reward,[8,10] it can be extremely difficult to stop. It is also common for dog owners to have difficulty accepting that their mild-mannered pet could do so much damage to another animal. Domestic livestock of all types are common victims of dog attacks. Poultry tend to bunch up, compounding the extent of the problem because of smothering or bruising. Cats are often killed because they are shaken. Larger ungulate injuries typically involve the tearing of parts out of the rear limbs, the neck, or the head.

Dogs that are involved in predation of livestock are usually unsuspected by their owner. Dogs are responsible for greater than 90% of most livestock attacks.[68] Even the very shy dog will become very different when it joins at least one other as a pack member.[26,155] Of investigated attacks involving 59 incidences of livestock predation, 20 involved single dogs, 32 were done by pairs of dogs, and 7 involved packs of 3 to 7 dogs.[37] Problem dogs are usually owned dogs that are allowed to run free for part of the day,[68] with half never confined and the other half confined only at night or during the day.[37] Thus, almost all the incidences occur within 3.7 miles of the dog's home.[37]

Initially the dog pack chases the other animals, causing them to lose weight, and inflicts minor injuries on them. Over time, the proficiency of attacking increases so that injuries become crippling or fatal. Fatality rates can be as high as 80%.[68] Two dogs were reported to have killed over 90 sheep in a month's time.[37] In the United States, dogs kill approximately 58,000 individuals of domestic livestock species per year, for an estimated loss of over $2.5 million.[62] In a typical year, dogs may kill 20,000 deer over a 32-state area,[62] but it can be even worse, as was experienced in New York State in 1981, where approximately 24,000 deer were killed by dogs.[116] Dogs may or may not eat part of the animal they have downed. If they do not, it is probably because the chase serves as its own reward.

For the same reasons that dogs chase livestock and wildlife, they may also chase cars, joggers, children running, or children on skates or bicycles.[8,10,155] Anything that moves away rapidly can trigger prey chasing. If it makes a high-pitched noise too, it is an even better target.[26]

Stopping unacceptable prey chasing can be extremely difficult. The only two methods that are guaranteed to work are (1) keeping the dog restrained so that it never has access to potential prey,[10,155] and (2) as wildlife officials and livestock owners have done, eliminating the dog. Because the internal reward is so difficult to overcome, long-term success in any behavior modification program is very limited. Punishment would have to occur each and every time and be severe enough so that each occurrence was unpleasant and unrewarding.[10]

For the dog that chases livestock, the most successful treatment has been to force the dog to live surrounded by the species that it attacks while being constrained in such a way that it cannot attack. This could mean continuous exposure to a young kitten that has not learned to run away yet or being confined in a pen with lambs all around the outside.[54,115] The initial excitement, by the end of a few weeks, should subside as the dog becomes used to the other animals.[14,32] Some have suggested tying a dead victim or part of it into the dog's mouth or around its neck until the prey decays.[14,32] Even then, the dog really cannot be trusted. If the lamb, calf, or cat starts running, the chase might occur again. For the livestock producer, management of the potential victims can also reduce fatalities. Penning the animals near an occupied house with a night-light and having another dog serve as a warning dog can be effective deterrents.[68]

Taste aversion, with or without emesis, has also been suggested as a means of stopping predation. It is usually easily learned. Most commonly used is lithium chloride—either 4 g/500 g baited meat or 30 g in 50 ml of water per 25 lb of dog body weight laced into the meat of a carcass.[30,32,51,70] Other products also have been tried against predatory canids, including estradiol,[120] thiabendazole,[67,164] antimony potassium,[85] capsaicin,[85] and vanillamide.[85] Results are mixed and generally less than desirable. At best, these compounds may inhibit the eating of a carcass, but they generally have minimal to no effect on the chase-and-kill parts of predation.[28,51,155] The dogs also may continue to eat the laced vomitus,[149] or just the untreated meat, probably using their sense of smell to make that determination.[67] That indicates there is a "taste of potentiation of odor."[18]

For dogs that chase joggers, adults on bicycles, or cars, the approach to stop the behavior can be somewhat modified. Prey normally do not chase back, so when a person stops moving away and moves toward the dog instead, confusion in the dog becomes apparent.[8] The person in a car can accomplish the same thing by stopping the car, jumping out, and chasing the dog with noisemakers or by throwing water balloons or cans at the dog or spraying mace at it.[10,14] The success rate is guarded (less than 50%). The internal reward must be great, because over half the dogs actually hit by a car while chasing one will chase again.[8,10,14]

## Other Oral Behavior Problems

A few other types of problems belong in this chapter—vomiting being one. A common cause of vomiting, or regurgitation, is overeating. Too much intake can cause the dog to vomit. Vomiting also is associated with plant or grass eating, as discussed earlier. Psychogenic vomiting is often mistaken for physical illness and becomes a diagnosis only after the more traditional causes of vomiting are ruled out.[11] Occasionally a good history may provide a key to the diagnosis if it includes a description of the vomiting occurring at a specific time each day, in a certain location, or in association with a particular event. Also, the owner's response to each episode may actually be rewarding the behavior if the owner has been picking up the dog or giving it a lot of attention when it vomits.

Treatment for psychogenic vomiting depends on the causative factors. Certainly the dog's behavior should not be rewarded with attention, and if the behavior is predictable, the owner may be able to distract the dog before any signs start at all. Other related factors should be changed to set the dog up for distraction.

Dietary protein has specifically been linked to two undesirable behaviors: fear aggression and territorial aggression. Both behaviors decrease when dietary protein is lowered from 32% to 25% or less.[45,46] It is hypothesized that low-protein diets facilitate the conversion of tryptophan to serotonin, which in turn reduces the impulsivity of fearful dogs.[45]

Food guarding is another type of aggression that really represents material protective aggression (see Chapter 4). It has been shown to be hierarchal. Almost 60% of dogs will guard rawhides, and just over 50% will protect the human food they receive.[84] Approximately 50% of dogs show protection of bones and toys. Lower are guarding of a dog biscuit, then dog food, and finally about 8% will guard their water bowl.[84]

Gastric dilation and volvulus is typically associated with large, deep-chested breeds of dogs. Owners are usually counseled to feed multiple meals to try to prevent the condition. One study showed that in giant breeds, a high activity level and a high level of "happiness" decreased the risk of this condition occurring.[64]

Self-nursing occurs in rare individuals. Although this could be a remnant of a problem common in orphan puppies, it may spontaneously appear in older dogs too. In those cases, the behavior probably began as a comfort behavior. The sucking can result in the stimulation of milk flow, which then forms an oral reward, in addition to the internal reward. Treatment consists of physically preventing the nursing behavior and replacing the inner drive with exercise and environmental stimulation.

# References

1. AAHA pet owner survey results. Trends Mag 1993; IX(2):32.
2. Amtsberg G, Drochner W, Meyer H: Influence of food composition on the intestinal flora of the dog. In Anderson RS (ed): Nutrition of the Dog and Cat. Oxford, England: Pergamon Press, 1978, p. 181.
3. Anderson BC, Barrett DP, Lane VM, et al: Dog bite-induced perineal lacerations in beef cows. Agri Pract 1983; 4(8):45.
4. Anderson RS: Obesity in the dog and cat. In Grunsell CSG, Hill FWG (eds): The Veterinary Annual 1973. Bristol, England: John Wright and Sons, 1974, p. 182.
5. Ballarini G: Animal psychodietetics. J Small Anim Pract 1990; 31(10):523.
6. Bamberger M, Houpt KA: Signalment factors, comorbidity, and trends in behavior diagnoses in dogs: 1,644 cases (1991-2001). J Am Vet Med Assoc 2006; 229(10):1591.
7. Barnett BD, Rudd RL: Feral dogs of the Galapagos Islands: Impact and control. Int J Stud Anim Probl 1983; 4(1):44.
8. Beaver B: Therapy of behavior problems. In Kirk RW (ed): Current Veterinary Therapy VIII: Small Animal Practice. Philadelphia: Saunders, 1983, p. 58.
9. Beaver BV: Grass eating by carnivores. Vet Med Small Anim Clin 1981; 76(7):968.
10. Beaver BV: Why dogs chase cars. Vet Med Small Anim Clin 1982; 77(8):1178.
11. Beaver BV: Psychosomatic behaviors in dogs and cats. Vet Med Small Anim Clin 1982; 77(11):1594.
12. Beaver BV: Feline Behavior: A Guide for Veterinarians. Philadelphia: Saunders, 2002.
13. Beaver BV: Owner complaints about canine behavior. J Am Vet Med Assoc 1994; 204(12):1953.
14. Beaver BV: The Veterinarian's Encyclopedia of Animal Behavior. Ames: Iowa State University Press, 1994.
15. Beaver BV: Behavior development and behavioral disorders. In Hoskins JD (ed): Veterinary Pediatrics: Dogs and Cats from Birth to Six Months of Age, 2nd ed. Philadelphia: Saunders, 1995, p. 23.
16. Beaver BV, Fischer M, Atkinson CE: Determination of favorite components of garbage by dogs. Appl Anim Behav Sci 1992; 34(1-2):129.
17. Bellows RT: Time factors in water drinking in dogs. Am J Physiol 1939; 125:87.
18. Bernstein IL: Taste aversion learning: A contemporary perspective. Nutrition 1999; 15(3):229.
19. Blackshaw JK: Abnormal behaviour in dogs. Aust Vet J 1988; 65(12):393.
20. Bleicher N: Behavior of the bitch during parturition. J Am Vet Med Assoc 1962; 140:1076.
21. Bleicher N: Physical and behavioral analysis of dog vocalizations. Am J Vet Res 1963; 24:415.
22. Blum SR: Behavioral vices in dogs: Hot sauce prevents coprophagy. Mod Vet Pract 1985; 66(12):1010.
23. Bomson L, Parker CHL: Effect of fenfluramine on overweight spayed bitches. Vet Rec 1975; 96:202.
24. Borchelt PL, Voith VL: Dominance aggression in dogs. Compend Contin Educ 1986; 8(1):36.
25. Boulcott SR: Feeding behaviour of adult dogs under conditions of hospitalization. Br Vet J 1967; 123:498.
26. Bowen J: Miscellaneous behaviour problems. In Horwitz DF, Mills DS, Heath S (eds): BSAVA Manual of Canine and Feline Behavioural Medicine. Quedgeley, Gloucester, England: British Small Animal Veterinary Association, 2002, p. 119.
27. Bradshaw JWS: The evolutionary basis for the feeding behavior of domestic dogs (*Canis familiaris*) and cats (*Felis catus*). J Nutr 2006; 136(7):1927S.
28. Burns RJ: Evaluation of conditioned predation aversion for controlling coyote predation. J Wildl Manage 1980; 44:938.
29. Campbell W: Destructive chewing. Mod Vet Pract 1973; 54(6):55.
30. Campbell WE: Calf-killing dogs. Mod Vet Pract 1974; 55(3):162.
31. Campbell WE: Rote solutions. Mod Vet Pract 1976; 57(9):740.
32. Campbell WE: Fowl play. Mod Vet Pract 1977; 58(3):202.
33. Campbell WE: Effects of training, feeding regiments, isolation and physical environment on canine behavior. Mod Vet Pract 1986; 67:239.

34. Chao ET: Hedonic scaling of sugars using concurrent operant schedules with dogs. Neurosci Biobehav Rev 1984; 8(2):225.

35. Chapman B, Voith V: Dog owners and their choice of a pet. American Veterinary Society of Animal Behavior meeting, Atlanta, July 20, 1986.

36. Cizek LJ, Semple RE, Huang KC, et al: Effect of extracellular electrolyte depletion on water intake in dogs. Am J Physiol 1951; 164:415.

37. Coman BJ, Robinson JL: Some aspects of stray dog behaviour in an urban fringe area. Aust Vet J 1989; 66(1):30.

38. Coppinger R, Glendinning J, Torop E, et al: Degree of behavioral neoteny differentiates canid polymorphs. Ethology 1987; 75:89.

39. Coppinger R, Zuccotti J: Kennel enrichment: Exercise and socialization of dogs. J Appl Anim Welfare Sci 1999; 2(4):281.

40. Crawford MA, Kittleson MD, Fink GD: Hypernatremia and adipsia in a dog. J Am Vet Med Assoc 1984; 184(7):818.

41. Crowell-Davis SL, Barry K, Ballam J, et al: The effect of caloric restriction on the behavior of dogs. Appl Anim Behav Sci 1994; 39:184.

42. Crowell-Davis SL, Barry K, Ballam JM, et al: The effect of caloric restriction on the behavior of pen-housed dogs: Transition from unrestricted to restricted diet. Appl Anim Behav Sci 1995; 43(1):27.

43. Crowell-Davis SL, Barry K, Ballam JM, et al: The effect of caloric restriction on the behavior of pen-housed dogs: Transition from restriction to maintenance diets and long-term effects. Appl Anim Behav Sci 1995; 43(1):43.

44. Davenport G, Kelley R, Altom E, et al: Effect of diet on the hunting performance of English pointers. Am Vet Soc Anim Behav Proc 2001:9.

45. Dodman NH, Reisner I, Shuster L, et al: The effect of dietary protein content on aggression and hyperactivity in dogs. Appl Anim Behav Sci 1994; 39:185.

46. Dodman NH, Reisner I, Shuster L, et al: Effect of dietary protein content on behavior in dogs. J Am Vet Med Assoc 1996; 208(3):376.

47. Drews JE: Effect of temperature on food consumption, body weight and stool condition of dogs. Wayne Res Rep, September 12, 1980.

48. Dry dog food takes 59% of total pet food market. Feedstuffs 1975; 47:1.

49. Durrer JL, Hannon JP: Seasonal variations in caloric intake of dogs living in an arctic environment. Am J Physiol 1962; 202(2):375.

50. Edney ATB: Management of obesity in the dog. Vet Med Small Anim Clin 1974; 69(1):46.

51. Ellins SR, Catalano SM: Field application or the conditioned taste aversion paradigm to the control of coyote predation on sheep and turkeys. Behav Neural Biol 1980; 29:532.

52. Ferrell F: Effects of restricted dietary flavor experience before weaning on postweaning food preference in puppies. Neurosci Biobehav Rev 1984; 8(2):191.

53. Ferrell F: Preference for sugars and nonnutritive sweetners in young beagles. Neurosci Biobehav Rev 1084; 8(2):199.

54. Fox MW: Psychogenic polyphagia (compulsive eating) in a dog. Vet Rec 1962; 74(38):1023.

55. Fox MW: Canine Behavior. Springfield, IL: Charles C Thomas, 1965.

56. Fox MW: Ontogeny of prey-killing behavior in Canidae. Behavior 1969; 35:259.

57. Fox MW: Understanding Your Dog. New York: Coward, McCann & Geoghegan Inc, 1972.

58. Fox MW: The Dog: Its Domestication and Behavior. New York: Garland STPM Press, 1978.

59. Fox MW, Beck AM, Blackman E: Behavior and ecology of a small group of urban dogs (*Canis familiaris*). Appl Anim Ethol 1975; 1(2):119.

60. Franklin B: Personal communication, December 14, 2001.

61. Fuller JL, Fox MW: The behaviour of dogs. In Hafez ESE (ed): The Behaviour of Domestic Animals, 2nd ed. Baltimore: Williams & Wilkins, 1969, p. 438.

62. Gentry C: When Dogs Run Wild: The Sociology of Feral Dogs and Wildlife. Jefferson, NC: McFarland & Co Inc, 1983.

63. Ginsburg BE, Zamis MJ: Hunting and herding behaviour in dogs. Anat Rec 1949; 105:507.

64. Glickman LT, Glickman NW, Schellenberg DB, et al: Non-dietary risk factors for gastric dilatation-volvulus in large and giant breed dogs. J Am Vet Med Assoc 2000; 217(10):1492.

65. Grace J, Russek M: The influence of previous experience on the taste behavior of dogs towards sucrose and saccharin. Physiol Behav 1969; 4(4):553.

66. Griffin RW, Beidler LM: Studies in canine olfaction, taste and feeding: A summing up and some comments on the academic-industrial relationship. Neurosci Biobehav Rev 1984; 8(2):261.

67. Gustavson CR, Gustavson JC, Holzer GA: Thiabendazole-based taste aversions in dingoes (*Canis familiaris dingo*) and New Guinea wild dogs (*Canis familiaris hallstromi*). Appl Anim Ethol 1983; 10:385.

68. Hagstad HV, Hubbert WT, Stagg LM: A descriptive study of dairy goat predation in Louisiana. Can J Vet Res 1987; 51:152.

69. Hand MS, Armstrong PJ, Allen TA: Obesity: Occurrence, treatment, and prevention. Vet Clin North Am [Small Anim Pract] 1989; 19(3):447.

70. Hansen I, Bakken M, Braastad BO: Failure of LiCl-conditioned taste aversion to prevent dogs from attacking sheep. Appl Anim Behav Sci 1997; 54(2-3):251.

71. Hart BL: Problems with feeding behavior. Canine Pract 1976; 3(4):10.

72. Hart BL: Maternal behavior in the twentieth century. Canine Pract 1979; 6(6):18.

73. Hart BL: Postparturient maternal responses and mother-young interactions. Canine Pract 1980; 7(1):10.

74. Hornung DE, Enns MP: Odor-taste mixtures. Ann N Y Acad Sci 1987; 510:86.

75. Horwitz D: The behavior of good nutrition: The good, the bad, and the obese. Vet Forum February 1994:18.

76. Hoskins JD, Rothschmitt J: Hypernatremia thirst deficiency in a dog. Vet Med Small Anim Clin 1984; 79(4):489.

77. Houpt K: Ingestive behavior problems of dogs and cats. Vet Clin North Am [Small Anim Pract] 1982; 12(4):683.

78. Houpt KA: Feeding and drinking behavior problems. Vet Clin North Am [Small Anim Pract] 1991; 21(2):281.

79. Houpt KA, Beaver B: Behavioral problems of geriatric dogs and cats. Vet Clin North Am [Small Anim Pract] 1981; 11(4):643.

80. Houpt KA, Coren B, Hintz HF, et al: Effect of sex and reproductive status on sucrose preference, food intake, and body weight of dogs. J Am Vet Med Assoc 1979; 174(10):1083.

81. Houpt KA, Davis PP, Hintz HF: Effect of peripheral anosmia on dogs trained as flavor validators. Am J Vet Res 1982; 43(5):841.

82. Houpt KA, Hintz H: Obesity in dogs. Canine Pract 1978; 5(2):54.

83. Houpt KA, Hintz H: Palatability and canine food preferences. Canine Pract 1978; 5(6):29.

84. Houpt KA, Zicker S: Dietary effects on canine and feline behavior. Vet Clin North Am [Small Anim Pract] 2003; 33(2):405.

85. Houpt K, Zgoda JC, Stahlbaum CC: Use of taste repellents and emetics to prevent accidental poisoning of dogs. Am J Vet Res 1984; 45(8):1501.

86. Hunthausen WL: Giving new puppy owners practical tips to curb unruly behavior can save lives. DVM July 1990; 21:29.

87. Hunthausen WL: The causes, treatments, and prevention of canine destructive chewing. Vet Med 1991; 86(10):1007.

88. Hunthausen WL: Identifying and treating behavior problems in geriatric dogs. Vet Med (Suppl) 1994; 89:688.

89. James WT: The effect of satiation on the sucking response in puppies. J Comp Physiol Psychol 1957; 50:375.

90. James WT: The development of social facilitation of eating in puppies. J Genet Psychol 1960; 96:123.

91. James WT, Gilbert TF: The effect of social facilitation on food intake of puppies fed separately and together for the first 90 days of life. Br J Anim Behav 1955; 3:131.

92. James WT, McCay CM: A study of food intake, activity, and digestive efficiency in different type dogs. Am J Vet Res 1950; 11:412.

93. Janowitz HD, Grossman MI: Effect of variations in nutritive density on intake of food in dogs and rats. Am J Physiol 1949; 158:184.

94. Janowitz HD, Grossman MI: Some factors affecting the food intake of normal dogs and dogs with esophagostomy and gastric fistula. Am J Physiol 1949; 159:143.

95. Kitchell RL: Taste perception and discrimination by the dog. Adv Vet Sci Comp Med 1978; 22:287.

96. Kleiman DG, Eisenberg JF: Comparisons of canid and felid social systems from an evolutionary perspective. Anim Behav 1973; 21:637.

97. Lawson DC, Schiffman SS, Pappas TN: Short-term oral sensory deprivation: Possible cause of binge eating in sham-feeding dogs. Physiol Behav 1993; 53(6):1231.

98. Lehner PN, Krumm R, Cringan AT: Tests for olfactory repellents for coyotes and dogs. J Wildl Manage 1976; 40:145.

99. Levitsky DA: Obesity and the behavior of eating. Gaines Dog Research Progress (Winter) 1973:4.

100. Lewis LD: Obesity in the dog. J Am Anim Hosp Assoc 1978; 14:402.

101. Lindell EM: Diagnosis and treatment of destructive behavior in dogs. Vet Clin North Am [Small Anim Pract] 1997; 27(3):533.

102. Linden A, Eriksson M, Carlquist M, et al: Plasma levels of gastrin, somatostatin, and cholecystokinin immunoreactivity during pregnancy and lactation in dogs. Gastroenterology 1987; 92:578.

103. Lohse CL: Preferences of dogs for various meats. J Am Anim Hosp Assoc 1974; 10(2):187.

104. Lohse CL, Selcer RR, Suter PF: Hepatoencephalopathy associated with situs inversus of abdominal organs and vascular anomalies in a dog. J Am Vet Med Assoc 1976; 168(8):681.

105. Lupfer-Johnson G, Ross J: Dogs acquire food preferences from interacting with recently fed conspecifics. Behav Processes 2007; 74:104.

106. Malm K: Regurgitation in relation to weaning in the domestic dog: A questionnaire study. Appl Anim Behav Sci 1995; 43(2):111.

107. Malm K, Jensen P: Regurgitation as a weaning strategy—A selective review on an old subject in a new light. Appl Anim Behav Sci 1993; 36(1):47.

108. Malm K, Jensen P: Weaning in dogs: Within- and between-litter variations in milk and solid food intake. Appl Anim Behav Sci 1996; 49(3):223.

109. Marder A, Engel J: Behavior problems after adoption. AVSAB Ann Symp Anim Behav Res 2002: Meeting Proc:6.

110. Markwell PJ, Thorne CJ: Early behavioural development of dogs. J Small Anim Pract 1987; 28(11):984.

111. Marshall DA, Doty RL: Taste responses of dogs to ethylene glycol, propylene glycol, and ethylene glycol-based antifreeze. J Am Vet Med Assoc 1990; 197(12):1599.

112. Mason E: Obesity in pet dogs. Vet Rec 1970; 86:612.

113. McKeown DB, Luescher UA, Halip J: Stereotypies in companion animals and obsessive compulsive disorder. Purina Specialty Review in Behavioral Problems in Small Animals 1992:30.

114. Mech LD: Hunting behavior in two similar species of social canids. In Fox MW (ed): The Wild Canids. Their Systematics, Behavioral Ecology and Evolution. New York: Van Nostrand Reinhold, 1975, p. 363.

115. Merrill GG: Breaking the killing habit in dogs by inhibiting the conditioned reflex. J Am Vet Med Assoc 1945; 107:69.

116. NACA News 1982; 4(3):6.

117. Neilson J: Personal communication, March 2, 2007.

118. Neilson JC: Unruly and annoying behaviors in dogs and cats. http://www.avma.org/conv/cv2002/cvnotes/CAn_AnB_UAB_NeJ.asp, 7/3/2002.

119. Neilson JC: Unruly and annoying behaviors in dogs and cats. Wild West Vet Conf Vet Syllabus 2002:597.

120. Nicolaus LK, Herrera J, Nicolaus JC, et al: Ethinyl estradiol and generalized aversions to eggs among free-ranging predators. Appl Anim Behav Sci 1989; 24(4):313.

121. Norris MP, Beaver BV: Application of behavior therapy techniques to the treatment of obesity in companion animals. J Am Vet Med Assoc 1993; 202(5):728.

122. Obesity in pet dogs. Mod Vet Pract 1970; 51(10):60.

123. Oftedal OT, Gittleman JL: Patterns of energy output during reproduction in carnivores. In Gittleman JL (ed): Carnivore Behavior, Ecology and Evolution. Ithaca, NY: Comstock Publishing Associates, 1989, p. 355.

124. Olsen SJ: Origins of the Domestic Dog: The Fossil Record. Tucson: University of Arizona Press, 1985.

125. Oppenheimer EC, Oppenheimer JR: Certain behavioral features in the pariah dog *(Canis familiaris)* in West Bengal. Appl Anim Ethol 1975; 2(1):81.

126. Overall K: How to stop even well-trained dogs from ingesting foreign objects. DVM 1996; 27(1):6S.

127. Overall KL: Anorexia can be distinguished as behavioral disorder in some dogs. DVM 1996; 27(7):6S.

128. Pal SK: Parental care in free-ranging dogs, *Canis familiaris*. Appl Anim Behav Sci 2005; 90:31.

129. Perlson J: The Dog: An Historical, Psychological and Personality Study. New York: Vantage Press, 1968.

130. Pet food sales on the rise; Dry dog food leads the pack. DVM 1979; 10(2):15.

131. Ramsay DJ, Reid IA: Some central mechanisms of thirst in the dog. J Physiol (Lond) 1975; 253(2):517.

132. Ramsay DJ, Rolls BJ, Wood RJ: Thirst following water deprivation in dogs. Am J Physiol 1977; 232(3):R93.

133. Rashotte ME, Smith JC, Austin T, et al: Twenty-four-hour free-feeding patterns of dogs eating dry food. Neurosci Biobehav Rev 1984; 8(2):205.

134. Robinson EA, Adolph EF: Pattern of normal water drinking in dogs. Am J Physiol 1943; 139:39.

135. Rosen BS, Cook KS, Yaglom J, et al: Adipsin and complement factor D activity: An immune-related defect in obesity. Sci 1989; 244:1483.

136. Rubin HD, Beck AM: Ecological behavior of free-ranging urban pet dogs. Appl Anim Ethol 1982; 8(1-2):161.

137. Satinoff E, Stanley WC: Effect of stomach loading on sucking behavior in neonatal puppies. J Comp Physiol Psychol 1963; 56(1):66.

138. Scott MD, Causey K: Ecology of feral dogs in Alabama. J Wildl Manage 1973; 37(3):253.

139. Share I, Martyniuk E, Grossman MI: Effect of prolonged intragastric feeding on oral food intake in dogs. Am J Physiol 1952; 169:229.

140. Simpson B: Personal communication, November 10, 1999.

141. Slater MR, Robinson LE, Zoran DL, et al: Diet and exercise patterns in pet dogs. J Am Vet Med Assoc 1995; 207(2):186.

142. Smith HW: The development of the flora of the alimentary tract in young animals. J Pathol Bact 1965; 90:495.

143. Smith JC, Rashotte ME, Austin T, et al: Fine-grained measures of dogs' eating behavior in single-pan and two-pan tests. Neurosci Biobehav Rev 1984; 8(2):243.

144. Stauffer VD, Swails GG: Abnormal canine behavior and the foreign body syndrome. Mod Vet Pract 1977; 58(3):241.

145. Sueda KC, Hart BL, Cliff KD: Plant eating in domestic dogs *(Canis familiaris)*: Characterization and relationship to signalment, illness, and behavior problems. In Mills D, Levine E, Landsberg G, et al (eds): Current Issues and Research in Veterinary Behavioral Medicine. West Lafayette, IN: Purdue University Press, 2005, p. 230.

146. Taylor A, Luescher UA: Animal behavior case of the month. J Am Vet Med Assoc 1996; 208(7):1026.

147. Teranishi R, Murphy EL, Stern DJ, et al: Chemicals useful as attractants and repellents for coyotes. Worldwide Furbearer Conference Proceedings 1981; 3:1839.

148. The Compleat Angler: Friskies Research Digest (Fall)1973:13.

149. Thorne C: Feeding behaviour of domestic dogs and the role of experience. In Serpell J (ed): The Domestic Dog: Its Evolution Behaviour and Interactions with People. Cambridge, England: Cambridge University Press, 1995, p. 103.

150. Towbin EJ: Gastric distension as a factor in the satiation of thirst in esophagostomized dogs. Am J Physiol 1949; 159:533.

151. Uvnäs-Moberg K: Release of gastrointestinal peptides in response to vagal activation induced by electrical stimulation, feeding, and suckling. J Auton Nerv System 1983; 9:141.

152. Uvnäs-Moberg K, Eriksson M: Release of gastrin and insulin in response to suckling in lactating dogs. Acta Physiol Scand 1983; 119:181.

153. Uvnäs-Moberg K, Stock S, Eriksson M, et al: Plasma levels of oxytocin increase in response to suckling and feeding in dogs and sows. Acta Physiol Scand 1985; 124:391.

154. Voith VL: Destructive behavior in the owner's absence. Canine Pract 1975; 2(3):11.

155. Voith VL: Behavioral disorders. In Ettinger S (ed): Textbook of Veterinary Internal Medicine. Philadelphia: Saunders, 1989, p. 227.

156. Vollmer PJ: Puppy rearing—7: Chewing. Vet Med Small Anim Clin 1979; 74(1):43.

157. Vucetich JA, Peterson RO, Waite TA: Raven scavenging favours group foraging in wolves. Anim Behav 2004; 67(6):1117.

158. Walker AD: Taste preferences in the domestic dog and cat. Gaines Dog Research Progress (Summer)1975:1.

159. Waterhouse HN, Fritsch CW: Dog food palatability tests and sources of potential bias. Lab Anim Care 1967; 17(1):93.

160. Weldon PJ: Personal communication, 1988.

161. Weldon PJ, Fagre DB: Responses by canids to scent gland secretions of the Western Diamondback Rattlesnake *(Crotalus atrox)*. J Chem Ecol 1989; 15(5):1589.

162. Wolski TR, Riter R, Houpt KA: The effectiveness of animal repellents on dogs and cats in the laboratory field. Appl Anim Behav Sci 1984; 12(1-2):131.

163. Wood RJ, Rolls BJ, Ramsay DJ: Drinking following intracarotid infusions of hypertonic solutions in dogs. Am J Physiol 1977; 232:R88.

164. Ziegler JM, Gustavson CR, Holzer GA, et al: Anthelmintic-based taste aversions in wolves *(Canis lupus)*. Appl Anim Ethol 1983; 9:373.

## Additional Readings

Anderson JR: Encounters between domestic dogs and free-ranging non-human primates. Appl Anim Behav Sci 1986; 15:71.

Baldwin Jr. CH: Provide dog with own territory. Mod Vet Pract 1985; 66(12):1011.

Bellinger LL, Williams FE: The effect of portal and jugular infused glucose, mannitol, and saline on food intake in dogs. Physiol Behav 1989; 46(4):693.

Boulcott SR: Eating habits of hospitalized dogs. J Am Vet Med Assoc 1968; 152(10):1516.

Campbell WE: Which dog breeds develop what behavioral problems? Mod Vet Pract 1972; 53(10):31.

Campbell WE: The stool-eating dog. Mod Vet Pract 1974; 56(8):574.

Chapman BL, Voith VL: Behavioral problems in old dogs: 26 cases (1984-1987). J Am Vet Med Assoc 1990; 196(6):944.

Cheney CD, Miller ER: Effects of forced flavor exposure on food neophobia. Appl Anim Behav Sci 1997; 53(3):213.

Darke PGG: Obesity in small animals. Vet Rec 1978; 102:545.

Della-Fera MA, Baile CA, McLaughlin CL: Feeding elicited by benzodiazepine-like chemicals in puppies and cats: Structure-activity relationships. Pharmacol Biochem Behav 1980; 12(2):195.

Devenport JA, Devenport LD: Time-dependent decisions in dogs *(Canis familiaris)*. J Comp Psychol 1993; 107(2):169.

Downey RL, Kronfeld DS, Banta CA: Diet of Beagles affects stamina. J Am Anim Hosp Assoc 1980; 16(2):273.

Exaggerated cost of feeding a Great Dane: Vet Med Small Anim Clin 1977; 72(4):513.

Fox MW: Spontaneous displacement activities, compulsive behaviour and abnormal social behaviour in the dog. Vet Rec 1964; 76(31):840.

Green PL, Rashotte ME: Demonstration of basic concurrent schedules effects with dogs: Choice between different amounts of food. Neurosci Biobehav Rev 1984; 8(2):217.

Griffin RW, Scott GC, Cante CJ: Food preferences of dogs housed in testing-kennels and in consumers' homes: Some comparisons. Neurosci Biobehav Rev 1984; 8(2):253.

Haglund WD, Reay DT, Swindler DR: Canid scavenging/disarticulation sequence of human remains in the Pacific Northwest. J Forensic Sci 1989; 34(3):587.

Hetts S, Estep DQ: Behavior management: Preventing elimination and destructive behavior problems. Vet Forum November 1994:60.

Houpt KA: What the technician should know about feeding behavior of dogs and cats. Compend Contin Educ Anim Health Tech 1980; (1):43.

Houpt KA, Smith SL: Taste preferences and their relation to obesity in dogs and cats. Can Vet J 1981; 22(4):77.

Janowitz HD, Hanson ME, Grossman MI: Effect of intravenously administered glucose on food intake in the dog. Am J Physiol 1949; 156:87.

Joshua JO, Taylor DR: Unusual behavior in the bitch. Vet Rec 1972; 90(6):163.

Kitchell RL: Dogs know what they like. Friskies Research Digest 1972; 8:1.

Landry SM, Van Kruiningen HJ: Food habits of feral carnivores: A review of stomach content analysis. J Am Anim Hosp Assoc 1979; 15(6):775.

Lawler DF: Impact of nutrition on geriatric patients. http://www.avma.org/conv/cv2002/cvnotes/CAn_Ger_ING_LaD.asp, 7/3/2002.

Lawson Jr RC: Behavioral vices in dogs: Change of environment causes problems. Mod Vet Pract 1985; 66(12):1011.

Levine AS, Sievert CE, Morley JE, et al: Peptidergic regulation of feeding in the dog (*Canis familiaris*). Peptides 1984; 5:675.

Lindberg S, Strandberg E, Swenson L: Genetic analysis of hunting behaviour in Swedish flatcoated retrievers. Appl Anim Behav Sci 2004; 88:289.

Martin P: The meaning of weaning. Anim Behav 1984; 32:1257.

Melese P: How to stop chewing problems in puppies. Vet Med 1999; 94(2):157.

Monks of New Skete: The Art of Raising a Puppy. Boston: Little, Brown and Co, 1991.

Moore RA: Behavioral vices in dogs: Educate owners. Mod Vet Pract 1985; 66(12):1010.

Mugford RA: The influence of nutrition on canine behaviour. J Small Anim Pract 1987; 28(11):1046.

Myers LJ, Boddie R, May K: Electrophysiological and innate behavioral responses of the dog to intravenous application of sweet compounds. Ann N Y Acad Sci 1987; 510:519.

Overall KL, Dunham AE: Clinical features and outcome in dogs and cats with obsessive-compulsive disorder: 126 cases (1989-2000). J Am Vet Med Assoc 2002; 221(10):1445.

Pappas TN, Melendez RL, Strah KM, et al: Cholecystokinin is not a peripheral satiety signal in the dog. Am J Physiol 1985; 249(Gastrointest Liver Physiol 12):G733.

Rashotte ME, Foster DF, Austin T: Two-pan and operant lever-press tests of dogs' preference for various foods. Neurosci Biobehav Rev 1984; 8(2):231.

Rashotte ME, Smith JC: Operant conditioning methodology in the assessment of food preferences: Introductory comments. Neurosci Biobehav Rev 1984; 8(2):211.

Rogers VP, Hartke GT, Kitchell RL: Behavioral technique to analyze a dog's ability to discriminate flavors in commercial food products. In Hayashi Y (ed): Olfaction and Taste II Japan. Oxford, England: Pergamon, 1967, p. 353.

Romsos DR, Ferguson D: Regulation of protein intake in adult dogs. J Am Vet Med Assoc 1983; 182(1):41.

Russek M, Lora-Vilchis MC, Islas-Chaires M: Food intake inhibition elicited by intraportal glucose and adrenaline in dogs on a 22-hour fasting/2-hour feeding schedule. Physiol Behav 1980; 24(1):157.

Smith JC, Rashotte ME, Austin T, et al: An apparatus for making fine-grained measurements of canine eating behavior. Neurosci Biobehav Rev 1984; 8(2):239.

Smith SL, Kronfeld DS, Banta CA: Owners' perception of food flavor preferences of pet dogs in relation to measured preferences of laboratory dogs. Appl Anim Ethol 1983; 10:75.

Smith JC, Rashotte ME, Austin T, et al: An apparatus for making fine-grained measurements of canine eating behavior. Neurosci Biobehav Rev 1984; 8:239.

Sweeney PA: Some observations on behavior of Greyhounds. J Small Anim Pract 1972; 13:679.

Tortora DF: Animal behavior therapy: Destructive behavior in dogs. Compend Contin Educ Anim Health Tech 1980; 1(5):229.

Voith VL: Destructive behavior in the owner's absence. Canine Pract 1975; 2(4):8.

Vollmer PJ: The chewing response in dogs—Various causes and treatments. Vet Med Small Anim Clin 1978; 73(4):420.

Ward A: The fat-dog problem: How to solve it. Vet Med Small Anim Pract 1984; 79(6):781.

Wolf AV: Osmometric analysis of thirst in man and dog. Am J Physiol 1950; 161:75.

Würbel H, Stauffaeher M: Age and weight at weaning affect corticosterone level and development of stereotypies in ICR-mice. Anim Behav 1997; 53:891.

# Canine Eliminative Behavior

Except perhaps when housetraining a puppy, owners often take their dog's eliminative behaviors for granted. They assume that a normal dog will ask to go out to urinate or defecate, "do its business," and return to the happy environment inside. Unfortunately, sometimes one or more of these assumptions breaks down, and the dog is no longer trustworthy in the house. The owner becomes unhappy and may actually complicate the problem with another set of incorrect assumptions. Understanding normal eliminative behaviors would be a big help in preventing problems in the first place.

## ELIMINATIVE BEHAVIOR DEVELOPMENT

As with most other behaviors, those associated with elimination change as the dog matures from birth into adulthood. Behaviors present at birth are gone by 3 months of age, and the new ones may completely change again in another 3 months.

### Puppy Behaviors

At birth, a puppy cannot urinate or defecate on its own. The bitch stimulates the puppy's elimination by licking the caudal abdomen and perineal regions (Fig. 8-1). Her licking triggers the anogenital reflex, resulting in urination or defecation. The anogenital reflex ensures that the bitch is present to ingest the puppy's waste and keep the nest area clean. While not particularly important in the pet, this behavior helps minimize attraction of potential predators and insect pests to the area in the wild, and it reduces the risk of disease.[15,45] Around 2 weeks of age, puppies will start to eliminate on their own, even though the bitch still ingests most of the urine and feces. By 16 to 18 days of age, the anogenital reflex disappears, and maternal stimulation is no longer needed.[15,50] Even so, the bitch may continue

to catch the puppy's urine for up to 5.5 weeks and feces up to 9.5 weeks.[73]

By 3 weeks of age, the puppy is mobile enough to walk to one corner of the nest box or leave it altogether before eliminating.[32,73] The location used by puppies of 3 to 5 weeks old is a general area.[32,73] Then, by 9 weeks, they use a specific area for eliminations, and in the right situation, this is the same area also used by the bitch.[73] The tendency to go to a specific elimination area by 9 weeks is useful in housetraining puppies, and it is apparently a genetically acquired trait.[35] In addition to location preferences, substrate, or surface, preferences are learned about the same time.[60,73]

By 2 months of age, a sexual dimorphism appears in eliminative postures used by puppies.[35,73] Females change from a slight squat to a deep squatting posture that remains pretty much unchanged into adulthood (Fig. 8-2).[35,56] The very slight squat of a male puppy changes gradually to the male juvenile urination posture.[35] This posture is one with the weight shifted slightly forward and rear feet spread somewhat apart (Fig. 8-3).[32,35,36,56,73] Around the time of sexual maturity, generally 5 to 8 months of age, the adult male urination posture appears, with the lifted leg and slightly rotated body, allowing the dog to urinate on vertical objects (Fig. 8-4). The scratching behavior that occasionally follows defecation may also begin about this time.[56,66] Most owners believe their male dog finally learns to lift his leg for urination, but research indicates the behavior is hormonally controlled and appears when testosterone levels rise.[14,31]

Experimentally, about half of intact female and neutered female puppies showed leg lifting for urination at 65 to 70 days of age when testosterone injections were started at 3 days of age.[4,56] Male puppies showed leg lifting at day 39 when injected with testosterone starting at day 3.[31,56] Without the

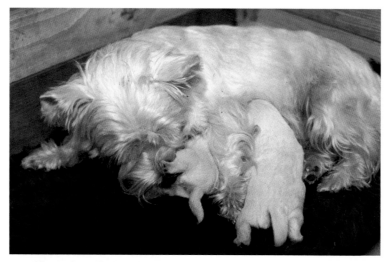

**Figure 8-1.** The dam stimulates a neonate's elimination by licking the perineum.

injections, the leg-lifting behavior in male puppies was expressed at an average of 173 days of age.[56] Castration after 4 months of age does not change this behavior, but earlier surgery resulted in periodic regression to the immature male posture.[4,14,56] Androgens given to the immature male will result in a leg lift, but the leg is more flexed in an adult.[14] The behavior reverts to that of the immature dog when testosterone is stopped.[73]

Occasionally females, especially neutered females, will lift a leg for urination.[73] This is usually an abbreviated lift and quite distinct from the typical male posture. Testosterone is produced by male puppies shortly before birth and is responsible for masculinizing the brain to respond to later testosterone elevations. It has been theorized that these female puppies were positioned next to or between male puppies in utero and thus exposed to some level of testosterone.[73]

## Housetraining

Because puppies have a natural tendency to eliminate in specific locations by 9 weeks of age, housetraining a newly acquired puppy is generally quite easy. The primary ingredients needed are *patience*, praise, confinement, and schedule.[11]

Patience is necessary because puppies do not become housebroken overnight. They will have

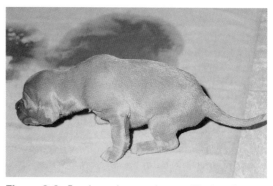

**Figure 8-2.** Female puppies use a deep squatting (squat) posture for urination.

accidents for even the most dedicated owner. Some puppies are also slower about learning what is expected, so the owner cannot necessarily expect carpets to be safe after just a few weeks of even concerted effort. Some dogs take a year of consistent handling before they finally become house-safe, and a few others never seem to learn. It is important, however, that owners be consistent in their housetraining program, because deviations can confuse the young dog and delay the learning even more.[11] The same holds true for dogs that have been adopted from an animal shelter. Consistency in the training, so that the dog will succeed, and patience

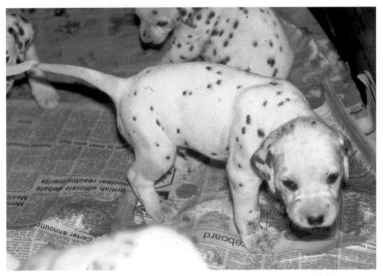

**Figure 8-3.** Male puppies use a slight squatting (flex) posture for urination.

while it does are important. Initially just under 75% of the adoptees are housetrained, making soiling the most common postadoption problem.[55] A brief counseling session increases the owner's ability to housetrain their dog in 1 month from 86.4% to 98.1% compared to just handing out educational materials.[39]

Supervision is the second recommendation for housetraining a dog. Puppies need to be supervised at all times. That either means the owner is actually watching them, or the puppy is confined. Activity triggers eliminative behaviors, so keeping the puppy still is an important management tool. Because puppies have a small urinary bladder and do not concentrate urine well in the kidneys, they generally cannot retain urine after 4 to 5 hours.[49] As a rule of thumb a puppy can hold urine for 1 hour for each month of age plus one.[38] Therefore, a 3-month-old puppy will need to urinate every 4 hours. They should not be left confined longer than this time, or they will not be able to avoid soiling their bed area. Special arrangements should be made if the owner must be gone for longer times.

Dog crates are ideal confinement areas and, if used properly, become a safe area instead of a punishment location. The crate should be big enough so that the puppy can lie fully extended in lateral

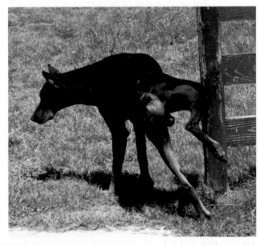

**Figure 8-4.** The leg-raised (elevate) posture is typically associated with adult male dog urination.

recumbency. It should be tall enough so that the puppy can stand and wide enough so that the puppy can easily turn around. The crate should not, however, be so big that the puppy can become active. For large dogs, it may be necessary to use two or three different sized crates as the puppy grows, or at least to block off part of a large crate at first. The goal of confinement is to discourage activity because it can trigger eliminative behaviors. When active movement is allowed, the puppy needs to be taken to the chosen elimination site to prevent it from soiling unacceptable locations.

The owner who must be gone more than 4 hours should look for alternatives to prolonged crate confinement. It may be possible to leave the puppy in a fenced yard, in a garage, or at a friend's home. Another alternative would be to keep the pup in an area two or three times larger than a crate, such as a bathroom or a wire- or plywood-framed indoor kennel. In this way the bed area can be separate from a newspaper-covered elimination area.[28,37] Any area larger than this, such as the whole house, is not conducive to successful house training.[37] When the owners are home, they should take the puppy outside at times when the probability of elimination is high.[37]

Surfaces used in elimination areas also need to be considered in confinement. Surface preferences are learned between 9 and 24 weeks, so it is best to start the puppy on the same surface type that will be used for the adult dog.[11] For most dogs this is grass. It is important that the mats in a crate have a different texture than that of the carpets in the house. Shag throw rugs are out.[11] The paper-trained puppy may be fine in a high-rise apartment, but expecting it to change its eliminations to grass a few years later after a move into a house is not realistic. It is also impractical to paper-train the puppy that will grow up to become a 50-lb dog because of the volume and associated odor of the excreta. It is possible to train a dog to use a litterbox for elimination using the same housetraining process. Special litters are available commerically,[30,46] but most people will line the litterbox with sod or a disposable pad.

The schedule is the third element of housetraining. Timing is critical, so the schedule used for a puppy becomes important. Puppies normally eliminate when they wake up, after they eat, after activity or excitement, approximately every 2 hours when awake,[46] and before bed.* These are the times a puppy should be taken to the elimination site. Because puppies sleep several times a day, they wake up often. They eat three or four meals a day, which

should be offered at the same time each day.[22,74] Dogs are prandial drinkers, so water intake is associated with meals.[46] They then need to urinate 20 to 30 minutes later.[46] Thus, more than four trips to the elimination site will be required in the beginning.

For the very young dog, it is desirable to have the owners take the puppy to the elimination site once during the middle of the night. This small investment of a few minutes each night minimizes the risk of accidental soiling when the puppy is least able to hold large volumes of urine and when it does not sleep through the night. After 3 to 4 weeks, the owner can gradually get up 30 to 45 minutes later each night until the puppy can last through an entire night without needing to eliminate. A 7-day-a-week schedule should be maintained for several months so that the expected pattern becomes firmly established. [19,21,67] Owners should never expect their dog, especially a puppy, to ask to go out to eliminate. That behavior can be taught, but not all dogs will pick it up on their own. By using the timing of a schedule, owners are less likely to have problems with housesoiling.

The fourth element of housetraining is praise, not punishment. It is important that the owner go outside with the dog each time, not to interact with it but to be able to give instant praise and treats for elimination. Punishment does not work well and is confusing to the dog. The puppy can not understand why it is being punished for a normal behavior. It has no concept of acceptable or unacceptable locations.

If a pet door is going to be used, it is best to start the puppy under supervision as already described, so that it learns what the preferred site and surface is. Once these patterns are well established, then the young dog can be taught how to use the door. The exception would be if an older dog is present that uses the pet door. In this case, the puppy will follow its older companion and usually pick up acceptable behaviors because it is in the right place at the right time.

To teach a dog to indicate a desire to go outside, an owner can use a shaping technique. If the typical routine to go out for eliminations involves calling the dog to the door, this behavior is rewarded with praise and a small food treat. A bell is hung from

---

*References 7, 19, 41, 67, 73, 75.

the doorknob so that it can be easily reached by the dog. After the dog learns that it will get a food treat, the owner should bring the treat close to the bell before the dog takes it and goes out. The next step is to move the treat into a position where the dog must bump the bell in order to reach the treat. Eventually the dog will have to ring the bell before getting the treat and getting let out. Finally, the connection will be made between ringing the bell and being let out, if the ringing is always associated with the opening of the door.

## ADULT URINATION

Dogs deposit a lot of urine on the ground each year in the United States. From an estimated dog population of 61.6 million, there is an average urine production of 30 ml/lb (60 ml/kg). Assuming an average dog weight of 25 lb (11.4 kg),[13] that amounts to approximately 10.5 million gallons (42.1 million liters) of urine voided each day.

People typically think of three urinary postures in dogs—the squat used by females, the leg-lift with partial squat used occasionally by females, and the male's raised-leg posture. Sprague and Anisko described eight elimination postures plus another four combination postures (Fig. 8-5).[68] Of the twelve, nine have been associated with urination (eight with females and four with males).[2,68]

In female dogs, 68% of the urinary postures are the squat.[16,54,68] Another 19.3% involve a squat and raise, in which the rear limb is raised off the ground but not as high as the horizontal plane.[68] Females are more apt to use that posture when away from their home area.[76] The raise alone occurs 4.6% of the time, and a slight stifle flex plus a raised rear limb (flex-raise) occurs 3.1% of the time.[68] In the elevated position (2.3% of urinary postures), the limb is lifted above the horizontal, necessitating pelvic rotation.[68] Other minor postures used by females include a handstand, a flex, and a lean at 1.9%, 0.4%, and 0.4%, respectively.[68] For males

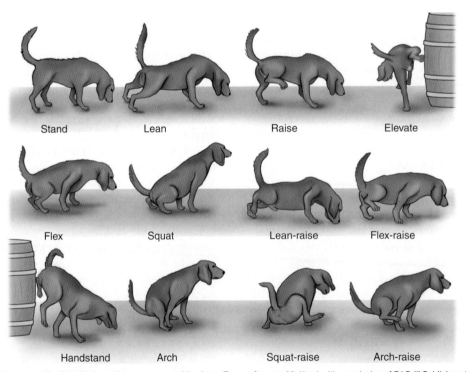

**Figure 8-5.** The 12 elimination postures used by dogs. (From reference 68. Used with permission of EJ Brill Publishers.)

97% of the urinary postures involve the typical male posture of elevation.[16, 54, 68] An occasional male will use a raised posture (2.1%), a squat-raise posture (0.6%), or a lean-raise posture (0.3%).[68]

Male urinations are directed toward vertical targets 97.6% of the time, but 15% of the time the dog urinates on the ground for at least a while.[68] Males that urinate on the ground instead of vertical objects use an elevated leg posture only 9% of the time; the rest of the time they use a raised-leg posture (52%) or some variant of the raised-leg posture (lean-raise 13% and squat-raise 26%).[68] When a male dog does use a raised-leg posture or a variant of it, he urinates on the ground instead of against a vertical object 60% of the time.[68] Males almost always sniff the ground or an object before and/or during urinating.[2,68] They also urinate where another male has urinated.[68] When not on leashes, male dogs are responsible for most urinations in public places,[64] because they urinate three to four times more often than do females. Castration decreases the frequency to approximately that of a female.[2,14,54,56] Males that are sick, anxious, or stressed may temporarily use a squatting posture for urination.[31,32]

For female dogs, the urinations are usually on the ground, except for the 11.6% that are oriented against a vertical object.[68] Of the female dogs, 13.2% urinate on a vertical object at least once, and 3.8% never urinate on the ground at all.[68] Females urinate less often than males and probably use urination mainly to empty their urinary bladder.[35,56] At least in certain breeds, female urinations may have a significant marking function.[76] The frequency increases during estrus.[2]

In both sexes, "pseudourination" motions may be made during which all the behaviors of urination are performed but no urine voided.[68] In males, the behavior is called a *raised-leg display*.[54] Both males and females are less active in urination when another dog is in view, but both hold a posture longer without actual urination. The female squat-urinates longer, and the male may remain in a squat-raise posture longer.[54]

Submissive urination occurs when the dog is showing one or more body postures associated with submission. In this case, the dog is not in a typical eliminative posture, but instead may be standing, crouching, or even lying down. Submissive urination is commonly shown by puppies and very submissive dogs to a dominant person. Punishment is inappropriate, because it usually makes the behavior worse—the dog is already showing submission.[10] Instead the best approach is to ignore the behavior.[72] Other techniques to use with these dogs include greeting the dog outdoors where the behavior will not soil the house, avoiding the situations that produce the behavior, redirecting the dog's attention from the greeting to playing with a ball, keeping the greeting low key, ignoring the behavior, or using food to countercondition the dog to stand.[10,69,70,72] Phenylpropanolamine may be useful to tighten the urinary bladder sphincter,[10,46] but most dogs will outgrow submissive urination by sexual maturity.[10,70] The incidence of the behavior can be reduced by regular handling of puppies from birth to 16 weeks of age.[79]

Outside factors influence eliminative behavior. Although the size of an area the dog stays in has minimal effect on where it eliminates, structural irregularities, such as exposed pipes, have an effect.[58] Dogs eliminate near them. They also have a tendency to eliminate as far from food and water as confinement allows.[58] Other stimuli for urination include fresh urine of another dog, excreta from birds and other animals, oil, tobacco,[25] and anise oil.[58] Stress and anticipation of a reward cause an increase in arterial blood pressure and a preglomerular resistance, with a resulting decrease in urine flow rate.[52,63]

Urine marking is another form of urination, but it is intended to call attention to a location or cover over another scent rather than empty the bladder. Some species, like cats, use a unique posture to leave the odor at nose height. In dogs, the elevated leg posture of male urination already accomplishes that. As most intact male dogs tend to urinate more often than other dogs and void small amounts each time instead of completely emptying their bladder in one location, urine marking probably is part of each urination.[35]

Marking is also a male sexually dimorphic behavior.[27,35] Females in estrus show an increased tendency to urine mark also.[27] When male dogs roam free, they routinely check certain scent posts daily, but they do not appear to systematically mark territorial boundaries.[35] These dogs do not show fearful responses to urine marks from other dogs, so the purpose of a urine mark is apparently for individual identification, much like a calling card, or for orientation within an area, keeping track of different individuals within an area, sexual stimulation, or giving familiarity to an area.[35,51,73] When a dog is put in a pen that previously contained other dogs, the new dog will urinate almost 25 times in the first 2 hours.[35] For the next few days thereafter, the frequency of urination is reduced to between two and five marks per 2-hour period.[35] When presented with its own urine, urine from a known male, or urine from an unknown male, the dog being tested will spend two times longer with the known male urine and four times longer with the unknown sample than with their own urine.[29] Male dogs often will urinate in sight of each other and then investigate the other dog's urine scent.[73] They also tend to mark a couple of times over the urine of a familiar male versus four times over that of a stranger.[73]

## ADULT DEFECATION

Dog feces is a major contaminant in a community and a public health concern. The average fecal output per dog is 0.75 lb (0.35 kg) per day in two or three defecations, and feces takes approximately 1 week to decompose.[8,13] Thus 46,200,000 lb (21,600,000 kg) of dog feces are deposited each day, most of which is not picked up, for a weekly accumulation of 161,700 tons (150,900,000 kg). A single fly can deposit up to 588 eggs (the average is 144),[13] so if one fly lays its eggs on each new fecal pile, that represents a hatch of approximately 26,600,000,000 new flies per day. Dog feces is second only to garbage as a source of flies.[13]

Unlike urination postures, defecation postures are more consistent between the sexes. At first, the dog shows a preliminary behavioral series that includes sniffing the ground, walking in a certain area or pattern, and assuming a stiff-legged, wide-base stance as the back becomes arched (Fig. 8-6). Among female dogs, 96.8% defecate with the arch posture, as do 79.5% of the males.[68] The remaining 3.2% of the females use a leg-elevated posture

for defecation.[68] Among male dogs, 10.2% use the leg-elevated posture, 5.1% use a combination arch-raise posture, and 2.6% each use either a leg-raised posture or a standing one.[68] An occasional dog uses the handstand posture to deposit feces approximately 1.5 feet up a tree trunk, probably an odor-marking behavior.[35] About 23% of the defecations made by male dogs are directed toward a fence, and at least 29% of males defecate on a fence.[68]

Urban dogs are most likely to defecate in public places while accompanied by their owner, especially when allowed off lead.[64] An inverse correlation exists between the number of visits made by dogs on a lead to the feces density.[64]

Defecation patterns of dogs vary with age, activity levels, and diet. Young dogs defecate more often than adults, active more than inactive, and those on higher fiber diets more than those on highly digestible ones. Typically these defecations will occur after waking, within 20 minutes of eating, and before bedtime. What many people do not recognize is that each bout of defecation can consist of a series of several eliminations, with some sniffing and walking in between. A problem can occur if the owner does not allow the dog to complete the entire defecation series before bringing the animal back into the house. Careful observation will show that when a dog actually finishes defecation, the last piece of feces that passes has a smooth, usually

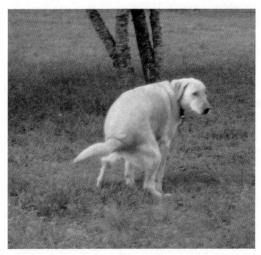

**Figure 8-6.** The defecation (arch) posture used by dogs.

tapered end. Before that, fecal pieces have a blunted or broken end instead.

Feral dogs have been observed to cover feces and urine with sand at certain stages of the reproductive cycle,[26] but domestic dogs usually eliminate and move on. Occasionally they will scrape the ground with all four feet after urination or defecation. This scraping behavior also occurs in wolves and jackals, but their behavior is not a covering one, either.[62] Ground scratching is regarded as a marking behavior that leaves a visual marker and may spread scent, too.[68] The behavior is more likely to be shown by males after urination, but females, particularly spayed females, may also demonstrate ground scraping after defecation, as well as after urination.[68,76] It tends to occur more often in new locations, in the presence of other dogs, and when first let out in the mornings, perhaps because the intensification of odors in the still morning air.

## ELIMINATIVE BEHAVIOR PROBLEMS

### Housesoiling

Problem behaviors associated with elimination are common and regarded by most owners as very serious. In owner surveys, 6.4% to 7.4% mentioned some form of housesoiling by their dog, making it the sixth most common annoying behavior after aggression, excessive vocalization, destructive chewing, digging, and begging for food.[3,9,72] Of owners reporting they had talked to their veterinarian about a behavior problem, 37.3% complained of housesoiling; it was the most common complaint.[1] Of calls to ask a behaviorist for help, 22.3% were for eliminative problems.[71] In referral cases seen by behavior specialists, however, housesoiling is only the second or third most common problem, representing 5.5% to 20.6% of the cases.*

Intact males have a higher incidence of housesoiling than do castrated males or females. The incidence in intact males alone is almost 60%,[44,71] and is associated with their tendency to urine mark. A breed predilection for housesoiling may exist as

well,[18] with Beagles and Bichon Frises reported to have a higher incidence than expected.[3] Whether this predilection changes over time, as breed popularity changes, or differs by geographic locations has not been studied. Owners with dogs that become housetrained in a few days cite significantly fewer problems later than do those whose dogs took several months to accomplish the same feat.[20]

Housesoiling, whether by urination, defecation, or both, can be related to many things, and a good historical and diagnostic workup is necessary because of all the possible causes (Boxes 8-1 and 8-2). These include many medical causes of housesoiling that must be ruled out.[61] It is common for owners

| BOX 8-1 | Differential diagnoses for dogs urinating in the house |
|---|---|

Canine cognitive dysfunction
Confinement
Degenerative joint disease
Excitement
Fear-inducing situations
Incomplete urination
Lack or of incomplete housetraining
Pollakiuria
    Neoplasia
    Urinary tract infection
    Uroliths
Polyuria
    Diabetes insipidus
    Diabetes mellitus
    Drug-induced
    Hepatic insufficiency
    Hyperadrenocorticism
    Hypercalcemia
    Hypoadrenocorticism
    Hypokalemia
    Neoplasia
    Psychogenic
    Pyometra
    Renal insufficiency
Psychogenic polydipsia
Separation anxiety
Submissive urination
Tenesmus/dyschezia
Urinary incontinence
    Anomalies
    Estrogen-responsive
    Neurogenic
Urine marking

Data from references 46, 53, 61, 69, 70, 71, 74.

---

*References 3, 9, 23, 44, 77, 78.

| BOX 8-2 | Differential diagnoses for dogs defecating in the house |
|---|---|

Canine cognitive dysfunction
Confinement
Degenerative joint disease
Diarrhea
Fear-induced
Fecal incontinence
Feces marking
Incomplete defecation
Lack of or incomplete housetraining
Malabsorption
Separation anxiety
Tenesmus/dyschezia

Data from references 46, 53, 61, 72, 74.

to say that the dog "knows it has done wrong," or that they can always tell when there is a mess somewhere in the house because the dog meets them with "a guilty look." The guilty look is submissive body language that the dog has learned to show in response to a specific situation.[11,72,74] Geriatric dogs that have recently started soiling often show this expression even when they seem unaware that they have just urinated or defecated.[47]

In multidog households it is important to identify the dog with the problem, rather than to assume it was a specific dog because of its "guilty look." If direct observation of defecation is not possible, a child's nontoxic color crayons can be broken into little pieces, with a different color fed to each dog.[46] When urination is the problem, a small amount of aspirin (5 mg/15-20 kg dog) will result in mopped up urine turning burgundy when ferric chloride is added to it.[46]

Once the problem dog has been identified for sure, specific treatment protocols can be started. Regardless of cause, the first step is to educate the owner that the dog does not recognize the concept of guilt. It has learned to respond submissively to the combined presence of excreta and owner. The dog has been home all day alone with the urine or feces without showing a "guilty" look. It can be with the owner alone without showing this behavior. But after a couple of times where the odor of urine or feces and the harsh tones of the owner are paired, the dog quickly learns to associate the two.

## Canine Cognitive Dysfunction

Veterinarians have become aware of a syndrome in dogs that resembles some of the mentally incapacitating diseases in humans. Clinically, these dogs seem to forget things they previously knew well, and at times seem to totally forget housetraining or which house to come back to. Their sleep-wake cycle is changed, and they become excessively vocal. Researchers have identified amyloidosis, meningeal fibrosis, and accumulations of ubiquitin-protein conjugates in these dogs but without the tangles typical of human Alzheimer's disease.[48,65] A more complete discussion of cognitive dysfunction is found in Chapter 2.

## Confinement

A common cause of dogs urinating or defecating in the house is that they are physically blocked from going out when it is physiologically necessary. This problem can take many forms. For crated dogs, it is necessary to take them out at times before the soiling is expected. If this involves a puppy, it could mean a trip outside at 2:00 in the morning or a trip home at noon. Confinement can also be the problem when people are gone for an extended period, if they accidentally forget to unlock a dog door, or if the dog is accidentally locked in the house. When the problem continues several days and is not an isolated incident, careful evaluation of the timing of the inappropriate urination or defecation and of other aspects of the dog's and the owner's routine may offer insight into the reasons for the problem. Suggestions can then be offered to circumvent the contributing factors.

## Degenerative Joint Disease

In older dogs that have been well housetrained for years and start urinating or defecating in the house, degenerative joint disease has been shown to be a major contributing factor.[24,25,48] It may be difficult to get to the normal toileting area.[42] Posturing attempts are usually made but are incomplete or not held long enough. These dogs, then, do not finish eliminating when outside. Eventually, the dog must finish eliminating, and often that happens in the wrong place. As would be expected, these dogs have some days that are better or worse than others. Treatment for the primary musculoskeletal problem, whether as symptomatic pain relief or surgical correction, is necessary to correct the housesoiling.

## Excitement

Exciting situations can be associated with urination at times and in places that are not typically associated with eliminative behaviors, especially in young dogs. This may represent a form of submissive urination.[67] Control of excitement urination is best done by avoiding the stimuli. The problem also can be treated by habituation or counterconditioning so that the stimulus loses its ability to excite.[70,74] As an example, the dog that becomes very excited when people visit can be made less excited by having a lot of people over with everyone completely ignoring the dog until it is calm. Then the dog is made to sit before being petted. Any increase in the excitement level means the dog is ignored again until it calms down.

## Fear-Inducing Situations

Extremely fear-inducing situations can cause urination, defecation, or expression of the anal sacs as a dog tries to escape. Although this response is most common in young dogs, it can occur at any age, especially if the dog has a submissive personality. A young dog being chased by a very dominant, older dog during their first encounter is one common scenario. Most dogs will outgrow this extreme expression of submission, but for those that do not, avoiding situations where the response is likely to be evoked is best.

## Incomplete Urination/Defecation

One of the most common causes of housesoiling is associated with inclement weather or owners being in a hurry. Owners usually put the dog outside in the morning, assuming that while they are getting ready for work or school the dog is urinating and defecating. On rainy, snowy, or very chilly days, the dog tends to stay by the back door instead of going out into the yard. Within a few hours of being let back into the house, the dog can no longer stop the urge to eliminate. If this type of weather continues for several days, the dog may end up

being presented as a behavior problem because of housesoiling. It is important that the veterinarian consider past weather factors and try to correlate the problem behavior with them, because owners seldom make the connection. This same pattern can occur if the dog is distracted from its eliminative behavior by chasing a bird, following a scent, or playing with another dog. Treatment goes back to the basics of having the owner go out with the dog until it finishes eliminating.

Even owners who go out with their dog can bring a dog back into the house too soon if they are in a hurry or they fail to recognize that the dog has not finished eliminating. This problem is most apt to happen with defecations and with male dog urinations. The typical history indicates that the dog either did not eliminate outside at all and "waited" until it got inside, or that the dog urinated/defecated outside but did so again after getting back inside. Successful management of such a case involves client education about normal eliminative behaviors. Owners should remain outside until the dog has finished eliminating, regardless of how long that is. This way they can reward the appropriate behavior instead of giving attention, even though it is negative, for unacceptable behavior.

## Incontinence

Urinary incontinence in young dogs, ovariohysterectomized females, and geriatric dogs can be misdiagnosed as other medical or behavioral problems; the same is true for fecal incontinence, especially in dogs older than 10 years of age.[34] A lack of appropriate posturing suggests a problem with incontinence, and a medical workup is appropriate.

## Lack of Complete Housetraining

One consideration in any case of housesoiling is how well housetrained the dog was before the problem started. A behavioral history may uncover that the dog never was completely trustworthy,[70] and a change in circumstances has suddenly made this fact important. For example, the dog might have occasionally urinated or defecated in the house, but now the owners have new carpeting and the old behavior is no longer acceptable. As another example, owners might try one housebreaking method for a few days, but if it "doesn't work," they try a second technique for the next few days, and then a third technique, and so on. Eventually, the puppy is so confused that it cannot learn the acceptable behavior.

Incomplete training or inconsistency in training techniques often results in a dog with problem behavior and is the leading cause of housesoiling problems. Incomplete housebreaking accounts for a high percentage of referral cases,[78] emphasizing the importance of proper counseling of new dog owners. Soiling in the house because of poor training can occur with or without the owner being home.[69] Some dogs can be helped by going back to the techniques of basic housetraining consistently applied over a long period to give the dog every opportunity to succeed. The desired behavior is rewarded instead of the wrong one being punished—a punishment the dog does not understand anyway.[70] Going back to basic housetraining techniques has a success rate of over 80%.[78]

Difficulty in house training is common for very small breeds. These breeds were originally developed to retain the characteristics of puppies. Although the appearance of the domed head and small size is considered desirable, other less desirable juvenile features also have been retained. One of these is the resistance to being housebroken. In small dogs, housetraining can be a difficult, long-term problem. Some owners will go so far as to keep diapers on the dog to make it an acceptable house pet.

Another alternative for dogs that are not completely housetrained is to make them yard dogs. This alternative has the advantage of not letting the dog soil in the house, and over time the dog can learn that grass or dirt is the preferred surface. Owners must be careful that these dogs get adequate human interaction and are not simply forgotten except at feeding time. The dog can still be allowed inside at regular times for supervised interaction with its people.

Converting a dog that was trained to eliminate on papers to one that eliminates on grass can be difficult to impossible if the paper-training lessons were well learned in the beginning. It may be necessary for the owner to very gradually move the papers closer to the door, so that the dog learns to eliminate on papers in different locations. The next step will be to move the papers out the door and then into the yard and eventually to an acceptable elimination area. It is important that the owner take the dog to the papers so that it can eliminate on the same schedule it used indoors. Several weeks must be allowed for the dog to get used to voiding on the papers in a specific outdoor location. The size of the paper is gradually reduced by a few square inches a day, so the dog will gradually get used to touching ground instead of paper. As the paper approaches a $6 \times 6$-inch square, the owner can try removing it entirely. The best chance for this technique to work, if it does at all, is to take an extra long time at each phase rather than hurry through the process.

Occasionally a person might want to reverse the training of a geriatric dog to have it eliminate in the house in an easily accessible area.[43] The general process is the same. The owner should first incorporate a piece of lawn sod (or other surface being used at the time) into the location to be used and be sure the dog is taken to the new area at times it is most likely to eliminate. It will need to be under confinement or close supervision at all times to ensure it is in the right place at the right time. There will be accidents in other locations, but the owner must be careful not to punish the dog for the accident or else they will generalize the punishment with indoor elimination. If a particular leash or collar excites the dog about going out, it is best to avoid those cues and use different ones during the training process.[43]

## Marking

Urine marking is a common problem for owners of male dogs because it is a sexually dimorphic behavior. The problem dogs are usually young adults between 1 and 2 years of age. An initial trigger may be involved, such as the visit of a house guest, a disrupted schedule, or a new dog added to the house. These events might be viewed by the dog as invasions of its territory or interference with its owner-directed interactions. Less obvious but just as likely to cause marking by an intact male is an estrous bitch somewhere within a several-block radius. On rare occasions, marking has been correlated with the menstrual cycle of a woman in the household.[17]

The first recommended treatment for urine-marking dogs is castration. After surgery, 30% of the dogs will show a rapid decline in the behavior, 20% a gradual decline over a few months, and 50% no change.[40] The results are the same regardless of the age at which the surgery was done.[40,59,74] If castration alone has not helped, progestins can be tried,[33,74] keeping in mind their many potential side effects. If stress is involved, benzodiazepines, tricyclic antidepressants, or selective serotonin reuptake inhibitors might be needed.

In addition to drug therapy, behavioral therapy and environmental manipulation can be useful. If the standard routine has been upset, it may be necessary to reestablish the old pattern and gradually begin a transition to the newer one.[5] Punishment at the very beginning of each and every marking episode can stop the problem, too.[74] The owner should look for ways to prevent access to the favored locations or to make those locations aversive.[74] A large sheet of plastic can be draped over the object so it is covered or so the dog might have to walk on plastic before getting to the spot. Large mats are available commercially that give mild shocks when touched. The owner can scare the dog several times by popping a balloon whenever the animal approaches the spot to mark it. After a few of these lessons, balloons can be hung by the location where the dog urinates, and the dog will avoid the area completely. A remote switch that turns on when a light beam is broken can be connected to a pistol-type hair dryer that then blasts the approaching dog with a rush of air and a loud noise.

Marking with feces occurs occasionally. In a typical history, the dog has been shut out of a specific location where it used to be allowed, and it may also be receiving less human interaction. As an example, the dog has been shut outside because a house guest does not like dogs or because the owners do not want the old black dog tracking in dirt and leaving black hairs on the new white carpet. Dogs accept gradual changes better than abrupt ones, and owners may need to be reminded of this fact. It may be necessary for the owner to decide whether the guest or white carpet has priority over the dog. By selecting what is important in their lives, owners can then look at the options that are most appropriate for them.

## Psychogenic Elimination

Stress can be internalized by dogs to the point that abnormal behaviors appear. Psychogenic polyuria, psychogenic polydipsia, psychogenic diarrhea, and psychogenic constipation are examples.[6] Show dogs seem particularly predisposed to psychogenic diarrhea, perhaps in part because of schedule changes, strange handlers, large numbers of dogs around, limited access to water, and the use of high-protein baits. Diagnosis of a psychogenic problem is usually made after medical causes of urination/defecation have been ruled out. Occasionally the cyclic nature of sick-at-the-home/well-in-the-hospital history is the first clue of a psychogenic problem. Environmental manipulation, whether by maintaining a very rigid schedule that includes a large amount of human attention or by providing access to old areas, is needed. Anxiolytic drugs, such as the tricyclic antidepressants or selective serotonin reuptake inhibitors, can help the animal adjust to the stress. Drug therapy in combination with environmental manipulation and large amounts of exercise to use up excess energy can be useful.

## Separation Anxiety

Separation anxiety in dogs was discussed in Chapter 4. One sign of this problem can be elimination in the house, and it may even be the only visible sign of this problem. Dogs with separation anxiety represented 39% of housesoiling cases in one study.[78] Because saliva can dry before the owner returns and whining is not heard, owners may need to videotape the dog's behavior when they are not home to see what behaviors occur too. In the typical history of a dog with separation anxiety, the housesoiling problem occurs only when the owner is not home, and it occurs regardless of whether the owner is gone 5 minutes or 5 hours.[69]

## Submissive Urination

In the presence of a highly dominant person or dog, a young dog may urinate as it shows a submissive greeting. Because this is a normal behavior and a submissive one, neither physical nor verbal punishment is appropriate. Such punishments only deepen the submissive response. It is important to separate this behavior from other eliminative problems because the cause is so different from most. Submissive urination was discussed earlier in the chapter.

## Odor Removal

Odors play an important role in canine site selection for elimination; however, to think that an odor can be made undetectable to a dog is probably unrealistic. The intensity of an odor can at least be minimized to deemphasize the attractiveness of a location. First it is necessary to locate urine-soaked areas, which are not always obvious. A cane-like moisture detector is commercially available, and fluorescein stain can be administered so an ultraviolet lamp will light up problem areas.[57] Cleanup should not depend on ammonia-based products.[5,67] Products that work at modifying the odor molecules or that break down bacterial/enzyme source odors are most effective.[12,57] Several good commercial, enzymatic odor eliminators are now on the market. The key to their successful use is that the product must both reach the source of the odor and be a sufficient amount to work on the entire spot.

## References

1. AAHA pet owner survey results. Trends Mag 1993; IX(2):32.
2. Anisko J: Communication by chemical signals in Canidae. In Doty RL (ed): Mammalian Olfaction, Reproductive Processes and Behavior. New York: Academic Press, 1976, p. 283.
3. Bamberger M, Houpt KA: Signalment factors, comorbidity, and trends in behavior diagnoses in dogs: 1,644 cases (1991-2001). J Am Vet Med Assoc 2006; 229(10):1591.
4. Beach FA: Effects of gonadal hormones on urinary behavior in dogs. Physiol Behav 1974; 12(6):1005.
5. Beaver B: Therapy of behavior problems. In Kirk RW (ed): Current Veterinary Therapy VIII: Small Animal Practice. Philadelphia: Saunders, 1983, p. 58.
6. Beaver BV: Psychosomatic behaviors in dogs and cats. Vet Med Small Anim Clin 1982; 77(11):1594.
7. Beaver BV: Housebreaking a puppy. Vet Med Small Anim Clin 1983; 78(5):670.
8. Beaver BV: The role of veterinary colleges in addressing the surplus dog and cat problem. J Am Vet Med Assoc 1991; 198(7):1241.
9. Beaver BV: Owner complaints about canine behavior. J Am Vet Med Assoc 1994; 204(12):1953.
10. Beaver BV: The Veterinarian's Encyclopedia of Animal Behavior. Ames: Iowa State University Press, 1994.
11. Beaver BV: Behavior development and behavioral disorders. In Hoskins JD (ed): Veterinary Pediatrics: Dogs and Cats From Birth to Six Months of Age, 2nd ed. Philadelphia: Saunders, 1995, p. 23.
12. Beaver BV, Terry ML, Lasagna CL: Effectiveness of products in eliminating cat urine odors from carpet. J Am Vet Med Assoc 1989; 194(11):1589.
13. Beck AM: The Ecology of Stray Dogs: A Study of Free-Ranging Urban Animals. Baltimore: York Press, 1973.
14. Berg IA: Development of behavior: The micturition pattern in the dog. J Exp Psychol 1944; 34(5):343.
15. Bleicher N: Behavior of the bitch during parturition. J Am Vet Med Assoc 1962; 140:1076.
16. Bradshaw JWS, Nott HMR: Social and communication behaviour of companion dogs. In Serpell J (ed): The Domestic Dog: Its Evolution, Behaviour and Interactions with People. Cambridge, England: Cambridge University Press, 1995, p. 115.
17. Campbell W: Household micturition. Mod Vet Pract 1973; 54(8):58.
18. Campbell WE: Which dog breeds develop what behavioral problems? Mod Vet Pract 1972; 53:31.
19. Campbell WE: A rapid approach to animal behavior problem solving. Mod Vet Pract 1977; 58(10):879.
20. Campbell WE: Effects of training, feeding regimens, isolation and physical environment on canine behavior. Mod Vet Pract 1986; 67:239.
21. Campbell WE: Housetraining puppies: Part 1: The three most violated principles. Mod Vet Pract 1987; 68 (1l-12):579.
22. Campbell WE: Housetraining puppies: Part 2: Teaching control of the urge. Mod Vet Pract 1988; 69(3):185.
23. Chapman B, Voith V: Dog owners and their choice of a pet. American Veterinary Society of Animal Behavior meeting, Atlanta, July 20, 1986.
24. Chapman B, Voith VL: Geriatric behavior problems not always related to age. DVM 1987; 18(3):32.
25. Chapman BL, Voith VL: Behavioral problems in old dogs: 26 cases (1984-1987). J Am Vet Med Assoc 1990; 196(6):944.
26. Clutton-Brock J, Jewell P: Origin and domestication of the dog. In Evans HE (ed): Miller's Anatomy of the Dog, 3rd ed. Philadelphia: Saunders, 1993, p. 21.
27. Connolly PB: Reproductive behaviour problems. In Horwitz DF, Mills DS, Heath S (eds): BSAVA Manual of Canine and Feline Behavioural Medicine. Quedgeley, Gloucester, England: British Small Animal Veterinary Association, 2002, p. 128.
28. Crowell-Davis S: House-breaking puppies. NAVC Clinician's Brief 2005; 3(1):44.
29. Dunbar IF, Carmichael M: The responses of male dogs to urine from other males. Behav Neural Biol 1981; 31:465.
30. Eig J: Behind the tense race to create dog litter with the right stuff. Wall Street Journal February 23, 2000; CV(38):A1.
31. Fox MW: Canine Behavior. Springfield, IL: Charles C Thomas, 1965.
32. Fuller JL, Fox MW: The behaviour of dogs. In Hafez ESE (ed): The Behaviour of Domestic Animals, 2nd ed. Baltimore: Williams & Wilkins, 1969, p. 438.
33. Gerber HA, Sulman FG: The effect of methyloestrenolone on oestrus, pseudo-pregnancy, vagrancy, satyriasis and squirting in dogs and cats. Vet Rec 1964; 76(39):1089.

34. Guilford WG: Fecal incontinence in dogs and cats. Compend Contin Educ 1990; 12(3):313.

35. Hart BL: Normal behavior and behavioral problems associated with sexual function, urination and defecation. Vet Clin North Am 1974; 4(3):589.

36. Hart BL: Gonadal hormones and behavior of the female dog. Canine Pract 1975; 5(2):8.

37. Hart BL: Toilet training and problems with elimination. Canine Pract 1979; 6(1):7.

38. Haug, L: Personal communication, September 2002.

39. Herron ME, Lord LK, Hill LN, et al: Effects of preadoption counseling for owners on house-training success among dogs acquired from shelters. J Am Vet Med Assoc 2007; 231(4):558.

40. Hopkins SG, Schubert TA, Hart BL: Castration of adult male dogs: Effects on roaming, aggression, urine marking, and mounting. J Am Vet Med Assoc 1976; 168(12):1108.

41. Horwitz DF: A practitioner's guide to housebreaking puppies. Vet Med 1999; 94(2):165.

42. Horwitz DF: Behavior problems in senior dogs. http://www.avma.org/conv/cv2002/cvnotes/Can_Ger_BPS_HoD.asp, 7/3/2002.

43. Horwitz DF: Reverse house-training. NAVC Clinician's Brief September 2003:43.

44. Houpt KA: Disruption of the human-companion animal bond: Aggressive behavior in dogs. In Katcher AH, Beck AM (eds): New Perspectives on Our Lives with Companion Animals. Philadelphia: University of Pennsylvania Press, 1983, p. 197.

45. Houpt KA: Feeding and drinking behavior problems. Vet Clin North Am [Small Anim Pract] 1991; 21(2):281.

46. Houpt KA: House soiling by dogs. In Horwitz DF, Mills DS, Heath S (eds): BSAVA Manual of Canine and Feline Behavioural Medicine. Quedgeley, Gloucester, England: British Small Animal Veterinary Association, 2002, p. 90.

47. Houpt KA, Beaver B: Behavioral problems of geriatric dogs and cats. Vet Clin North Am [Small Anim Pract] 1981; 11(4):643.

48. Hunthausen W: Identifying and treating behavior problems in geriatric dogs. Vet Med (Suppl) 1994; 89:688.

49. Hunthausen WL: Giving new puppy owners practical tips to curb unruly behavior can save lives. DVM 1990; 21:29.

50. Johnson CA, Grace JA: Care of newborn puppies and kittens. Forum 1987; 6(1):9.

51. Kleiman D: Scent marking. Symp Zool Soc Lond 1966; 18:167.

52. Koepke JP, Light KC, Obrist PA, et al: Vasopressin and urine now rate responses to stress in conscious dogs. Am J Physiol 1984; 247(2,II):F213.

53. Landsberg GM: Veterinarians as behavior consultants. Can Vet J 1990; 31:225.

54. Macdonald DW: The carnivores: Order Carnivora. In Brown RE, Macdonald DW (eds): Social Odours in Mammals, vol 2. Oxford, England: Clarendon Press, 1985, p. 619.

55. Marder A, Engel J: Behavior problems after adoption. AVSAB Annual Symposium on Animal Behavior Research 2002. Meeting Proceedings 2002:6.

56. Martins T, Valle JR: Hormonal regulation of the micturition behavior of the dog. J Comp Physiol Psychol 1948; 41:301.

57. Melese P: Detecting and neutralizing odor sources in dog and cat elimination problems. Appl Anim Behav Sci 1994; 39:188.

58. Meyers L: Elimination patterns of dogs in 3 types of confinement. Am Soc Vet Anim Behav meeting, July 18, 1988.

59. Neilson JC, Eckstein RA, Hart BL: Effects of castration on problem behaviors in male dogs with reference to age and duration of behavior. J Am Vet Med Assoc 1997; 211(2):180.

60. Overall KL: Preventing behavior problems: Early prevention and recognition in puppies and kittens. Purina Specialty Review Behavioral Problems in Small Animals 1992:13.

61. Overall KL: Medical differentials with potential behavioral manifestations. Vet Clin North Am [Small Anim Pract] 2003; 33(2):213.

62. Perlson J: The Dog: An Historical, Psychological and Personality Study. New York: Vantage Press, 1968.

63. Rader RD, Stevens CM: Telemetered renal responses in dogs during detection of explosives. Biotelemetry 1975; 2(5):265.

64. Reid JB, Chantrey DF, Davie C: Eliminatory behaviour of domestic dogs in an urban environment. Appl Anim Behav Sci 1984; 12(3):279.

65. Ruehl WW: Personal communication, 1994.

66. Scott JP, Fuller JL: Genetics and the Social Behavior of the Dog. Chicago: The University of Chicago Press, 1965.

67. Seksel K: Inappropriate defecation and urination in dogs. Proc 75th Jubilee New Zealand Veterinary Association 1998:109.

68. Sprague RH, Anisko JJ: Elimination patterns in the laboratory beagle. Behavior 1973; 47:257.

69. Voith VL: Differential diagnoses of canine elimination behavior problems. Mod Vet Pract 1981; 62(10):794.

70. Voith VL: Behavioral disorders. In Ettinger S (ed): Textbook of Veterinary Internal Medicine. Philadelphia: Saunders, 1989, p. 227.

71. Voith VL: Elimination problems in dogs. American Veterinary Medical Association meeting, Boston, August 1, 1992.

72. Voith VL, Borchelt PL: Diagnosis and treatment of elimination behavior problems in dogs. Vet Clin North Am [Small Anim Pract] 1982; 12(4):637.

73. Voith VL, Borchelt PL: Elimination behavior and related problems in dogs. Compend Contin Educ 1985; 7(7):537.

74. Voith VL, Marder AR: Canine behavioral disorders. In Morgan R (ed): Handbook of Small Animal Practice. New York: Churchill Livingstone, 1988, p. 1033.

75. Vollmer PJ: Puppy rearing—5: Housetraining. Vet Med Small Anim Clin 1978; 73(11):1369.

76. Wirant SC, McGuire B: Urinary behavior of female domestic dogs (Canis familiaris): Influence of reproductive status, location, and age. Appl Anim Behav Sci 2004; 85:335.

77. Wolski TR: Preventing canine behavior problems. In Kirk RW (ed): Current Veterinary Therapy VIII: Small Animal Practice. Philadelphia: Saunders, 1983, p. 52.

78. Yeon SC, Erb HN, Houpt KA: A retrospective study of canine house soiling: Diagnosis and treatment. J Am Anim Hosp Assoc 1999; 35(2):101.

79. Young MS: The influence of early handling on submissive urination in Cocker Spaniels. Animal Behavior Society meeting, Knoxville, TN, June 1981.

## Additional Readings

Beaver BVG: Understanding of canine urinary behavior patterns, desirable and undesirable. Southwest Vet 1974; 27(3):225.

Brunner F: Typical and abnormal urination by dogs. Mod Vet Pract 1972; 53(3):43.

Campbell WE: Housetraining—A natural method. Mod Vet Pract 1974; 55(1):53.

Campbell WE: Rote solutions. Mod Vet Pract 1976; 57(9):740.

Canine geriatric behavior changes established. Vet Forum June 25, 1998:18.

Dunbar I: The control of anti-social behavior in dogs. Appl Anim Ethol 1982; 9(1):98.

Fox MW: The Dog: Its Domestication and Behavior. New York: Garland STPM Press, 1978.

Hart BL: Anthropomorphism: Two perspectives. Canine Pract 1978; 5(3):12.

Hart BL: Toilet training and problems with elimination. Canine Pract 1979; 6(1):7.

Hart BL: Indications for progestin therapy for problem behavior in dogs. Canine Pract 1979; 6(5):10.

Horwitz DF: Puppy training and problem prevention. http://www.avma.org/conv/cv2002/cvnotes/CAn_Ped_PTP_HoD.asp, 7/3/2002.

Houpt KA: Companion animal behavior: A review of dog and cat behavior in the field, the laboratory and the clinic. Cornell Vet 1985; 75:248.

Kantrowitz Z, Shamaun M: Paraplegic dogs: Urinary bladder evacuation with direct electric stimulation. SCI 1963; 139:115.

Lawson Jr RC: Change of environment causes problems. Mod Vet Pract 1985; 66(12):1011.

Mestel R: Ascent of the dog. Discover October 1994:90.

Monks of New Skete: The Art of Raising a Puppy. Boston: Little, Brown and Co, 1991.

Moore RA: Behavioral vices in dogs: Educates owners. Mod Vet Pract 1985; 66(12):1010.

Moreau PM, Lees GE, Hobson HP: Simultaneous cystometry and uroflowmetry for evaluation of micturition in two dogs. J Am Vet Med Assoc 1983; 183(10):1084.

Sessions B: Re-housebreaking the mature dog. Dog Fancy 1974; 5(3):10.

Voith VL, Borchelt PL: Housebreaking. What is a new puppy owner to do? Vet Tech 1985; 6(6):288.

Vollmer PJ: Submissive urination. Vet Med Small Anim Clin 1977; 72(9):1435.

Vollmer PJ: Puppy rearing—4: Crate-training the pup. Vet Med Small Anim Clin 1978; 73(10):1265.

Whited S: Housebreaking puppies. Vet Tech 1992; 13(2):126.

# Canine Locomotive Behavior

Some dogs are couch potatoes. Others are in perpetual motion. Regardless of whether they are resting or moving, they display a wide variety of locomotive behavior. Prenatal development of locomotor activities in dogs is not well studied, as it is in the cat, but progressive changes from birth onward are. Many of the movements begin as weak or incomplete forms of adult patterns. Others are present early and then go away.

## INFANT GROWTH AND MOVEMENTS

Behavior changes that puppies go through are associated with their ability to interact with their environment. In many ways, then, the development of locomotor behaviors is almost equal to development of the senses in the environmental component of a dog's personality. The extensive locomotor changes that occur so early in life parallel those in the central nervous system.

### Prewalking Movements

Because of its immature state of development at the time of birth, a puppy depends on a number of different reflexes for protection. Those involving sensory perception were discussed in Chapter 2 and summarized in Table 2-1. Those for locomotor skills, plus or minus sensory input, are summarized in Table 9-1. A new puppy moves with circular and side-to-side movements. While doing so, it uses its head in side-to-side scanning-like motions and as a lever against anything rigid enough to push against.[22,27,72,94] The front limbs make awkward paddling-like movements, while the rear limbs make right-left pushing attempts.[72]

Several motor reflexes are present at or near birth. Some persist into adulthood; others decrease over time. If a newborn puppy is gently suspended by its neck, the back flexes, and the puppy curls up (Fig. 9-1). This excess of the vertebral flexor response is present from birth to day 4 and is called *flexor dominance*.[57,59,60,96,105] If the head is extended dorsally, the forelimbs extend, and the rear ones flex; if the neck is flexed, the rear limbs extend.[27]

The *pinna reflex* is present from birth until 2 to 3 weeks of age.[11,56] To demonstrate this reflex, hold the puppy so that its vertebral column is parallel to the floor and dorsal relative to the rest of the puppy. The long axis of the body is rotated 90 degrees. As soon as the tilting of the head begins, the upper pinna will rise dorsally away from the body until its external surface falls toward the top of the puppy's head and the external auditory canal is exposed. The lower pinna will point toward the ground.[11,55,56]

The *abdominal reflex* is present in 80% of young puppies but only 1% of adults.[56] Stroking of the abdomen results in a contraction of the abdominal muscles. This reflex tends to disappear around 6 months of age.[56] In 94% of male puppies, the *preputial reflex* results in the penis being withdrawn when the puppy is stroked cranial to the prepuce. This reflex remains in 30% of adult dogs.[56] The *cutaneous muscle (panniculus), scratch,* and *superficial anal reflexes* are present in 94% to 100% of all dogs regardless of age, although they may strengthen as the dog gets older.[56,57] The *Magnus reflex* is another reflex present from birth, and it lasts approximately 21 days.[57,60,105] When the head is turned to one side, the fore and rear limbs on the side toward which the head is turned will extend, and the opposite limbs will flex (Fig. 9-2).[27,60]

The *placing responses* also appear in very young puppies. When a forelimb touches an edge, a puppy will begin placing it on top of the edge at 2 to 4 days of age.[57,59,60] The capability to support weight, and thus walk, comes later. Around 4 days of age, the dominance of the vertebral flexors is rather quickly

| **TABLE 9-1** | Motor response development in puppies | | |
|---|---|---|---|
| | Age at appearance | Adult-like | Age at disappearance |
| **Head** | | | |
| Pinna reflex | Birth | | 2-3 weeks |
| **Trunk** | | | |
| Abdominal reflex | 1-7 days | | 6 months |
| Cutaneous muscle (panniculus) | Birth | 19 days | |
| Extensor dominance | 4 days | | 21 days |
| Flexor dominance | Birth | | 3-4 days |
| Preputial reflex | Birth | | 6 months |
| **Forelimb** | | | |
| Forelimb bracing | 21 days | | |
| Forelimb placing | 2-4 days | | |
| Hopping reflex | 2.5-3 weeks | | |
| Postural support reflexes | 3 weeks | | |
| Weight support (direct) | 6-10 days | | |
| Weight support (suspended) | 5-6 days | | |
| **Hindlimb** | | | |
| Hopping | 5-6 weeks | | |
| Postural support reflexes | 4-5 weeks | | |
| Rear limb bracing | 4-5 weeks | | |
| Rear limb placing | 6-8 days | | |
| Weight support (direct) | 11-16 days | | |
| Weight support (suspended) | 7-10 days | | |
| **Total body** | | | |
| Landau reflex | 18-21 days | | |
| Magnus reflex (tonic neck reflexes) | Birth-1 day | 18-21 days | |
| Moving backward | 12 days | 17 days | |
| Seal reflex | 2 weeks | | |
| Spontaneous righting | 1 day | | |
| Standing alone | 21 days | | |
| Supporting reaction | 2 weeks | | |
| Tail-drop reflex | 2-3 days | | |
| Turning to face upward on an incline | 4 days | 25 days | |
| Walking | 21 days | | |

Data from references 11, 27, 55, 56, 59, 60, 65, 95.

replaced by *extensor dominance* (Fig. 9-3). In this typically quick transition, the vertebral extensors overpower the flexors when the puppy is gently suspended by its neck. The resulting arched-back response will continue until the puppy is almost 21 days old.[60,96,105]

The *seal reflex* is somewhat similar, but it starts around 2 weeks of age and gradually disappears.

If the puppy is held vertically by grasping it just caudal to the forelimbs, it becomes opisthotonic, with the hind limbs extended caudally, the toes spread, and the neck extended.[11,27] If the puppy is held vertically, with the head down instead of up, a slight opisthotonos will also occur, called a *supporting reaction*.[55] In another supporting reaction, puppies placed on a 25-degree incline have a strong

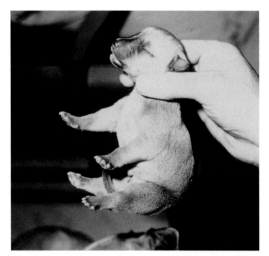

**Figure 9-1.** In flexor dominance, the vertebral flexors overpower the extensors.

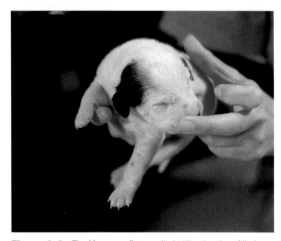

**Figure 9-2.** The Magnus reflex results in (1) extension of limbs on the side to which the head is turned and (2) contralateral flexion.

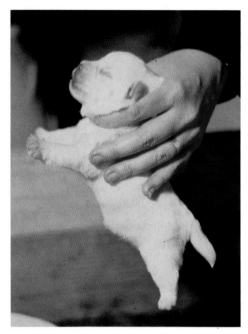

**Figure 9-3.** In extensor dominance, the vertebral extensors overpower the flexors.

tendency to orient upward. They will squirm and use distress vocalizations if pointed downward, whereas they will sleep if pointed upward. As soon as they are physically strong enough, as early as 4 days, they will pull themselves around.[95] By day 25, a puppy can actually rotate its body a full 180 degrees by pivoting on its rear end.[95]

## Walking and Other Later Movements

The initial movements a puppy makes are paddling-like, and they make little forward progress. Support of body weight on the forelimbs does not begin until 7 to 14 days of age,[59,60,96] with heavier puppies taking longer (Fig. 9-4). A puppy can move backward once it can hold its forelimbs under its body, even though weight support may not be possible yet.[94] This ability to back away appears about day 12, although it may take up to 5 days later than that for surfaces that are not flat.[55,94,95] Rear limb support begins at 14 or more days,[57,59,60,94] and standing occurs by 21 days.[57,59] Initially, walking is very unsteady, but by 21 days, puppies are quite mobile and move well in a straight line.[55,94,96]

Bracing itself when pushed is another type of postural support that a puppy develops over time. A puppy will brace or show lateral stepping with the forelimbs at approximately 3 weeks of age.[27] In the rear, the ability for this type of support begins at 4 to 5 weeks.[27] From then on, motor skills rapidly mature; and, with the parallel sensory development, puppies can orient on distant littermates and objects.[65] Puppies that stay with their mother until they are 6 to 10 weeks old are influenced by her and have significantly better developed motor ability and agility than those that are separated from her at 6 weeks.[51]

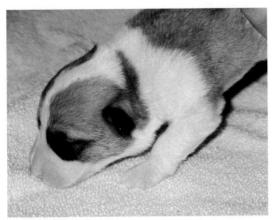

**Figure 9-4.** First attempts at forelimb support.

Once the puppy is capable of moving and is old enough to go to its new home, puppy behaviors can become potential problems. When left alone, puppies that are acquired from private sources, not from dog breeders, show more exploratory behavior, but the actual amount is affected by its age.[36]

## ADULT MOVEMENTS

Studies of adult, laboratory-raised dogs show several types of activity patterns. This is divided into 2.9 hours of movement, 4.3 hours of wakeful resting, and 3.7 hours in transitional behaviors.[146] They may sleep for the remaining 13 hours. Those housed in outdoor kennels show significantly higher activity levels, increased frequency of moving, and lower frequency of passive behavior.[134]

Dog owners describe their adult pets as being very (48%) to moderately (46%) active,[132] and studies have shown that the actual number of steps taken does correlate with the owner's perception.[37] It also correlates to the activity of their owners.[37] The average owner takes the dog on a leash walk or jog between three and seven times a week for exercise.[132] The dog is exercised off leash about as often, with 84% of the dogs doing some or a lot of running during this free time.[132] Overall activity levels in dogs are quite variable,[43] probably because much of a dog's movement tends to be reactive rather than spontaneous.[45] This was collaborated in laboratory dogs, regardless of cage size.[31]

Activity levels in giant breed dogs have been linked to health in an interesting way. Giant dogs with high activity levels and a "high level of happiness" are at a reduced risk for gastric dilation-volvulus.[69] This correlation does not hold true for large-breed dogs.

Aging can result in a greater decline in curiosity, exploration, and responses to novel stimuli than to activity.[131] Even after consideration of degenerative orthopedic conditions, though, activity levels in older dogs tend to be reduced.[91,131] Old dogs spend more time awake and in slow-wave sleep and less time in rapid eye movement (REM) sleep than do young adult dogs.[135] It has been observed in racing sled dogs that activity levels are diurnal, tending to increase around sunrise and sunset, and are independent of ambient temperatures.[45]

### Walking

The *walk* of a dog is a four-beat gait in which each foot touches the ground at a different time (Fig. 9-5). Each hind foot is placed less than one quarter of a cycle before the forelimb on the same side.[93] In the walk, there are typically two or three feet on the ground at anyone time. Three feet on the ground at one time is the most common and at no time are there less than two on the ground.[8] In a really slow walk, all four feet may touch the ground at a time but briefly. The gait is described as symmetric because the movements during the second half of a complete stride are a mirror image of those during the first half. The actual footfall pattern remains the same for all dogs. The timing of each foot striking the ground is relative to that of another specific foot, and it varies among dogs and at different speeds.

The vertical force exerted on the pads of the front feet of a walking dog is approximately equal to the dog's body weight.[92] It is less on the rear limb pads, approximating 0.8 of the body weight.[92] Ground contact time for the front pads is about 1.5 times longer than for the rear limbs.[92]

### Ambling

The *amble,* also called the *slow pace* or the *running walk,* is also a four-beat, symmetric gait that has the same footfall pattern as the walk (see Fig. 9-5). The difference between the amble and the walk is a visual one. In the amble, the limbs on each side of the body appear to be moving forward at almost the same time, with the rear limb touching the ground slightly before the front limb touches it. The slower version includes a segment in which all four limbs have ground contact at the same time.

## Trotting

The *trot* is a two-beat, symmetric gait (see Fig. 9-5). The contralateral fore and hind feet move forward in unison, landing at the same time. Usually a suspension phase exists between the lifting of one alternate pair of limbs and the landing of the next pair. In a very slow trot, there will be a very short period in which all four limbs are in contact with the ground instead of being suspended above it.

The trot is probably the most popular gait for dogs. It allows them to cover a lot of ground quickly, but it does not use much energy. The stride frequencies at preferred trotting speeds are approximately 0.85 those of the galloping frequency.[10] As the diaphragm moves forward and backward twice during each full stride cycle, the frequency of breathing during trotting is 1.7 times that during galloping.[10] When a forepaw is on the ground, the thorax on that side is also compressed, so that between diaphragmatic action and thoracic compression, ventilation during the trot can be regarded as asynchronous.[10,25]

## Pacing

The *pace* is another two-beat, symmetric gait (see Fig. 9-5). Here the limbs on the same side of the body move forward in unison. Because the body's center of gravity shifts from right to left and back, the dog has a sideways rocking motion. All four feet make ground contact at the slowest expression of the pace. The most typical faster pace has a suspension phase. Dogs that pace tend to have a slightly elevated center of gravity as they perform this gait. They also tend to have a short back-relative-to-leg length. As a result of this conformation, they may have learned to modify their trot into a pace to avoid interference between feet on the same side.

## Galloping/Running

The *gallop* is the fastest of the dog's gaits, being a four-beat and asymmetric movement. During the slowest form of the gallop, the *canter,* between one and three feet maintain ground contact (see Fig. 9-5). As the dog goes faster, the canter changes to the single-suspension form of the gallop. Here the vertebral column is extended and the body is suspended in the air ("floating phase"[93]) between the time the rear limbs push off and the forelimbs touch down again.[66] The fastest gallop is the double-suspension version, with a second suspension phase occurring as the forelimbs leave the ground. There is enough forward push to lift the body off the ground for a brief period before the rear limbs touch down. The total amount of time a dog is suspended approximates one third of the total time for one complete stride.[83] This phase of second suspension is possible only because of a very flexible vertebral column that allows the rear limbs to overreach and land in front of the spot where the front feet were.[66] Using a double suspension, a racing Greyhound can achieve speeds approximating 40 miles per hour.[78]

At all speeds of the gallop, a careful observer can notice that one forelimb and one rear limb land before the contralateral limb. The second limb of the pair is then placed slightly forward from the first. If the second foot to land of the front and rear pairs is the left foot, the dog is said to have a "left lead" in front and behind. Dogs often switch their lead foot as they run. They will commonly *cross-canter* (also called a "rotatory gallop"[93]) by using the opposite lead in the front from that in the rear. The relative lateral rigidity of horses makes it important for them to use an inside lead as they gallop around a corner. In other words, if a horse is galloping in a circle to its left, it is most stable if it is in the left-lead front and rear. Because most dogs are very flexible and have a low center of gravity, leads are less important for them from a safety standpoint.

Breathing during the gallop is at a ratio of one breath to one stride.[24] The aerobic work capacity of the diaphragm averages 23% and is constant as the workload increases.[124] Only when the phrenic venous oxygen tension gets below a certain point do problems occur.[124]

## Jumping

In dogs, *jumping* tends to take two forms. In the first, the dog springs straight up into the air from a push by both rear limbs. This dog might be trying to see out the window, reach a doorknob, or grab a tasty morsel off a counter. As the dog leaves the ground, the forelimbs are accelerated against the body, and the center of gravity shifts.[140] During the floating phase, there is no activity in the muscles of the rear limbs,[140] but they absorb the shock as the dog lands on both rear limbs first. The second type of jumping is from one location to another across a space. Examples would include a dog jumping over a hurdle, across a mud hole, or onto a sofa. The dog pushes off with the rear limbs, either with both at the same time from a standing start, or with one slightly before the other if galloping. It lands on the front feet with one forelimb touching down first and slightly behind where the second will land.

Muscles, tendons, ligaments, and bones take a tremendous beating during jumping activities.[9] That holds true regardless of whether the jump covers a long distance or a vertical height.

## Swimming

The paddling movements associated with a dog *swimming* are made in a rhythmic pattern rather than by random thrashing. The movements occur in the same sequence as those of the trot—contralateral fore and rear limbs moving in unison. This combination offers many of the same advantages in the water as it does on land. Equal force on right and left sides establishes lateral stability and allows minimal exertion for distance gained.

## Retrieving

The tendency to chase moving things is connected with skills needed for hunting. In canids, the usual outcome of a chase is to eat the downed prey at the location of the kill. When young canids are to be fed at a distant location, food is carried in the stomach and disengorged secondary to begging by the young. When young do get to join the adults at kill sites, they might carry small pieces from the carcass to a nearby quiet spot. Puppies generally do not have innate behaviors to capture prey and bring it back to a home base for eating, called *retrieving*.

Retrieving behaviors have developed for other reasons. The thrill of the chase comes to be associated with returning the object so that the chase can occur again. Bringing the object to a person is rewarded by the chase that follows. Selective breeding for this tendency in the retriever breeds has allowed the behavior to be refined to the extent that a dog can be sent after an object it never even got to chase.

## Digging

*Digging* is a normal locomotive behavior that can also become an unacceptable one. In this normal behavior, a dog alternates use of the forelimbs while its rear feet are relatively immobile in an attempt to move dirt or some other barrier. Breeds selectively developed to go after burrowing vermin are very efficient diggers. Other dogs may dig in moist soil to have a damp spot to lie in for conductive cooling on a hot summer day. Digging can also occur in unacceptable locations or to excess and be considered a problem, as discussed later in the chapter.

## Paw Dominance

Many house dogs will use one foot to paw at their bedding as they rearrange it before lying down or to scratch at a door when asking to go out. Studies in *paw dominance* (also called "laterality") are not always easy to set up in an objective way because of environmental and positional influences. Yet, paw dominance is a subject of much interest, especially to schoolchildren looking for science fair projects. Controlled studies have shown that approximately 57% of dogs show a preference for their right paw,[136] and female dogs are more likely to show this right-paw preference.[123] Another 18% show a left-paw preference, leaving 25% as ambidextrous.[136] Of all dogs tested, 75% show a strong preference too, especially if it is in favor of the right paw.[136]

Paw dominance turns out to be slightly more complicated than left paw–right paw. Paw dominance, or factors relating to it, also affects immunity. Left-pawed individuals have a higher percentage and absolute number of lymphocytes.[123] They also have a lower percentage of granulocytes and number of γ-globulins than either right-pawed or ambidextrous dogs.[123] There is also a correlation between laterality of a dog and its response to immunization.

Dogs that are left-pawed develop lower immuno-globulin G antibody titers and interferon-γ serum levels following a rabies vaccination than do right-pawed or ambidextrous dogs.[122] The interleukin-10 responses do not differ.

Reaction to noise may also be related to paw dominance, or rather to the lack of it. There is a positive correlation between ambidextrous dogs and noise phobia.[26]

A study looking at brain anatomy and paw dominance concluded that there is no correlation between either cerebral asymmetry or fissures and a dominant paw.[137] These findings are consistent with similar comparisons in humans.[137]

## Unusual Patterns of Locomotion

Some uncommon locomotor behaviors have been reported. The Dalmatian provides one example. This breed has been associated with fire engines and before that with horse-drawn coaches. The tendency for these dogs to choose a specific position beneath the coach or fire engine has a strong genetic basis, with 70% of the dogs choosing a safe position.[141]

Newspaper articles or television news shows have highlighted other unusual locomotor behaviors. Dogs have been featured that surf, water-ski, dive underwater, play pool, walk on sheep, ride motorcycles, walk only on their hind legs or front legs, pull carts, get pulled in wagons, ride horses or cattle, and balance on top of moving pickup trucks. The variety is limited only by what individual dogs are willing to learn and owners are willing to teach.

## Homing/Roaming

One of the more sensational types of news stories is about a dog that is lost but manages to find its way home. The idea was popularized by the story "Lassie, Come Home." In general, dogs have an un-usually good sense of direction to start them randomly searching in a general direction.[120] If they then encounter familiar odors from other dogs with which they share overlapping home ranges, the search pattern can be narrowed. This was probably the explanation that brought a blind Cocker Spaniel 45 miles to within a few miles of her home.[125] Documentation of actual cases of returned dogs must depend on rabies tags, microchips, or names on collars, because physical appearances, even un-usual features, and behaviors have fooled more than one owner.

Studies of path integration, or the dog's ability to update information of direction and distance traveled relative to a starting point, suggest dogs are not accurate.[128] They tend to overestimate turn angles and underestimate return distances. This probably explains why there are over 7 million pets lost each year that never return home.[125]

Of dogs that stay outside, 10% run loose, 71% are kept in a fenced yard, 15% stay in a kennel, and 4% are tied.[132] Twenty percent of dog owners admit to having dogs that roam free or escape regularly.[2] Approximately 46% of dogs are outside at least 11 hours each day, and another 32% are out 3 to 10 hours.[132] The number of dogs that are free ranging tends to peak around 7:00 in the morning and 5:00 in the afternoon,[19] suggesting that the animals have recently been turned out by their owners.

The daily numbers of roaming dogs tends to increase as temperatures grow warmer, peaking at around 91° F (23° C). Most traveling during those days is restricted to the morning hours and resting is saved for later in the day.[19] Feral dogs show a similar pattern of traveling more during the coolest part of the day (the morning); these dogs are most active at night, regardless of the season.[127] A feral pack will travel 0.3 to 5.1 miles (0.5 to 8.2 km) in a 24-hour period.[127] The tendency to stray continues after adoption too. It is more common in dogs that were strays before adoption than in those adopted that had been surrendered as unwanted.[148] Roaming is a male sexually dimorphic behavior because it is most commonly shown by intact male dogs, and it can be eliminated or dramatically reduced in 94% of these male dogs after castration.[86]

## Dog Parks

The development of fenced dog parks for off-leash exercise has become an international, urban trend (Fig. 9-6). Both dog owners and politicians look for ways to ensure maximum enjoyment of a dog with minimal inconvenience to the citizens. There is no single pattern that works for the "perfect" dog park, but the positives need to outweigh the negatives.

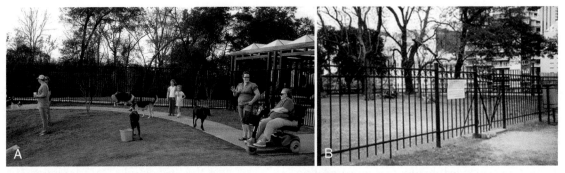

**Figure 9-6.** Dog parks are available in many cities around the world, from College Station, Texas **(A)**, to Buenos Aires, Argentina **(B)**.

Benefits for dogs include exercise, social interaction with other dogs and people, and environmental stimulation. Owners benefit from quality time with their dog, exercise, and interaction with other people. The community can benefit from having community activism, reduced illegal off-leash use, and improved esthetics of underused land.[12]

There are negatives and other factors to consider in setting up a dog park. First is public safety, which is currently not reported to be an issue.[12] Dog fights can happen, so special areas are needed to separate small and large dogs, and rules must ensure that the wrong elements of society are not allowed to use the park for dog fighting. The costs of a park are ongoing from the original fencing and signs, to upkeep of grass and shade, to waste management.[12]

## Activity Patterns in Laboratory Dogs

With the passage of federal legislation and the adopting of rules on cage sizing and exercise requirements for laboratory-housed dogs, there has been strong interest in whether a dog's activity is affected by cage size. The standard size has been calculated as follows:

$$(\text{length of the dog} + 6 \text{ inches}) \times (\text{length}$$
$$\text{of the dog} + 6 \text{ inches}) \times (\text{height of the}$$
$$\text{dog} + 6 \text{ inches})$$

This formula could, however, be modified by exercise or social groupings.[79]

A number of conclusions can be drawn from published studies. Neither physiologic capabilities nor activity levels vary significantly among dogs kept in different-sized cages.* More activity occurs when dogs are housed with other dogs and when people or toys are present.[86,87,88,89] When comparing Beagles exercised alone or with other Beagles that were not exercised or only caged, there is no difference in the overall health of the dogs nor in the development of abnormal behaviors.[39] Social isolation may be more important than spatial restrictions relative to the well-being of laboratory dogs.[80,88]

In work done at Texas A&M University, laboratory Beagles kept in runs were videotaped over several different 24 consecutive-hour periods and their activities calculated to 0.1 second. Though kept individually in the runs, all the dogs could see each other and could touch adjacent dogs through the chain-link fence. The average time spent in various activities is presented in Tables 9-2 and 9-3. This information can be used as a reference point for evaluating dogs kept in different environments.

## RESTING BEHAVIORS

Dogs show a number of resting behaviors, including sitting, lying down but being alert, slow-wave sleeping, and REM sleeping.

In the specific postures used for sitting, the dog rests on its perineum and ischiatic tuberosities. The legs typically point forward (Fig. 9-7). Minor variations occur in which legs are directed to one side or the other or the back is arched so that the dog

---

*References 18, 38, 82, 89, 114, 139.

| TABLE 9-2 | Average 24-hour activity patterns of normal laboratory Beagles | |
|---|---|---|
| | Time in seconds | Time in minutes |
| Grooming | 1214 | 20 |
| Walking | 16,653 | 278 |
| Standing | 4966 | 83 |
| Sitting | 3785 | 63 |
| Lying | | |
|   Sternal recumbency | 11,993 | 200 |
|   Lateral recumbency | 15,761 | 263 |
|   Combined sternal and lateral | 31,765 | 529 |
|   On back | 246 | 4 |

| TABLE 9-3 | Average number of activity changes made in 24 hours by normal laboratory Beagles |
|---|---|
| Activity | Number |
| Stretches | 2 |
| Urinations | 9 |
| Defecations | 3 |
| Jumps | 60 |
| Position changes | 490 |
| Average number of activity changes in 24 hours | 564 |

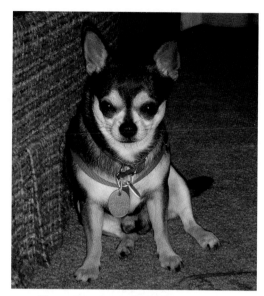

**Figure 9-7.** The sitting posture of a Chihuahua.

sits flatter on the perineum. These variations may indicate orthopedic or neurologic problems, especially if they show up in an older dog.

When a dog lies down, it uses one of four postures. The posture used most frequently when alertness is important is that of *sternal recumbency* (Fig. 9-8). Here the sternum and ventral midline touch the ground. The forelimbs are directly in front of the dog and the rear limbs are either flexed directly below its normal position or extended behind the dog. In *lateral recumbency* the dog lies with either the right or left side touching the ground (Fig. 9-9). This posture allows complete relaxation for deep sleep. A combination of sternal and lateral recumbency is a posture commonly used by resting dogs (Fig. 9-10). Although not all dogs lie on their back, a few will (Fig. 9-11). Puppies are more likely than older dogs to rest this way, and small, broad-backed

dogs are more likely than long-legged slimly built dogs. This lying on the back posture can be used for resting or it can be a submissive posture, as for a "tummy rub." In the latter case, the eyes are usually wide open and the tongue may be flicked in and out occasionally.

The Beagle study at Texas A&M University showed that the run-housed dog averaged 1 hour a day sitting and 16.6 hours lying in one of the various positions (see Table 9-2). Other researchers have noticed a difference in the percent of time spent sitting or lying based on cage size. Beagles kept in standard cages spend 12.7% of their day sitting and 6.6% of their time lying. Those in large cages sit 9.4% of the time and lie down 8.3% of the day.[82]

Where a dog rests varies with individuals. Many house dogs will lie near an owner, or they have favorite spots if the owner is not home. This preferred location could be on a tile floor for coolness or on a sofa or owner's bed. Some outdoor dogs like to rest on top of their doghouse roof, perhaps to be able to keep an eye on neighborhood activities. Kennelled dogs and some house pets prefer a nest box sleeping environment. A relatively confined space with soft bedding that can be washed is ideal. There is also some evidence to suggest that provision of such a

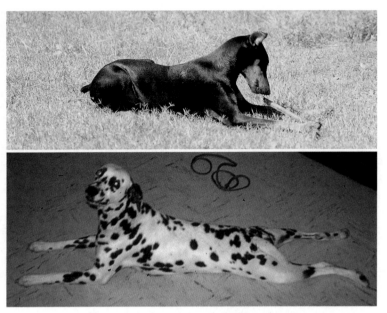

**Figure 9-8.** Two variations of sternal recumbency.

sleeping arrangement in each kennel will reduce the overall noise in a kennel.[30]

Young puppies sleep in a heap during their first few weeks of life (Fig. 9-12). As they begin developing thermoregulation at around 3 weeks of age, the puppies gradually begin to lie parallel to each other (Fig. 9-13).[65] When the individual can maintain its own body temperature, it becomes more likely to sleep alone or with just one or two littermates.

During puppyhood, changes in sleep patterns occur, documented both by electroencephalograms (EEGs) and behavioral observations. At birth, puppies tend to abruptly alternate between wakefulness and activated sleep, such that the EEGs show little change.[61,64] At 2 weeks, slow-wave sleep patterns first appear on the EEG.[64] The amount of wakefulness increases, and activated sleep decreases so that by 3 weeks, they are about equal.[64] At this time, it is uncommon for the puppy to go directly from wakefulness to activated sleep.[61,62] By 4.5 weeks, the puppies are alert more than 50% of the time, and the amount of quiet sleep becomes greater than that of activated sleep.[64] Activated sleep has decreased significantly in 5-week-old puppies.[64] By 8 weeks, differences between sleep and wakefulness are adult-like.[55]

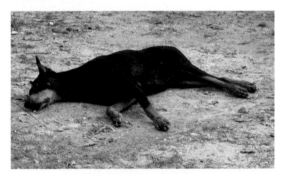

**Figure 9-9.** A Doberman pinscher in lateral recumbency.

Sleep patterns in adult dogs will vary somewhat because of light/dark cycles, surrounding activities, and familiarity of surroundings. In 12-hour light/dark cycles, laboratory dogs have one peak sleep period from 2100 to 0400 hours, and many also show a tendency to sleep from 1300 to 0500.[4,77,104] The adult dog goes from wakefulness, to drowsiness, to slow-wave sleep, to REM (rapid eye movement or active) sleep, and then back to slow-wave sleep again or to arousal. Alertness gradually decreases for the first hour after the lights go out, and a gradual increase begins approximately 1 hour before the lights come on again.

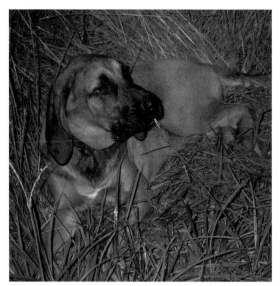

**Figure 9-10.** A combination lying posture of sternal recumbency in front and lateral recumbency behind.

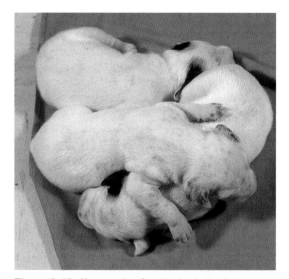

**Figure 9-12.** Young puppies often sleep in a heap to help conserve body heat.

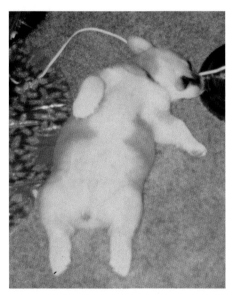

**Figure 9-11.** A tired puppy sleeps on its back.

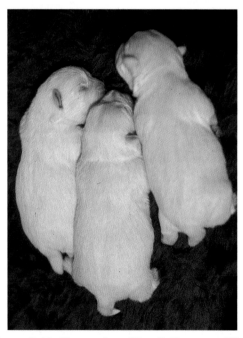

**Figure 9-13.** Warm puppies and those that have some ability to conserve body heat tend to lie parallel.

In slow-wave sleep, the animal will lie down or crouch, close its eyes, and breathe regularly. Although it may shift positions occasionally, the dog is relatively unresponsive to the environment.[76]

In REM sleep, the EEG is almost the same as when the dog is awake, but there is a motor paralysis of the skeletal muscles.[77] Complete relaxation of the neck and back muscles results from active inhibition of spinal motor neurons, possibly by activation of acetylcholine-containing neurons in the causal brainstem, releasing a chain of events that results in the postsynaptic inhibition.[111] Respiration is irregular. Phasic movements of the distal digital, facial, extraocular, and tail muscles occur.[76,77] Dogs appear to paddle with all four limbs, and they may vocalize, as air is irregularly forced through the larynx.[76,77] In humans, dreaming occurs during REM sleep.[4,133] Because dogs also have REM sleep, it is possible that they might be able to dream, but this theory is impossible to prove.[77,133] Although a new habitat will suppress REM sleep for a night, the deficit will be made up during the next 2 nights.[5]

Dogs average 23 sleep-wake episodes per hour during an 8-hour period.[5,6,7] Each episode consists of a sleep period of 5 to 16 minutes followed by a 5-minute awake period. Active sleep, presumed to be REM sleep, occurs in 0.2 to 1.0 sessions per hour, each lasting 2.1 to 9.7 minutes.[7] These sessions are followed by either more slow-wave sleep or spontaneous arousal.[5] Dogs in REM sleep can be aroused almost instantly by external stimuli.[76] In 24 hours, the average dog spends 9.7 hours in quiet sleep (3.6 to 5.9 hours in light, slow-wave sleep; 4.6 to 7.0 hours in deep, slow-wave sleep) and between 2.3 and 3.3 hours in active, REM sleep.[146]

The active sleep-quiet sleep cycle takes 20 minutes in dogs versus 90 minutes in humans.[50,77,104] The average sleep-wake cycle is 79 to 83 minutes, with 39 to 45 minutes of sleep episodes, 38 to 40 minutes of a mean wake period, and two REM episodes per sleep-wake cycle.[4,104,121] A normal pet dog spends 44% to 48% of its time awake, 19% to 21% drowsy, 22% to 23% in slow-wave sleep, and 9% to 12% in REM sleep.[40,103,104,121] These sleep patterns can be affected by drugs in dogs just as in humans.[145]

Components of REM are initiated by catecholamine mechanisms in the lateral pontine reticular area.[133] The muscular atonia is associated with that area's locus coeruleus.[133] The movements that are so characteristic of REM sleep occur as the result of monophasic spike clusters originating in the pons.[133] People are more easily aroused from REM sleep than from slow-wave sleep, and it is generally believed that this is true for animals as well.[6]

One trait that dog owners appreciate is being warned about potential danger, so they would like the dog to be responsive to appropriate stimuli at all times. Tests of a dog's responsiveness to auditory stimuli show a weak startle response during sleep beginning at about 18 days of age in puppies.[59] As might be expected, a dog is significantly more responsive when it is awake than when it is asleep,[6] and there is no difference in responsiveness to auditory stimuli during slow-wave sleep versus REM sleep.[6] Dogs bark at 29% of the auditory stimuli, and they are more likely to bark or be alert to a barking sound than to any other stimuli.[6] In groups of dogs, one individual is usually more likely to bark than the others, and barking in response to a stimulus is more apt to occur when dogs are kept in a group than when they are kept alone.[6]

# LOCOMOTOR BEHAVIOR PROBLEMS

Lameness is the typical problem thought of in association with locomotor activities; however, there are many other problems that involve different forms of movement. Problems can range from the extremes of the hyper syndrome to narcolepsy.

## Hyper Syndrome

Excessive activity in dogs has many causes, so the word *hyper* really describes a syndrome rather than a specific diagnosis. Overall, the generic category of *hyper syndrome* accounts for approximately 4% of canine problem behaviors.[85]

### Overactivity

Most cases of excessive activity involve normal dogs that have an abundance of energy because of genetic, nutritional, or environmental factors. The overactive dog is often from a breed with a high energy level, such as the sporting or working breeds. It is common for Weimaraners, Irish Setters, Dalmatians, Border Collies, and Labrador Retrievers to be on the go all the time. These dogs learn normally and they rest as normal dogs do. Their activity has a purpose, which means they can concentrate on a task.[23] If the environment limits the amount of exercise a dog can get, especially if the dog is naturally high in energy, behavior problems are likely to occur. Add a high-energy diet, and the problem can worsen.

Treatment for these dogs includes large amounts of exercise. A regular (not high-energy) diet should be advocated to prevent problems from starting and as part of a program to stop any problem that has already begun. Environmental enrichment helps channel mental activity, so agility coursing and flyball work well. Owners should also be careful that they do not reward attention-seeking behavior because that will reinforce the inappropriate behaviors.[23]

### Food-Related Hyper Behavior

Food can be related to excess activity in dogs.[17] Several years ago this was a popular diagnosis in children, as in pets,[49] but research did not seem to validate the diagnosis for a while. Further research has shown that allergies can be related to hyper behaviors in children, but in those children, the condition is related to multiple coexisting allergies. In overactive dogs seen at Texas A&M University, the problem generally started when the dog was over 1 year of age, was on a diet of more than 30% protein, and historically may have gotten worse or better with changes in brands of commercial dog food. Another study of "hyper" dogs did not find a correlation between high-protein diets, low-protein diets, or low-protein diets supplemented with tryptophan and the activity level.[46] Hyper behavior because of food or other allergies should be considered rare but must be included as a differential diagnosis for dogs with excess energy.

### Hyperthyroidism

Increased activity levels can be associated with hyperthyroidism in dogs. This condition is usually secondary to thyroid neoplasia or excessive doses of synthetic thyroid hormone.[52] The occasional presence of this condition underscores the importance of a thorough physical examination and laboratory screen in cases of hyper syndrome.

### Hyperactivity/Hyperkinesis

In human medicine, the terms *hyperactivity* and *hyperkinesis* are used interchangeably. In veterinary medicine, the two can be differentiated on the basis of response to therapy.[17] The hyperactive dog will return to normal activity levels in response to mild tranquilization. The hyperkinetic dog calms down when given a stimulant. The presenting complaint for both the hyperactive and hyperkinetic dog typically includes unruliness; doing poorly in obedience class, especially on a "stay" command; excessive barking; and disruptive nocturnal activities. In the examination room, affected dogs tend to be thin, have an elevated heart rate and respiratory rate, salivate excessively, be unable to settle down, and appear overreactive to noises without being able to habituate to them.[33,34] Some dogs appear to have a stereotypic or obsessive-compulsive disorder. A few do not show excessive locomotion, but instead demonstrate an extreme personality type, such as an overly fearful one. A hyper component is suggested by an excessively alert attitude. The hyper syndrome, including hyperactivity and hyperkinesis, is discussed in Chapter 2.

### Separation Anxiety

Dogs with separation anxiety may show continued activity when the owner is gone. In this case, the activity is secondary to the loss of the owner. Thus, it is important to address the problem relative to the stress, not to dwell specifically on the excess activity.[143] Separation anxiety is discussed in Chapter 4.

### Psychomotor Epilepsy

Seizures in animals can be manifested in a number of different ways, depending on what part of the brain is affected. Continuous or sporadic pacing can be the presenting sign.[42,44] Other behavioral signs of seizures may be present, such as staring into space, excessive licking, and fly snapping.[42,44] Although obsessive-compulsive disorders and stereotypies are fashionable diagnoses, repetitive disorders can be psychomotor epilepsy. Most are controllable with phenobarbital or other antiseizure medications

### Narcolepsy

Narcolepsy is a spontaneous REM sleep disorder with episodes of sleepiness and cataplexy in dogs.[75,76,98,130] It has been reported in dogs of at least 16 breeds and in mixed-breed dogs, but its appearance in inbred strains of Poodles, Doberman Pinschers, Labrador Retrievers, and Dachshunds suggests a genetic factor.[77,109,111] In the Doberman and the Labrador Retriever, the trait is autosomal recessive with full penetrance,[53,111] but the genetics of narcolepsy in other breeds may differ.[53] In affected individuals, narcoleptic events are often triggered by excitement, such as with food, play, social interaction, or sexual behavior.[77,109,130] Signs of narcolepsy can occur as early as 4 weeks of age in Dobermans and 14 weeks in Labrador Retrievers and Poodles.[53,111] Overall, 62% of affected dogs show signs before 6 months of age and 82% by 2 years. No obvious relationship exists between the age of onset and the severity of the condition.[53]

A partial cataplectic attack begins as progressive weakness in the rear limbs so that the dog slowly sits. It gradually becomes immobile, with a glassy-eyed stare.[109] A complete attack is characterized by totally flaccid muscles; the eyes remain open and will blink, and swallowing can occur. If the attack is long enough in duration, full REM activity can occur.[109,111] Narcoleptics have a latency-to-sleep onset of 0.8 to 3.8 minutes, compared with that in a nonaffected dog of 6.5 to 28.5 minutes.[111] REM sleep often is not preceded by slow-wave sleep in narcoleptic dogs.[111]

A great deal of speculation exists about the underlying mechanisms of narcolepsy. Cholinergic, noradrenergic, and perhaps dopaminergic transmitters are involved.[53,111,130] A number of different drugs have been tried for treating the condition, with stimulants like dextroamphetamine and methylphenidate used most often. The condition in mildly affected dogs often can be reversed by petting or loud noises.[53,109] Severely affected dogs generally do not make suitable pets.

### Atypical Narcolepsy

Veterinarians will occasionally see a dog presented for a routine visit during which the client remarks that the dog has a predictable but unusual behavior. This is the typical, "Oh, by the way, why does my dog do this?" presentation. The behavior is described as follows: The owner presents a bowl of food, and the dog barks for a short time after looking at the bowl but before eating. Occasionally, a dog may shake its head instead of barking, even to the point of developing an aural hematoma. One dog barked, ate some, and then barked again before finishing the meal. Studies have not been done on these dogs because they are more of a curiosity than a problem, so the actual cause of their unusual behavior is unknown. It is speculated that these dogs are borderline narcoleptics and have learned how to minimize their attack as it is being precipitated by the presence of food.[17] The excitement developed by the barking may be enough to get them through the meal without being further affected.

## Locomotor Stereotypies

A *stereotypic behavior* has been broadly defined as a repetitive action that is constant in form and serves no obvious purpose.[107] They are considered to be internally motivated behaviors that appear in stressful situations.[41] The classic stereotypic behavior of a caged animal pacing back and forth at the front of its cage with a head flip at each end is a locomotor pattern. Many patterns are shown by dogs. A dog may pace in a certain area, walk in a figure eight or circle, jump in place, snap at imaginary flies, run along a fence line, dig, scratch at the floor, circle, whirl, or not move at all (freeze).[13,107,119] In the early stages of its development, the form of the repetitive behavior varies more than it does later. As discussed in Chapter 2, not all stereotypical behaviors can be treated the same way, and this is true as well for locomotor stereotypies. They are a symptom of which the exact causes are unknown. Stress is thought to play a role in their development, but genetic predispositions are most apt to be precipitated during conflicts.[107,119] Results of drug therapy indicate that many conditions can be behaviorally expressed in the same or similar ways. For example, the tail chasing/circling/whirling behavior may represent a single manifestation of three or more causes.

## Tail Chasing/Circling/Whirling

Mild forms of tail chasing can occur, especially in Labrador Retrievers, that are not stereotypic. There is a good correlation between this behavior, excess energy, and the lack of control or poor communication by the owner.[67] Severe forms of tail chasing are very frustrating stereotypies. Most affected dogs walk in a tight circle as if trying to catch their tail.

A few dogs run in this tight circle. Others go after their tail in such a tight circle that they are sitting as much as standing.

The tail chasing/circling/whirling behavior can occur in mixed-breed and purebred animals and has become a significant problem in German Shepherds and Bull Terriers.[21,67,81,110,117] In Bull Terriers, a possible relationship with white colors is suggested.[21] One of the earliest conditions identified as being related to tail chasing/circling/whirling was epilepsy, with the whirling behavior being the locomotor manifestation of the seizure. The seizure may be triggered by excitement or stress as might be produced when people approach a dog's cage,[47,48] stare at the dog, or call its name in an excited tone. For many of these dogs, the circling manifestation of the seizures is controllable with traditional medications, primarily phenobarbital. Thioridazine, a phenothiazine derivative, has been shown to have a treatment potential, too.[97]

Several other etiologies have been associated with tail chasing/circling/whirling. Dogs with high energy levels, including hyperactivity and hyperkinesis, may begin the circling behavior to work off excess energy.[58,63,116] Over time, the pattern becomes more rigid and eventually becomes a stereotypy. The list of differential diagnoses should also consider the effects of lack of attention, excitement, lack of environmental stimulation, very restricted early environments, nutritional deficiencies, anxiety, thwarted escape behavior, attention seeking, hormonal abnormalities, endocrine disease, metabolic disease, neoplasia, food allergies, and inappropriate play behavior.[63,108,118,138]

Occasionally, a dog will actually chew on the tail or on their rear limb enough to damage the skin. Even repeated tail amputations do not stop the behavior when damage occurs. Localized neurologic disease must be considered, because it can cause a tail chasing/circling/whirling behavior. Mild intervertebral disk herniation, tumors of the spinal canal, lumbosacral instability, impingement on spinal nerves (including the cauda equina syndrome), granulomatous meningoencephalomyelitis, post–tail-docking neuromas, rabies, and chronic anal saculitis must be ruled out by a thorough diagnostic workup. All these conditions have been found in dogs presented as behavior problems where tail chasing/circling/whirling was the primary manifestation.

Hydrocephalus is another differential diagnosis for tail chasing/circling/whirling. In small dogs, it remains the diagnosis of choice, unless another cause is found, because of its common occurrence and its association with seizures and abnormal behaviors of all types. Of particular interest is the common finding of some degree of hydrocephalus in circling Bull Terriers.[21,47,48] Whether this is a cause-and-effect relationship is unknown at this time.[47]

Other Bull Terriers that circle may have a stereotypy as indicated by their response to narcotic antagonists.[21] As we currently understand stereotypies, they can be made worse by dopamine agonists like amphetamine and can be inhibited by dopamine antagonists such as haloperidol and opioid antagonists.[28,126] The opioid antagonists, like naloxone and naltrexone, block central endorphin receptors and thus may prevent an internal reward associated with the stereotypy. Taking away the reward reduces the desirability of performing the behavior.

Tail chasing/circling/whirling may also be an obsessive-compulsive disorder, because some dogs will perform the whirling behaviors until they are exhausted. For many of these dogs, the circling begins as an occasional action that can escalate over a period of a few months to one so severe that even physical restraint is difficult. Until we understand more about the biochemical etiology, dogs showing the extreme manifestation will continue to have a very guarded prognosis. The tricyclic antidepressant and selective serotonin reuptake inhibitor drugs commonly used for obsessive-compulsive disorders may need 4 to 6 weeks before serotonin levels are high enough at the neurotransmitter junctions to have a major impact on behavior—if they work at all. There is reported to be at least a 75% improvement in 75% of terriers with compulsive tail chasing.[110] The addition of memantine or dextromethorphan may improve the response to fluoxetine.[106] It is also important to work on environmental enrichment so that the dog can focus on other activities instead.

A particularly extreme manifestation is expressed as self-mutilation, usually of the rear limb or tail. This form has a sudden onset that is extreme and continuous.[117] For owners of dogs showing extreme manifestations, especially dogs engaging in self-mutilations, 1 week is an eternity to wait for a meaningful response to drug therapy, much less 1 month. These patients need a complete neurologic workup. The syndrome is not well understood and the prognosis is poor.

Dealing with the primary etiology is important to controlling the problem. The long-term prognosis is often not good unless the dog shows a good response to a specific treatment.

## Riding in a Car

Dogs can be very anxious when traveling in a car. Some will pant, whine, bark, and run back and forth nonstop from the time they get in until they can get out again. Even if the animal is restrained in a crate or carrier, in the back seat, or behind a wire panel, the activity is still distracting for owners. When the dog is not restrained and can run over the owner's lap or under his or her legs, or lean out the window of the driver's door, the activity is potentially accident-inducing. Veterinarians may not be aware of this problem unless the owner requests tranquilizers for an upcoming trip or unless the dog's body temperature is noted to be excessively high during a routine visit.

Tranquilizers are not the answer for this problem for several reasons. Phenothiazine tranquilizers affect motor skills so that the dog is less able to move, but they do not affect the mental state of the dog. The end result is a masking of signs as the dog gets worse. Also, the effects of these drugs are not consistent when given orally, so oversedation or undersedation is common. Owners usually do not try different doses before travel to find what works best, or they do not give the drug far enough ahead of leaving for it to really take effect. More significantly, tranquilization can interfere with a dog's ability to regulate its body temperature, so hyperthermia or hypothermia can occur.

For puppies the problem may start as the result of motion sickness. They cannot see out the window and may experience a response similar to what some people describe when confined below deck on a ship. For dogs with motion sensitivity, diphenhydramine or dimenhydrinate would be appropriate.

Aromatherapy using the scent of lavender has been studied in dogs that show travel-induced excitement. Dogs spend significantly less time moving and vocalizing and more time resting and sitting when exposed to the lavender than they do before the odor is used.[147]

For most dogs, a few training sessions are easy to do and can make a significant improvement in how the dog rides in the car. Puppy owners can start with short, fun car trips so that negative experiences are not the only association made with travel. Visits to a park, puppy socialization classes, or friends' homes work well.

For the adult dog, a desensitization and counterconditioning program teaches a gradual association with positive experiences and cars. The owner should use whatever reward is most significant to the dog—food, praise, or both. During the first lesson, the owner should walk the dog on a heel command toward the car but stop before the dog shows any anticipation about going to the car. If signs of such anticipation occur 15 feet away, the first training session would occur at 25 feet from the car. The dog is commanded to sit and lavishly rewarded for a correct response. The dog is then walked away from the car on a "heel" command and rewarded again with a fun session of some kind.

The second lesson will bring the dog closer, say, 20 feet from the car. Again it is told to "sit" and is rewarded. The third lesson has the dog sit at 10 feet from the car, and the fourth lesson brings the dog right beside the car. When the dog freely moves to the side of the car and works quickly for its reward, lesson five will have the dog come to the car on a "heel" command and stand until the door is opened. The dog is then told to "sit," is rewarded, the door is shut, and the dog is taken away on a "heel" without even entering the car.

In lesson six, the dog comes to the car, the door is opened, the dog gets in the back seat or crate and sits on command. The reward is given, and the dog gets out before the door is shut. Lesson seven has the dog get in. The dog is put on a "sit-stay." The door is shut and opened right away, the dog is rewarded, and then the dog is taken away. In lesson eight, the dog has to sit-stay longer with the door closed before the reward is given. It is usually a good idea to repeat this lesson several times, gradually increasing the length of confinement each time. During lesson nine, the dog is in a sit-stay in the closed car, the engine is turned on and then immediately off again, the door opened, and the sit-stay is rewarded. After several sessions in which the engine is on for longer periods but the car is immobile, the car is moved back and then forward again a few yards in lesson ten. A second person can liberally drop food treats near the dog for acceptable behaviors. Subsequent lessons involve short trips around the block, to a park, or to a friend's home where fun interactions can occur when the dog gets out of the car. All lessons must be small steps and must be repeated several times before going on to the next lesson, to be sure the dog remains relaxed.

## Digging as a Problem Behavior

Digging is a common problem behavior in dogs (Fig. 9-14). According to owner interviews, the incidence varies considerably—from 8.7% to 83%.[3,16] Yet, digging represents no more than 5% of the problem behaviors seen by a behaviorist.[16,20] Other than a significant correlation between large dogs and digging, no correlations have been found—not for age, sex, length of hair, exercise area, exercise frequency, feeding time, or whether a family member is home during the day.[3] The holes are usually singular, although dogs do have favorite sites and will repeat digging bouts in these sites.[3]

Owners may blame the problem on a number of factors that could or could not be significant,[3] and they may try a number of generic remedies to stop the digging. They fill in holes only to have them dug out again. They put mousetraps, feces, pepper, bricks, or water in the holes only to have the dog move over a few feet and try again. They bury the dog almost completely in the hole for varying periods of time or hold the dog's head under water in the hole. They also use electric shocks. None of these tactics has been successful in the long run, because none addresses the cause of the digging behavior. Although some dogs do stop the digging, another

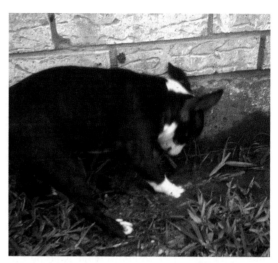

**Figure 9-14.** Digging near a building can indicate that the dog needs increased social interaction.

problem such as barking or fence climbing soon emerges to take its place. *Where* and *when* dogs dig often provide valuable clues about *why* they dig.[32]

Body temperature regulation is an important causative factor when environments are very hot or cold, especially for very young and geriatric dogs.[17] The outdoor dog with a black hair coat needs supplemental cooling in August, especially in the southern part of the United States where both humidity and temperatures are high. Dogs will usually dig in locations that are shady in the afternoon. Areas that are occasionally watered, and therefore moist, are an added bonus. Keeping a child's wading pool with clean water in a shady location is often sufficient to meet the dog's cooling needs. Another tactic is to provide a certain shady location for the dog with loose dirt inside the site to encourage its use instead of an unpreferred location. The loose dirt is dampened occasionally and replaced as needed.

Indoor dogs that are too hot may dig through carpet or flooring in an attempt to cool themselves. Leaving a box fan blowing where they can get to it or lowering the thermostat for more air conditioning solves that problem. Very cold environments can also cause a dog to dig as it prepares a site where it can curl up to minimize the loss of body heat. Cold temperatures can be hard on indoor dogs, especially short-haired breeds on drafty floors.

Raising the thermostat setting or even wrapping the dog loosely in a blanket is usually sufficient.

It is generally believed that outdoor dogs will use their doghouse on rainy or wintry days; however, owners frequently observe that their dogs fail to use the doghouse even in the coldest weather. One reason may be that the people-oriented dog chooses to be closer to the family rather than isolated in the doghouse. In some cases, the inside of the doghouse is poorly kept. Bedding gets dirty, is packed down, grows mold, or supports a healthy flea, tick, or mosquito population. The result is a doghouse that is very undesirable. Instead, the dog digs a hole in which to curl up for warmth.

Another reason dogs dig is for activity, and where they dig often points to what is going on. Digging will be along the fence closest to attractive forms of activity such as a neighboring yard with an active dog, children playing, or a cat walking on the fence. If children are playing near the front yard, the hole may be located near a gate or section of the fence leading to the front. When the dog is isolated from the family and receives minimal interaction with people or other dogs, the holes are usually near doors or windows.

As it is not possible to control the activity in the neighboring yard, the owner may choose to restrict the times when the dog is in the backyard to those when nearby activity is less likely. Another approach is to keep the dog from the part of the yard closest to the activity. As an example, a yard may be divided in half by a fence and the dog kept in the part farthest from the problem area. The dog that digs out but just goes to the front yard or nearby yards, or the one that digs near the house, especially when the owners are home, is often one that is relatively socially isolated from people. The front yard may have better visibility of events in the neighborhood. It will be important to address the social needs of the dog to solve this attention-seeking problem. Dogs like this are often confined to the yard and more or less forgotten except for the few minutes when they are fed.[15]

Some dogs dig for exercise. Active dogs, including those from breeds that were developed to dig, large-breed hunting dogs, and dogs from the working breeds, may dig to get rid of excess energy.

These dogs usually dig inside a yard rather than by the fence and often pick locations where the dirt is loose, such as flower beds, gardens, or former dig sites that the owner filled back in. Dogs that dig to go after ground-dwelling animals like gophers also dig within the yard rather than at fences. In this situation, however, the holes are often in the lawn instead of soft-dirt areas.

In consideration of the different conditions that can be manifested by digging, separation anxiety and obsessive-compulsive disorders need to be ruled out. Hyperactive and hyperkinetic individuals should be treated appropriately before treating the digging problem because the problem may stop with appropriate treatment. Stressful environments also should be changed to eliminate or minimize their impact on the dog.

## Stair-Climbing Fear

It is fairly common for dogs to be afraid of climbing and descending stairs, and there are probably multiple reasons. In some cases, the dog may have poor depth perception, having difficulty determining how far down a step is or how long the total flight of steps might be. This is especially true for puppies. In other cases, open-backed stairways can give the impression of little support or poor differentiation to individual stair treads. Puppies that have a bad experience can quickly learn to avoid stairs completely.

It is best to start young dogs on stairs limited to one or two closed steps until they can comfortably negotiate them. Gradually progress to three, four, and five steps. Practice sessions should include stopping midway up, so that the dog learns to go slowly and not bolt in either direction.

For older dogs, the concept is to start with one or two steps and progress to an additional step only after the dog is comfortable handling that number. When stairways have open treads, another technique can be used. First the dog is taught to walk the length of a carpet runner on flat ground. The carpet runner is then draped over a single step and the dog practices the one step until it is comfortable. The runner is then draped over a two-step stairway, then three, and so on, repeating each stairway several times until the dog is comfortable. Liberal praise and food treat rewards are appropriate.

## Climbing as an Escape Behavior

Dogs may climb over fences and gates as an escape behavior instead of just digging under the obstacle. Some will use props like a nearby stack of firewood or the roof of their doghouse. Others can successfully jump high enough to get a paw hold on the top and then pull themselves up and over. Still others successfully get paw holds to climb up the side, much as a rock climber would, especially when the fence is chain link.

Owners typically try physically preventing the climbing by tying the dog so that it cannot reach the fence, confining the dog to a kennel, punishing the behavior with an electric wire at the top, and thwarting the escape by putting a top of inwardly pointing fencing section over the problem area. As with digging, it is important to understand the forces that are causing the behavior and address those. Social isolation, excessive energy, and the drive for mating are most common. Hunger or an internal reward from predation may occasionally be involved.

## Chasing Cars and Bicycles

Dogs that chase cars and bicycles are a safety hazard to themselves and to drivers. As was discussed in Chapter 7, the basic instinct of predation is to chase things that move away. Predatory instinct and defense of territory are the probable reasons for car/bicycle chasing.[14,17] The internal reward that comes with the abbreviated chase or successfully driving off the intruder usually ensures that the behavior will continue and probably escalate. It becomes extremely difficult to stop the behavior problem in any way other than physically preventing the dog from getting to the moving car, lawn mower, wheelbarrow, skater, bike rider, or other target.

Of dogs that have survived being hit by a car, approximately half will continue to chase them if given the opportunity. Therefore, punishment, even when severe, is not very successful.[14] For those owners who must try some type of retraining, the dog must be restricted from cars at all times except during the training period. Owners must understand that intermittent success is a very strong reinforcer for the behavior to continue. Then a number of techniques can be tried. The owner can be a passenger in the car that slowly drives by. The instant the dog starts running forward, the car suddenly stops as the owner jumps out, yelling, screaming, making tremendous noise, and running at the dog, As an alternative, owners may try using mace spray, throwing water balloons, or using some other extreme but instantaneous and severe punishment. This punishment must happen with each and every attempt to chase. Another technique uses a very long rope or line attached to the dog, so that as soon as the car chase begins, the owner can rapidly pull the animal back while yelling and making lots of noise, Some dogs learn to associate the rope and presence of the owner with being dragged back, so the owner may need to hide until the dog starts after the car. The success rate for these training techniques is low, making physical restraint the most effective method to prevent car chasing.

## Difficult to Control on Leash

Dogs that are difficult to control when they are on a leash are common. In fact, 57% of dog owners complain about this problem. The dog pulls, the owner pulls harder, the dog pulls harder still. This negative cycle tends to lead to the use of severe methods of restraints like prong collars, and these lead to pain and fear. The owner tensing on the leash also can send a message of "concern ahead" to a dog, which then increases its arousal level. Even dogs that respond well to commands at home tend to ignore them completely if their focus of attention shifts away from the owner.

Treatment is multifaceted. The dog is not taken to an area where many things vie for its attention. Instead it is worked on leash in the house or backyard. Head halters (head collars) allow gentle refocusing of attention to the owner and that refocusing is quickly rewarded with a food treat and a praise reward. A number of head halters are currently on the market, with some working better than others.[74] The Gentle Leader works particularly well and has the advantage that it can be fitted to remain on the dog even when the dog and owner are not working. It is also a favorite for working with aggressive dogs because of the amount of head control it offers. A professional dog trainer who uses head halters and positive training techniques can be a very valuable part of this process. A good trainer can ensure the owner uses the head halter correctly, has good reward timing, and knows how to give commands. Basic obedience commands are practiced and rewarded over and over again. As the dog perfects the basic obedience, the owner then moves the work area to a location with a few mild distractions—the front yard perhaps. The obedience work is repeated again and again in the second location, and when consistently done well, the dog and owner move on to a third location with a few extra distractions.

There are occasional dogs that fight head halters almost worse than they fought the leash in the first place. For these dogs there are harnesses that work quite well, such as the Gentle Leader Easy Walk Harness and the TopNotch Harness.

## Roaming and Running Away

Dogs that do not stay home or that run away from the owner were reported to be a problem for 5.8% to 6.4% of surveyed dog owners.[1,16] Twenty-seven percent of owners complain that their dog runs away when off leash.[102] Wolf behavior shows that individual pack members may occasionally take off alone and return a few days later, so this behavior in dogs should not be totally surprising.[73] Understanding the inducements to run away can be helpful in understanding the problem and devising ways to stop it from happening. The reproductive drive is strong, and roaming in response to it is significant, especially for intact male dogs.[73] Dogs also roam in search of food or special treats and for social interaction.[73] When dogs get insufficient exercise, running and resisting the owner's attempts at capture are rewarded internally and may be thought of as play by the dog. These dogs will eventually allow capture after their energy has been expended. Chasing things that move away is also internally rewarding.

For intact male dogs, roaming is significantly reduced with castration or progesterones.[68,73,84] Good-quality food in specific daily meals makes it more likely that a dog will stay at home, at least during those specific times. The owner can also reward the dog's presence by giving a food treat every 15 minutes throughout the day. On the third day,

the reward time is varied to 15 to 45 minutes between treats. Gradually, the between-treat interval is increased and occasional rewards given with social interaction instead.[73]

Punishment for running away seldom works because it conveys the message that proximity to the owner means a negative interaction. Ambivalent behavior toward the dog is best.[73] Confinement is the surest technique for preventing a dog from running off; however, even then, 28% of confined dogs manage to escape on at least one occasion.[2] These dogs can somehow crawl through the tiniest of spaces that if not actually seen would never be believed. If confinement is used, it is important to meet the dog's needs for exercise and social contact so supervision and leash control are important. Prevention of roaming or running away ultimately depends on preventing the opportunity and reducing the incentives.

## Attacking the Phone or Door

Certain dogs get very excited when the phone or doorbell rings, even to the point of attacking the object. With the exception of a rare individual that is having a seizure, this behavior is learned in association with excitement. Typically, the involved family has teenage children who run to grab the ringing telephone or see who is at the door. The dog gradually learns to share in the excitement and will attack the phone or door if it gets there first. Occasionally, the excitement is redirected toward a nearby person or dog instead.[129]

A learned behavior can be extinguished over time if the inherent reward is eliminated. To accomplish extinction, access to the object must be controlled. When the owners are not home, it may be necessary to restrain the dog in another part of the house, put the phone up high, or unplug it from the jack. When the owner is home, the dog can be habituated to the noise stimulus. Have a friend call so that the phone rings a long time without anyone even answering it, much less running for it. The unanswered call sequence is repeated several times until the dog no longer pays attention to the ring. From then on, family members should no longer run or get excited about answering the phone. Extension telephones or an answering machine may help.

When the dog attacks the door, the same principles of habituation can be used. At first, a family member can sneak outside and ring the doorbell several times until the dog calms down. It is important that the dog not be able to see who is at the door, so it may be necessary to cover up nearby windows. The doorbell sequence is repeated in several sessions over multiple days until the dog no longer reacts.

Another way to work on this problem is to teach the dog to "heel" to the door, "sit," and "stay" on a throw rug placed near the door for short periods. The dog is given the "heel" command to leave the area. This is repeated several times until the dog quickly sits and is quiet on the throw rug. The dog should drag a leash from its collar so that the owner can quickly grab it to enforce the behavior at the door. Have one family member ring the doorbell once and another make the dog respond to the "sit" on the throw rug, rewarding the dog when it is quiet. This is repeated many times until the dog remains quiet, realizing no one is coming in. Then move on to lesson three, where the doorbell is rung a second time after the dog has settled down, but still the door is not opened. When the dog learns to sit quietly for a reward, lesson four has the doorbell ringer opening the door and standing still. The dog must sit quietly before it is rewarded. This ring doorbell-open door sequence is repeated until the dog will sit quietly before moving on to lesson five. Now the doorbell ringer opens the door and moves near the dog. When the dog sits quietly, the dog is rewarded. Excitement is the enemy.

As the dog masters the sit and stay commands in this situation, a friend becomes the doorbell ringer. Gradually, the dog learns to temper excitement and to expect a certain routine. Whenever there is a relapse, the routine is repeated until the dog gets it correct again. Acquaintances and finally strangers are introduced to the dog this way in turn. All the time the dog is learning appropriate door manners, it is important that the doorbell does not ring at other times than during training sessions so that unwanted behavior is not reinforced.

If the problem dog has been showing redirected aggression toward a person or another dog as part of the behavior pattern due to the excitement, the initial training sessions should occur without the usual victim being present. Once the dog learns the accepted behavior, the last set of lessons has the dog repeat the "heel-sit-stay" in the presence of the previous victim until there is no suggestion of attention being given toward the usual victim.

## Jumping on People

In surveys, the complaint that the dog jumps on people was mentioned by 6.1% of owners.[16] This behavior may have originated from the wolf behavior of face licking as a greeting.[112,113,144] The face of a person is high enough that the dog cannot reach it without jumping. Owners often reward the behavior in puppies by bending over and petting the excited youngster. The puppy, then, is alternately rewarded for jumping up and punished if it happens when the owner has good clothes on—a distinction the young dog cannot make.

Many techniques have been advocated that do not work particularly well. Stepping on the back feet sounds reasonable until you try it. The feet are not easy to find when a dog is jumping up, and even if they are found, the timing is so long after the jump was started that the effectiveness of the punishment is lost. Putting a knee in the chest usually teaches the dog to jump on the person's side instead of the front. Squeezing the paw or showing the nail clippers may be effective for jumping up, but it makes foot handling and nail trimming significantly more difficult. There are other techniques that can be useful instead.

Dealing with a dog that jumps on people requires time for retraining the dog and for the use of consistent signals by everyone who interacts with the dog. Because a dog cannot jump and sit at the same time, the "sit" command is given as the dog approaches. The dog should know this command well, and then the owner does not interact with the dog until it does sit.[90,144] Then the "no jump" lesson is started. If necessary, the person can even turn and walk away if there is no response to the "sit" command. Turning toward the dog again, the owner should repeat the "sit." Only after the dog sits should it be rewarded.

An alternative to use to teach the dog not to jump up is to have the person continue walking forward into the dog. This throws the dog off balance and, if done every time while paired with the words "no jump," will teach the dog to inhibit the behavior.

## Injuries

Cats have the ability to right themselves during falls and to survive falls from great heights. They have only occasional run-ins with cars. Dogs, on the other hand, are involved in 87% of the trauma cases typically seen in veterinary emergencies.[100] When hit by a car, 12.5% of the dogs die,[99] 32% receive injuries to the bones of the pelvic limb, and 9.8% receive injuries to the thoracic limb.[99] The types of injuries received by dogs that fall from a particular height are similar to those received by cats falling from the same height.[71] Injuries sustained in falls of less than three stories are usually limb fractures, and those from greater heights are more commonly spinal injuries.[71] When the beginning of the fall is witnessed, observers report that 75% of the dogs actually jump—as if to chase a squirrel, go after a departing owner, or respond to a thunderstorm.[71] Approximately one third of the dogs fall from a window and another one third come off the roof of a building.[71]

## Sleep Disorders

Behavioral disorders during sleep are apparently rare in dogs.[142] These are most likely to occur during the REM phase, as is typical of sleep problems in humans. The abnormal behavior could be locomotor or seizure-like activity.[29] In one very unusual report, the dog would suddenly and explosively awaken and run into another room to attack the other dogs in the household.[115] That dog did well on fluoxetine and environmental management that kept it away from the other dogs until it was awake. Disturbances in the sleep-wake cycle occur in geriatric dogs and may be associated with cognitive dysfunction.[35] Encouraging daytime activities and providing a nightlight may be sufficient to ease the dog's switch. Melatonin use also has been suggested.

## Other Locomotor Behavior Problems

Sympathy (psychogenic) lameness and paw raising are ploys used by some dogs for attention.[54,58] The behavior usually is learned following a real lameness when the owner gives the dog a lot of extra attention. As the actual cause of lameness goes away, the dog may again start limping or holding up its paw to get more attention. Some dogs are very convincing actors until they accidentally show the lameness on the wrong limb. The treatment is simple—ignore the lameness and divert the dog's attention by getting it actively involved in activities it enjoys. The hardest part of treatment, though, is convincing the owners that they are not going to harm the dog by ignoring the lameness, so an extensive diagnostic workup may be indicated to rule out musculoskeletal conditions in the owner's mind.

Fly-snapping behavior is another problem of motion.[101] Like tail chasing, it can have multiple etiologies. Seizure disorders are commonly involved, but differential diagnoses must also consider ocular abnormalities, attention seeking, hyperactivity, hyperkinesis, lack of exercise, stereotypic behavior, and obsessive-compulsive disorders. Successful treatment depends on determining the cause and treating it appropriately.

Responses to fearful situations are individual in nature. Fearful dogs tend to increase visual and auditory exploration, but other than that, individuals may increase or decrease their activity levels.[70] Fear of thunderstorms, as discussed in Chapter 2, is a good example. Some dogs will hide in a closet, impossible to get out. Others will break out of a house or yard and be found wandering far away from home.

## References

1. AAHA pet owner survey results. Trends Mag 1993; IX(2):32.
2. Adams GJ, Clark WT: The prevalence of behavioural problems in domestic dogs: A survey of 105 dog owners. Aust Vet Pract 1989; 19(3):135.
3. Adams GJ, Grandage J: Digging behaviour in domestic dogs. Aust Vet J 1989; 66(4):126.
4. Adams GJ, Johnson KG: Sleep and nocturnal behaviour in domestic dogs. Aust Vet Pract 1991; 21(3):144.
5. Adams GJ, Johnson KG: Sleep-wake cycles and other night-time behaviours of the domestic dog *Canis familiaris*. Appl Anim Behav Sci 1993; 36(2-3):233.
6. Adams GJ, Johnson KG: Behavioural responses to barking and other auditory stimuli during the night-time sleeping and waking in the domestic dog *(Canis familiaris)*. Appl Anim Behav Sci 1994; 39:151.

7. Adams GJ, Johnson KG: Sleep, work and the effects of shift work in drug-detector dogs *Canis familiaris*. Appl Anim Behav Sci 1994; 41(1-2):115.

8. Adrian MJ, Roy WE, Karpovich PV: Normal gait of the dog: An electrogoniometric study. Am J Vet Res 1966; 27(116):90.

9. Alexander RM: Mechanics of jumping by a dog *(Canis familiaris)*. J Zool Lond 1974; 173:549.

10. Alexander RM: Breathing while trotting. SCI 1993; 262(5131):196.

11. Bahrs AM: Notes on the reflexes of puppies in the first six weeks after birth. Am J Physiol 1927; 82:51.

12. Bain MJ: The role of dog parks in society and the impact on behavior. Am Vet Med Assoc Convention Proceedings, 2006.

13. Beaver B: Therapy of behavior problems. In Kirk RW (ed): Current Veterinary Therapy VIII: Small Animal Practice. Philadelphia: Saunders, 1983, p. 58.

14. Beaver BV: Why dogs chase cars. Vet Med Small Anim Clin 1982; 77:1178.

15. Beaver BV: The digging dog. Southwest Vet 1987; 38(1):35.

16. Beaver BV: Owner complaints about canine behavior. J Am Vet Med Assoc 1994; 204(12):1953.

17. Beaver BV: The Veterinarian's Encyclopedia of Animal Behavior. Ames: Iowa State University Press, 1994.

18. Bebak J, Beck AM: The effect of cage size on play and aggression between dogs in purpose-bred Beagles. Lab Anim Sci 1993; 43(5):457.

19. Berman M, Dunbar I: The social behaviors of free-ranging suburban dogs. Appl Anim Ethol 1983; 10(1-2):5.

20. Blackshaw JK: Abnormal behaviour in dogs. Aust Vet J 1988; 65(12):393.

21. Blackshaw JK, Sutton RH, Boyhan MA: Tail chasing or circling behavior in dogs. Canine Pract 1994; 19(3):7.

22. Bleicher N: Behavior of the bitch during parturition. J Am Vet Med Assoc 1962; 140(10):1976.

23. Bowen J: Miscellaneous behaviour problems. In Horwitz DF, Mills DS, Heath S (eds): BSAVA Manual of Canine and Feline Behavioural Medicine, Quedgeley, Gloucester, England: British Small Animal Veterinary Association, 2002, p. 119.

24. Bramble DM, Carrier DR: Running and breathing in mammals. SCI 1983; 219:251.

25. Bramble DM, Jenkins Jr FA: Mammalian locomotor-respiratory integration: Implications for diaphragmatic and pulmonary design. SCI 1993; 262(5131):235.

26. Branson N: Landmark study: How does handedness affect behaviour? http://www.ava.com.au/news.php?action+show&news_id=246&c=O&PHPSESSID=aoaflc09e5228f741ac8668)a4543968, 6/14/2007.

27. Breazile JE: Neurologic and behavioral development in the puppy. Vet Clin North Am 1978; 8(1):31.

28. Brown S, Crowell-Davis S, Malcolm T, et al: Naloxone-responsive compulsive tail chasing in a dog. J Am Vet Med Assoc 1987; 190(7):884.

29. Bush WW, Barr CS, Stecker MM et al: Diagnosis of rapid eye movement sleep disorder with electroencephalography and treatment with tricyclic antidepressants in a dog. J Am Anim Hosp Assoc 2004; 40(6):495.

30. Cameron DB: Canine bedding preferences. E-mail communication, June 26, 2001.

31. Campbell SA, Hughes HC, Griffin HE, et al: Some effects of limited exercise on purpose-bred Beagles. Am J Vet Res 1988; 49(8):1298.

32. Campbell WE: Digging dogs. Mod Vet Pract 1973; 54(7):53.

33. Campbell WE: Behavioral modification of hyperkinetic dogs. Mod Vet Pract 1973; 54(13):49.

34. Campbell WE: Canine hyperkinesis. Mod Vet Pract 1974; 55(4):313.

35. Canine geriatric behavior changes established. Vet Forum June 25, 1998:18.

36. Cannas S, Frank D, Minero M, et al: Puppy behaviours when left home alone. In Landsberg G, Malliello S, Mills D (eds): Proceedings of the 6th International Veterinary Behaviorists Meeting & European College of Veterinary Behavioural Medicine-Companion Animal European Society of Veterinary Clinical Ethology. Brescia, Italy: Fondazione Iniziative Zooprofilattiche e Zootecniche, 2007, p. 29.

37. Chan CB, Spierenburg M, Ihle SL, et al: Use of pedometers to measure physical activity in dogs. J Am Vet Med Assoc 2005; 226(12):2010.

38. Clark JD, Calpin JP, Armstrong RB: Influence of type of enclosure on exercise fitness of dogs. Am J Vet Res 1991; 52(7):1024.

39. Clark JD, Rager DR, Crowell-Davis S, et al: Housing and exercise of dogs: Effects on behavior, immune function, and cortisol concentration. Lab Anim Sci 1997; 47(5):500.

40. Copley MP, Jennings DP, Mitler MM: A study of continuous 48-hour sleep-waking recordings in five dogs. Sleep Res 1970; 5:94.

41. Coppinger R, Zuccotti J: Kennel enrichment: Exercise and socialization of dogs. J Appl Anim Welfare Sci 1999; 2(4):281.

42. Crowell-Davis S: A case of psychomotor epilepsy responsive to environmental stimuli. American Veterinary Society of Animal Behavior, Las Vegas, July 22, 1985.

43. Crowell-Davis SL, Barry K, Ballam JM, et al: The effect of caloric restriction on the behavior of pen-housed dogs: Transition from unrestricted to restricted diet. Appl Anim Behav Sci 1995; 43(1):27.

44. Crowell-Davis SL, Lappin M, Oliver JE: Stimulus-responsive psychomotor epilepsy in a Doberman Pinscher. J Am Anim Hosp Assoc 1989; 25:57.

45. Delude LA: Activity patterns and behaviour of sled dogs. Appl Anim Behav Sci 1986; 15(2):161.

46. DeNapoli JS, Dodman NH, Shuster L, et al: Effect of dietary protein content and tryptophan supplementation on dominance aggression, territorial aggression, and hyperactivity in dogs. J Am Vet Med Assoc 2000; 217(4):504.

47. Dodman NH, Bronson R, Gliatto J: Tail chasing in a Bull Terrier. J Am Vet Med Assoc 1993; 202(5):758.

48. Dodman NH, Bronson R, Gliatto J: Tail chasing in a Bull Terrier. Appl Anim Behav Sci 1993; 37(1):86.

49. Dodman NH, Reisner I, Shuster L, et al: The effect of dietary protein content on aggression and hyperactivity in dogs. Appl Anim Behav Sci 1994; 39:185.

50. Elgar MA, Pagel MD, Harvey PH: Sleep in mammals. Anim Behav 1988; 36:1407.

51. Falt L, Wilsson E: The effect of maternal deprivation between 6 and 10 weeks of age upon the behaviour of Alsatian puppies. Appl Anim Ethol 1979; 5(3):299.

52. Forrester SD, Monroe WE: Diseases of the thyroid gland. In Leib MS, Monroe WE (eds): Practical Small Animal Internal Medicine. Philadelphia: Saunders, 1997, p. 1027.

53. Foutz AS, Mitler MM, Dement WC: Narcolepsy: Vet Clin North Am [Small Anim Pract] 1980; 10(1):65.

54. Fox MW: Observations on paw raising and sympathy lameness in the dog. Vet Rec 1962; 74(33):895.

55. Fox MW: Conditioned reflexes and innate behaviour of the neonate dog. J Small Anim Pract 1963; 4(2):85.

56. Fox MW: Development and clinical significance of superficial reflexes in the dog. Vet Rec 1963; 74(14):378.

57. Fox MW: The clinical behavior of the neonatal dog. J Am Vet Med Assoc 1963; 143(12):1331.

58. Fox MW: Spontaneous displacement activities, compulsive behaviors and abnormal social behaviour in the dog. Vet Rec 1964; 76(31):840.

59. Fox MW: The ontogeny of behaviour and neurologic responses in the dog. Anim Behav 1964; 12:301.

60. Fox MW: Canine Pediatrics: Development, Neonatal and Congenital Diseases. Springfield, IL: Charles C Thomas, 1966.

61. Fox MW: Postnatal development of the EEG in the dog. II. Development of electrocortical activity. J Small Anim Pract 1967; 8:77.

62. Fox MW: Postnatal development of the EEG in the Dog. III. Summary and discussion of development of canine EEG. J Small Anim Pract 1967; 8:109.

63. Fox MW: Understanding Your Dog. New York: Coward, McCann & Goeghegan, Inc, 1972.

64. Fox MW, Stanton G: A developmental study of sleep and wakefulness in the dog. J Small Anim Pract 1967; 8:605.

65. Fuller JL, Fox MW: The behaviour of dogs. In Hafez ESE (ed): The Behaviour of Domestic Animals, 2nd ed. Baltimore: Williams & Wilkins, 1969, p. 438.

66. Gambaryan PP: How Mammals Run. New York: John Wiley & Sons, 1974.

67. Gaultier E, Pageat P: Ethological and clinical study of dogs performing tail-chasing. Proceedings Am Vet Soc Anim Behav poster presentations, Denver, 2003:51.

68. Gerber HA, Sulman FG: The effect of methyloestrenolone on oestrus, pseudo-pregnancy, vagrancy, satyriasis and squirting in dogs and cats. Vet Rec 1964; 76(39):1089.

69. Glickman LT, Glickman NW, Schellenberg DB, et al: Non-dietary risk factors for gastric dilatation-volvulus in large and giant breed dogs. J Am Vet Med Assoc 2000; 217(10):1492.

70. Goddard ME, Beilharz RG: The relationship of fearfulness to, and the effects of, sex, age and experience on exploration and activity in dogs. Appl Anim Behav Sci 1984; 12(3):267.

71. Gordon LE, Thacher C, Kapatkin A: High-rise syndrome in dogs: 81 cases (1985-1991). J Am Vet Med Assoc 1993; 202(1):118.

72. Hart BL: Postparturient maternal responses and mother-young interactions. Canine Pract 1980; 7(1):10.

73. Hart BL: Training dogs not to roam. Canine Pract 1980; 7(5):10.

74. Haug LI, Beaver BV, Longnecker MT: Comparison of dogs' reactions to four different head collars. Appl Anim Behav Sci 2002; 79:53.

75. Hendricks JC, Hughes C: Treatment of cataplexy in a dog with narcolepsy. J Am Vet Med Assoc 1989; 194(6):791.

76. Hendricks JC, Lager A, O'Brien D, et al: Movement disorders during sleep in cats and dogs. J Am Vet Med Assoc 1989; 194(5):686.

77. Hendricks JC, Morrison AR: Normal and abnormal sleep in mammals. J Am Vet Med Assoc 1981; 178(2):121.

78. Herron MR: Personal communication, 1997.

79. Hetts S: Psychologic well-being. Conceptual issues, behavioral measures, and implications for dogs. Vet Clin North Am [Small Anim Pract] 1991; 21(2):369.

80. Hetts S, Clark JD, Calpin JP, et al: Influence of housing conditions on Beagle behaviour. Appl Anim Behav Sci 1992; 34:137.

81. Heywood S: Chasing one's own tail? An example of self-pursuit in a Red Setter. Perception 1977; 6(4):483.

82. Hite M, Hanson HM, Bohidar NR, et al: Effect of cage size on patterns of activity and health of Beagle dogs. Lab Anim Sci 1977; 27(1):60.

83. Hollenbeck L: The Dynamics of Canine Gait: A Study of Motion. Erie, PA: A-K-D Printing Co, 1971.

84. Hopkins SG, Schubert TA, Hart BL: Castration of adult male dogs: Effects on roaming, aggression, urine marking, and mounting. J Am Vet Med Assoc 1976; 168(12): 1108.

85. Houpt KA: Disruption of the human-companion animal bond: Aggressive behavior in dogs. In Katcher AH, Beck AM (eds): New Perspectives on Our Lives with Companion Animals. Philadelphia: University of Pennsylvania Press, 1983, p. 197.

86. Hubrecht RC: Behaviour of kennelled dogs. Appl Anim Behav Sci 1991; 31(3-4):294.

87. Hubrecht RC: A comparison of social and environmental enrichment methods for laboratory housed dogs. Appl Anim Behav Sci 1993; 37(4):345.

88. Hubrecht RC, Serpell JA, Poole TB: Correlates of pen size and housing conditions on the behaviour of kennelled dogs. Appl Anim Behav Sci 1992; 34:365.

89. Hughes HC, Campbell S, Kenney C: The effects of cage size and pair housing on exercise of Beagle dogs. Lab Anim Sci 1989; 39(4):302.

90. Hunthausen WL: Giving new puppy owners practical tips to curb unruly behavior can save lives. DVM 1990; 21:29.

91. Hunthausen WL: Identifying and treating behavior problems in geriatric dogs. Vet Med (Suppl) 1994; 89:688.

92. Hutton WC, Freeman MAR, Swanson SAV: The forces exerted by the pads of the walking dog. J Small Anim Pract 1969; 10:71.

93. Jayes AS, Alexander RM: Mechanics of locomotion of dogs (Canis familiaris) and sheep (Ovis aries). J Zool Lond 1978; 185:289.

94. James WT: Observations on the behavior of new-born puppies: II. Summary of movements involved in group orientation. J Comp Physiol Psychol 1952; 45:329.

95. James WT: The geotropic reaction of newborn puppies. J Genet Psychol 1956; 89:127.

96. Johnson CA, Grace JA: Care of newborn puppies and kittens. Forum 1987; 6(1):9.

97. Jones RD: Use of thioridazine in the treatment of aberrant motor behavior in a dog. J Am Vet Med Assoc 1987; 191(1):89.

98. Knecht CD, Oliver JE, Redding R, et al: Narcolepsy in a dog and cat. J Am Vet Med Assoc 1973; 162(12):1052.

99. Kolata RJ, Johnston DE: Motor vehicle accidents in urban dogs: A study of 600 cases. J Am Vet Med Assoc 1975; 167(10):938.

100. Kolata RJ, Kraut NH, Johnston DE: Patterns of trauma in urban dogs and cats: A study of 1000 cases. J Am Vet Med Assoc 1974; 164(5):499.

101. Lane JG, Holmes RJ: Auto-induced "fly-catching" on the King Charles Spaniel. Br Vet J 1972; 128(9):4 77.

102. Lindell E: Control problems in dogs. In Horwitz DF, Mills DS, Heath S (eds): BSAVA Manual of Canine and Feline Behavioural Medicine. Quedgeley, Gloucester, England: British Small Animal Veterinary Association, 2002, p. 69.

103. Lucas EA, Foutz AS, Dement WC, et al: Sleep cycle organization in narcoleptic and normal dogs. Physiol Behav 1979; 23(4):737.

104. Lucas EA, Powell EW, Murphree OD: Baseline sleepwake patterns in the pointer dog. Physiol Behav 1977; 19(2):285.

105. Markwell PJ, Thorne CJ: Early behavioural development of dogs. J Small Anim Pract 1987; 28(11):984.

106. Maurer BM, Dodman NH: Animal behavior case of the month. J Am Vet Med Assoc 2997; 231(4):536.

107. McKeown DB, Luescher UA, Halip J: Stereotypies in companion animals and obsessive compulsive disorder. Purina Specialty Review in Behavioral Problems 1992:30.

108. Messonneir S: An unusual case of self-mutilation in a dog. Texas Vet Med J 1989; 51(3):13.

109. Mitler MM, Soave O, Dement W: Narcolepsy in seven dogs. J Am Vet Med Assoc 1976; 168(11):1036.

110. Moon-Fanelli AA, Dodman NH: Description and development of compulsive tail chasing in terriers and response to clomipramine treatment. J Am Vet Med Assoc 1998; 212(8):1252.

111. Morrison AR: Contributions of animal models to sleep disorders medicine. Lab Anim 1996; 25(2):22.

112. Neilson JC: Unruly and annoying behaviors in dogs and cats. http://www.avma.org/conv/cv2002/cvnotes/CAn_AnB_UAB_NeJ.asp, 7/3/2002.

113. Neilson JC: Unruly and annoying behaviors in dogs and cats. Wild West Vet Conf Vet Syllabus, 2002:597.

114. Newton WM: An evaluation of the effects of various degrees of long-term confinement on adult Beagle dogs. Lab Anim Sci 1972; 22(6):860.

115. Overall K: Personal communication, March 30, 2005.

116. Overall KL: Part 3: A rational approach: Recognition, diagnosis, and management of obsessive-compulsive disorders. Canine Pract 1992; 17(4):39.

117. Overall KL: Dealing with tail-chasing behavior in a 3-year-old German shepherd. Vet Med 2002; 97(3):185.

118. Overall KL: Medical differentials with potential behavioral manifestations. Vet Clin North Am [Small Anim Pract] 2003; 33(2):213.

119. Overall KL, Dunham AE: Clinical features and outcome in dogs and cats with obsessive-compulsive disorder: 126 cases (1989-2000). J Am Vet Med Assoc 2002; 221(10): 1445.

120. Perlson J: The Dog: An Historical, Psychological and Personality Study. New York: Vantage Press, 1968.

121. Powell EW, Lucas EA, Murphree OD: Influence of human presence on sleep-wake patterns of nervous Pointer dogs. Physiol Behav 1978; 20(1):39.

122. Quaranta A, Siniscalchi M, Frate A, et al: Lateralised behaviour and immune response in dogs: Relations between paw preference and interferon-γ, interleukin-10 and IgG antibodies production. Behav Brain Res 2006; 166(2):236.

123. Quaranta A, Siniscalchi M, Frate A, et al: Paw preference in dogs: Relations between lateralized behaviour and immunity. Behav Brain Res 2004; 153:521.

124. Reid MB, Johnson Jr RL: Efficiency, maximal blood now, and aerobic work capacity of canine diaphragm. J Appl Physiol 1983; 54(3):763.

125. Sadie returned to her home. Canine Pract 1994; 19(2):20.

126. Schwartz S: Naltrexone-induced pruritus in a dog with tail-chasing behavior. J Am Vet Med Assoc 1993; 202(2):278.

127. Scott MD, Causey K: Ecology of feral dogs in Alabama. J Wildl Manage 1973; 37(3):253.

128. Seguinot V, Cattet J, Benhamou S: Path integration in dogs. Anim Behav 1998; 55(4):787.

129. Seward RJ, Hart BL: Aggressive behavior. Canine Pract 1985; 12(1):27.

130. Siegel JM, Nienhuis R, Fahringer HM, et al: Neuronal activity in narcolepsy: Identification of cataplexy-related cells in the medial medulla. SCI 1991; 252:1315.

131. Siwak CT, Tapp PD, Milgram NW: Age-associated changes in non-cognitive behaviours in a canine model of ageing. Proceedings of the Third International Congress on Veterinary Behavioural Medicine. Wheathampstead, Hertfordshire, England: Universities Federation for Animal Welfare, 2001, p. 133.

132. Slater MR, Robinson LE, Zoran DL, et al: Diet and exercise patterns in pet dogs. J Am Vet Med Assoc 1995; 207(2):186.

133. Snyder F: Towards an evolutionary theory of dreaming. Am J Psychiatry 1966; 123(2):121.

134. Spangenberg EMF, Björklund L, Dahlborn K: Outdoor housing of laboratory dogs: Effects on activity, behaviour and physiology. Appl Anim Behav Sci 2006; 98:260.

135. Takeuchi T, Harada E: Age-related changes in sleep-wake rhythm in dogs. Behav Brain Res 2002; 136:193.

136. Tan U: Paw preference in dogs. International J Neurosci 1987; 32:825.

137. Tan U, Caliskan S: Asymmetries in the cerebral dimensions and fissures of the dog. International J Neurosci 1987; 32:943.

138. Thompson WR, Melzack R, Scott TH: "Whirling behavior" in dogs as related to early experience. SCI 1956; 123:939.

139. Tipton CM, Carey RA, Eastin WC, et al: A submaximal test for dogs: Evaluation of effects of training, detraining, and cage confinement. J Appl Physiol 1974; 37(2):271.

140. Tokuriki M: Cinematographic and electro myographic analysis of vertical standing jump in the dog. J Exp Biol 1979; 83:271.

141. Trimble HC, Keeler CE: Preference of Dalmatian dogs for particular positions in coach running, and inheritance of this character. Nature 1939; 144(3650):671.

142. UF DVMs treat dog with sleeping disorder. DVM Newsmagazine May 2001:13S.

143. Voith VL, Marder A: Overactivity. In Morgan R (ed): Handbook of Small Animal Practice. New York: Churchill Livingstone, 1988, p. 1036.

144. Vollmer PJ: Puppy rearing—8: Jumping up. Vet Med Small Anim Clin 1979; 74(2):159.

145. Wauquier A: Drug effects on sleep-wakefulness patterns in dogs. Neuropsychobiol 1983; 10(1):60.

146. Wauquier A, Verheyen JL, van den Broeck WAE, et al: Visual and computer-based analysis of 24 H sleep-waking patterns in the dog. Electroenceph Clin Neurophysiol 1979; 46:33.

147. Wells DL: Aromatherapy for travel-induced excitement in dogs. J Am Vet Med Assoc 2006; 229(6):964.

148. Wells DL, Hepper PG: Prevalence of behaviour problems reported by owners of dogs purchased from an animal rescue shelter. Appl Anim Behav Sci 2000; 69(1):55.

## Additional Readings

Adams GJ, Johnson KG: Guard dogs: Sleep, work and the behavioural responses to people and other stimuli. Appl Anim Behav Sci 1995; 46(1-2):103.

Ballarini G: Animal psychodietetics. J Small Anim Pract 1990; 31:523.

Bergman L: Anxious athletes: Treating behavior problems in performance dogs. Am Vet Med Assoc Convention Proceedings, July 2006.

Bouvier M, Hylander WL: In vivo bone strain on the dog tibia during locomotion. Acta Anat 1984; 118(3):187.

Breazile JE, Thompson WD: Motor cortex of the dog. Am J Vet Res 1967; 28(126):1483.

Campbell WE: Which dog breeds develop what behavior problems? Mod Vet Pract 1974; 55(3):229.

Campbell WE: Rote solutions. Mod Vet Pract 1976; 57(9):740.

Cavagna GA, Heglund NC, Taylor CR: Walking, running, and galloping. Mechanical similarities between different animals. In Pedley TJ (ed): Scale Effects in Animal Locomotion. London: Academic Press, 1977, p. 111.

Dodman NH, Shuster L: Pharmacologic approaches to managing behavior problems in small animals. Vet Med 1994; 89(10):960.

Downey RL, Kronfeld DS, Banta CA: Diet of Beagles affects stamina. J Am Anim Hosp Assoc 1980; 16:273.

Fox MW: Canine Behavior. Springfield, IL: Charles C Thomas, 1965.

Haddad GG, Jeng HJ, Lee SH, et al: Rhythmic variations in R-R interval during sleep and wakefulness in puppies and dogs. Am J Physiol 1984; 247(1):H67.

Hart BL: Behavioral aspects of canine narcolepsy. Canine Pract 1975; 2(1):8.

Hart BL: Animal behavior and the fever response: Theoretical considerations. J Am Vet Med Assoc 1985; 187(10):998.

Hildebrand M: Analysis of tetrapod gaits: General considerations and symmetrical gaits. In Herman RM, Grillner S, Stein PSG, et al (eds): Neural Control of Locomotion. New York: Plenum, 1976, p. 203.

Kiley-Worthington M: The tail movements of ungulates, canids and felids with particular reference to their causation and function as displays. Behavior 1976; LVI(1-2):69.

Komareck JV: Fallbericht: Verfolgung der Rute beim Hund-Cauda-equina-syndrom. Kleintierpraxis 1988; 33(1):25.

Mason GJ: Stereotypies: A critical review. Anim Behav 1991; 41:1015.

Murphee OD: Inheritance of human aversion and inactivity in two strains of the Pointer dog. Biol Psychiatry 1973; 7-8:23.

Overall KL: Use of clomipramine to treat ritualistic, stereotypic motor behavior in three dogs. J Am Vet Med Assoc 1994; 205(12):1733.

Pollack R: Scuba dog: Retriever hounds master to go underwater. Houston Chronicle, November 11, 1993: 1OC.

Redding RW, Prynn B, Colwell RK: The phenomenon of alternate sleep and wakefulness in the young dog. J Am Vet Med Assoc 1964; 144(6):605.

Roy WE: Examination of the canine locomotor system. Vet Clin North Am [Small Anim Pract] 1971; 1(1):53.

Shik ML, Orlovskii GN: Biophysics of complex systems and mathematical models: Co-ordination of the limbs during running of the dog. Biofizika 1965; 10(6):1037.

Takahashi Y, Ebihara S, Nakamura Y, et al: An automatic device for forced wakefulness in dogs. Neurosci Lett 1979; 13(1):1.

The sensational surfer of Hilton Head: The Friskies Research Digest 1974; 10(2):8.

Thrall DE, Bovee KC, Biery DN: Demonstration of a "position and relief" in dogs with lesions of the stomach or small bowel. J Am Anim Hosp Assoc 1978; 14:343.

VanValkenburgh B: Locomotor diversity in past and present guilds of large predator mammals. Paleobiology 1985; 11:406.

VanValkenburgh B: Skeletal indicators of locomotor behavior in living and extinct carnivores. J Vertebr Paleontol 1987; 7:162.

Voith VL: Teaching the down-stay. Mod Vet Pract 1982; 63(5):425.

# Canine Grooming Behavior

Grooming is a maintenance behavior in dogs that is important for good health as well as good looks. Good health in a dog is reflected in a shiny coat that is maintained on a daily basis. When things go wrong, not only can the hair coat look bad, but the dog may actually mutilate its own skin.

## GROOMING FUNCTIONS

The obvious function of grooming is to maintain healthy hair and skin, but grooming has several other functions as well. For example, dogs will lick to clean wounds. Canine saliva has been shown to be bactericidal against *Escherichia coli* and *Streptococcus canis,* two common wound contaminants.[18] These two organisms are also the main pathogens implicated in neonatal septicemia, so maternal licking of young puppies protects as well as grooms. Maternal licking also stimulates puppies' urination and defecation.[18]

Grooming is an effective method for removing ectoparasites such as fleas and ticks.[17] Heavy infestations of these blood-sucking parasites can severely incapacitate a dog, making outside intervention necessary to restore the animal's health. Although much of the understanding of the role of grooming relative to ectoparasite infestations has been done in exotic animals, the concepts learned appear to apply to domestic pets as well. Animals that are physically restrained so that they cannot self-groom have significantly higher parasite loads and do not thrive.

A couple of times each year, most dogs will go through major hair-shedding bouts. Grooming helps remove this loose hair and keep the underlying skin healthy. Long-haired breeds often need human assistance. Breeds like the Old English Sheepdog, Komondor, Poodle, and Collie will get hair mats if not occasionally groomed by their owners, and the underlying skin then becomes unhealthy, even to the point of having infestations of maggots.

Evaporative cooling is an important heat-regulatory function of licking. Exact figures have not been determined for dogs, but as much as a third of a cat's evaporative cooling is achieved by licking of the hair and skin. As dogs tend to spend less time grooming than cats, they are more apt to depend on environmental aids to help them cool off, such as moist soil, a lake, or a wading pool.

Dispersion of stress or relief from tension is another purpose of grooming.[3,41] A displacement activity is a normal behavior shown at an inappropriate time, thus appearing out of context. When confronted with a very dominant dog, the submissive one might show a grooming activity, a sexual posture, or excessively submissive posture. The inappropriateness of the behavior helps defuse the tensions. In dogs, grooming as a displacement activity is more apt to eventually become excessive, as compared to cats. Then it becomes a problem behavior.

## GROOMING PATTERNS

The two broad categories of grooming patterns shown by dogs are self-grooming and mutual grooming. The former serves the functions already described. Mutual grooming does as well, but in addition, it is important for maintaining social bonds.

### Self-Grooming

Oral grooming is the most common type of self-grooming. A dog will lick its limbs, the area immediately around its mouth, and areas of short hair, such as the anogenital area (Fig. 10-1).[3] Injuries are also licked, especially if they are bloody or have serum oozing from them. Teeth can also be used as a tool for oral grooming. They are used more in areas of longer hair to remove burrs and mats.

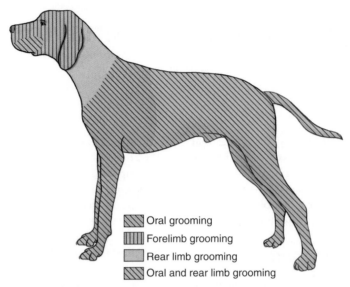

| | Oral grooming |
| --- | --- |
| | Forelimb grooming |
| | Rear limb grooming |
| | Oral and rear limb grooming |

**Figure 10-1.** Areas groomed in various manners by a dog.

Dogs will also chew on their nails and will use their teeth to relieve any itchy spots caudal to the thoracic limbs.

The nails of the pelvic limbs are important grooming tools. The back limbs are used to groom most of those areas inaccessible to the mouth.[3] Generally these are the areas that extend from just behind the thoracic limb and forward, including the neck, head, and ears. Depending on the agility of the individual and its body length compared to leg length, some dogs can successfully scratch most of the thorax as well.

Dogs use their forepaws as grooming tools for the head. They will wipe their face with the medial aspect of the manus, especially around the eyes and ears.[3] Following a wiping bout, they will lick the accumulated matter off their paws and perhaps repeat the sequence.

Rolling is another form of self-grooming used by dogs, and it is usually seen in three different situations.[3] In one situation an individual may roll on the ground or on an object. Sometimes the dog just rubs along the ground instead. This type of rolling/rubbing does not seem to be associated with scent marks, because it can involve parts of the body without well-developed scent glands. Also, the dog does not smell the area before rubbing over it.[3]

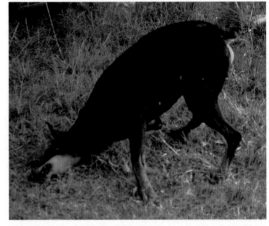

**Figure 10-2.** A dog showing the rubbing behavior used after being dipped in a strong-smelling flea-control product. (From reference 3. Used with permission of Veterinary Medicine Publishing Group.)

A second type of rolling/rubbing behavior is shown after exposure to a strong odor, like skunk spray or flea dips (Fig. 10-2).[3] The intention here is probably to eliminate or dilute the odor, and the rubbing is frequently associated with sneezing and running.[3]

Rolling on odors is the third form this behavior takes, and it is often associated with a "pleasure face"

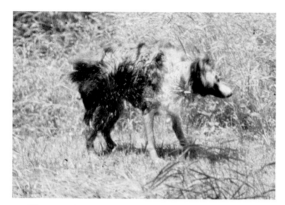

**Figure 10-3.** A dog shakes its whole body after a swim.

(see Chapter 3, Fig. 3-5). Many times the material rolled on is considered unpleasant or malodorous by humans.[3,37] This material includes animal feces, garbage, or decaying, dead animal parts. Why dogs roll on such things is unknown, but various theories attempt to explain it. The first is that the dog is attempting to take on the odor, much as we would put on perfume or cologne, and although the odor is unacceptable to us, dogs have different aesthetics.[3] This would make the behavior socially rewarding.[37] A second theory is that the amount of odor is too great to be able to cover it up with a urine mark, so the dog attempts to cover it with the entire body surface instead.[2] The acquisition of an odor may serve to reduce the novelty of that odor because of the long duration of exposure, or it might help increase the amount of social investigation by conspecifics.[37]

Total body shaking is a behavior commonly used by dogs to remove excess water from their hair coats (Fig. 10-3). The behavior typically begins at the head and gradually progresses caudally To maintain balance, the front and back halves of the dog tend to be rotating in opposite directions at any one time.

## Mutual Grooming (Allogrooming)

Technically, allogrooming is one individual grooming another, with or without reciprocal grooming behavior, whereas mutual grooming would imply that both animals are grooming each other. Both of these behaviors are done by individuals closely

associated to each other. Licking, with occasional teeth nibbling, is the typical method for this grooming.[3] Subordinate dogs may lick the muzzle of a more dominant dog. Although in the technical sense this represents allogrooming, it is more significant to the dog as a social function. "Nitting" is the nibbling behavior by a dog directed at a person, and in this case, it would represent a type of allogrooming. There has been discussion whether nitting is more common in Greyhounds.[22]

## GROOMING BEHAVIOR PROBLEMS

Before the latest generation of flea control products, excessive grooming behaviors were primarily associated with that parasite. There still is a strong relationship with medical conditions, but the incidence has been significantly reduced. Currently about 9% of cases seen by a behaviorist are grooming-related.[1]

### Normal Behavior as a Problem

Owners may complain about the loudness of their dog's licking. This usually is associated with the dog's nighttime activity of grooming at times of limited physical activity. The distraction to the owner is a result of the quiet in the home after bedtime being broken suddenly by the sound of a loud slurp. As grooming is a normal behavior and the lack of other stimuli makes nighttime perfect for the activity, it is unreasonable to expect the dog to stop. Instead, the problem is best managed by looking for alternatives. For the dog that sleeps in the bedroom, having it sleep in another room puts wall barriers between the person and the animal. This could be the room of a child who sleeps through almost anything, or it could be an unused room so the dog now has its own room. Older dogs or those used to sleeping with the owner may need to first get used to sleeping in their own bed for a while. Gradually that bed is moved farther from the human's bed until it is in the new dog room.

Another technique is to put the dog in its new room for the night and use a barrier, like a child's gate. If the dog whines or barks, it is ignored so that the behavior is not rewarded by human attention, and the dog is encouraged to learn the new rules. The nighttime use of a box-style muzzle, after the dog has been gradually introduced to it, is another technique that can be tried.

## Medical Problems Associated with Excessive Grooming

Most, but not all, of the medical problems associated with excessive grooming in dogs are skin conditions, often pruritic ones. Pruritus is closely intertwined with the other sensations of pain and touch.[35] These sensations are all carried on the same fibers and terminate in various brain centers, including the thalamus and cortex.[35] Central factors can also amplify or reduce the perception of any of these cutaneous sensations.[35] The classic mediator for pruritus is histamine. Other mediators, such as proteases, peptides, substance P, opiate peptides, prostaglandins, and leukotrienes, may work directly or may liberate histamine's pruritic properties instead.[35]

In addition to the standard treatment of the underlying cause of pruritic conditions, the use of tricyclic antidepressants may be helpful.[30] These drugs have antihistaminic, anticholinergic, and centrally mediated analgesic effects that appear to be independent of their antidepressant activity.[15] If used early in the excessive grooming condition, tricyclic antidepressants may help prevent progression to stereotypic or obsessive-compulsive disorders.[30]

Several other medical conditions should be considered as differential diagnoses for excessive grooming. Referred pain or phantom pain is one possibility, although it is difficult to prove.[41] Others include neuritis; sensory neuropathy; encephalitis, especially after distemper; and psychomotor epilepsy.[23] Hyperadrenocorticism also has been reported to be associated with pruritus and hair chewing.[6]

## Psychogenic Dermatoses

Several conditions in the dog can be classified as psychogenic dermatoses, which are self-inflicted skin disorders initiated or intensified by non-organic causes.[44] Included in this list of related conditions are psychogenic alopecia, acral lick dermatitis, flank sucking, psychogenic dermatitis, foot licking, anal licking, foot biting, tail biting, allonursing, and tail sucking.[36,44] For any of these, a diagnosis cannot be made until organic and medical causes have been ruled out and any type of pain or distress eliminated.

The development of psychogenic dermatoses tends to fall into one of three categories. It may be important to determine the category to treat the problem successfully. Psychogenic causes, the first category, are learned problems, as when a wound heals but the licking continues.[44] The second category is social interaction, and here the owners reinforce the behavior by paying attention to the dog as it grooms.[44] Worse yet, the reinforcement is actually intermittent, making the learned behavior more difficult to stop.[44] How a dog is maintained, the third category, can also result in the development of psychogenic disorders.[44] Environments that lack stimuli, like chain-link runs, are frequently where problem dogs are kept. Licking is one activity a dog could use to provide mental stimulation.

## Psychogenic Alopecia

As was mentioned earlier in this chapter, grooming is one of the most common displacement activities. Because it is related to conflict or other anxiety-producing situations, resolution of this psychogenic problem depends on identifying and addressing the underlying cause. Dogs affected with psychogenic alopecia will lick one spot until the hair is gone. When they get to the point of injuring the skin, some will just widen the area of alopecia. Others start licking on a new spot, and a few continue working on the original spot until the condition progresses to acral lick dermatitis. For dogs with psychogenic alopecia, increased exercise is often helpful, probably because of associated endorphin release. Tightening up the dog's schedule of human interaction and daily events is another generic recommendation. Stress for dogs often comes as a result of subtle changes for owners. These changes can include new deadlines at work; an illness, death, or wedding in the family; examinations at school; or business trips. Once these measures are started to reduce the stress or the dog adapts to a new schedule, psychogenic alopecia usually stops being a problem.

## Flank Sucking

Flank sucking is a behavior almost exclusively restricted to Dobermans. The dog puts its open mouth on its lateral abdomen and holds that position for extended periods (Fig. 10-4). Although the hair may become wet, there is generally no harm done to the skin or general condition of the dog.[16] Often the behavior is not shown until the dog undergoes some type of stressful event, and it tends to stop again as the schedule and environment return to normal. This behavior occurs in certain family lines, indicating the strong possibility of a genetic base.[2,14,19] It could be a genetic problem precipitated by stress or excitement.[2,28,41] Increased exercise and a rigid daily schedule are usually sufficient to control the flank sucking; however, some owners and handlers rely on small crates to physically prevent the behavior. Antianxiety drugs are probably a better choice than physical restraint when the problem is initially addressed to help break the pattern of behavior, but long-term control should depend more on environmental management than on drug therapy.

## Acral Lick Dermatitis (Lick Granuloma)

The excessive grooming behavior that receives the most attention is acral lick dermatitis, also called *lick granuloma, acral pruritic nodule,* and *neurodermatitis.*[12,33,44] This problem licking can be directed at the tail, but is usually done on the limbs, especially the forelimbs (Fig. 10-5). In affected dogs, 70% of the acral lick lesions are on the left side of the body; especially the left forelimb.[32,43]

Several inciting factors have been named and, as will be discussed later, some may be more significant than others in the development of long-term problems. Preexisting wounds or localized pain are likely to be the initial reason the dog's attention became focused on the area. Certain medical conditions have been reported to mimic acral lick dermatitis. These include nevus, lymphoma, mast cell tumors, an orthopedic pain, deep pyoderma, leishmaniasis, and sporotrichosis.[8] Others—acute moist dermatitis, allergies, hormonal dermatitis, hypothyroidism, hyperadrenocorticism, and hyper behavior—are medical problems that can contribute to the start or continuance of acral lick dermatitis.[30] It is also important to rule out the possibility that the dog uses the behavior to get attention.[30] A behavior of psychogenic origin can be facilitated by stresses, including changes in schedules or even the lack of environmental stimuli.[12,27,30] Dysfunction of sensory innervation in the affected area is another possible etiology.[12,30,39] Dogs may be programmed to lick excessively on a periodic

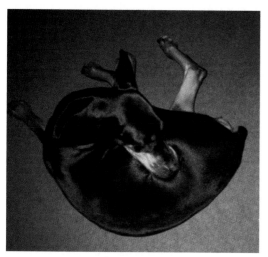

**Figure 10-4.** Flank-sucking behavior. (From reference 2. Used with permission of Veterinary Medicine Publishing Group.)

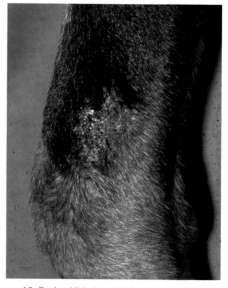

**Figure 10-5.** Acral lick dermatitis is usually on the left forelimb.

basis, as has been suggested in an ungulate grooming model.[12,17] The lick-irritation cycle can also maintain a positive feedback mechanism through endogenous opioids in the brain.[12,43] Finally acral lick dermatitis may be a canine manifestation of an obsessive-compulsive disorder.[12,13,20,30,33]

Dogs with acral lick dermatitis can be grouped according to the duration of the problem; thus the condition can be acute or chronic.[32,34] The length of time needed for a dog to move from the acute to the chronic group is not well defined, but about 6 weeks has been suggested. The dogs in each group differ in their response to treatment; their exploratory, sleep, and eating behaviors; and related activities.

Dogs in both groups are more likely to have reduced exploratory behavior than normal dogs; 89% of chronic cases and 42% of acute cases show reduced exploration.[32] About 37% of dogs with short-term acral lick dermatitis show a reduction in the duration of sleep bouts and an increased frequency in waking up.[32] The rate is twice as high for chronically affected dogs.[32] Dogs affected with a short-term problem tend to have many disruptions in their feeding behavior. Those in the chronic group are more likely to have alternating periods of anorexia and polyphagia.[32]

Acral lick dermatitis is associated with changes within a dog's territory 91% of the time in chronic cases and 63% of the time in acute cases.[32] The condition is associated with a change in daily schedule 78% of the time in chronic cases and 18% of the time in acute cases.[32] Dogs with chronic problems are more likely to be big dogs, particularly Dobermans and Labrador Retrievers, perhaps indicating a genetic component.* Approximately 57% of affected dogs are male,[31,33] and males tend to start developing acral lick dermatitis problems at an earlier age than do females—4.2 ± 3.0 years versus 6.1 ± 2.3 years.[33]

Affected dogs are more likely to have had the initial behavior triggered by local trauma.[37,40] Stress also has been associated with the onset of acral lick dermatitis.[24,34,40,43] Chronically affected dogs have

significantly lower amplitudes on evoked sensory nerve action potentials of the radial and ulnar nerves of affected limbs.[38,39] The electromyogram of the affected limb is abnormal in 56% of affected dogs.[38] The development of this polyneuropathy may determine whether an acute condition becomes chronic.

Dogs in the acute phase may stop on their own,[32] or they tend to respond to a number of treatment regimens. Antianxiety drugs and local treatments tend to be very helpful. A wide range of antianxiety drugs have been tried with some success, including the benzodiazepines, progestins, and phenothiazines.[34] Success with the tricyclic antidepressants, especially when it occurs after only a few days of treatment, is as likely to be the result of their antihistamine actions as to their serotonin effects. Also used are topical products like Synotic-Banamine,[34] intralesional injections of corticosteroids or cobra venom,[5,12,24,29] taste aversion with topical products,[12,44] acupuncture,[5,9,25] and physical restraints like bandaging and Elizabethan collars.[12]

Once owners are alerted to the early stages of acral lick dermatitis, they may be able to prevent development of the typical lesion by increasing the amount of exercise the dog is getting; tightening up the dog's schedule, including times of exercise and human interaction; and identifying stressors in their own lives that might also be affecting the dog.[4,34] In college towns, student-owned dogs with tendencies for acral lick dermatitis are most likely to begin licking during the week of final examinations. Initially, owners will claim there have been no changes in their lives, but once the suggestion has been made that there might have been a change, it is usually easy for them to recognize the connection between the dog's behavior and the human event that affects the dog.

At some point, acute acral lick dermatitis becomes chronic if it is not cured. Based on response to therapy, this chronic category may actually represent two different derivations of the same problem. For several years, dogs that were chronically affected were treated as if they had developed a "bad habit."[34] The lesion was allowed to heal by whatever means necessary, and the dog was distracted whenever it started

---

*References 20, 24, 30, 33, 34, 36, 43, 44.

licking the problem area. When unsupervised, the dog would wear a full muzzle or Elizabethan collar. Exercise for the dog was increased dramatically, too. Although this approach can be effective in eventually eliminating the problem, it is difficult for owners to implement. The behavior may create its own internal reward by stimulating the release of endogenous opioids that act on the pleasure centers of the central cortex. Consequently, disruption of this sensation or punishment greater than the reward is necessary to stop the behavior.[10,12]

A shock collar set at medium (13.2 ms) has been used successfully to stop the licking associated with acral lick dermatitis.[11,12] As with any punishment, to be effective it must be delivered each and every time the behavior occurs, coincident with or immediately following the behavior, and it must be sharp and intense enough to be meaningful.[12] If the dog will show the licking behavior in the clinic, a trial injection of a narcotic antagonist like naltrexone or nalmefene can be tried to see if the behavior stops or is at least reduced.[10,26,42,43] Unfortunately, long-acting narcotic antagonists are not available currently. Clients are faced with the inconvenience of using an injectable product or with the reduced efficacy of an oral product that is only a partial antagonist, like Talwin NX.

The second group of dogs with chronic acral lick dermatitis may have the canine equivalent of an obsessive-compulsive disorder. The histories of many of these dogs reveal a time when the behavior seemed to change from an occasional happening to an almost constant one. At one time the dog could be distracted from the behavior; now the dog is difficult to distract. Drugs that cause increases in serotonin buildup at the neurotransmitter level are showing some promise for treating these dogs.[13,20,27,33,36]

Acupuncture has also been tried on dogs with acral lick granulomas. The points described are He Gu and Qu Chi.[5]

## Acral Mutilation

A nonrelated but extreme condition, often called acral lick dermatitis, can be seen in dogs. Affected dogs seem to attack their tail or one of their limbs, usually a rear limb, creating a severe wound in a

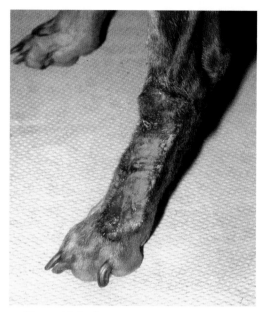

**Figure 10-6.** Severe acral mutilation of the rear limb.

relatively short period of time (Fig. 10-6). The first assessment is that the condition is an extreme form of acral lick dermatitis, and that certainly is one differential; however, the rapidity of onset, extreme manifestation, and caudal location suggest a different problem. It is likely that this dog truly perceives "something," meaning the condition is not an obsessive-compulsive disorder. It is unlikely that selective serotonin reuptake inhibitors will impact the condition, and the seriousness will not allow the luxury of time to confirm that something needs to be done immediately. Neurologic problems, such as the cauda equina syndrome, disc disease, and neoplasia must be ruled out with a magnetic resonance imaging (MRI) workup.

If no neurologic diagnosis can be determined, behavioral therapy is of little long-term benefit. Preventing access to the damaged body part, usually with sedation, will stop the damage but not the urge to do harm. Generally owners come to feel the quality of life is so poor that euthanasia is indicated.

## Acral Mutilation and Analgesia

Acral mutilation and analgesia is a rare, recessively inherited condition in English Short-Haired Pointers that can progress to the point of autoamputation of the digits.[7] This condition is first characterized by insufficient development and then a slow, progressive postnatal degeneration of primary sensory neurons.[7]

## Lethal Acrodermatitis

Bull Terrier puppies as young as 4 weeks of age can begin to show behavior changes associated with lethal acrodermatitis.[21] The abnormal behaviors include extreme aggression toward littermates, diminished responses to external stimuli, shorter play periods with increased sleeping time, and prolonged periods of staring at objects.[21] In addition, the puppies show retarded growth, progressive acrodermatitis, chronic pyoderma, diarrhea, and bronchopneumonia.[21] The median survival time is 7 months, and death is usually associated with respiratory infections.[21]

## References

1. Bamberger M, Houpt KA: Signalment factors, comorbidity, and trends in behavior diagnoses in dogs: 1,644 cases (1991-2001). J Am Vet Med Assoc 2006; 229(10):1591.
2. Beaver BV: The genetics of canine behavior. Vet Med Small Anim Clin 1981; 76(10):1423.
3. Beaver BV: Canine and feline grooming behaviors. Vet Med Small Anim Clin 1982; 77(5):713.
4. Beaver BV: The Veterinarian's Encyclopedia of Animal Behavior. Ames: Iowa State University Press, 1994.
5. Bullock JE: Acupuncture treatment of canine lick granuloma. Calif Vet 1978; 32:14.
6. Chastain CB: Hair chewing associated with suspected hyperadrenocorticism in a dog. J Am Vet Med Assoc 1978; 172(5):573.
7. Cummings JF, deLahunta A, Winn SS: Acral mutilation and nociceptive loss in English Pointer dogs: A canine sensory neuropathy. Acta Neuropathol 1981; 53:119.
8. Denerolle P, White SD, Taylor TS, et al: Organic diseases mimicking acral lick dermatitis in six dogs. J Am Anim Hosp Assoc 2007; 43(4):215.
9. Dodd R: Lick granuloma therapies. Am Vet Soc Anim Behav listserve 9/18/2001.
10. Dodman NH, Shuster L, White SD, et al: Use of narcotic antagonists to modify stereotypic self-licking, self-chewing, and scratching behavior in dogs. J Am Vet Med Assoc 1988; 193(7):815.
11. Eckstein R: Use of electronic stimulation to treat acral lick dermatitis. American Veterinary Medical Association meeting, San Francisco, July 10, 1994.
12. Eckstein RA, Hart BL: Treatment of canine acral lick dermatitis by behavior modification using electronic stimulation. J Am Anim Hosp Assoc 1996; 32(3):225.
13. Goldberger E, Rapoport JL: Canine acral lick dermatitis: Response to the antiobsessional drug clomipramine. J Am Anim Hosp Assoc 1991; 27(2):179.
14. Griffiths AO: Flank sucking. American Veterinary Society of Animal Behavior meeting, Chicago, IL, July 20, 1987.
15. Gupta M, Gupta AK, Ellis CN: Antidepressant drugs in dermatology: An update. Arch Dermatol 1987; 123:647.
16. Hart BL: Three disturbing behavioral disorders in dogs: Idiopathic viciousness, hyperkinesis, and flank sucking. Canine Pract 1977; 4(6):10.
17. Hart BL, Hart LA, Mooring MS, et al: Biological basis of grooming behaviour in antelope: The body-size, vigilance and habitat principles. Anim Behav 1992; 44:615.
18. Hart BL, Powell KL: Antibacterial properties of saliva: Role in maternal periparturient grooming and in licking wounds. Physiol Behav 1990; 48(3):383.
19. Houpt KA: Feeding and drinking behavior problems. Vet Clin North Am [Small Anim Pract] 1991; 21(2):281.
20. Jerome R: A model of good grooming. The Sciences September/October 1992:5.
21. Jezyk PF, Haskins ME, MacKay-Smith WE, et al: Lethal acrodermatitis in Bull Terriers. J Am Vet Med Assoc 1986; 188:833.
22. Juarbe-Díaz SV: Personal communication, March 19, 2007.
23. Landsberg GM: Veterinarians as behavior consultants. Can Vet J 1990; 31:225.
24. Lick granuloma. Mod Vet Pract 1974; 55:139.
25. Lindsay MC: Lick granuloma therapies. Am Vet Soc Anim Behav listserve, 9/18/2001.
26. Marder AR: Naltrexone for the treatment of acral lick dermatitis in dogs. Am Vet Soc Anim Behav Newsletter 1987; 10(3):7.
27. McKeown DB, Luescher UA, Halip J: Stereotypies in companion animals and obsessive compulsive disorder. Purina Specialty Review in Behavioral Problems1992:30.
28. Moses JD: A behavior comment. Canine Pract 1978; 5(1):6.
29. Neibert HC: Orgotein treatment of canine lick granuloma. Mod Vet Pract 1975; 56:529.
30. Overall KL: Part 3: A rational approach: Recognition, diagnosis, and management of obsessive-compulsive disorders. Canine Pract 1992; 17(4):39.
31. Overall KL, Dunham AE: Clinical features and outcome in dogs and cats with obsessive-compulsive disorder: 126 cases (1989-2002). J Am Vet Med Assoc 2002; 221(10):1445.
32. Pageat P: Personal communication, April 22, 1994.
33. Rapoport JL, Ryland DH, Kriete M: Drug treatment of canine acral lick: An animal model of obsessive-compulsive disorder. Arch Gen Psychiatry 1992; 49:517.
34. Scott DW, Walton DK: Clinical evaluation of a topical treatment for canine acral lick dermatitis. J Am Anim Hosp Assoc 1984; 20:565.
35. Shanley K, Overall K: Psychogenic dermatoses. In Kirk RW, Bonagura JD (eds): Current Veterinary Therapy XI: Small Animal Practice. Philadelphia: Saunders, 1991, p. 552.
36. Shanley KJ: Pathophysiology of pruritus. Vet Clin North Am [Small Anim Pract] 1988; 18:971.
37. Simpson BS: Canine communication. Vet Clin North Am [Small Anim Pract] 1997; 27(3):445.

38. Steiss JE, Bradley DM, Macdonald J, et al: Letters to the editor. Vet Dermatol 1995; 6(2):115.

39. van Ness JJ: Electrophysiological evidence of sensory nerve dysfunction in 10 dogs with acral lick dermatitis. J Am Anim Hosp Assoc 1986; 22(2):157.

40. Veith L: Acral lick dermatitis in the dog. Canine Pract 1986; 13:15.

41. Voith VL, Marder AR: Canine behavioral disorders: Excessive grooming and self-licking. In Morgan R (ed): Handbook of Small Animal Practice. New York: Churchill Livingstone, 1988, p. 1038.

42. White SD: Treatment of acral lick dermatitis with the endorphin blocker naltrexone. In Advances in Small Animal Medicine and Surgery 1989; 1(12):6 [Excerpt from Proceed Am Coil Vet Derm (April) 1988:37].

43. White SD: Naltrexone for treatment of acral lick dermatitis in dogs. J Am Vet Med Assoc 1990; 196(7):1073.

44. Young MS, Manning TO: Psychogenic dermatoses. Derm Rep 1984; 3(2):1.

## Additional Readings

AAHA pet owner survey results. Trends Mag 1993; IX(2):32.

Blackshaw JK: Abnormal behaviour in dogs. Aust Vet J 1988; 65(12):393.

Haggerty AJ: Flank sucking behavior. Canine Pract 1978; 5(2):11.

Doering GG: Acral lick dermatitis: Medical management. Canine Pract 1974; 1:21.

Mease C, Reisner I: Behavioral problems in cats and dogs. Vet Forum June 1994:22.

Moses JD: Flank sucking behavior. Canine Pract 1978; 5(2):11.

Niebuhr BR, Nobbe DE: Flank-sucking behavior causes. Canine Pract 1978; 5(4):6.

Roe DJ, Sales GD: Welfare implications of ultrasonic flea collars. Vet Rec 1992; 130(7):142.

Urmanski A: Canine acral lick dermatitis. Newsl Soc Vet Hosp Pharm 1995; 14(3):1.

# Psychotropic Drug Formulary

| Drug and trade names | Action and precautions | Usual dose | Range of doses and references |
|---|---|---|---|
| Acepromazine maleate<br>  Acepromazine | Phenothiazine tranquilizer | 0.55-2.2 mg/kg PO | 0.22-2.2 mg/kg PO q8-36h<br>0.055-1.1 mg/kg IV, IM, SC<br>(1, 3, 8, 13, 19, 20, 26) |
| Alprazolam<br>  Xanax | Benzodiazepine<br>(Useful in panic states)<br>(Start at lower doses)<br>(Best not to exceed<br>  4 mg/day) | 0.1-0.5 mg/kg PO | 0.025-0.1 mg/kg PO q8h<br>0.125-1.0 mg/kg PO<br>  q12-24h<br>(3, 15, 19, 20) |
| Amitriptyline HCl<br>  Elavil<br>  Etrafon<br>  Limbitrol | TCA<br>(Bitter taste)<br>(Caution with thyroid<br>  medication)<br>(Not with MAOIs) | 2.2-4.4 mg/kg PO q24h | 1.0-2.0 mg/kg PO q12-24h<br>(6, 8, 10, 12, 13, 15, 19,<br>  24, 25) |
| Bethanechol Cl<br>  Urecholine | Increase urinary bladder<br>  constriction<br>(Increase gastric motility) | 5-15 mg PO q8h | 5.0-25 mg PO q8-12h<br>2.5-15.0 mg SC q8-12h<br>(13, 19, 20, 26) |
| Buspirone HCl<br>  BuSpar | Azapirone | 1.0 mg/kg PO q24h | 0.5-2.0 mg/kg PO q8-24h<br>2.5-10.0 mg q8-12h<br>(3, 8, 10, 11, 13, 15, 19, 25) |
| Clomipramine HCl<br>  Clomicalm<br>  Anafranil | TCA<br>(Caution with thyroid<br>  medication)<br>(Not with MAOIs) | 1.0-3.0 mg/kg PO q24h<br>(Start at ½ dose for 1 week) | 0.5-1.5 mg/kg PO q12h<br>(3, 8, 11-15, 19, 25) |
| Clonazepam<br>  Klonopin | Benzodiazepine | 0.1-0.5 mg/kg PO q12h | 0.01-1.0 mg/kg PO q8-12<br>(2, 18, 23) |
| Clorazepate<br>  dipotassium<br>  Tranxene | Benzodiazepine | 0.55-2.2 mg/kg PO q24 | 0.125-2.0 mg/kg PO<br>  q12-24h<br>11.25-22.5 mg PO q8-24h<br>(1, 8, 13, 19) |
| Dextroamphetamine<br>  Adderall<br>  Dexedrome<br>  Dextrostat | Amphetamine<br>  sympathomimetic<br>  stimulant | 0.2-1.0 mg/kg PO q24h | 0.2-1.3 mg/kg PO as<br>  needed<br>(3, 13, 14, 27) |

| Drug and trade names | Action and precautions | Usual dose | Range of doses and references |
|---|---|---|---|
| Dextromethorphan<br>Benylin | NMDA receptor<br>antagonist<br>(OCD that responds<br>poorly to SSRIs)<br>(Not with MAOIs<br>or SSRIs)<br>(Can cause histamine<br>release) | 2.0 mg/kg PO q8-12h | 0.5-2.0 mg/kg PO q6-8h<br>20.0 mg/kg PO q8-12h<br>(9, 19) |
| Diazepam<br>Valium | Benzodiazepine | 0.5-2.2 mg/kg PO as<br>needed | 0.25-2.2 mg/kg PO as<br>needed<br>0.5-2.0 mg/kg PO q8h<br>2.5-20.0 mg PO<br>(1, 3, 8, 13, 20, 26) |
| Diethylstilbestrol | Synthetic estrogen<br>(Caution; bone marrow<br>suppression) | 0.1-1.0 mg q24h for 3-5 days,<br>then 1.0 mg PO q2-7d | (13, 20) |
| Diphenhydramine<br>Benadryl<br>Hydramine | Antihistamine,<br>antidepressant,<br>sedative | 2.0-4.0 mg/kg PO q8h | 2.0-4.0 mg/kg PO q8-12h<br>25-50 mg PO q8h<br>(19, 20, 26) |
| Doxepin HCl<br>Adapin<br>Sinequan | TCA<br>(Not with MAOIs) | 3.0-5.0 mg/kg PO q12h | 0.5-10.0 mg/kg PO q12-24h<br>(3, 8, 11-13, 24) |
| Fluoxetine<br>Reconcile<br>Prozac | SSRI<br>(Not with MAOIs) | 1.0 mg/kg PO q24h | 0.5-1.0 mg/kg PO q12-24h<br>(3, 8, 11, 13, 24) |
| Fluvoxamine<br>Luvox | SSRI<br>(Not with MAOIs) | 1.0 mg/kg PO q12-24h | (17) |
| Haloperidol | Neuroleptic<br>butyrophenone | 1-4 mg/kg PO q24h | 0.5-4.0 mg/kg PO q12-24h<br>(16, 17) |
| Hydroxyzine HCl<br>Atarax | Piperazine<br>antihistamine | 1.0-2.0 mg/kg PO q6-8h | (12, 19) |
| Imipramine HCl<br>Tofranil | TCA<br>(Not with MAOIs) | 2.2-4.4 mg/kg PO q12-24h | (6, 8, 10, 12, 13) |
| Levoamphetamine<br>sulfate | Amphetamine<br>sympathomimetic<br>stimulant | 1.0-4.0 mg/kg PO as<br>needed | (13, 27) |
| Lithium carbonate | Antidepressant<br>(Toxic dose close<br>to therapeutic dose) | 650-730 mg/m² PO | 0.6 mg/kg PO q12h<br>(21, 26) |
| Medroxyprogesterone<br>acetate<br>Depo-Provera | Synthetic progestin<br>(Numerous side effects<br>with repeated use) | 5.0-10.0 mg/kg SC | 5.0-20.0 mg/kg IM, SC<br>(3, 4, 8, 13, 14, 24, 28) |
| Megestrol acetate<br>Ovaban<br>Megase | Synthetic progestin<br>(Numerous side effects<br>with long-term use) | 2.0 mg/kg PO q24h for<br>7 days, then 1.0 mg/kg<br>PO q24h for 7 days | 1.1-5.0 mg/kg PO q24h for<br>2-14 days<br>(1, 5, 8, 13, 24, 28) |

*Continued*

| Drug and trade names | Action and precautions | Usual dose | Range of doses and references |
|---|---|---|---|
| Memantine<br>Axura<br>Namenda | NMDA receptor antagonist<br>(OCD that responds poorly to SSRIs) | 0.4-1.0 mg/kg PO q12h<br>(Start with lower dose) | (9) |
| Methylphenidate HCl<br>Ritalin | Amphetamine surrogate sympathomimetic stimulant | 0.5-2.0 mg/kg PO q12-24h<br>(Start with low dose) | 0.05-4.0 mg/kg PO q12-24h<br>5.0-40.0 mg PO q24h<br>(1, 13, 14, 27) |
| Mirtazapine<br>Remeron | TCA<br>(Appetite stimulant)<br>(Not with MAOIs) | 3.75 mg PO q24h, small dog<br>7.5 mg PO q24h, 20-35 lb<br>15.0 mg PO q24h, 40-60 lb<br>22.5 mg PO q24h, 75 lb<br>30.0 mg PO q24h, 100+ lb | (7) |
| Naloxone HCl<br>Narcan | Narcotic antagonist | 11.0-22.0 µg/kg SC, IM, IV | (11, 12, 13, 19, 24) |
| Naltrexone<br>Trexan | Narcotic antagonist | 2.2 mg/kg PO q24h | 1.0-4.0 mg/kg PO q12-24h<br>(3, 6, 8, 11-13, 24) |
| Oxazepam<br>Serax | Benzodiazepine | 0.2-1.0 mg/kg PO q12-24h | (17, 18, 19) |
| Paroxetine<br>Paxil | SSRI | 0.5-1.0 mg/kg PO q24h | (17, 19, 21) |
| Phenobarbital | Barbiturate, hypnotic sedative | 2.0-4.0 mg/kg PO q12-24h | 2.0-6.6 mg/kg PO q12-24h<br>(12, 13, 19, 20, 26) |
| Phenylpropanolamine HCl | Sympathomimetic amine, antihistamine, bronchodilator | 1.0-2.0 mg/kg PO q8h | 12.5-50.0 mg PO q8-12h<br>(8, 13, 17, 19, 26) |
| Promazine HCl<br>Sparine | Phenothiazine tranquilizer | 1.0-4.0 mg/kg PO as needed | (13) |
| Propranolol<br>Inderal<br>Inderide | Nonselective beta-adrenergic receptor blocker | 0.5-1.0 mg/kg PO q8h | 0.5-2.0 mg/kg PO q8h<br>5.0-40.0 mg PO q8h<br>(3, 13, 19, 26) |
| Selegiline (L-deprenyl)<br>Anipryl<br>Eldepryl | MAOI<br>(Not with TCAs, SSRIs, or other MAOIs) | 0.25-0.5 mg/kg PO q24 | 0.25-0.5 mg/kg PO q12-24h<br>1.0-2.0 mg/kg PO q24h (start low)<br>(19, 22) |

*IM,* Intramuscular; *IV,* intravenous; *MAOI,* monoamine oxidase inhibitor; *NMDA,* N-methyl-D-aspartate; *OCD,* over-the-counter drug; *PO,* per os (by mouth); *SC,* subcutaneous; *SSRI,* selective serotonin reuptake inhibitor; *TCA,* tricyclic antidepressant.

# References

1. Burghardt Jr WF: Using drugs to control behavior problems in pets. Vet Med 1991; 86(11):1066.
2. Curtis TM: Treating dogs with Klonopin (clonazepam). DACVB listserve, 10/28/04.
3. Dodman NH, Shuster L: Pharmacologic approaches to managing behavior problems in small animals. Vet Med 1994; 89(10):960.
4. Hart BL, Hart LA: Canine and Feline Behavioral Therapy. Philadelphia: Lea & Febiger, 1985.
5. Joby R, Jemmett JE, Miller ASH: The control of undesirable behaviour in male dogs using megestrol acetate. J Small Anim Pract 1984; 25:567.
6. Mandelker L: Uncovering many new psychotherapeutic agents. Vet Forum August 1990:28.
7. Mandelker L: Mirtazapine dose for appetite stimulation in dogs. VIN Message Board Archive, 10/11/2006.
8. Marder AR: Psychotropic drugs and behavioral therapy. Vet Clin North Am [Small Anim Pract] 1991; 21(2):329.
9. Maurer BM, Dodman NH: Animal behavior case of the month. J Am Vet Med Assoc 2007; 231(4):536.
10. Overall KL: Recognition, diagnosis, and management of obsessive-compulsive disorders. Part 1: A rational approach. Canine Pract 1992; 17(2):40.
11. Overall KL: Recognition, diagnosis, and management of obsessive-compulsive disorders. Part 2: A rational approach. Canine Pract 1992; 17(3):25.
12. Overall KL: Recognition, diagnosis, and management of obsessive-compulsive disorders. Part 3: A rational approach. Canine Pract 1992 17(4):39.
13. Overall KL: Practical pharmacological approaches to behavior problems. St. Louis: Purina Specialty Review, Behavioral Problems in Small Animals, 1992. 36.
14. Overall KL: Use of clomipramine to treat ritualistic stereotypic motor behavior in three dogs. J Am Vet Med Assoc 1994; 205(12):1733.
15. Overall KL: Diagnosing separation anxiety can be difficult for practicing veterinarians. DVM 1996; 27(4):145.
16. Overall KL: Pharmacologic treatments for behavior problems. Vet Clin North Am [Small Anim Pract] 1997; 27(3):637-665.
17. Overall KL: Behavioral Pharmacology. American Animal Hospital Association Proceedings, April 2000:65.
18. Overall KL: Step 3: Dealing with dogs affected by separation anxiety. Vet Forum 2001; 40-46:48-53.
19. Papich MG: Saunders Handbook of Veterinary Drugs, 2nd ed. St. Louis, Saunders, 2007.
20. Plumb DC: Veterinary Drug Handbook, Pocket Edition. White Bear Lake, MN: Pharma Vet Publishing, 1991.
21. Reisner IR: Canine aggression: Neurobiology, behavior and management. Friskies PetCare Symposium: Small Animal Behavior 19-31, October 4, 1998.
22. Ruehl WW: Personal communication, 1995.
23. Seibert L: Treating dogs with Klonopin (clonazepam). DACVB listserve, 10/29/04.
24. Shanley K, Overall K: Psychogenic dermatoses. In Kirk RW, Bonagura JD (eds): Current Veterinary Therapy XI. Philadelphia: Saunders, 1992, p. 552.
25. Shanley K, Overall K: Rational selection of antidepressants for behavioral conditions. Vet Forum November 1995:30.
26. Texas A&M University: Formulary of the Texas A&M University Texas Veterinary Medical Center Veterinary Teaching Hospital. College Station: Texas A&M University, 1990.
27. Voith VL: Hyperactivity and hyperkinesis. Mod Vet Pract 1980; 61(9):787.
28. Voith VL, Marder AR: Behavioral disorders: Introduction. In Morgan RV (ed): Handbook of Small Animal Practice. New York: Churchill Livingstone, 1992,

# Index

Page numbers followed by *f* indicate figures; *t*, tables; *b*, boxes.